This important new publication provides a comprehensive and up-to-date consensus on a variety of aspects of clinical nutrition. The volume has been prepared to mark ten years of The Leeds Course in Clinical Nutrition, which has established itself as the major clinical nutrition course in the UK and Europe. An international and authoritative team of contributors has been drawn together to reflect the strength of the Leeds Course and provide a self-contained publication which will benefit all professionals involved in the nutritional management of patients. One of the special features of the publication is that in addition to providing practical advice on nutritional management, it also encompasses the basic scientific background, including physiology, biochemistry and immunology. In addition there are helpful and practical chapters on individual clinical states in which nutrition is often a problem.

CONSENSUS IN CLINICAL NUTRITION

CONSENSUS IN CLINICAL NUTRITION

Edited by
RICHARD V. HEATLEY,
J. HILARY GREEN
and MONTY S. LOSOWSKY
Department of Medicine, St James's University Hospital, Leeds, UK

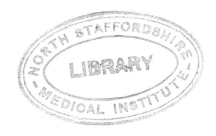

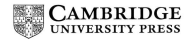

CAMBRIDGE
UNIVERSITY PRESS

Published by the Press Syndicate of the University of Cambridge
The Pitt Building, Trumpington Street, Cambridge CB2 1RP
40 West 20th Street, New York, NY 10011-4211, USA
10 Stamford Road, Oakleigh, Melbourne 3166, Australia

First published 1994

Printed in Great Britain at the University Press, Cambridge

A catalogue record for this book is available from the British Library

Consensus in clinical nutrition/edited by Richard V. Heatley, J.
Hilary Green, Monty S. Losowsky.
   p.   cm.
Includes index.
ISBN 0-521-44134-X (hc)
1. Diet therapy. I. Heatley, Richard. II. Green, J. Hilary.
III. Losowsky, M. S.
[DNLM: 1. Enteral Nutrition. 2. Parenteral Nutrition. 3. Diet
Therapy. WB 400 C755 1994]
RM216.C675 1994
615.8′54—dc20
DNLM/DLC
for Library of Congress 93-42563 CIP

ISBN 0 521 44134 X hardback

Contents

List of contributors   *page* ix

Preface   xiii

1 Measurement of body composition in clincal practice
   S. A. Jebb and M. Elia   1

2 Assessment of energy requirements   *J. H. Green*   22

3 Amino acid requirements in health and disease
   P. J. Garlick, M. A. McNurlan and M. F. Fuller   38

4 Mineral and vitamin metabolism   *A. Shenkin*   56

5 Nutritional immunology   *A. Animashaun and
   R. V. Heatley*   72

6 Physiology of nutrient absorption: a decade of
   advance in formulation of enteral diets
   G. K. Grimble   95

7 Enteral and parenteral nutrition   *C. R. Pennington*   130

8 Is nutritional support worthwhile?   *R. L. Koretz*   158

9 Enteral feeding and food intolerance in paediatrics
   A. MacDonald   192

10 Neonatal intravenous feeding   *I. W. Booth*   224

11 Nutrition and the surgical patient   *N. Everitt and
   M. McMahon*   239

12 Perioperative feeding   *M. M. Meguid and
   A. C. L. Campos*   256

13 How I feed the starving patient   *S. P. Allison*   307

14 Intensive care management   *I. T. Campbell and
   R. A. Little*   319

15 The role of the liver in nutrition   *M. S. Losowsky
   and P. N. Bramley*   333

16 Nutritional deficiencies in inflammatory bowel disease
   P. Duane and R. V. Heatley   350

17 Short bowel syndrome   *J. E. Lennard-Jones*   370
18 Nutrition in cystic fibrosis   *J. M. Littlewood and*
   S. P. Wolfe   388
19 Diet, lipids and lipoproteins   *J. P. Miller and*
   A. Naylor   420
20 Diet and blood pressure   *J. D. Swales*   444
21 Obesity   *J. Garrow*   460
22 Eating disorders   *L. F. Pieri and A. C. P. Sims*   473
Index   488

List of contributors

S. P. Allison
University Hospital, Queen's Medical Centre, Nottingham NG7 2UH, UK

A. Animashaun
York District Hospital, Wigginton Road, York YO3 7HE, UK

I. W. Booth
Institute of Child Health, Francis Road, Birmingham B16 8ET, UK

I. T. Campbell
University Department of Anaesthesia, Withington Hospital, Manchester M20 8LR, UK

A. C. L. Campos
Surgical Metabolism and Nutrition Laboratory, Department of Surgery, University Hospital, SUNY Health Science Center, Syracuse, NY, USA

P. Duane
Withybush General Hospital, Haverfordwest, Pembrokeshire, Dyfed SA61 2PZ, UK

M. Elia
MRC Dunn Nutrition Centre, 100 Tennis Court Road, Cambridge, UK

N. Everitt
Department of Surgery, Leeds General Infirmary, Leeds LS1 3EX, UK

M. F. Fuller
The Rowett Research Institute, Greenburn Road, Bucksburn, Aberdeen AB2 9SB, UK

P. J. Garlick
The Rowett Research Institute, Greenburn Road, Bucksburn, Aberdeen AB2 9SB, UK. Present address: Department of Surgery, Health Sciences Center, SUNY at Stony Brook, Stony Brook, New York 11794-8191, USA

J. Garrow
Rank Department of Human Nutrition, University of London, Charterhouse Square, London EC1M 6BQ, UK

J. H. Green
Aacademic Unit of Medicine, Department of Clinical Medicine, St James's University Hospital, Leeds LS9 7TF, UK

G. K. Grimble
Department of Gastroenterology and Nutrition, Central Middlesex Hospital, Acton Lane, London NW10 7NS, UK

R. V. Heatley
Department of Medicine, St James's University Hospital, Leeds LS9 7TF, UK

S. A. Jebb
MRC Dunn Nutrition Centre, 100 Tennis Court Road, Cambridge, UK

R. L. Koretz
Division of Gastroenterology, Olive View Medical Center, Sylmar, California and Professor of Medicine, University of California, Los Angeles, California

J. E. Lennard-Jones
University of London and St Mark's Hospital, London, UK

R. A. Little
Research Centre, University of Manchester M13 9PL, UK

J. M. Littlewood
Regional Cystic Fibrosis Unit, St James's University Hospital, Leeds, UK

M. S. Losowsky
Academic Unit of Medicine, St James's University Hospital, Leeds, UK

A. MacDonald
Children's Hospital, Ladywood Middleway, Birmingham B16 8ET, UK

M. McMahon
Department of Surgery, Leeds General Infirmary, Leeds LS1 3EX, UK

M. A. McNurlan
The Rowett Research Institute, Greenburn Road, Bucksburn, Aberdeen AB2 9SB, UK. Present address: *Department of Surgery, Health Sciences Center, SUNY at Stony Brook, Stony Brook, New York 11794-8191, USA*

M. M. Meguid
Surgical Metabolism and Nutrition Laboratory, Department of Surgery, University Hospital, SUNY Health Science Center, Syracuse, NY, USA

J. P. Miller
Department of Medicine, University Hospital of South Manchester, Manchester M20 8LR, UK

A. Naylor
Department of Dietetics, University Hospital of South Manchester, Manchester M20 8LR, UK

C. R. Pennington
Ninewells Hospital, Dundee DD2 1UB, UK

L. F. Pieri
Department of Psychiatry, St James's University Hospital, Leeds LS9 7TF, UK

A. Shenkin
Department of Clinical Chemistry, University of Liverpool, Prescot Street, PO Box 147, Liverpool L69 3BX, UK

A. C. P. Sims
Department of Psychiatry, St James's University Hospital, Leeds LS9 7TF, UK

J. D. Swales
Department of Medicine, University of Leicester, UK

S. P. Wolfe
Regional Cystic Fibrosis Unit, St James' University Hospital, Leeds, UK

Preface

The nutritional sciences have their origins in antiquity. Nevertheless, the development of clinical nutrition has largely been limited to the latter part of this century. As equipment and techniques have become more available, so has interest in nutritional treatment increased within clinical medicine. Other speciality groups, including nursing and pharmacy staff, have developed interests within this field, and clinical nutrition has now undoubtedly become truly multidisciplinary.

We started The Leeds Course in Clinical Nutrition over ten years ago to reflect these developments and to act as a forum for the various interest groups which exist within clinical nutrition. Over the years, The Leeds Course in Clinical Nutrition has become widely accepted within this country and overseas. Well over 1000 delegates and about a tenth of that number of distinguished lecturers have attended the Course, from more than a dozen countries.

We have chosen to mark the first decade of The Leeds Course in Clinical Nutrition with this volume, which we hope will become the first of others to represent a consensus in clinical nutrition.

We have been most fortunate in receiving the support of so many over this time. We are very grateful to those who have so freely given their time and effort in these endeavours, and we hope they will continue to support us in the future. We gratefully acknowledge the assistance and encouragement we have received from Peter Silver and colleagues at Cambridge University Press who have helped considerably in bringing this work to fruition.

Leeds,
July, 1993

R. V. Heatley
J. H. Green
M. S. Losowsky

1

Measurement of body composition in clinical practice

S. A. JEBB AND M. ELIA

Why measure body composition?

Human curiosity has been an important influence on the early attempts to assess what the human body consists of, and how it changes during the human life span. The development of the foetus to a baby and its subsequent growth and development into adulthood has been the focus of much scientific discussion over many centuries. There are also very practical reasons for measuring body composition. Epidemiological studies suggest that weight for height is an important predictor of morbidity and mortality. However, indices of weight and height do not provide the best measure of body composition and so more direct measurements are required to improve the prediction of morbidity and mortality. Longitudinal changes in body composition may be useful in monitoring the effects of a disease and its treatment, in obese individuals undergoing weight reduction or in athletes during training. Changes may be related to body performance or tissue function, e.g. in athletes or obese individuals undergoing different training and dietary regimes.

There are many other specific examples in which a knowledge of body composition may be important. For example, in studies of energy metabolism, estimates of fat-free mass are important in relation to the assessment of energy requirements. In the clinical field, knowledge of the metabolically active component of body weight (uncomplicated by excess fat or water) may allow more rational methods of prescribing drugs, particularly anaesthetics and hormones, than current estimates which are based on body weight or surface area.

There is also clinical interest in specific body constituents. For example, osteoporosis, which leads to vertebral collapse and fractured neck of femur, is a common cause of morbidity in old age. The assessment of bone mineral content and the effects of specific therapeutic measures

Table 1.1. *Gross com-*
position of reference man[a]

	kg
Weight	70.00
Fat	15.00
Fat-free mass:	55.00
Water	40.15
Protein	10.86
Glycogen	0.50
Mineral	3.49

[a] In this reference man the hydration of fat-free mass is 73%, the density of fat-free mass is 1.1 kg/l and 21% of the body weight is fat.

that attempt to prevent bone mineral loss are clearly of importance here.

The concept of a reference body

Our direct understanding of the gross composition of man is based on a limited number of chemical analyses of cadavers (Brozek *et al.*, 1963). These studies provide the basis for many of the principles which sustain *in vivo* investigations today. It is apparent that, in normal subjects, the fat-free body, although of heterogeneous composition, shows a remarkable degree of constancy in terms of the proportion of its constituents. Secondly, the amount of fat in the body varies enormously between individuals.

From these data a so-called 'reference man' has been constructed whose composition reflects that of a normal male subject (Table 1.1). However, in practice, individuals do not accurately fit this model and the extent of deviation from reference man, for a given individual will determine the magnitude of the error and thus define the relative accuracy of different techniques which make different fundamental assumptions.

The original division of the body into two compartments – fat and fat-free mass – is the basis of most of the classical reference methods for the measurement of body composition (densitometry, water dilution and total body potassium). More recently it has been possible to separate out the contributions to fat-free mass of water (using dilution techniques) and/or bone (using dual energy X-ray absorptiometry, DXA, or measurements of total body calcium by *in vivo* neutron activation analysis, IVNAA) to give three or four compartment models. IVNAA also offers the possibility of dividing the body into several of its constituent elements.

The measurement of additional compartments will reduce the error in the estimation of body fat but, in some cases, part of this improvement in accuracy may be offset by the propagation of measurement errors. The magnitude of both precision and accuracy are functions of the relative size of each compartment. In practice, the choice of method depends not only on the accuracy and precision required but also on the simplicity, availability, and cost of different methods.

This chapter will describe the principle of some of the basic body composition techniques and illustrate the potential uses of methods in combination with each other to produce complex models of the body. For a fuller account of multi-compartment models see Elia (1992).

'Reference' methods

Although reference methods are mostly reserved for specialised research projects, it is important to have an overall understanding of these methods as they form the basis of the bedside techniques, which are more commonly used for the measurement of body composition in clinical practice.

Body density

The principles of densitometry to make measurements of body composition were first described by Behnke, Feen & Welham in 1942. The method assumes that the body is composed of two compartments: fat and fat-free mass, each of which has a known and constant density. Conventionally, these are taken to be 0.9 kg/l for fat and 1.1 kg/l for fat-free mass, thus by measuring the density of the body the proportion of body fat may be calculated from Siri's equation (1956).

$$\% \text{ fat} = \left[\frac{(4.95)}{d} - 4.50 \right] \times 100$$

where d = body density.

There is little dispute over the assumption of a constant density of the homogeneous fat mass. However, fat-free mass is a very heterogeneous compartment comprising protein, water, bone and glycogen. If the fat-free mass has a constant density, its constituents must exist in a fixed proportion to each other in all individuals, at all times, which is clearly incorrect. For example, water balance is known to fluctuate at different times of day and to change rapidly in situations such as exercise, or following excessive alcohol. Bone mass and density also vary with sex, race and age (see Elia, 1992 for changes in the density of fat-free mass during growth and development).

The density of a body is equivalent to the mass of that body in air divided by its volume. The mass of the subject in air can be simply and accurately measured, but a more elaborate procedure is necessary to calculate volume. This may take the form of a body volumeter in which the volume of water displaced is measured directly using a tilted burette attached to the side of the tank of water in which the subject is submerged. Alternatively, weight may be used which is generally more accurately measured than volume, by weighing the subject underwater and subtracting this from body weight in air. In both cases the aim is to measure the volume of body tissues and so the volume of the lungs must be measured and subtracted. Gut volume is not measured, but radiological studies suggest that for a fasted subject it is approximately 100 ml, which must be deducted from the measured body volume (Buskirk, 1961).

There are obvious practical limitations to this technique. Many subjects are unable to co-operate with the rigorous procedure; it is unsuitable for the very young, old or infirm and appropriate facilities and trained investigators are required. However, experience in our laboratory has shown that the method is well accepted by most subjects, including a number of patient groups.

The technique may be refined by improving the estimation of the density of fat-free mass, by making separate measurements of body water (isotope dilution) and bone mineral (dual energy X-ray absorptiometry) to produce a multi-compartment model (Elia, 1992).

Total body water (TBW)

This method is again a two-compartment model (fat and fat-free mass) in which it is further assumed that the fat compartment is anhydrous and that the fat-free compartment is hydrated to a known and constant extent, usually between 71% and 74% (based on the results of the limited human cadaver analyses and animal desiccations). Thus, if total body water can be measured, lean tissue mass can be calculated and hence fat mass by difference from body weight.

Total body water can be measured by a variety of dilution techniques requiring a minimum of subject co-operation although the analysis frequently requires access to sophisticated facilities (e.g. mass spectrometry for analysis of ^{18}O). The subject drinks a dose of the labelled water and, after equilibration with body water, a sample of body fluid (blood, saliva or urine) is taken to measure the extent of dilution of the administered dose. The dilution principle may be simplified to: Amount of dose given = Amount of dose found. Today, the tracers of choice are $^{2}H_2O$ or $H_2^{18}O$ which are stable and non-radioactive. The former is more commonly used than the latter on account of the cost differential. Total body water may be estimated either by calculating the intercept of an isotope disappearance curve measured over several days or by sampling body water at a fixed time after the dose, when equilibration has occurred and assuming the existence of a plateau of isotope enrichment. However, $^{2}H_2O$ also exchanges with some non-aqueous hydrogen (Culebras *et al.*, 1977), mainly in the form of free hydroxyl groups on proteins and glycogen and the amino groups on proteins. This leads to an overestimation of body water of the order of 3–4%, which must be included in the calculation of water volume.

One of the greatest errors incurred in this method lies in the assumption that the fat-free mass has a constant and a known hydration fraction. The hydration of lean tissue is extremely variable, both within and between individuals. In one study (Fuller *et al.*, 1992), the hydration fraction in normal men (mean 73.32%) and women (mean 74.49%) was found to vary from 69.41 to 78.37%. In the clinical environment, many patients will have abnormalities of water balance which are manifest as oedema or dehydration, and these patients are likely to represent more extreme ends of this range. Adipose tissue is known to contain a small amount of water and as the degree of adiposity increases its water content increasingly contributes to that of the body. Further errors in the actual measurement of total body water relate to the impossibility of defining the point of equilibration in what is a dynamic system with continual water losses (urine, sweat, etc.) and intermittent water additions (eating and drinking).

Total body potassium (TBK)

In the body there is a natural gamma-emitting isotope of potassium: ^{40}K. Its presence can be measured *in vivo* using a whole-body counter, to give an estimate of total body potassium (Sievert, 1951). It is then assumed that potassium exists only in lean tissue and not in fat and that ^{40}K represents a fixed proportion of total body potassium. Thus, having measured ^{40}K, lean tissue mass may be calculated and hence body fat, by difference from body weight.

However, potassium is not evenly distributed throughout lean tissues (Widdowson & Dickerson, 1960) with more found in muscle than other lean tissues (Snyder et al., 1975). Its concentration also varies with age, both during growth and development (Dickerson & Widdowson, 1960) and after maturity (Womersley et al., 1976). Its concentration varies with adiposity such that, in obese subjects, the concentration of potassium in lean tissue is lower than in their lean counterparts (Colt et al., 1981). The concentration, also tends to be higher in subjects with a high proportion of fat-free mass (Morgan & Burkinshaw, 1983). Forbes, Gallup & Hursh (1961) suggest a value of 68.1 mmol/kg, but this is widely disputed. Boddy et al. (1973), in a review of the literature, claim that average values for men and women are 3% and 15% lower, respectively. There may also be substantial changes in potassium concentration with disease, e.g. patients receiving diuretics (Morgan, Burkinshaw and Davidson, 1978). A major reduction in the potassium content of the brain has been reported in protein-energy malnutrition (Garrow, 1967).

The precision of the counting procedure is related to specific aspects of the design of individual counters, both in terms of hardware (e.g. number of counting crystals) and software (e.g. calibration equations). Furthermore, the number of counts recorded for an obese subject will be fewer than for a lean subject for the same amount of potassium, as the adipose tissue exerts a shielding effect over the body. To overcome this, appropriate calibration of each individual counter is required using the ^{42}K isotope.

Practically, the measurement of total body potassium is not straightforward. Few centres have access to whole-body counters and the measurement takes time to perform (over one hour in some whole-body counters) during which the subject is enclosed in a well-shielded counter connected only by an intercom to the observer. It is therefore not suitable for all subjects.

Dual energy X-ray absorptiometry (DXA)

This is a scanning device which emits X-rays at two different energies, typically 40 and 80 keV. A detector system measures the attenuation of

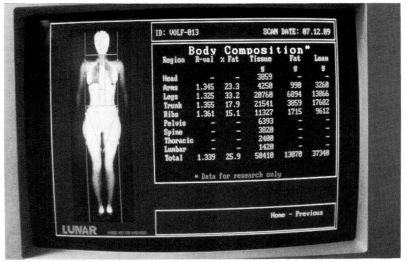

Fig. 1.1. Body composition analysis using DXA.

the rays as they are transmitted through the body. Using the two different wavelengths, it is possible to solve simultaneous equations to calculate two compartments: bone and soft tissue. More recently, the same principles have been extended to resolve the non-bony compartment into fat and fat-free mass (Mazess, Peppler & Gibbons, 1984). Body composition analysis of a typical patient is shown in Fig. 1.

The technique is reproducible with coefficients of variation for bone mineral of less than 1% and fat-free mass of approximately 0.8%. Several studies have shown good agreement between measurements of body composition by DXA and other reference methods within groups (e.g. Hassanger *et al.*, 1989; Heymsfield *et al.*, 1989; Van Loan & Maycli, 1992*a*, *b*) although, for individuals, body fat mass may differ by almost 3 kg (2SD) from densitometry (Fuller *et al.*, 1992). Large errors may be anticipated in patients with abnormal hydration status since the attenuation of water is similar to that of fat-free mass. An advantage of this technique is the ability to divide the body into segments e.g. trunk, right and left legs, which gives an indication of regional body composition (Mazess *et al.*, 1990). This may be useful, for example, in assessing fat distribution as a predictor of coronary heart disease. Furthermore, it can provide useful information on the muscle mass of limbs which allows a reasonable prediction of the total musculature, since the limbs represent around 75% (Heymsfield *et al.*, 1990; Fuller, Laskey & Elia, 1992).

In practice, the procedure is straightforward and non-invasive. Subjects lie still on a bed as the scanning arm passes over them, which takes approximately 20 minutes. As the radiation dose is minimal (approximately equal to a day's background radiation), this procedure is eminently suitable for most subjects and for longitudinal studies in which a number of measurements are required. However, DXA has not been used for studies in pregnant women. The necessary equipment is available in an increasing number of hospitals and, in such cases, it can readily be applied to patients.

Other techniques

IVNAA provides useful information about the elemental composition of the body, e.g. nitrogen (as an index of protein), potassium, calcium, etc., but it is associated with much more radiation than other techniques (Beddoe, Streat & Hill, 1986). It is being increasingly used, either alone or in combination with other techniques (Elia, 1992) as a standard against which to validate other techniques. Computerised axial tomography (CT) can provide information about organ size and adipose tissue mass and distribution, but it also exposes the subject to a significant radiation dose (Foster et al., 1988; Ross et al., 1991). Nuclear magnetic resonance (NMR) provides similar information to CT scanning and does not involve radiation (Foster et al., 1988; Ross et al., 1992). All these three techniques are restricted to specialised centres. The last two are mainly employed for clinical diagnosis, and their use for body composition analysis has been very limited.

Precision

The estimated methodological precision of each of these methods is shown in Table 1.2. DXA is associated with the greatest precision in terms of the reproducibility of the method, although this may not reflect its absolute accuracy. Density and total body water are associated with intermediate precision which varies between laboratories. In general, TBK is the least reproducible of the reference techniques, varying with specific aspects of the hardware.

Bedside techniques

Although one or more of these methods may be available for some clinical studies, their application is often restricted by access to such facilities,

Table 1.2. *Precision in the basic measurement and estimates of body fat (adapted from Elia, 1992)*

Method	Precision Raw measurement (%CV)	Body fat[a] (kg)	Reference
Reference methods:			
Density	0.21–0.23	0.73–0.79	Siri, 1961; Durnin & Taylor, 1960
Total body water	1.0–2.0	0.55–1.10	Murgatroyd & Coward, 1989; Fuller *et al.*, 1992
Total body potassium	2.0–3.0	1.1–4.7	Shukla *et al.*, 1973; Forbes *et al.*, 1968
DXA	–	0.45	Fuller, Laskey & Elia, 1992
Bedside techniques:			
BMI[b]	0.8	0.15	Fuller *et al.*, 1991
Skinfold thickness[c]	9.0	0.65	
Resistance[d]	1.2	0.35	
NIRI[e]	5.9	0.60	

[a] Assuming 20% fat in a 70 kg reference man.
[b] Calculated from equation of Black *et al.* (1983), which uses the body mass index.
[c] Calculated from Durnin & Wormersley (1974).
[d] Caclulated from manufacturers' equations (Valhalla equation):

(% fat = 9.07 + [0.603 × weight (kg)] − [0.581 Height^2/Resistance (Ω)]

[e] Calculated from manufacturers' equations (Futrex 5000):

% fat (men) = 54.172 − 4.2 od2 + 0.1232 weight (kg) − 0.11693 height (cm) − 14.9 od1 − 139.4 activity score.

% fat (women) = 60.228 − 4.2 od2 + 0.1232 weight (kg) − 0.11693 height (cm) − 14.9 od1 − 139.4 activity score.

CV = coefficient of variation.

time or cost. There is a great need for body composition studies either at the bedside or for large field studies for screening or epidemiological studies. For such studies a range of simple techniques is available which enables an estimate to be made of body composition using a prediction equation. Such methods have been mainly based on measurements of body density, TBW or TBK and not on DXA, imaging techniques of IVNAA. However, it is apparent that, since even reference methods are associated with significant errors, there is little scope to compromise convenience for accuracy.

The precision of these prediction techniques is also shown in Table 1.2. In this format they compare favourably with the precision of reference methods, but this reflects only the methodological precision of the technique, to which must be added the errors of the method from which it was derived. In addition, it is important to note the large coefficient of variation of the raw measurement which is not always reflected in the precision of the body fat estimate. This gives an indication of the extent to which factors other than that actually measured contribute to the final estimate of fat mass.

Weight and height

Weight and height may be simply and, with due care, accurately measured. A variety of simple prediction equations have been published which use weight and height to estimate body fat (see Elia, 1992). For cross-sectional purposes these may be as good, or almost as good, as other bedside body composition techniques. However, obvious errors arise in patients who are abnormally hydrated or kyphotic. Errors may also occur in patients who have muscle wasting. Changes in body weight give little indication of the component that has changed its mass, although large daily fluctuations are likely to reflect changes in fluid balance.

Skinfolds

Large studies in which such measurements of fat folds at one or more sites have been compared to estimates of body fat by densitometry have resulted in a variety of prediction equations in which skinfold thicknesses can be used to predict total body fat. Such methods assume first that subcutaneous fat is a constant proportion of total body fat and secondly that the chosen measurement sites have a known relationship to total body fat. Differences in fat distribution either between individuals, or in one individual studied on several occasions will lead to errors.

The interpretation of skinfold thicknesses depends on previously derived prediction equations which, in order to account for differences in the density of fat-free mass and fat distribution, are age, sex and population specific. In Britain the most commonly employed equations are probably those of Durnin & Womersley (1974), which are based on measurements made at four sites: triceps, biceps, subscapular and suprailiac. A logarithmic transformation of the sum of four skinfold thicknesses, produces a linear relationship with body density which is age and sex specific.

Such a method is cheap, simple, non-invasive and can be performed outside the confines of a laboratory. However, there are some practical problems. The correct anatomical site may be difficult to establish and in some cases the site may be inaccessible due to burns, bandages, etc. The extent of skin compressibility varies, leading to unstable readings particularly in the obese, where a further problem is that the jaws of the calipers may not be wide enough to encompass the fat fold. One of the major criticisms of the technique is that measurements made by different observers may have a coefficient of variation of 9%, giving a precision on the measurement of fat of 5% (Fuller *et al.*, 1991). The question of inter-observer error should not be confused with considerations regarding the accuracy of the method, in terms of its relationship to reference methods. Our group has suggested that the estimation of body fat by skinfold thicknesses is probably better than other simple prediction techniques, as shown by a series of our studies in normal subjects (Elia, Parkinson & Diaz, 1990; Fuller *et al.*, 1992).

Impedance/resistance

The use of whole body impedance to estimate body composition depends on the principle that fat is a relatively poor conductor of an applied current of electricity, whereas lean tissue with its water and electrolyte content is highly conductive. At low frequencies (approximately 1 kHz) the current travels solely through extracellular water, whilst at higher frequencies (greater than 50 kHz) it is able to overcome the capacitance of cell membranes and thus penetrates the entire body water pool. Currently, relatively little work has been carried out at low frequencies or at multiple frequencies, although there is increasing interest in these approaches (Van Loan & Mayclin, 1992a, b; Pullicino, Coward & Elia, 1992; Thomas, Ward & Cornish, 1993).

Whole-body impedance methods have been extensively validated against measurements of total body water made by isotopic dilution techniques (Hoffer, Meadow & Simpson, 1969; Kushner & Schoeller, 1986; Lusaki *et al.*, 1986) and there is a firm relationship between the measured impedance and total body water (with an appropriate height correction). The standard error of the estimate of total body water made in this way is approximately 2 litres. This reflects the complex geometry of biological systems which cannot be adequately described by this simple formula.

The precision of the basic measurement is good, although this error must be added to those already described when total body water measurements are translated into estimates of fat and fat-free mass.

The measurement is simple and rapid to perform. A tetrapolar surface electrode system is used (to minimise differences in skin conductivity) and the voltage drop across the body measured when an alternating current (typically 800 μamp, 50 kHz) is passed between the hand and foot on the ipsilateral part of the body. A large number of regression equations are available to calculate body composition from the measurement of impedance and resistance (see Elia, 1992) and these may give substantially different estimates of body composition, despite the same observed impedance/resistance measurement.

An important consideration is that the contribution of different segments of the body to whole-body impedance is extremely variable, as a result of differences in body geometry and particularly cross-sectional area. For example as shown in Fig. 1.2, an arm represents only 4% of body weight yet contributes as much as 46% of the total body impedance, whereas the trunk which is 46% of body weight contributes 10% to total body impedance. This is particularly important when measuring changes in body composition and changes in fluid balance. Changes in fluid in the trunk (e.g. pleural fluid or ascites) are expected to have little influence on the change in whole-body impedance whereas changes in fluid in the limbs will have a much greater effect. Changes in electrolyte concentration will also affect the results as it is ions which are responsible for the conduction of the current through the fat-free body (Jebb & Elia, 1991).

Near infra-red interactance

This technique involves irradiating body tissues with a beam of near infra-red radiation (Conway, Norris & Bodwell, 1984). The pattern of the reflected radiation is influenced by the specific absorption characteristics of the underlying tissue. Again the method is cheap, simple and non-invasive to perform. A commercial instrument is available (Futrex 5000) which employs two wavelengths of light at 940 and 950 nm. Prediction equations are used to interpret the optical density measurements to produce an estimate of body fat. Using the equations supplied by the manufacturer, measurements are made at a single site at the midpoint of the upper arm over the biceps muscle. It must therefore be assumed that this local tissue composition reflects that of the whole body, which may not be true. The measured optical density depends to some extent on the

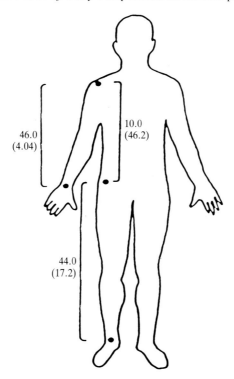

Fig. 1.2. Percentage distribution of segmental impedance at 50 kHz (and % body weight).

pressure exerted by the observer. Furthermore, the prediction equations employ weight, height, sex and a subjective assessment of activity in order to calculate body composition, such that the optical density measurement makes a relatively small contribution to the final estimate of body fat.

Comparison with reference methods

A variety of studies have compared the results obtained from bedside methods with those from a selection of reference techniques. Accumulated data from our laboratory (Table 1.3) suggests that of the prediction methods, skinfold thicknesses show the best agreement with measurements made from body density or total body water and near infra-red interactance the poorest agreement. The results from bioelectrical impedance and weight for height indices vary with the prediction equation employed, but the examples shown here have an intermediate error.

Table 1.3. *Comparison of bedside methods with reference techniques (kgfat): Bias (±2 SD)*

	Reference method				
	1 Densitometry (n = 24)	2 Densitometry (n = 29)	3 Total body water (n = 55)	4 3-Compartment model (n = 28)	5 4-Compartment model (n = 28)
BMI[a]	1.9 (5.2)	2.3 (5.3)	1.4 (5.8)	−0.20 (6.54)	0.54 (6.34)
Skinfold thicknesses[b]	1.9 (4.9)	1.8 (4.8)	1.3 (4.6)	−0.54 (4.04)	0.20 (3.88)
Resistance[c]	3.5 (4.4)	3.6 (4.7)	2.4 (4.2)	—	—
Impedance[d]	−3.1 (3.8)	−3.1 (4.6)	−4.1 (4.9)	1.69 (6.43)	2.43 (6.04)
NIRI[e]	—	2.5 (5.4)	—	−0.03 (6.39)	0.71 (5.84)

[a] Calculated from equation of Black *et al.*

[b] Calculated from Durnin & Womersley (1974).

[c] Calculated from manufacturers' equations (Valhalla equation):

$(\% \text{ fat} = 9.07 + [0.603 \times \text{weight (kg)}] - [0.581 \text{ Height}^2/\text{Resistance} (\Omega)]$.

[d] Calculated from manufacturers' equation (Holtain):

$\text{TBW (kg)} = 0.585 \text{ Height}^2/\text{Impedance} + 1.825; \text{ LBM} = TBW/0.73$

[e] Calculated from manufacturers' equations (Futrex 5000):

$\% \text{ fat (men)} y = 54.172 - 4.2 \text{ od2} + 0.1232 \text{ weight (kg)} - 0.11693 \text{ height (cm)} - 14.9 \text{ od1} - 139.4 \text{ activity score.}$

$\% \text{ fat (women)} = 60.228 - 4.2 \text{ od2} + 0.1232 \text{ weight (kg)} - 0.11693 \text{ height (cm)} - 14.9 \text{ od1} - 139.4 \text{ activity score.}$

1 Fuller & Elia (1989).
2 Elia, Parkinson & Diaz (1990).
3 Pullicino *et al.* (1990).
4 Fuller *et al.* (1992).
5 Fuller *et al.* (1992).

Accuracy and precision

To validate the true accuracy of a method requires comparison with cadaver analysis, but in view of the difficulties with this practice, methods are often compared with each other and conclusions regarding their relative merits are sought. The accuracy of *in vivo* techniques is limited more by the errors involved in the assumptions about the composition of fat-free mass than by the technical measurement imprecision; it is not uncommon for measurements of body composition made by different methods to disagree.

The statistical comparison of two or more methods most commonly takes the form of correlation analysis. However, this only denotes a relationship between the methods and not agreement. Fig. 1.3 shows a hypothetical set of results which compares two methods, A and B, to measure body fat, with a correlation coefficient of 0.99. More usefully, a statistical technique described by Bland and Altman (1986) can be employed in which the mean results of the two methods are compared with the difference between each pair of values (Fig. 1.3). The mean is the best estimate it is possible to make without making any assumptions regarding the relative merit of each technique, whilst the difference represents the deviation of individual points from the mean. In this way the mean difference between pairs of points will indicate the bias of one method relative to the other, and the standard deviation of the differences will indicate the amount of scatter. The narrower these limits and the smaller the bias implies a closer agreement between methods. Furthermore, by plotting a regression line through the points it is possible to examine whether the bias is related to the magnitude of the measurement. Fig. 1.3 shows that as the body fat mass increases, the difference between the two methods also increases, such that in subjects with more than 40 kg fat, method A underestimates by over 5 kg compared to method B.

Often it is not essential to know the absolute body fat or fat-free mass of an individual, but rather it is more important to know how the composition changes in response to a change in diet, exercise or disease. If the aim is to assess the accuracy of methods to measure a change in body energy stores, energy and nitrogen balance studies can provide an appropriate independent standard. Furthermore, such balances can be performed with an accuracy infinitely superior to that of any of the indirect body composition methodologies. Such studies have demonstrated the superiority of multi-compartment models of body composition (Jebb & Elia, 1993).

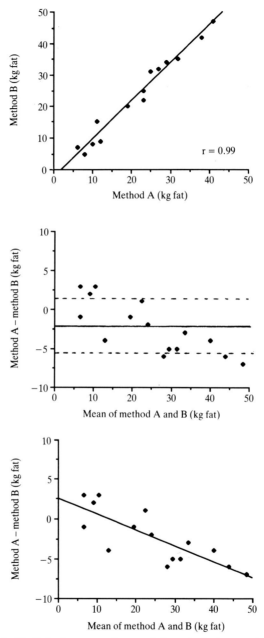

Fig. 1.3. Statistical comparison of two techniques. (*a*) Correlation analysis; (*b*) Bland and Altman (1986); (*c*) regression of mean versus difference plot.

Table 1.4. *Inter-observer measurement variability for bedside body composition techniques* (*adapted from Fuller* et al., *1991*)

Method	Residual CV (%)	
	Raw measurement	Calculated body fat (kg)
Weight (kg)	0.001⎫	
Height (cm)	0.4 ⎭	0.8[a]
Skinfold thicknesses[b] (mm)		
Triceps	11	4.6[b]
Biceps	16	
Subscapula	13	
Suprailiac	18	
Resistance[c] (Ω)	1.2	2.6[c]
Near infra-red interactance[d]		
Optical density 1	5.6	4.2[d]
Optical density 2	6.2	

[a] Calculated from equation of Black *et al.* (1983) which uses the body mass index.
[b] Calculated from Durnin and Womersley (1974).
[c] Calculated from manufacturers' equations (Valhalla equation):

$$(\% \text{ fat} = 9.07 + [0.603 \times \text{weight (kg)}] - [0.581 \text{ Height}^2/\text{Resistance } (\Omega)].$$

[d] Calculated from manufacturers' equations (Futrex 5000):

$$\% \text{ fat (men)} = 54.172 - 4.2 \text{ od2} + 0.1232 \text{ weight (kg)} - 0.11693 \text{ height (cm)}$$
$$- 14.9 \text{ od1} - 139.4 \text{ activity score.}$$
$$\% \text{ fat (women)} = 60.228 - 4.2 \text{ od2} + 0.1232 \text{ weight (kg)} - 0.11693 \text{ height (cm)}$$
$$- 14.9 \text{ od1} - 139.4 \text{ activity score.}$$

CV = coefficient of variation.

Observer error

Observer error is a component of the precision of body composition measurements, although it is independent of its absolute accuracy. However, it is pertinent to note that in some cases the error on the estimate of body composition may be compromised more by the extent of observer variability, than by the inaccuracy of the methodology. In studies which involve more than one observer, it is therefore essential to pay due consideration to such errors at an early stage during the design of a study.

The reproducibility of a method by a single observer is often quoted, but there is far less information on inter-observer error and particularly the observer error of one method relative to another. Objective methods such as DXA, density or total body water are considered to be relatively free of such errors, but problems arise with many of the prediction methods which incorporate a degree of subjectivity when making the measurement. In a study by Fuller *et al.* (1992) the extent of observer variability was greater for skinfold thicknesses (where there is a contribution to the error from determining the correct anatomical site), and near infra-red interreactance (where observer differences in the pressure exerted on the instrument can yield different results) than for biolectrical impedance analysis (Table 1.4).

References

Beddoe, A. H., Streat, S. J. & Hill, G. L. (1986). Clinical body composition assessment using *in-vivo* neutron activation analysis (IVNAA). In *In vivo Body Composition Studies*, ed. K. J. Ellis, S. Yasumura and W. D. Morgan. United States Department of Energy. Brookhaven National Laboratory, Associated Universities Inc.

Behnke, A. R., Feen, B. G. & Welham, W. C. (1942). The specific gravity of healthy men. Body weight/volume as an index of obesity. *Journal of the American Medical Association*, **118**, 495–8.

Black, D., James, W. P. T., Besser, G. M. *et al.* (1983). Obesity. A report of the Royal College of Physicians. *Journal of the Royal College of Physicians, London*, **17**, 5–65.

Bland, J. M. & Altman, D. G. (1986). Statistical methods for assessing agreement between two methods of clinical measurement. *Lancet*, **i**, 307–10.

Boddy, K., King, P. C., Womersley, J. & Durnin, J. V. G. A. (1973). Body potassium and fat-free mass. *Clinical Science*, **44**, 622–5.

Brozek, J., Grande, F., Anderson, T. & Keys, A. (1963). Densitometric analysis of body composition: revisions of some quantitative assumptions. *Annals of the New York Academy of Sciences*, **110**, 113–40.

Buskirk, E. R. (1961). Underwater weighing and body density: a review of procedures. In *Techniques for Measuring Body Composition*, ed. J. Brozek and H. Henschel. National Academy of Sciences – National Research Council, Washington DC.

Colt, E. W. D., Wang, J., Stallone, F., Van Itallie, T. B. & Pierson, R. N. (1981). A possible low intracellular potassium in obesity. *American Journal of Clinical Nutrition*, **34**, 367–72.

Conway, J. M., Norris, K. H. & Bodwell, C. E. (1984). A new approach for the estimation of body composition: infra-red interactance. *American Journal of Clinical Nutrition*, **40**, 1123–30.

Culebras, J. M., Fitzpatrick, G. F., Brennan, M. F., Boyden, C. M. & Moore, F. D. (1977). Total body water and the exchangeable hydrogen II. A review of comparative data from animals based on isotope dilution and desiccation, with a report of new data from the rat. *American Journal of Physiology*, **232**, R60–5.

Dickerson, J. W. T. & Widdowson, E. M. (1960). Chemical changes in skeletal muscle with development. *Biochemical Journal*, **74**, 24–57.

Durnin, J. V. G. A. & Taylor, A. (1960). Replicability of measurements of density of the human body as determined by underwater weighing. *Journal of Applied Physiology*, **15**, 142–4.

Durnin, J. V. G. A. & Womersley, J. (1974). Body fat assessed from total body density and its estimation from skinfold thickness: measurements on 481 men and women aged 16–72 years. *British Journal of Nutrition*, **32**, 77–97.

Elia, M., Parkinson, S. A. & Diaz, E. (1990). Evaluation of near infra-red interactance as a method for predicting body composition. *European Journal of Clinical Nutrition*, **44**, 113–21.

Elia, M. (1992). Body composition analysis: an evaluation of 2 component models, multicomponent models and bedside techniques. *Clinical Science*, **11**, 114–27.

Forbes, G. B., Gallup, J. & Hursh, J. B. (1961). Estimation of total body fat from potassium-40 content. *Science*, **133**, 101–2.

Forbes, G. B., Shultz, F., Cafarrelli, C. & Amirhakimi, G. H. (1968). Effect of body size on potassium-40 measurement in the whole-body counter. *Health Physics*, **15**, 142–4.

Foster, M. A., Fowler, P. A., Fuller, M. F. & Knight, C. H. (1988). Non-invasive methods for assessment of body composition. *Proceedings of the Nutrition Society*, **47**, 375–85.

Fuller, N. J. & Elia, M. (1989). Potential use of bioelectrical impedance of the 'whole-body' and of body segments for the assessment of body composition: comparison with densitometry and anthropometry. *European Journal of Clinical Nutrition*, **43**, 779–91.

Fuller, N. J., Jebb, S. A., Goldberg, G. R. *et al.* (1991). Inter-observer variability in the measurement of body composition. *European Journal of Clinical Nutrition*, **45**, 43–9.

Fuller, N. J., Jebb, S. A., Laskey, M. A., Coward, W. A. & Elia, M. (1992). Four-component model for the assessment of body composition in humans: comparison with alternative methods and evaluation of the density and hydration of fat-free mass. *Clinical Science*, **82**, 687–93.

Fuller, N. J., Laskey, M. A. & Elia, M. (1992). Assessment of major body regions by dual energy X-ray absorptiometry (DEXA), with special reference to limb muscle mass. *Clinical Physiology*, **12**, 1–15.

Garrow, J. S. (1967). Loss of brain potassium in kwashiorkor. *Lancet*, **ii**, 643–5.

Hassanger, C., Sølvesten, S., Sørensen, S., Nielson, B. & Christiansen, C. (1989). Body composition measurement by dual photon absorptiometry: comparison with body density and total body potassium measurements. *Clinical Physiology*, **9**, 353–60.

Heymsfield, S. B., Wang, J., Heshka, S., Kehayias, J. J. & Pierson, R. N. (1989). Dual-photon absorptiometry: comparison of bone mineral and soft tissue mass measurements *in vivo* with established methods. *American Journal of Clinical Nutrition*, **49**, 1283–9.

Heymsfield, S. B., Smith, R., Aulet, M. *et al.* (1990). Appendicular skeletal mass measurement by dual-photon absorptiometry. *American Journal of Clinical Nutrition*, **52**, 214–18.

Hoffer, E. C., Meadow, C. K. & Simpson, D. C. (1969). Correlation of whole-body impedance and total body water. *Journal of Applied Physiology*, **27**, 531–4.

Jebb, S. A. & Elia, M. (1991). Assessment of changes in total body water in patients undergoing renal dialysis using bioelectrical impedance analysis. *Clinical Nutrition*, **10**, 81–4.

Jebb, S. A., Murgatroyd, P. R., Goldberg, G. R., Prentice, A. M. & Coward, W. A. (1993). *In-vivo* measurement of changes in body composition:

description of methods and their validation against 12-day continuous whole-body calorimetry. *American Journal of Clinical Nutrition*, **58**, 455–62.

Kushner, R. F. & Schoeller, D. A. (1986). Estimation of total body water by bioelectrical impedance analysis. *American Journal of Clinical Nutrition*, **44**, 417–24.

Lusaki, H. C., Bolonchuk, W. W., Hall, C. B. & Siders, W. A. (1986). Validation of tetrapolar impedance method to assess human body composition. *Journal of Applied Physiology*, **60** (4), 1327–32.

Mazess, R. B., Peppler, W. W. & Gibbons, M. (1984). Total body composition by dual-photon (153 Gd) absorptiometry. *American Journal of Clinical Nutrition*, **40**, 834–9.

Mazess, R. B., Barden, H. S., Bisek, J. P. & Hanson, J. (1990). Dual energy X-ray absorptiometry for total-body and regional bone mineral and soft tissue composition. *American Journal of Clinical Nutrition*, **51**, 1106–12.

Morgan, D. B., Burkinshaw, L. & Davidson, C. (1978). Potassium depletion in heart failure and its relation to long term treatment with diuretics: a review of the literature. *Postgraduate Medical Journal*, **54**, 72–9.

Morgan, D. B. & Burkinshaw, L. (1983). Estimation of non-fat body tissues from measurements of skinfold thickness, total body potassium and total body nitrogen. *Clinical Science*, **65**, 407–14.

Murgatroyd, P. R. & Coward, W. A. (1989). An improved method for estimating changes in whole-body fat and protein mass in man. *British Journal of Nutrition*, **62**, 311–14.

Pullicino, E., Coward, W. A., Stubbs, J. & Elia, M. (1990). Bedside and field methods for assessing body composition: comparison with the deuterium dilution technique. *European Journal of Clinical Nutrition*, **44**, 753–62.

Pullicino, E., Coward, W. A. & Elia, M. (1992). The potential use of dual frequency impedance in predicting total body water in health and disease. *Clinical Nutrition*, **11**, 69–74.

Ross, R., Leger, L., Guardo, R. & de Guise, J. (1991). Adipose tissue volume measured by magnetic resonance imaging and computerized tomography in rats. *Journal of Applied Physiology*, **70** (5), 2164–72.

Ross, R., Leger, L., Morris, D., de Guise, J. & Guardo, R. (1992). Quantification of adipose tissue by MRI: relationship with anthropometric variables. *Journal of Applied Physiology*, **72** (2), 787–95.

Shukla, K. K., Ellis, K. J., Dombrowski, C. S. & Cohn, S. H. (1973). Physiological variation of total body potassium in man. *American Journal of Physiology*, **224**, 271–4.

Sievert, R. M. (1951). Measurements of gamma radiation from the human body. *Archives Fysik*, **3**, 337–56.

Siri, W. S. (1956). The gross composition of the body. In *Advances in Biological and Medical Physics*, ed. T. H. Lawrence and C. A. Tobias. Academic Press, New York.

Siri, W. S. (1961). Body composition from fluid spaces and density: analysis of methods. In *Techniques for Measuring Body Composition*, ed. J. Brozek and H. Henschel. National Academy of Sciences – National Research Council, Washington DC.

Snyder, W. S., Cook, M. J., Nasset, E. S., Karhausen, L. R., Parry Howells, G. & Tipton, I. H. (1975). *Report of the Task Group on Reference Man*. Pergamon Press, Oxford.

Thomas, B. J., Ward, L. C. & Cornish, B. H. (1933). Bioelectric impedance analysis for measurements of body fluid volumes. *Journal of Clinical Engineering.* In press.

Van Loan, M. D. & Mayclin, P. L. (1992*a*). Body composition assessment: dual-energy X-ray absorptiometry (DEXA) compared to reference methods. *European Journal of Clinical Nutrition*, **46**, 125–30.

Van Loan, M. D. & Mayclin, P. L. (1992*b*). Use of multifrequency bioelectrical impedance analysis for the estimation of extracellular fluid. *European Journal of Clinical Nutrition*, **46**, 117–24.

Widdowson, E. M. & Dickerson, J. W. T. (1960). The effect of growth and function on the chemical composition of soft tissues. *Biochemical Journal*, **77**, 30–43.

Womersley, J., Durnin, J. V. G. A., Boddy, K. & Mahaffey, M. (1976). Influence of muscular development, obesity and age on the fat-free mass of adults. *Journal of Applied Physiology*, **41**, 223–9.

2

Assessment of energy requirements

J. H. GREEN

The assessment of energy requirements is an important, and often central, component of both basic scientific and clinical studies concerning nutrition. An understanding of energy requirements is of interest in various clinical contexts, including diseases involving weight loss (such as anorexia nervosa, cirrhosis, the emphysematous type of chronic obstructive pulmonary disease and cancer) or weight gain (such as obesity), diseases associated with malabsorption (such as Crohn's disease and cystic fibrosis), diseases of the thyroid gland, sepsis, trauma, burns, pregnancy, lactation, growth and ageing, as well as in patients requiring nutritional support.

A report by the FAO/WHO/UNU in 1985 suggested that energy requirements should be related to the basal metabolic rate instead of body weight, as previously recommended (WHO, 1973). This has been substantiated in a study of the energy requirements for physical tasks, with the energy cost of activity being more closely related to the basal metabolic rate than to body weight (Lawrence, 1988). More recently, the sedentary daily energy expenditure has been found to more closely predict energy requirements than even the basal metabolic rate (Webb & Sangal, 1991). This is perhaps not surprising, because the sedentary energy expenditure (which includes resting energy expenditure and the thermic effect of food) would be expected to more closely approximate to the total energy requirements than basal metabolic rate. The only other component of daily energy expenditure is exercise, and this is variable both within and between individuals and, moreover, is often negligible in hospital patients. Therefore, the measurement of energy expenditure, as a means of assessing energy requirements, will be the focus of the present chapter.

The human body obeys the first law of thermodynamics, in that it converts chemical energy into mechanical work and heat. Chemical energy is provided by the dietary intake of carbohydrate, fat and protein. The energy released from the aerobic and, to a lesser extent, anaerobic breakdown of these nutrients, is used to perform mechanical work (membrane transport, synthesis of the stored form of nutrients, or muscular contraction) with the concomitant release of heat. Thus, an individual's energy requirements may be assessed either by measuring the input of the system (oxygen consumption) or by measuring the output of the system (heat). For a detailed account of the biochemistry of energy expenditure see Flatt (1978), and for a comprehensive account of the laboratory methods for measuring energy expenditure see McLean & Tobin (1987).

Methods for assessing energy requirements

Direct calorimetry

Chamber method

The earliest method for assessing energy requirements measured heat production using the technique of direct calorimetry. The first report of a calorimeter chamber to measure heat production in man was published in the last century, but the basic technique, although modified over the years, remains in use. The subject is studied in an insulated chamber and the heat generated is measured directly. These chambers are usually quite small, for example, 1.08 m long, 1.22 m wide and 1.95 m high (Dauncey & Murgatroyd, 1978; Dauncey, Murgatroyd & Cole, 1978). There are two types of direct calorimeter, one in which no heat from the subject is transferred to the outside of the chamber and which, in principle, behaves like an adiabatic bomb calorimeter. In the second type, heat from the subject is transferred to the outside of the chamber, either through the walls or through a circulating medium. Direct calorimetry measures conductive, convective and radiant heat losses, with evaporative heat loss being measured separately. Under some circumstances, such as during physical exercise, the amount of heat stored in the body must also be accounted for. This is done by measuring the change in mean body temperature and multiplying by the body mass and the specific heat of the body tissues, assumed to be 3.47 J/g.

The heat dissipated by the subject is attributed to the oxidation of nutrients. Fat and carbohydrate are oxidised to CO_2 and H_2O. There is no residual potential energy in CO_2 because the carbon atoms are oxidised or, in H_2O, because the hydrogen atoms are oxidised. However, the end products of protein metabolism (urea, uric acid and creatinine) do still contain potential energy in their chemical bonds, and this energy must be accounted for. This method is not practical for most clinical studies, as the subject is required to be in the chamber for several hours, if not days. However, the method has been used extensively in dietary studies involving both healthy volunteers and obese individuals (e.g. Pittet, Gygax & Jéquier, 1974; Pittet *et al.*, 1976; Dauncey, 1980).

Suit method

In the suit method, the subject wears a water-cooled garment which acts as a heat exchanger, with heat loss being calculated from the mass flow rate of water and temperature change across the suit (Webb, Annis & Troutman, 1972). The suit may be worn for 36–48 hours, keeping the subject in a thermoneutral state, even during physical exercise. It was this method which was used to show that sedentary daily energy expenditure is more precise than the basal metabolic rate for predicting energy requirements (Webb & Sangal, 1991).

Infra-red thermography method

Infra-red thermography has recently been adapted to measure heat loss (Shurun & Nelson, 1991). With this method, infrared thermography images are digitised and mean body surface temperature is computed. These data are then used to derive heat loss. The measurements are made with the subjects standing, the negligible heat loss through the feet being ignored. The total heat loss measured over 24 hours has been found to agree well with measurements made by indirect calorimetry, both in healthy controls and post-surgical patients receiving total parenteral nutrition (Shurun & Nelson, 1991).

Although direct calorimetry provides accurate measurements of heat production (energy expenditure), it does not provide any information about the mixture of nutrients which are being oxidised. Such information does come from the technique of indirect calorimetry, and this method is described in the next section.

Indirect calorimetry

Assumptions of indirect calorimetry

Energy expenditure and fuel oxidation rates are calculated from measurements of respiratory gas exchange and urinary nitrogen production rate.

Table 2.1. *Respiratory gas exchange and fuel use*

	Protein (P)	Carbohydrate (C)	Fat (F)
VO$_2$ (litres O$_2$ consumed per g fuel)	0.966	0.746	2.03
VCO$_2$ (litres CO$_2$ produced per g fuel)	0.782	0.746	1.43
RQ (VCO$_2$/VO$_2$)	0.81	1.00	0.74

Magnus-Levy (1907).

Three basic assumptions are made. The first assumption is that since there are no appreciable oxygen stores in the body, oxygen consumption reflects the oxidation of nutrients for energy. The second assumption is that all chemical energy ultimately comes from the oxidation of carbohydrate, fat and protein and the third assumption is that the ratio of oxygen consumed and carbon dioxide produced for the oxidation of these nutrients, is fixed.

VO_2 and VCO_2

The amount of oxygen required, carbon dioxide produced and respiratory quotient of each metabolic fuel is first obtained by bomb calorimetry (Table 2.1). Most of the values which are in current use were derived over 50 years ago. Different laboratories have published different values for each of the calorific factors, and so derived heat production and fuel oxidation rates will vary according to which factors are used. To some extent, these differences depend on which compound was burned in the bomb calorimeter. Monosaccharides, disaccharides and polysaccharides each have different heats of combustion and oxygen consumption per g of fuel oxidised, as do the different fatty acids and amino acids. This problem is addressed in detail by Livesey & Elia (1988). The empirical data provided in the following tables are those currently used in the Academic Unit of Medicine at Leeds.

Protein oxidation rate (Po)

The amount of protein oxidised is calculated from the urinary nitrogen production rate (ṅ) assuming that, on average, nitrogen accounts for 16% of the weight of protein. Thus, for every g of nitrogen excreted, 6.25 g protein (100/16) are assumed to have been oxidised. Any change in the bicarbonate pool is accounted for by measuring the blood urea nitrogen and multiplying the change in blood urea nitrogen by the distribution volume for urea (assumed to be the same as for the total body water, namely 60% of body mass).

Table 2.1 can now be expanded to give the VO_2 and VO_2 per g urinary nitrogen:

$$VO_2 \text{ (litres } O_2 \text{ consumed per g } N_2) = 6.25 \times 0.966 = 6.04$$

$$VCO_2 \text{ (litres } CO_2 \text{ produced per g } N_2) = 6.25 \times 0.782 = 4.89$$

$$RQ = 4.89/6.04 = 0.809$$

Carbohydrate and fat oxidation (Co and Fo)

Using the information given in the previous two sections, the overall rates of oxygen consumption ($\dot{V}O_2$) and carbon dioxide elimination ($\dot{V}CO_2$) can be described:

$$\dot{V}O_2 \text{ (1/min)} = 0.746C + 2.03F + 6.04\dot{n}$$

$$\dot{V}CO_2 \text{ (1/min)} = 0.746C + 1.43F + 4.89\dot{n}$$

Where C = carbohydrate (g)

F = fat (g)

This pair of simultaneous equations is then resolved to derive the oxidation rates (g/min) of carbohydrate and fat.

$$Co = 4.55\dot{V}CO_2 - 3.21\dot{V}O_2 - 2.87\dot{n}$$

$$Fo = (1.67\dot{V}O_2 - \dot{V}CO_2) - 1.92\dot{n}$$

Table 2.2. *Energy equivalents for fuel use*

	Protein (P)	Carbohydrate (C)	Fat (F)
kJ/g fuel	17.5	15.65	39.75

Consolazio, Johnson & Pecora (1963).

Energy requirements due to oxidation of fuels

The energy equivalents of these fuel oxidation rates are derived from the empirical values using bomb calorimetry shown in Table 2.2

Therefore, the energy equivalents (kJ/min) for the fuel oxidation rates derived in the previous two sections are:

$$Pe = 6.25\dot{n} \times 17.15$$
$$Ce = 4.55\dot{V}CO_2 - 3.21\dot{V}O_2 - 2.87\dot{n} \times 15.65$$
$$Fe = (1.67\dot{V}O_2 - \dot{V}CO_2) - 1.92\dot{n} \times 39.75$$

Where Pe = Energy expended in protein oxidation (kJ/min)

Ce = Energy expended in carbohydrate oxidation (kJ/min)

Fe = Energy expended in fat oxidation (kJ/min)

Total energy expenditure

Total energy expenditure (EE) is calculated as the sum of energy expenditure for the three fuels:

$$EE = Pe + Ce + Fe$$
$$EE = 3.860\dot{V}O_2 + 1.156\dot{V}CO_2 - 3.345\dot{n}$$

Limitations

It is important to recognise that indirect calorimetry really measures the disappearance rates of substrates and does not take account of intermediary pathways.

Interpretive problems occur under certain metabolic situations, notably during times of net synthesis of nutrients when the rates of gluconeogenesis, ketogenesis and lipogenesis are raised. Problems also occur if the body bicarbonate does not remain stable during the period of study. This pool decreases during hyperventilation when carbon dioxide elimination exceeds that produced by metabolic activity. This results in a respiratory exchange ratio ($\dot{V}CO_2/\dot{V}O_2$) above 1.0 and a subsequent period of hypoventilation when carbon dioxide from metabolic activity is stored. Alternatively, if lactic acid accumulates, the associated accumulation of H^+ will displace CO_2 from the body's bicarbonate pool.

These problems are discussed in detail elsewhere (Frayn, 1983; Jéquier & Felber, 1987; Ferrannini, 1988; Elia & Livesey, 1988; Simonson & De Fronzo, 1990).

There are basically four methods of indirect calorimetry to which the above assumptions apply, and these are described below.

Respiration chamber method

Direct calorimeter chambers may double as respiration chambers (Dauncey *et al.*, 1978). The subject is confined in a chamber, with heat production being derived from the ventilation rate of the chamber and the gas compositions of the air entering and leaving the chamber.

Closed-circuit method

In closed-circuit indirect calorimetry, the subject breathes in and out of a closed system, commonly a spirometer, which is sealed to the room air. Oxygen, or a mixture of oxygen and nitrogen, is supplied to the spirometer at the rate at which it is consumed. Thus the rate at which oxygen is delivered is the same as oxygen consumption. Heat production may be estimated from oxygen consumption alone (Weir, 1949), in which case the carbon dioxide produced by the subject is absorbed, for example by soda lime within the closed breathing circuit. Alternatively, weight gain of the carbon dioxide absorber may be used to derive carbon dioxide production using this method. The method has found clinical application during mechanical ventilation in anaesthetised patients, although special problems relating to the anaesthetic gases are encountered (Engstrom, Herzoz & Norlander, 1961; Westenskow *et al.*, 1977).

Collection method (Fig. 2.1)

In the collection method the subject's air is collected, either in a bag or a tank, and its volume and gas composition are measured to derive heat

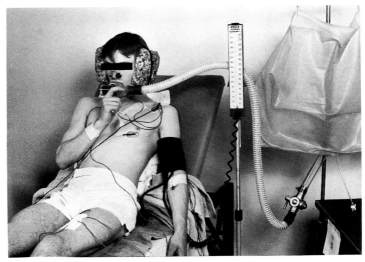

Fig. 2.1. Collection method of indirect calorimetry.

production. This method was originally described by Douglas in 1911, but still remains in use. Its major limitation is that the subject breathes through a mouthpiece or mask, which may cause hyperventilation, especially in individuals who are unaccustomed to the method.

Open-circuit method

There are two main systems of open-circuit indirect calorimetry. In one, the subject breathes in room air and expires directly into a circuit which includes a gas meter to determine pulmonary ventilation rate and gas analysers to determine composition. These methods may be portable, giving them applications to field studies of energy requirements (Humphrey & Wolff, 1977; Eley *et al.*, 1978).

The second method is flow-through calorimetry, and this is probably the most common technique for measuring human energy requirements today. Several types of flow-through method exist, but the ventilated hood method is perhaps the most common (Fig. 2.2). A clear plastic hood is placed over the subject's head and shoulders, and room air is blown or sucked through it at a known flow rate. The gas composition is measured by conventional oxygen and carbon dioxide analysers. The method has been available for over 50 years (Benedict, 1930), but its clinical application has become especially apparent in the last 10 years or so.

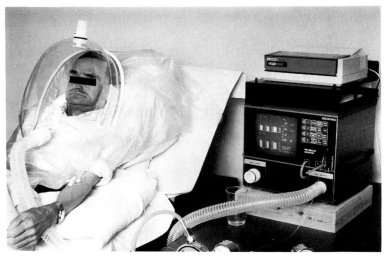

Fig. 2.2. Flow-through method of indirect calorimetry.

Flow-through indirect calorimetry is especially convenient for clinical use, since it is non-invasive and portable. The technique is commercially available from a number of manufacturers as a virtually automatic system, which includes a programmed microprocessor to derive values of energy expenditure and fuel oxidation rates. A potential difficulty with the method in the clinical setting is the measurement of urinary nitrogen and, when necessary, blood urea nitrogen which are not routine diagnostic tests and, therefore, may require the facilities and expertise of a research laboratory. For normal, healthy volunteers, equations are available to derive energy data without urinary nitrogen and yet with negligible error (Weir, 1949). These equations involve the assumption that energy expenditure from protein oxidation accounts for 12.5% of total energy expenditure. However, protein oxidation may greatly exceed normal values in many hospital patients, including those who are acutely ill and catabolic, with evidence of muscle wasting. Indeed, Bursztein *et al.* (1989) have reported that the range of urinary nitrogen excretion in acutely ill patients is 0–60 g/day; a typical normal value is of the order of 6 g/day. Despite these abnormalities in urinary nitrogen excretion, Bursztein *et al.*, (1989) have shown that the overall error in calculating energy expenditure without measuring urinary nitrogen in these patients is usually $< 2.0\%$ and rarely $> 3.0\%$.

Flow-through indirect calorimetry has been used to assess energy requirements in many clinical states. These include obesity (e.g. Ravussin *et al.*, 1988), weight loss (e.g. Kurpad, Kulkarby & Shetty, 1989), inflammatory bowel disease (e.g. Kushner & Schoeller, 1991), carcinoma (e.g. MacFie *et al.*, 1982), mental illness (e.g. Prentice *et al.*, 1989) and Parkinson's disease (Levi *et al.*, 1990), as well as in patients following surgery (e.g. Brandi *et al.*, 1988) and in acutely ill patients requiring nutritional support (e.g. Makk *et al.*, 1990). Studies using indirect calorimetry in Leeds have focussed on liver disease (Green, Bramley & Losowsky, 1991) and chronic obstructive pulmonary disease (Green & Muers, 1991, 1992).

Comparisons between direct and indirect calorimetry methods

When respiratory measurements are made in a chamber, which is also designed as a direct calorimeter, energy expenditure is often derived simultaneously by both methods (Pittet *et al.*, 1974, 1976; Dauncey, 1980). In the absence of any change in heat storage by the body, the direct and indirect methods should agree, since heat production equals heat loss during thermal energy balance. Under such conditions, a mean difference of 1.2% has been observed between the two methods during a 24-hour period (Dauncey, 1980).

A recent study which compared three methods of indirect calorimetry with each other (both open-circuit methods and the respiration chamber method) found no significant differences between them (Soares *et al.*, 1989).

Other indirect methods

Doubly labelled water method

The doubly-labelled water method, developed nearly 30 years ago (Lifson, 1966), has made it possible to assess energy requirements in free-living individuals. The subject is given a bolus of two stable isotopes of water, ^2H_2O and $H_2^{18}O$, either orally or intravenously. Deuterium is eliminated by the body only as water, whereas $H_2^{18}O$ is eliminated as water and in carbon dioxide. The difference in the turnover rates of these two stable isotopes can, therefore, be used to derive carbon dioxide production. By knowing the fuel mix, energy expenditure is derived. The fuel mix may be obtained from the food quotient using dietary records (Black, Prentice & Coward, 1986) or from indirect calorimetry. A single value for the energy equivalent of carbon dioxide is inappropriate, since it varies with diet as well as nutritional status (Elia, 1991). This method has been used to assess energy requirements in a variety of clinical conditions, including burns (Goran *et al.*, 1990), pregnancy, lactation, growth, malnutrition and obesity (Schoeller & Fjeld, 1991). However, it has been found to underestimate energy expenditure in obesity, with larger underestimates in heavier, fatter people compared with measurements made by indirect calorimetry using a respiration chamber (Ravussin, *et al.*, 1991).

Variables which correlate with energy expenditure

Both pulmonary ventilation (Durnin & Edwards, 1955) and, more commonly, heart rate (e.g. Booyens & Hervey, 1960; Spurr *et al.*, 1988) have been used as indices of energy expenditure. With the advent of portable heart rate monitors which are capable of storing data, the latter method offers a cheap, although less accurate, alternative to the doubly-labelled water method of assessing energy expenditure in free-living subjects (Spurr *et al.*, 1988; Heini *et al.*, 1991).

Predictive methods based on physical characteristics

Over 190 equations have been published to predict resting energy expenditure from the subject's physical characteristics (commonly age, height, weight and gender) (Foster *et al.*, 1987). The most widely used is the Harris–Benedict equation (Harris & Benedict, 1919). A major limitation of such predictive equations is that they do not take account of the lean body mass, which is the metabolically active cell mass. Therefore, the equations are not appropriate to predict the energy requirements of individuals with an abnormal body composition. An abnormal body composition is found in many clinical conditions, including obesity, diseases associated with wasting and diseases associated with fluid retention in the form of oedema or ascites.

Lean body mass has been found to be a better predictor of 24-hour energy expenditure than any other physical characteristic (Bogardus *et al.*, 1986), but its accurate assessment is difficult. It is most accurately assessed by the measurement of total body potassium (Jensen *et al.*, 1988) or by dual photon absorptiometry (Gotfredsen *et al.*, 1986), but these methods are not routinely available. Probably the most common bedside technique is the use of skinfold thickness (Durnin & Womersley, 1974), although the technique has been questioned for clinical purposes (Streat, Beddow & Hill, 1985). Alternatively, it can be derived from hydrostatic weighing (Goldman & Buskirk, 1961), but many patients would find water immersion unacceptable. Muscle mass, a major component of lean body mass, may be derived from measurements of urinary creatinine. This requires an accurately timed 3-day urine collection however, and the measurements are influenced by many factors including stress, the menstrual cycle and diet (especially meat consumption) (Heymsfield *et al.*, 1983), making it unsuitable for routine clinical use.

A more recent technique to derive lean body mass which has been used in conjunction with measurements of energy expenditure in healthy controls is bioelectrical impedance (Astrup *et al.*, 1990). This method is ideal in a clinical context, because it is portable, easy to use and does not require elaborate data analysis. Moreover, measurements of lean body mass by bioelectrical impedance analysis compare favourably with those made by dual energy X-ray absorptiometry in normal subjects (Stewart *et al.*, 1992). Furthermore, measurements made in an arm can be used to derive total body composition, making it a potentially useful method even for patients who are confined to bed or who have ascites (Stewart *et al.*, 1992). More studies are required to validate its use in patients with wasting and/or fluid retention.

The above discussion raises an important issue in the field of energy metabolism concerning the comparison of data derived from patients with normal values and/or unexpected values. Comparisons between patient data and established predictive equations based on weight, height, age and gender may be inappropriate if the patients have gained or lost weight, giving them an abnormal body composition. The alternative would be to study matched pairs of individuals, but the selection of an under- or overweight, albeit otherwise healthy, individual to act as a control would seem equally questionable in view of the well known metabolic adaptations to weight change.

Summary

In summary, there are several methods for assessing energy requirements in man. Direct calorimetry is used to determine energy expenditure, but indirect calorimetry is used when a knowledge of the mix of fuels being oxidised is also required. Direct and indirect calorimetry, as well as the doubly labelled water method, are more accurate than methods which involve the measurement of variables which correlate with energy expenditure, or those which use predictive equations. However, correlation and prediction methods are cheaper and technically easier to carry out, making them attractive for clinical purposes. A major limitation of predictive equations based on the physical characteristics of normal healthy volunteers, is that they are likely to produce erroneous results in patients with abnormal body composition.

References

Astrup, A., Thorbeck, G., Lind, J. & Isaksson, B. (1990). Prediction of 24 hour energy expenditure and its components from physical characteristics of body composition in normal-weight humans. *American Journal of Clinical Nutrition*, **52**, 777–83.

Benedict, F. G. (1930). Helmet for use in clinical studies of gaseous metabolism. *New England Journal of Medicine*, **203**, 150–8.

Black, A. E., Prentice, A. M. & Coward, W. A. (1986). Use of food quotients to predict respiratory quotients for the doubly-labelled water method of measuring energy expenditure. *Human Nutrition: Clinical Nutrition*, **40C**, 381–91.

Bogardus, C., Lillioja, S., Ravussin, E. *et al.* (1986). Familial dependence of the resting metabolic rate. *New England Journal of Medicine*, **315**, 96–100.

Booyens, J. & Hervey, G. R. (1960). The pulse rate as a means of measuring metabolic rate in man. *Canadian Journal of Biochemistry & Physiology*, **38**, 1301–9.

Brandi, L. S., Oleggini, M., Lachi, S. *et al.* 1988). Energy metabolism in surgical patients in the early postoperative period: a reappraisal. *Critical Care Medicine*, **16**, 18–22.

Bursztein, S., Saphar, P., Singer, P. & Elwyn, D. H. (1989). A mathematical analysis of indirect calorimetry measurements in acutely ill patients. *American Journal of Clinical Nutrition*, **50**, 227–30.

Consolazio, C. F., Johnson, R. E. & Pecora, L. J. (1963). *Physiological Measurements of Metabolic Functions in Man.* New York: McGraw-Hill.

Dauncey, M. J. & Murgatroyd, P. R. (1978). A direct and indirect calorimeter for studies on energy expenditure in man over 24 hour periods. *Journal of Physiology,* London, **284**, 7P–8P.

Dauncey, M. J., Murgatroyd, P. R. & Cole, T. J. (1978). A human calorimeter for the direct and indirect measurement of 24 h energy expenditure. *British Journal of Nutrition,* **39**, 557–66.

Dauncey, M. J. (1980). Metabolic effects of altering the 24 h energy intake in man using direct and indirect calorimetry. *British Journal of Nutrition,* **43**, 257–69.

Douglas, G. (1911). A method for determining the total respiratory exchange in man. *Journal of Physiology,* London, **42**. 17P–18P.

Durnin, J. V. G. A. & Edwards, R. G. (1955). Pulmonary ventilation as an index of energy expenditure. *Quarterly Journal of Experimental Physiology,* **40**, 370–7.

Durnin, J. V. G. A. & Womersley, J. (1974). Body fat assessed from total body density and its estimation from skinfold thickness: measurements on 481 men and women aged 16 to 72 years. *British Journal of Nutrition,* **32**, 77–92.

Eley, C., Goldsmith, R., Layman, D., Tan, G. L. E. & Walker, E. (1978). A respirometer for use in the field for the measurement of oxygen consumption. 'The Miser' a miniature indicating and sampling electronic respirometer. *Ergonomics,* **21**, 253–64.

Elia, M. (1991). Energy equivalents of carbon dioxide and their importance in assessing energy expenditure when using tracer techniques. *American Journal of Physiology,* **260** (*Endocrinology & Metabolism,* **23**), E75–88.

Elia, M. & Livesey, G. (1988). Theory and validity of indirect calorimetry during net lipid synthesis. *American Journal of Clinical Nutrition,* **47**, 591–607.

Engstrom, C. G., Herzoz, P. & Norlander, O. (1961). A method for the continuous measurement of oxygen consumption in the presence of inert gases during controlled ventilation. *Acta Anaesthesiologica Scandinavica,* **5**, 115–28.

FAO/WHO/UNU. (1985). Energy and protein requirements. Report of a joint FAO/WHO/UNU Expert Consultation. Tech. Rep. Ser. No. 724; WHO, Geneva.

Ferrannini, E. (1988). The theoretical bases of indirect calorimetry: a review. *Metabolism,* **37**, 287–301.

Flatt, J. P. (1978). The biochemistry of energy expenditure. In *Recent Advances in Obesity Research,* Volume 2. *Proceedings of the Second International Congress in Obesity,* ed. G. A. Bray. Newman Publishing Ltd, London.

Foster, G. D., Knox, L. S., Dempsey, D. T. & Mullen, J. L. (1987). Caloric requirements in total parenteral nutrition. *Journal of the American College of Nutrition,* **6**, 231–53.

Frayn, K. N. (1983). Calculation of substrate oxidation rates in vivo from gaseous exchange. *Journal of Applied Physiology: Respiratory Environmental & Exercise Physiology,* **55**, 628–34.

Goldman, R. F. & Buskirk, E. R. (1961). A method for underwater weighing and the determination of body density. In *Techniques for Measuring Body Composition,* ed. J. Brozek & A. Henschel, pp. 78–106, National Academy of Sciences, National Research Council, p. 16.

Goran, M. I., Peters, E. J., Herndon, D. N. & Wolfe, R. R. (1990). Total energy expenditure in burned children using the doubly labeled water technique.

American Journal of Physiology, **259** (*Endocrinology & Metabolism*), **22**), E576–85.

Gotfredsen, A., Jensen, J., Borg, J. & Christiansen, C. (1986). Measurement of lean body mass and total body fat using dual photon absorptiometry. *Metabolism*, **35**, 88–93.

Green, J. R., Bramley, P. N. & Losowsky, M. S. (1991). Are patients with primary biliary cirrhosis hypermetabolic? A comparison between patients pre- and post-liver transplantation and controls. *Hepatology*, **14**, 464–72.

Green, J. H. & Muers, M. F. (1991). The thermic effect of food in underweight patients with emphysematous chronic obstructive pulmonary disease. *European Respiratory Journal*, **4**, 813–19.

Green, J. H. & Muers, M. H. (1992). Comparisons between basal metabolic rate and diet-induced thermogenesis in different types of chronic obstructive pulmonary disease. *Clinical Science*, **83**, 109–16.

Harris, J. A. & Benedict, F. G. (1919). *A Biometric Study of Basal Metabolism in Man*. Publication No. 279, Carnegie Institute, Washington.

Heini, A., Schutz, Y., Diaz, E., Prentice, A. M., Whitehead, R. G. & Jéquier, E. (1991). Free-living energy and expenditure measured by two independent techniques in pregnant and non-pregnant Gambian women. *American Journal of Physiology*, **261** (*Endocrinology & Metabolism*, **24**), E9–17.

Heymsfield, S. B., Arteaga, C., McManus, C., Smith, J. & Moffitt, S. (1983). Measurement of muscle mass in humans: validity of the 24 hour urinary creatinine method. *American Journal of Clinical Nutrition*, **37**, 478–94.

Humphrey, S. J. E. & Wolff, H. S. (1977). The Oxylog. *Journal of Physiology, London*, **267**, 12P.

Jensen, M. D., Braun, J. S., Vetterr, J. & Marsh, H. M. (1988). Measurements of body potassium with a whole-body counter: relationship between lean body mass and resting energy expenditure. *Mayo Clinic Proceedings*, **63**, 864–8.

Jéquier, E. & Felber, J-P. (1987). Indirect calorimetry. *Ballière's Clinical Endocrinology and Metabolism*, **1**, 911–36.

Kurpad, A. V., Kulkarby, R. N. & Shetty, P. N. (1989). Reduced thermoregulatory thermogenesis in undernutrition. *European Journal of Clinical Nutrition*, **43**, 27–33.

Kushner, R. F. & Schoeller, D. A. (1991). Resting and total energy expenditure in patients with inflammatory bowel disease. *American Journal of Clinical Nutrition*, **53**, 161–5.

Lawrence, M. (1988). Predicting energy requirements: is energy expenditure proportional to the BMR or to body weight? *European Journal of Clinical Nutrition*, **42**, 919–27.

Levi, S., Cox, M., Lugon, M., Hodkinson, M. & Tomkins, A. (1990). Increased energy expenditure in Parkinson's disease. *British Medical Journal*, **301**, 1256–7.

Lifson, N. (1966). Theory of use of the turnover rates of body water for measuring energy and material balance. *Journal of Theoretical Biology*, **12**, 46–74.

Livesey, G. & Elia, M. (1988). Estimation of energy expenditure, net carbohydrate utilization and net fat oxidation and synthesis by indirect calorimetry: evaluation of errors with special reference to the detailed composition of fuels. *American Journal of Clinical Nutrition*, **47**, 608–28.

MacFie, J., Burkinshaw, L., Oxby, C., Holmfield, J. H. M. & Hill, G. L. (1982). The effect of gastrointestinal malignancy on resting metabolic expenditure. *British Journal of Surgery*, **69**, 443–6.

Magnus-Levy, A. (1907). In *Metabolism and Practical Medicine*, English Translation, First Edition, ed. C. Von Noorden, pp. 185–282. Heinemann, London.

Makk, L. J. K., McClave, S. A., Creech, P. W. *et al.* (1990). Clinical application of the metabolic cart to the delivery of total parenteral nutrition. *Critical Care Medicine*, **18**, 1320–7.

McLean, J. A. & Tobin, G. (1987). *Animal and Human Calorimetry*. Cambridge University Press.

Pittet, P. H., Gygax, P. H. & Jéquier, E. (1974). Thermic effect of glucose and amino acids in man studied by direct and indirect calorimetry. *British Journal of Nutrition*, **31**, 343–9.

Pittet, P. H., Chappuis, P. H., Acheson, K., de Techtermann, F. & Jéquier, E. (1976). Thermic effect of glucose in obese subjects studied by direct and indirect calorimetry. *British Journal of Nutrition*, **35**, 281–92.

Prentice, A. M., Leavesley, K., Murgatroyd, P. R. *et al.* (1989). Is severe wasting in elderly mental patients caused by an excessive energy requirement? *Age and Ageing*, **18**, 158–67.

Ravussin, E., Lillioja, S., Knowler, W. C. *et al.* (1988). Reduced rate of energy expenditure as a risk factor for body-weight gain. *New England Journal of Medicine*, **318**, 467–72.

Ravussin, E., Harper, I. T., Rising, R. & Bogardus, C. (1991). Energy expenditure by doubly labeled water. Validation in lean and obese subjects. *American Journal of Physiology*, **261** (*Endocrinology & Metabolism*, **24**), E402–9.

Schoeller, D. A. & Fjeld, C. R. (1991). Human energy metabolism: what have we learned from the doubly labeled water method? *Annual Review of Nutrition*, 355–73.

Shurun, M. & Nelson, R. A. (1991). Quantitation of energy expenditure by infrared thermography. *American Journal of Clinical Nutrition*, **53**, 1361–7.

Simonson, D. C. & De Fronzo, R. A. (1990). Indirect calorimetry: methodological and interpretive problems. *American Journal of Physiology*, **258** (*Endocrinology & Metabolism*, **21**), E399–412.

Soares, M. J., Sheela, M. L., Kurpad, A. V., Kulkarni, R. N. & Shetty, P. S. (1989). The influence of different methods on basal metabolic rate measurements in human subjects. *American Journal of Clinical Nutrition*, **50**, 731–6.

Spurr, G. B., Prentice, A. M., Murgatroyd, P. R., Goldberg, G. R., Reina, J. C. & Christman, N. T. (1988). Energy expenditure from minute-by-minute heart rate recording: comparison with indirect calorimetry. *American Journal of Clinical Nutrition*, **48**, 552–9.

Stewart, S. P., Bramley, P. N., Heighton, R. *et al.* (1992). Estimation of body composition from bioelectrical impedance of body segments: Comparison with dual energy X-ray absorptiometry. *British Journal of Nutrition* (in press).

Streat, S. J., Beddow, A. H. & Hill, G. L. (1985). Measurement of body fat and hydration of the fat-free body in health and disease. *Metabolism*, **34**, 509–18.

Webb, P., Annis, J. F. & Troutman, S. J. (1972). Human calorimetry with a water cooled garment. *Journal of Applied Physiology*, **32**, 412–18.

Webb, P. & Sangal, S. (1991). Sedentary daily expenditure: a base for estimating individual energy requirements. *American Journal of Clinical Nutrition*, **53**, 606–11.

Weir, V. de J. B. (1949). New methods for calculating metabolic rate with special reference to protein metabolism. *Journal of Physiology*, London, **109**, 109.

Westenskow, D. R., Johnson, C. C., Jordan, W. S. & Gehmlich, D. K. (1977). Instrumentation for measuring continuous oxygen consumption of surgical patients. *IEE Transactions on Biomedical Engineering*, **24**, 331–7.

WHO. (1973). *Energy and protein requirements.* Report of a joint FAO/WHO *ad hoc* expert committee. Tech. Rep. Ser. No. 522, WHO, Geneva.

3

Amino acid requirements in health and disease

P. J. GARLICK, M. A. McNURLAN
AND M. F. FULLER

Without an adequate supply of dietary protein, lean tissue, of which protein is the major component, is lost and body function is compromised. This dietary requirement for protein exists even in fully grown adults whose body protein content is in a steady state, but even higher amounts are needed during conditions which consume protein, such as growth or lactation. Moreover, protein consists of twenty or so different amino acids, which are present in each protein species in fixed proportions, leading to a separate metabolic requirement for each amino acid. Of these twenty, nine have been defined as essential (or indispensable) for man. Because mammals lack the enzyme pathways to synthesise these from simpler precursors, they must be supplied in the diet (Table 3.1). The others can be synthesised from simple carbon sources and non-specific nitrogen compounds and were originally designated non-essential (or dispensable). More recently it has been recognised that the synthesis of non-essential amino acids can, under certain circumstances, become limiting, leading to a third designation, conditionally essential (see below).

Physiological basis for amino acid requirements

The reason why dietary amino acids are required to maintain the body protein content, even in the absence of growth or lactation, is the presence of irreversible pathways that lead inevitably to net losses. If these minimal losses, termed obligatory losses, are not replaced from dietary sources or by endogenous synthesis from simpler precursors, there will be a net breakdown of body protein. Losses of amino acids occur through six principal routes (Table 3.2). Although these losses are small in relation to normal requirements, they can become significant with low dietary intake. Moreover, since the losses of some amino acids are greater

Table 3.1. *The major amino acids found in protein, their metabolic precursors and the major processes for which they are utilised*

	Precursor	Non-protein pathways
Essential amino acids		
L-threonine	—	n.i.
L-valine	—	n.i.
L-methionine	—	cysteine methylation, e.g. choline, creatine, polyamines, sulphations
L-isoleucine	—	n.i.
L-leucine	—	n.i.
L-phenylalanine	—	tyrosine
L-lysine	—	hydroxylysine, methyllysine, carnitine, pipecolic acid
L-histidine	—	histamine
L-tryptophan	—	serotonin, melatonin, NAD, NADP
Non-essential and conditionally essential		
L-cyst(e)ine	methionine	taurine, glutathione
L-tyrosine	phenylalanine	melanin, dopamine, catecholamines, thyroid hormones
L-arginine	citrulline/glutamine	urea, polyamines, creatine, nitric oxide
L-glycine	serine	haem, creatine, glutathione, nucleic acids
L-proline	glutamate	hydroxyproline (in collagen)
L-alanine	pyruvate (by transamination)	transamination, glucose/urea
L-aspartic acid	oxaloacetate (by transamination)	transamination, glucose/urea, nucleic acids
L-asparagine	aspartic acid	urea, nucleic acids
L-glutamic acid	α-ketoglutarate (by transamination)	transamination, glucose/urea
L-glutamine	glutamic acid	citrulline, alanine, ammonia, nucleic acids
L-serine	glycerol/ glycine	phospholipids, choline

n.i. none identified.

Table 3.2. *Routes of obligatory amino acid losses*

Urinary excretion
Irreversible modification
Synthesis of non-protein substances
Irreducible oxidation
Losses from the skin
Losses via the gastrointestinal tract

than others, obligatory losses have differential effects on amino acid requirements.

Small amounts of amino acids are excreted in the urine, some in free form, some in proteins. However, for most essential amino acids these losses are small, accounting for less than 5% of total requirements (Leverton, Waddill & Skellenger, 1959). The exceptions are those amino acids which are irreversibly modified and excreted in the urine. For example, some histidine residues in proteins such as actin and myosin are irreversibly methylated. When the protein is degraded, the methylhistidine cannot be reutilised for new protein synthesis and is therefore excreted in the urine. Similar processes occur for lysine and proline.

Most amino acids are obligatory precursors for the synthesis of non-protein substances. These are summarised in Table 3.1. The quantities of amino acids used for the synthesis of non-protein substances are difficult to estimate, but for most amino acids are thought to be small. Among the essential amino acids, one exception may be the sulphur amino acids. Methionine has many functions in the body. It is the only precursor for the synthesis of S-adenosyl methionine, the major methyl donor in the numerous methylation reactions throughout the body. However, these processes do not necessarily imply a net utilisation of methionine, since S-adenosyl homocysteine produced by the demethylation of S-adenosyl methionine can be remethylated to form methionine again. Methionine is also the source of the propylamine moiety in the synthesis of poly-amines, but in this case also the remaining part of the molecule may be recycled back to methionine (Edwards *et al.*, 1977). If the dietary supply of taurine (a non-protein amino acid which none the less appears to be required for normal body function) is inadequate, there may also be a requirement for methionine or cystine for its synthesis. Glycine is another amino acid of which the quantities involved in the synthesis of a wide range of metabolically important compounds may not be trivial. The glycine requirements for the synthesis of haem and creatine, for example, are substantial.

Normally, oxidation is a mechanism for disposing of amino acids in excess of other needs and for converting them into energy substrates. However, when the diet is deficient in an amino acid, there is a need to conserve it as fully as possible and the activity of the oxidative pathway is suppressed. However, amino acid oxidation does not cease altogether and this minimal rate of oxidation constitutes a further obligatory loss.

Finally, protein and amino acids are continually lost from body epithelia, both from the skin and via the gastrointestinal tract. There is little direct information on amino acid losses from the skin, but comprehensive measurements of skin nitrogen loss showed it to be sensitive to protein intake, with a minimum of approximately 120 mg/d in subjects on a protein-free diet (Calloway, Odell & Margen, 1971). This constitutes less than 5% of total nitrogen needs in the non-growing adult (i.e. at maintenance). Furthermore, only part of this loss is amino acid nitrogen. The most important amino acid losses are probably in the keratins of skin, hair and nails, which collectively account for the loss of approximately 300 mg of protein per day (Calloway *et al.*, 1971). Because of the high cystine content of keratin these dermal losses could account for some 5% of maintenance sulphur amino acid requirements. Amino acids are also lost via the gastrointestinal tract. Although much of the protein secreted into the gut is reabsorbed and recycled, some, such as mucin, is relatively resistant and either escapes digestion or is sequestered in the microbial biomass. These losses may be much greater than those via the external epithelia, especially for threonine (Fuller *et al.*, 1993). It should be noted that the amino acids appearing in the faeces originate from several sources. Some arise from undigested protein and some are in the mucous secretions. However, the major part is in bacteria, which have themselves obtained their nitrogen from the other two sources. Thus, there is no relationship necessary between the faecal amino acid composition and the actual losses of amino acids by the gastrointestinal route.

All these losses must be replaced by dietary intake (for essential amino acids), or by endogenous synthesis (for non-essential and conditionally essential amino acids). Because they involve non-protein pathways or the synthesis of proteins of atypical composition, rather than the net synthesis of body protein, the maintenance needs for individual amino acids bear little relationship to the average composition of body proteins (see Table 3.3). By contrast, the needs for amino acids for growth or lactation

Table 3.3. *Patterns of essential amino acids (g/16 g N) required for maintenance, expressed in proportion to the total nitrogen requirement (54 mg/kg) and the corresponding amino acid patterns of whole-body protein and of milk protein*

	Maintenance[a]	Body protein[b]	Milk protein[c]
Threonine	2.1	4.8	4.9
Valine	3.0	6.2	6.5
Methionine	n.e.	1.9	1.6
Methionine + cystine	3.9	4.3	3.7
Isoleucine	3.0	4.8	6.2
Leucine	4.1	7.7	9.8
Phenylalanine	n.e.	5.3	4.5
Phenylalanine + tyrosine	4.1	8.6	8.9
Lysine	3.6	8.2	6.9
Histidine	2.3–3.6	2.4	2.1
Tryptophan	1.0	1.4	1.6

n.e. not estimated.
[a] From FAO/WHO/UNU 1985.
[b] From Smith (1980).
[c] From Macy & Kelly (1961).

are approximately in proportion to the composition of the protein deposited or secreted.

Estimates of essential amino acid requirements

Maintenance needs

Because, in dietary amino acid deficiency, metabolic amino acid requirements are met from body protein breakdown, the primary criterion of amino acid adequacy has conventionally been the maintenance of nitrogen equilibrium (i.e. nitrogen balance). This was the criterion used in the pioneering studies on men by Rose and his co-workers and by Leverton and others (Table 3.4). In the interpretation of such studies, two difficulties arise. First, the intention is clearly to estimate the amino acid needs of the population as a whole. However, some authors have estimated the 'requirement' as the mean amino acid intake required to achieve nitrogen equilibrium in a group of subjects, whereas others have estimated the 'requirement' as the greatest amount required to attain nitrogen equilibrium in any subject, which clearly leads to higher estimates,

Table 3.4. *Estimates of the essential amino acid requirement*
(mg/d) for the maintenance of nitrogen equilibrium in adult men
and women

	Men[a]	Women[b] (recalculated[c])	FAO/WHO/UNU (1985)
Threonine	500	305 (375)	455
Valine	800	650 (622)	650
Methionine	165	180 (194)	n.e.
Methionine + cystine	1100	550 (700)	845
Isoleucine	700	450 (550)	650
Leucine	1100	620 (727)	910
Phenylalanine	300	220 (258)	n.e.
Phenylalanine + tyrosine	1100	n.e.	910
Lysine	800	500 (545)	780
Histidine	n.e.	n.e.	520–780
Tryptophan	250	157 (168)	228

n.e. not estimated.
[a] Rose (1957).
[b] Leverton *et al.* (1959).
[c] recalculated by Hegsted (1963).

more akin to 'safe' recommended dietary allowances. This might explain some of the discrepancies between published values. The second difficulty relates to the well-known tendency for nitrogen balance methods to overestimate the true retention of nitrogen in the body. This arises in part from failure to measure the integumental and other small incidental nitrogen losses mentioned above, and partly from the fact that intake tends to be overestimated and output underestimated, leading to an exaggerated estimate of nitrogen retention, which in turn leads to an underestimate of the amino acid requirement to maintain nitrogen equilibrium.

Current international reviews of the amino acid requirements of adults (FAO/WHO/UNU, 1985, see Table 3.4) are largely based on the classical nitrogen balance studies mentioned, and have been criticised because of the problems pointed out above. These estimates have recently been challenged by the results of studies in which rates of oxidation of single essential amino acids have been measured using isotopically labelled amino acids (Meguid *et al.*, 1986; Zhao *et al.*, 1986; Young *et al.* 1987, 1991; Cortiella *et al.*, 1992). From the relationship between the oxidation rate and dietary intake of a specific amino acid, the minimum oxidation rate was determined and taken to represent the requirement for balance. This approach is not itself without problems of interpretation (discussed by Millward & Rivers, 1988), specifically those associated with interpreting the stable isotope data obtained in terms of a model of whole body amino acid metabolism. However, these studies suggest, for those amino acids so far studied, a higher requirement than that currently recommended from nitrogen balance studies, and this would clearly be even higher if all other obligatory losses were included.

Requirements for growth, gestation and lactation

In addition to their maintenance needs, children and women who are pregnant or lactating require extra amino acids to form the proteins of body tissue or milk (Table 3.5). In each case, the quantity of amino acid needed daily depends on the rate of growth, the stage of gestation or the rate of milk secretion, each of which is affected by both genetic and environmental factors. In the utilisation of dietary amino acids for these processes, there are inevitably increased losses, both via the gastrointestinal tract and through oxidation. These depend on the digestibility and amino acid composition of the diet. The marginal efficiency of protein utilisation (i.e. improvement of protein retention as a proportion of the protein intake above maintenance) for these processes is estimated (FAO/WHO/UNU, 1985) to be around 0.7; a value which accords with more comprehensive estimates made in experimental animals.

Estimates of the amino acid needs of infants have, for the most part, been made from analyses of breast milk or of formula diets that supported satisfactory growth. For older children more direct experimental data are available, based again on nitrogen balance. These estimates are summarised in Table 3.5.

Similarly in gestation and lactation, although there is considerable information on protein requirements, there are no direct estimates of amino acid requirements. The values given in Table 3.5 have been calculated from information on protein needs and the pattern of amino acids utilised for each process.

Non-essential and conditionally essential amino acids

With the work of Rose and Colleagues (summarised by Rose, 1957), amino acids were regarded as non-essential if protein equilibrium (nitrogen balance) was maintained when these amino acids were omitted from the

Table 3.5. *Daily amino acid requirements (mg/kg body weight) during growth and adult life, and the additional requirements (g/d) for gestation and lactation*[a]

| | Daily requirements (mg/kg body weight) | | | | Additional requirements (g/d) | | | | | |
| | | | | | Gestation trimester | | | Lactation | |
Amino acid	3–4 months	2 years	10–12 years	Adult	1	2	3	0–6 months	6–24 months
Threonine	87	37	28	7	0.06	0.29	0.51	0.66	0.47
Valine	93	38	25	10	0.07	0.38	0.66	0.88	0.62
Methionine + cystine	58	27	22	13	0.05	0.26	0.46	0.49	0.35
Methionine	n.e.	n.e.	n.e.	n.e.	0.02	0.12	0.20	0.22	0.15
Isoleucine	70	31	28	10	0.06	0.29	0.51	0.84	0.59
Leucine	161	73	44	14	0.09	0.47	0.82	1.32	0.93
Phenylalanine + tyrosine	125	69	22	14	0.10	0.53	0.92	1.20	0.84
Phenylalanine	n.e.	n.e.	n.e.	n.e.	0.06	0.32	0.57	0.61	0.43
Lysine	103	64	44	12	0.10	0.50	0.88	0.93	0.66
Histidine	28	n.e.	n.e.	8–12	0.03	0.15	0.26	0.28	0.20
Tryptophan	17	12.5	3.3	3.5	0.02	0.09	0.15	0.22	0.15

n.e. not estimated.
[a] From FAO/WHO/UNU, 1985.

diet. The amino acids classified in this way were those indicated in Table 3.1. However, since this early work, the concept of non-essential amino acids has been extended by the concept of conditionally essential amino acids (Laidlaw & Kopple, 1987). This distinction recognises that amino acid requirements are not fixed but change with conditions. When the requirement for an amino acid exceeds the body's capacity for synthesis, the amino acid must be supplied from dietary sources, making it conditionally essential.

From this concept of conditionally essential amino acids, probably only alanine, glutamate and aspartate, which are made by simple transfer of an amino group (transamination) to intermediates in the tricarboxylic acid cycle (TCA), can be regarded as fully non-essential. Because the TCA cycle is highly active in cells throughout the body, the necessary intermediates, pyruvate, α-ketoglutarate and oxaloacetate, are plentiful and transamination occurs readily.

Cystine and tyrosine provide obvious examples of conditionally essential amino acids, because they are synthesised exclusively from methionine and phenylalanine and therefore depend on a plentiful supply of these precursors. Growth can precipitate a dietary requirement for a particular amino acid, which is not demonstrable in the non-growing adult. Thus, it has been suggested that glycine might become essential in milk-fed premature infants, because of the additional demands of its non-protein pathways (Jackson, 1989). As pointed out above, these pathways utilise a substantial amount of glycine, which must be met before net deposition of protein can occur. Arginine has also been shown to be required for optimal growth in a number of species, and appears to become essential after trauma (Visek, 1986). Similarly, glutamine requirements are believed to increase during infection and injury. Because of the extensive recent literature on the potential use of arginine or glutamine in a variety of clinical conditions, they are discussed separately in the next section.

Are there special needs during illness?

Infection, cancer and trauma cause a loss of lean body mass, particularly from skeletal muscle. The aim of nutritional support is to prevent this loss, to improve body function and to facilitate recovery. On the premise that the optimal pattern of amino acids for this purpose might differ from that for growth and maintenance in health, there have been a large number of studies examining the effects of supplements of specific amino acids on nutritional and metabolic parameters both in health and disease.

Branched chain amino acids (BCAA)

In the last 20 years there has been substantial interest in the BCAA, leucine, isoleucine and valine, as a possible way of minimising body protein wasting after trauma. This was stimulated by experiments on isolated animal muscles *in vitro*, which showed that elevated concentrations of BCAA could inhibit protein loss by stimulating protein synthesis and inhibiting protein degradation (Buse & Reid, 1975; Fulks, Li & Goldberg, 1975; Li & Jefferson, 1978). Moreover, supplements of leucine or BCAA have been shown to improve nitrogen balance in various groups of patients with muscle wasting (see reviews by Adibi, 1980; Smith & Elia, 1983; Walser, 1984; Brennan *et al.*, 1986). However, attempts to demonstrate a clinical, as opposed to a biochemical, benefit have not been successful. Thus, a Workshop sponsored by the American Society for Parenteral and Enteral Nutrition concluded that, as little major effect on outcome had yet been demonstrated, no widespread application of BCAA formulations could be endorsed (Brennan *et al.*, 1986).

The apparent discrepancies between the experimental and clinical studies might have a number of explanations. The early experiments on effects of BCAA were performed on isolated muscle, but when measurements have been made *in vivo*, effects of BCAA on muscle protein synthesis have not usually been detected (McNurlan, Fern & Garlick, 1982; Louard, Barrett & Gelfand, 1990). Also, the patients studied with BCAA were adult, whereas the animal work was performed in muscle from growing animals, in which the effects of BCAA might have been related more to growth than to the recovery from illness (Baillie & Garlick, 1992). Even when biochemical measurements have been made in trauma patients, there have been many conflicting responses to BCAA supplements (e.g. Cerra *et al.*, 1985; Hammarqvist *et al.*, 1990) and the Workshop on Clinical Uses of BCAA (Brennan *et al.*, 1986) concluded that positive benefits of BCAA on nitrogen metabolism had been shown only in the most severely ill patients.

The case for BCAA supplementation is clearer for hepatic encephalopathy (see Walser, 1984). When the liver function is compromised, the ability to oxidise amino acids such as the aromatics (phenylalanine and tyrosine) and methionine is reduced and their concentrations in the blood are increased. The BCAA, by contrast, continue to be oxidised in peripheral tissues and their concentrations decrease. As a result there are increases in the concentrations of aromatic amino acids and the neurotransmitters derived from them, methionine and various other metabolites in the brain. Although these changes were originally believed to be the cause of encephalopathy, it has been shown that the ratio of BCAA to aromatics is reduced in chronic liver failure, whether or not there is encephalopathy (see Walser, 1984).

Attempts to correct amino acid abnormalities by giving amino acid mixtures enriched in BCAA have had mixed success (see Walser, 1984). For example, there have been reports of clinical and/or biochemical improvements in patients with encephalopathy (e.g. Egberts *et al.*, 1981, Cerra *et al.*, 1985), whereas other studies have shown no benefit (e.g. McGhee *et al.*, 1983; Horst *et al.*, 1984). In a recent review, Fischer (1990) attempts to explain these discrepancies and concludes that when all the literature is taken into account, BCAA or a BCAA-enriched amino acid mixture give significant benefits, in terms of nitrogen equilibrium, wake-up from coma and mortality, compared with conventional therapy including no amino acids. Whether an amino acid mixture of more normal composition would be as successful as the BCAA mixtures, as suggested by Michel, Pomier-Layrargues & Aubin (1984), remains to be answered.

Glutamine

This amino acid is a normal constituent of protein, but is not included in the conventional amino acid mixtures for intravenous use, because it is not stable in solution. Until recently this has not been considered to be a problem, since it is classed as a non-essential amino acid. However, there is substantial depletion of muscle-free glutamine content after trauma (Vinnars, Bergström & Fürst, 1975) and there is also a correlation between low muscle glutamine and mortality (Roth *et al.*, 1982). These observations have stimulated a considerable interest in the possible benefits of supplements of glutamine or glutamine analogues in traumatised patients. These supplements have been shown to result in an improvement in muscle protein metabolism, as well as in whole-body nitrogen economy after trauma (Hammarqvist *et al.*, 1989; Stehle *et al.*, 1989; Vinnars *et al.*, 1990; Wernerman, Hammarqvist & Vinnars, 1990). Studies in animals have demonstrated a correlation between muscle protein synthesis rate and glutamine concentration in rat muscle (Jepson *et al.*, 1988), but it has not proved possible to restore protein synthesis to normal by infusion of glutamine in traumatised or starved animals (Jepson & Millward, 1991; Khan, Wusteman & Elia, 1991; Wusteman & Elia, 1991). Perhaps the existence of a correlation should not be taken to imply that altered glutamine levels caused the observed changes in muscle protein synthesis.

Skeletal muscle is the major producer of glutamine, which is utilised by a variety of other tissues. It is continuously transported by the blood to the splanchnic area to be used as an oxidative fuel in the intestine, the major part being converted to CO_2, ammonia, lactate or alanine (Windemueller & Spaeth, 1974). The most active glutamine-consuming cells in the intestine are enterocytes and immunocompetent cells (Ardawi & Newsholme, 1984; Souba, Smith & Wilmore, 1985). This has led to a large number of studies in animals showing better tolerance to burns, cortisol or cytostatic drugs (Souba *et al.*, 1990) when glutamine-supplemented total parenteral nutrition (TPN) is provided, although similar tolerance is shown by animals receiving ordinary food by the oral route. Beneficial effects of glutamine-supplemented TPN on nitrogen balance, the number of positive bacterial cultures, the need for blood transfusions and the length of hospital stay, have been shown in bone marrow transplant patients (Ziegler *et al.*, 1992).

The instability of glutamine in solution has led to the use of several glutamine analogues. Dipeptides, such as alanyl glutamine or glycyl glutamine and the keto acid of glutamine, α-ketoglutarate, have been shown to maintain the free glutamine level in muscle of critically ill patients (Hammarqvist *et al.*, 1990; Wernerman *et al.*, 1990; Petersson *et al.*, 1992). Amino acid solutions containing glutamine analogues will be available commercially, but more work still needs to be done to establish their value clearly.

Arginine

As shown in Table 3.1 the synthesis of several compounds of metabolic significance, including polyamines, creatine and nitric oxide, requires arginine as a precursor. Perhaps more than any other amino acid, arginine has been reported to have a wide range of potentially beneficial effects, including the stimulation of secretion of several hormones, improvement of wound healing and effects on tumour implantation and growth (see Table 3.6). Its impact on wound healing and tumour growth have been attributed to the ability of arginine supplements to enhance various aspects of the immune system. Detailed reviews of the biological effects of arginine are available (Visek, 1986; Barbul, 1986, 1990; Kirk & Barbul, 1990).

In traumatised animals, there is an involution of the thymus and a suppression of immune responses, and these effects have been shown to be reversed by the provision of arginine supplements (Barbul *et al.*, 1980). Also, weight loss is reduced (Seifter *et al.*, 1978) and nitrogen retention is

Table 3.6. *Some biological responses to dietary arginine supplements*

Immune responses
↑   Lymphocyte blastogenesis in healthy and injured animals and man
↑   NK and LAK cytotoxicity in animals and man
↑   Allograft rejection in animals

Recovery from surgery/sepsis
↑   Survival in septic animals
↑   Wound healing in animals and man
↑   N balance after surgery

Cancer
↓   Tumour induction by carcinogens in animals
↓   Latency period, incidence and growth of transplanted tumours in animals
↑ or ↓   Growth of tumour cells in culture
↑   Growth of transplanted tumours in athymic nude mice
↑   Protein synthesis and cell division in tumours of breast cancer patients

improved (Barbul *et al.*, 1981). Similarly, humans given supplements of arginine (15–25 g/d) have shown enhanced wound healing, improved immune responses and a reduction in nitrogen losses (Elsair *et al.*, 1978; Barbul *et al.*, 1990). These effects can be regarded as more pharmacological than nutritional, as they occur at high doses of about five times the normal dietary intake.

Arginine might also have a role in the treatment of cancer. A number of studies in experimental animals bearing implanted or induced tumours have shown that the growth or spread of the cancer is inhibited (Barbul, 1986). However, the only study on human tumours to date has shown the opposite effect, with tumour protein synthesis and cell proliferation being stimulated by arginine supplements of 30 g/d for 3 days in breast cancer patients (Park *et al.*, 1992). The difference between the human and animal tumours might be a consequence of arginine's stimulatory action on both the tumour and the immune system. In cultured tumour cells and in mice lacking a competent immune system, arginine can stimulate tumour growth, as in the human patients, suggesting that the patients might also lack effective immunity (Park *et al.*, 1990). Although this suggests caution when contemplating the use of arginine supplements in cancer, it has been suggested that arginine might be used to advantage by stimulating the tumour, to enhance its sensitivity to cell cycle specific chemotherapeutic agents (Park *et al.*, 1992).

The mechanism of these effects of arginine is not at present clear and there are several possibilities (Barbul, 1986; Kirk & Barbul, 1990): stimulation of hormone secretion, notably of growth hormone; increased supply of proline precursors, needed for collagen synthesis by the healing wound; as a precursor of polyamines, which are involved in cell division or as the precursor of nitric oxide, which has been shown to be involved in the activation of various components of the immune system. However, despite this lack of knowledge on its mechanism of action, products supplemented with arginine are becoming available for enteral feeding of traumatised patients. Until more is known about arginine's effects on tumours, however, its use for feeding cancer patients requires caution.

Other amino acids

Tyrosine and cysteine are also regarded as conditionally essential in man, because they rely on an adequate synthesis from phenylalanine and methionine, which might be insufficient in some patients (e.g. in liver failure). Also, they cannot be included in conventional amino solutions because tyrosine is insoluble and cysteine is unstable. Attempts are therefore being made to make derivatives of these two amino acids (e.g. dipeptides, *N*-acetyl derivatives), which can be included in intravenous feeds (Bässler, 1989).

Proline can also be regarded as a conditionally essential amino acid. Although sufficient proline can be synthesised to meet normal body needs, in severely burned patients, elevated proline oxidation and diminished *de novo* proline synthesis contribute to an enhanced requirement for dietary proline. In addition, proline is a major component of skin collagen, so there may also be an enhanced requirement associated with tissue repair (Jaksic *et al.*, 1991).

Conclusions

As can be seen from the preceding discussion, the subject of amino acid needs is still an active, and sometimes controversial, topic. The requirements of amino acids for optimum health, as opposed to protein balance, are not fully understood and a great deal of work still needs to be done on specific requirements in altered metabolic states, particularly for those amino acids previously regarded as non-essential. In particular, the last few years have seen an extremely active discussion in the clinical literature of the potential benefits of intravenous or oral supplementation of diseased or traumatised patients with specific amino acids. Although there is no clear consensus on their value at the present time, there is reason for optimism that improvements in our understanding of the altered needs for amino acids will lead to better survival and recovery.

Acknowledgements

The authors are grateful for the support of the Scottish Office Agriculture and Fisheries Department, and Grampian Research into Intestinal Disorders.

References

Adibi, S. A. (1980). Roles of branched-chain amino acids in metabolic regulation. *Journal of Laboratory and Clinical Medicine*, **95**, 475–84.

Ardawi, M. S. M. & Newsholme, E. A. (1984). Glutamine metabolism in lymphoid tissues. In *Glutamine Metabolism in Mammalian Tissues*, ed. D. Häussinger & H. Sies, pp. 235–46. Berlin, Springer-Verlag.

Baillie, A. G. S. & Garlick, P. J. (1992). Attenuated response of muscle protein synthesis to fasting and insulin in adult female rats. *American Journal of Physiology*, **262**, E1–5.

Barbul, A., Wasserkrug, H. L., Seifter, E., Rettura, G., Levenson, S. M. & Efron, G. (1980). Immunostimulatory effects of arginine in normal and injured rats. *Journal of Surgical Research*, **29-a**, 228–35.

Barbul, A., Sisto, D. A., Wasserkrug, H. L., Yoshimura, N. N. & Efron, G. (1981). Metabolic and immune effects of arginine in postinjury hyperalimentation. *Journal of Trauma*, **21**, 970–4.

Barbul, A. (1986). Arginine: biochemistry, physiology, and therapeutic implications. *Journal of Parenteral and Enteral Nutrition*, **10**, 227–38.

Barbul, A. (1990). Arginine and immune function. *Nutrition*, **6**, S56–62.

Barbul, A., Lazarou, S. A., Efron, D. T., Wasserkrug, H. L. & Efron, G. (1990). Arginine enhances wound healing and lymphocyte immune responses in humans. *Surgery*, **108**, 331–7.

Bassler, K. H. (1989). Metabolic basis for inclusion of tyrosine and cysteine in amino acid solutions. In *Nutrition in Clinical Practice*, ed. W. Hartig, G. Dietze, R. Weiner & P. Fürst, pp. 46–55. Karger, Basel.

Brennan, M. F., Cerra, F., Daly, J. M. *et al.* (1986). Branched chain amino acids in stress and injury. *Journal of Parenteral and Enteral Nutrition*, **10**, 446–52.

Buse, M. J. & Reid, S. S. (1975). Leucine: a possible regulator of protein turnover in muscle. *Journal of Clinical Investigation*, **56**, 1250–61.

Calloway, D. H., Odell, A. C. F. & Margen, S. J. (1971). Sweat and miscellaneous nitrogen losses in human balance studies. *Journal of Nutrition*, **101**, 775–86.

Cerra, F. B., Cheung, N. K., Fischer, J. E. *et al.* (1985). Disease-specific amino acid infusion (F080) in hepatic encephalopathy: a prospective, randomized, double-blind, controlled trial. *Journal of Parenteral and Enteral Nutrition*, **9**, 288–95.

Cortiella, J., Marchini, J. S., Branch, S., Chapman, T. E. & Young, V. R. (1992). Phenylalanine and tyrosine kinetics in relation to altered protein and phenylalanine and tyrosine intakes in healthy young men. *American Journal of Clinical Nutrition*, **56**, 517–25.

Edwards, C. H., Wade, W. D., Freeburne, M. M. *et al.* (1977). Formation of methionine from α-amino-n-butyric acid and 5′-methylthioadenosine in the rat. *Journal of Nutrition*, **107**, 1927–36.

Egberts, E.-H., Hamster, W., Jurgens, P. *et al.* (1981). Effect of branched chain amino acids on latent protal-systemic encephalopathy. In *Metabolism and Clinical Implications of Branched Chain Amino and Ketoacids*, ed. M. Walser & J. R. Williamson, pp. 453–64. Elsevier/North-Holland, New York.

Elsair, J., Poey, J., Issad, H., Reggabi, M., Bekri, T., Hattab, F. & Spinner, C. (1978). Effect of arginine chlorhydrate on nitrogen balance during the three days following routine surgery. *Biomedical Express*, **29**, 312–17.

FAO/WHO/UNU. (1985). *Energy and Protein Requirements. Technical Report Series No. 724*. Geneva, WHO.

Fischer, J. E. (1990). Branched-chain-enriched amino acid solutions in patients with liver failure: an early example of nutritional pharmacology. *Journal of Parenteral and Enteral Nutrition*, **14**, 249S–56S.

Fulks, R. M., Li, J. B. & Goldberg, A. L. (1975). Effects of insulin, glucose, and amino acids on protein turnover in rat diaphragm. *Journal of Biological Chemistry*, **250**, 290–8.

Fuller, M. F., Milne, A., Harris, C. I., Reid, T. M. & Keenan, R. (1993). Amino acid losses in ileostomy fluid on a protein-free diet. *Proceedings of the Nutrition Society*, in press.

Hammarqvist, F., Wernerman, J., Ali, R., von der Decken, A. & Vinnars, E. (1989). Addition of glutamine to total parenteral nutrition after elective abdominal surgery spares free glutamine in muscle, counteracts the fall in muscle protein synthesis, and improves nitrogen balance. *Annals of Surgery*, **209**, 455–61.

Hammarqvist, F., Wernerman, J., Ali, R. & Vinnars, E. (1990). Effects of an amino acid solution enriched with either branched chain amino acids or ornithine-α-ketoglutarate on the postoperative intracellular amino acid concentration of skeletal muscle. *British Journal of Surgery*, **77**, 214–18.

Hegsted, D. M. (1963). Variation in requirements of nutrient-amino acids. *Federation Proceedings*, **22**, 1424–30.

Horst, D., Grace, N., Conn, H. O., Schiff, E., Schenker, S., Viteri, A., Law, D. & Atterbury, C. E. (1984). Comparison of dietary protein with an oral, branched chain-enriched amino acid supplement in chronic portal-systemic encephalopathy: a randomized controlled trial. *Hepatology*, **41**, 279–87.

Jackson, A. A. (1989). Optimizing amino acid protein supply and utilization in the newborn. *Proceedings of the Nutrition Society*, **48**, 293–301.

Jaksic, T., Wagner, D. A., Burke, J. F. & Young, V. R. (1991). Proline metabolism in adult male burned patients and healthy control subjects. *American Journal of Clinical Nutrition*, **54**, 408–13.

Jepson, M. M., Broadbent, P., Bates, P. C. & Millward, D. J. (1988). The relationship between skeletal muscle glutamine concentration and protein synthesis in rats. *American Journal of Physiology*, **225**, E166–72.

Jepson, M. M. & Millward, D. J. (1991). Impact of glutamine infusions on muscle protein synthesis in fasted and endotoxin treated rats. *Clinical Nutrition*, **10** (Supplement), 43–6.

Khan, K., Wusteman, M. & Elia, M. (1991). The effect of severe dietary restriction on intramuscular glutamine concentrations and protein synthetic rate. *Clinical Nutrition*, **10**, 120–4.

Kirk, S. J. & Barbul, A. (1990). Role of arginine in trauma, sepsis, and immunity. *Journal of Parenteral and Enteral Nutrition*, **14**, 226S–9S.

Laidlaw, S. A. & Kopple, J. D. (1987). Newer concepts of the indispensable amino acids. *American Journal of Clinical Nutrition*, **46**, 593–605.

Leverton, R. M., Waddill, F. S. & Skellenger, M. (1959). The urinary excretion of five essential amino acids by young women. *Journal of Nutrition*, **67**, 19–28.

Li, J. B. & Jefferson, L. S. (1978). Influence of amino acid availability on protein turnover in perfused skeletal muscle. *Biochemica et Biophysica Acta*, **544**, 351–9.

Louard, R. J., Barrett, E. J. & Gelfand, R. A. (1990). Effect of infused branched-chain amino acids on muscle and whole-body amino acid metabolism in man. *Clinical Science*, **79**, 457–66.

Macy, I. G. & Kelly, H. J. (1961). Human milk and cow's milk in infant nutrition. In *Milk: the Mammary Gland and Its Secretion*, ed. S. K. Kon & A. T. Cowie, pp. 265–304. London, Academic Press.

McGhee, A., Henderson, J. M., Millikan, W. J. *et al.* (1983). Comparison of the effects of hepatic acid and a casein modular diet on encephalopathy, plasma amino acids, and nitrogen balance in cirrhotic patients. *Annals of Surgery*, **197**, 288–93.

McNurlan, M. A., Fern, E. B. & Garlick, P. J. (1982). Failure of leucine to stimulate protein synthesis *in vivo*. *Biochemical Journal*, **204**, 831–8.

Meguid, M. M., Matthews, D. E., Bier, D. M., Meredith, C. N. & Young, V. R. (1986). Valine kinetics at graded valine intakes in young men. *American Journal of Clinical Nutrition*, **43**, 781–6.

Michel, H., Pomier-Layrargues, G. & Aubin, J. P. (1984). Treatment of hepatic encephalopathy by infusion of a modified amino acid solution: results of a controlled study in 47 cirrhotic patients. In *Hepatic Encephalopathy in Chronic Liver Failure*, ed. L. Capocaccia, J. E. Fischer & F. Rossi-Fanelli, pp. 301–10. Plenum Press, New York.

Millward, D. J. & Rivers, J. (1988). The nutritional role of indispensable amino acids and the metabolic basis for their requirements. *European Journal of Clinical Nutrition*, **42**, 367–93.

Park, K. G. M., Heys, S. D., Blessing, K., Eremin, O. & Garlick, P. J. (1990). The effect of arginine on the growth of experimental tumours. *Proceedings of the Nutrition Society*, **49**, 168A.

Park, K. G. M., Heys, S. D., Blessing, K., Kelly, P., Eremin, O. & Garlick, P. J. (1992). The stimulation of human breast cancers by dietary *L*-arginine. *Clinical Science*, **82**, 413–17.

Petersson, B., Vinnars, E., Waller, S.-O. & Wernerman, J. (1992). Long-term changes in muscle-free amino acid levels after elective abdominal surgery. *British Journal of Surgery*, **79**, 212–16.

Rose, W. C. (1957). The amino acid requirements of adult man. *Nutrition Abstracts and Reviews*, **27**, 631–47.

Roth, E., Funovics, J., Mühlbacher, F. *et al.* (1982). Metabolic disorders in severe abdominal sepsis: glutamine deficiency in skeletal muscle. *Clinical Nutrition*, **1**, 25–41.

Seifter, E., Rettura, G., Barbul, A. & Levenson, S. M. (1978). Arginine: an essential amino acid for injured rats. *Surgery*, **84**, 224–30.

Smith, R. & Elia, M. (1983). Branched chain amino acids in stress and injury. *Journal of Parenteral and Enteral Nutrition*, **10**, 446–52.

Smith, R. H. (1980). Comparative amino acid requirements. *Proceedings of the Nutrition Society*, **39**, 71–8.

Souba, W. W., Smith, R. J. & Wilmore, D. W. (1985). Glutamine metabolism by the intestinal tract. *Journal of Parenteral and Enteral Nutrition*, **9**, 608–17.

Souba, W. W., Klimberg, S., Plumley, D. A. *et al.* (1990). The role of glutamine in maintaining a healthy gut and supporting the metabolic response to injury and infection. *Journal of Surgical Research*, **48**, 383–91.

Stehle, P., Zanders, J., Mertes, N., Albers, S., Puchstein, C., Lawin, P. & Fürst, P. (1989). Effect of parenteral glutamine peptide supplements on muscle glutamine loss and nitrogen balance after major surgery. *Lancet*, **i**, 231–3.

Vinnars, E., Bergström, J. & Fürst, P. (1975). Influence of the postoperative state on the intracellular free amino acids in human tissue. *Annals of Surgery*, **182**, 665–71.

Vinnars, E., Hammarqvist, F., von der Decken, A. & Wernerman, J. (1990). Role of glutamine and its analogs in posttraumatic muscle protein and amino acid metabolism. *Journal of Parenteral and Enteral Nutrition*, **14**, 125S–9S.

Visek, W. J. (1986). Arginine needs, physiological state and usual diets. A reevaluation. *Journal of Nutrition*, **116**, 36–46.

Walser, M. (1984). Therapeutic aspects of branched-chain amino and keto acids. *Clinical Science*, **66**, 1–15.

Wernerman, J., Hammarqvist, F. & Vinnars, E. (1990). Alpha-ketoglutarate and postoperative muscle catabolism. *Lancet*, **335**, 701–3.

Windmueller, H. G. & Spaeth, A. E. (1974). Uptake and metabolism of plasma glutamine by the small intestine. *Journal of Biological Chemistry*, **249**, 5070–9.

Wusterman, M. & Elia, M. (1991). Effect of glutamine infusions on glutamine concentration and protein synthetic rate in rat muscle. *Journal of Parenteral and Enteral Nutrition*, **15**, 521–5.

Young, V. R., Gucalp, C., Rand, W. M., Matthews, D. E. & Bier, D. M. (1987). Leucine kinetics during three weeks at submaintenance-to-maintenance intakes of leucine in men: adaptation and accommodation. *Human Nutrition: Clinical Nutrition*, **41C**, 1–18.

Young, V. R., Wagner, D. A., Burini, R. & Storch, K. J. (1991). Methionine kinetics and balance at the 1985 FAO/WHO/UNU intake requirement in adult men studied with L-[^{2}H$_3$-methyl-1-^{13}C]methionine as a tracer. *American Journal of Clinical Nutrition*, **54**, 377–85.

Zhao, X.-H., Wen, Z.-M., Meredith, C. N., Matthews, D. E., Bier, D. M. & Young, V. R. (1986). Threonine kinetics at graded threonine intakes in young men. *American Journal of Clinical Nutrition*, **43**, 795–802.

Ziegler, T. R., Young, L. S., Benfell, K. *et al.* (1992). Clinical and metabolic efficacy of glutamine-supplemented parenteral nutrition after bone marrow transplantation – a randomized, double-blind controlled study. *Annals of Internal Medicine*, **116**, 821–8.

4

Mineral and vitamin metabolism

A. SHENKIN

Introduction – consequences of an inadequate intake of vitamins

Throughout the evolution of the science of nutrition, the emphasis on vitamin and trace element requirements has focussed on the deficiency states which result from an inadequate intake. Thus, the major criterion used to determine adequacy of provision has been the amount of an individual micronutrient which will prevent the occurrence of deficiency signs and symptoms. These classical signs of deficiency are well described in standard text books of nutrition and medicine and will therefore not be summarised here.

Of greater interest in recent years has been the concept that micronutrient deficiency is not absolute, in terms of the presence or absence of these characteristic signs, but rather is a relative process, in which an individual may become progressively depleted. The characteristic deficiency symptoms are therefore the end result of a prolonged period of inadequate intake, during which the individual will pass through successive stages of deficit (Fig. 4.1). The duration within each of these phases will differ for each micronutrient, depending upon the extent of stores, adaptation of function, and the metabolic role of the trace element or vitamin in question.

In the early stages of an inadequate intake, there will be mobilisation of stores. For some nutrients, these can be quite substantial, lasting as much as 1–2 years (e.g. Vitamin A or Vitamin B_{12}), but for most water soluble vitamins and trace elements there are little or even no available stores. As depletion progresses, compensatory mechanisms may be invoked, such as to increase absorption from the diet (e.g. for iron or zinc), or to reduce urinary excretion, which is effective for elements such as magnesium or phosphorus.

A disturbance in intracellular metabolism may subsequently develop

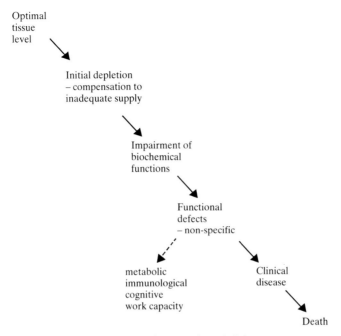

Fig. 4.1. Development of micronutrient deficiency.

as a result of impaired activity of enzymes requiring trace elements or vitamins as co-factors. Measurement of intracellular enzyme activity (e.g. red blood cell transketolase for Vitamin B_1, or red cell transaminase for Vitamin B_6), may reveal such abnormalities. However, specific biochemical indicators are available for only a few of the micronutrients (Fidanza, 1991).

At this stage there may be no obvious clinical consequences. A *subclinical deficiency state* can be defined as a state in which vitamin or trace element status is poor but with no overt symptoms of deficiency being present. Further depletion will lead to certain non-specific clinical symptoms, such as apathy, fatigue, anorexia, or cognitive or immunological abnormalities. These signs and symptoms are of special importance, since they may be the first indication of a sub-clinical deficiency. On the other hand, they are highly non-specific, and further evidence of a micronutrient deficiency would be required to confirm the diagnosis. The main evidence for the existence of such effects comes from biochemical evidence of impaired status of certain micronutrients in association with these symptoms, and from studies of supplementation of apparently healthy individuals, with trace elements or vitamins (Gaby *et al.*, 1991; Benedich & Butterworth, 1991).

Before exploring further the question of optimal intake, patient groups at risk of micronutrient depletion should first be considered.

'Healthy' individuals at risk of poor micronutrient status

Many adults are at risk of micronutrient depletion, even in the absence of a specific disease state influencing micronutrient requirements.

Poor dietary habits

Studies of free-living individuals in Western Societies, have revealed a variable proportion of individuals with poor dietary habits, usually resulting in excess refined carbohydrate intake, inadequate fibres, and variably inadequate intake of fruit, vegetables and milk, leading to insufficient intakes mainly of B vitamins and iron. None the less, any nutrient can be affected by ingestion of an unbalanced diet.

Adolescence

This is especially true during the adolescent period when the rapid growth spurt places heavy demands on provision of all nutrients. Of particular concern is the folate, Vitamin A and iron intake. It should also be remembered that this group is prone to unusual diets (e.g. reducing diets), which may exacerbate the problem.

Excess alcohol intake

Depending upon the proportion of energy derived from alcohol, there may be an inadequate intake of water soluble vitamins, phosphate, magnesium and other micronutrients. In addition, there may be impaired metabolism of Vitamin A, possibly related to inadequate zinc status. Alcoholic cirrhosis can affect both zinc absorption and urinary zinc excretion (Aggett, 1991). The most florid deficiency syndromes of Vitamin B_1, magnesium and phosphate in Western Societies, occur in this group.

Cigarettes

Smokers have significantly poorer status of several micronutrients. There is good evidence for an increased requirement of Vitamin C in smokers (Panel on Dietary Reference Values, 1991) and in addition both β carotene and Vitamin E status is impaired relative to non-smokers.

Elderly

Elderly individuals may have multiple nutritional problems, relating to inadequacy of the diet, dental problems, drug interactions, chronic illness, as well as economic factors. It is therefore not surprising that there is a high incidence of abnormalities, especially relating to Vitamin C, iron, zinc and folate status (Chandra, 1992).

Effects of disease on likelihood of micronutrient deficiency

Increased requirements due to metabolic demands

All acute disease states are associated with an increased requirement for micronutrients. This results from an increase in metabolic rate and protein turnover, associated with the metabolic response to injury or infection.

Micronutrients as cofactors in metabolism

Since a major function of water soluble vitamins and most trace elements is to facilitate intermediary metabolism, this will place additional requirements on the supply of these micronutrients. In studies on patients in Intensive Care, we have demonstrated an increased incidence of sub-clinical deficiency of thiamine and riboflavin, confirming an increased requirement (Cruickshank, Telfer & Shenkin, 1988; Shenkin, Cruickshank & Shenkin, 1989). For some vitamins, the requirement has been linked to the energy supply (e.g. 0.3 mg thiamine/1000 kcal, 5.5 mg niacin/1000 kcal); or to the protein intake (e.g. 15 µg vitamin B_6/g protein) (Panel on Dietary Reference Values, 1991). For others, the increase has not been accurately quantified and varying estimates of up to 10 fold have been proposed. It would, however, seem logical to relate the micronutrient requirement to the increase in metabolic rate (up to 2 fold) or protein turnover (2–3 fold).

Free radical scavenging mechanisms

The increased metabolic rate is associated with increased oxidative metabolism. An important consequence of this is an increased production of free radicals which are potentially damaging to cell membranes and to DNA (Dreosti, 1991). Free radicals have an unpaired electron which is highly unstable and tends to attack further molecules (e.g. polyunsaturated fatty acids or nucleic acids), by removing an electron from them. Subsequent reactions take place causing damage to the cellular structures. The antioxidants within the body can minimise the extent of this oxidative damage – most of these natural antioxidants are micronutrients, or depend on micronutrients for their activity:

- β carotene, Vitamin C and Vitamin E are all important nutrient antioxidants
- superoxide dismutase, a manganese metalloenzyme in mitochondria, and a copper/zinc metalloenzyme in cytoplasm, is important in removing superoxide radicals.
- glutathione peroxidase, a selenoenzyme, is involved in the removal of hydrogen peroxide.
- metallothionein, a low molecular weight cysteine-rich protein, which also has a high content of zinc and copper, may be a general antioxidant.

This remains an area of great controversy. The quantitative effects of free radical production and scavenging are not known, nor are there proven clinical benefits resulting from increased provision of these 'free radical scavengers'. The main debate centres on the extent to which free radicals are directly aetiological in causing tissue damage and disease, in contrast to their increased production in response to disease. Clinical trials with various mixtures of the above free radical scavengers are ongoing in many conditions associated with acute inflammation and sepsis, and in a number of chronic disease states such as atherosclerosis and cancer – the results of these are eagerly awaited.

Requirements due to growth and anabolism

It is inevitable that at times of rapid growth, there is an increased requirement for all micronutrients, e.g. zinc may be limiting to the growth and development of young children (Golden, 1989). In the comparable situation in adults, patients who have lost considerable lean body mass due to catabolic illness, may develop an acute deficiency state when there is a change to net anabolism and tissue regeneration. This will generally occur when the stimulus to release of catabolic mediators (interleukins and tumour necrosis factor) and of catabolic hormones, has been resolved (e.g. drainage of abscess). Thus, deficiency states are more likely to occur during the anabolic phase, which follows the resolution of a catabolic illness (Tasman-Jones, Kay & Lee, 1978).

Malabsorption

Malabsorption of micronutrients is rarely congenital, as in the in-born error of zinc absorption, acrodermatitis enteropathica. This is diagnosed early in infancy. Much more commonly in both infancy and adulthood, malabsorption of micronutrients is secondary to an acquired disease process. Any illness leading to reduction in absorptive surface area of the small intestine, will lead to malabsorption of any of the nutrients. This can be general (e.g. in short bowel syndrome), or specific (as in surgery to the distal ileum leading to impaired Vitamin B_{12} absorption).

Most commonly, fat malabsorption results from coeliac disease, pancreatic insufficiency, or Crohn's disease, which are associated with malabsorption of the fat soluble Vitamins A, D, E and K and in severe cases this will lead to clinical vitamin deficiency.

An interesting form of malabsorption is alteration in bioavailability, for example, excess fibre or phytate reduce zinc and calcium absorption. Furthermore, iron supplements can lead to impaired zinc or copper absorption, whereas excess oral copper can inhibit zinc absorption (O'Dell, 1984). Zinc supplements have been used in treatment of Wilson's disease, by inhibiting copper absorption. On the other hand, Vitamin C increases the absorption of oral iron. Care must therefore be taken when providing oral supplements of micronutrients, to consider any other effects which this may have on the overall absorptive process.

Increased losses

All body fluids are rich in trace elements and water soluble vitamins and hence, increased losses of any of these fluids will lead to micronutrient depletion. The commonest source of loss is gastrointestinal fluid, especially from diarrhoea or vomiting, but fistula losses and nasogastric aspirate should not be forgotten. Since manganese and copper are excreted in the bile, a biliary fistula will lead to substantial losses, whereas zinc is present in high concentration in pancreatic and gut secretions.

Haemodialysis is generally considered to be a potential source of loss, although most studies have demonstrated only a minor degree of depletion if any – folic acid deficiency being most likely (Kopple, 1988).

Of potential importance are losses through the skin, especially from exudate following severe burn injury. In a series of elegant studies, Berger and colleagues (1992*a, b*) have shown that losses of zinc, copper, and selenium in exudate are very much greater than the losses from urine or faeces. This is probably also the case for most other micronutrients present in plasma in significant amounts, e.g. water soluble vitamins and also those nutrients bound to carrier proteins. The amount of extra micro-nutrient required to meet these losses is not clear, although preliminary studies do suggest that provision of about 4–6 times the standard daily dose may be beneficial (Berger *et al.*, 1992*c*).

Optimisation of intake of micronutrients

The requirement for each micronutrient therefore depends upon two major factors:

1. The existing status of the micronutrient in the patient, especially with regard to the magnitude of any depletion.
2. The net daily requirement for that micronutrient to sustain metabolism and daily losses.

Since these vary between individuals, especially in illness, criteria are required to judge the adequacy of the intake.

Prevention of clinical symptoms

Clinical symptoms of micronutrient deficiency, such as skin rash in riboflavin, niacin or zinc deficiency, bleeding gums in Vitamin C deficiency, or muscle weakness in selenium deficiency, occur only after a prolonged period of inadequate intake. Hence the development of such a situation usually implies a failure, on the part of the patient's physician, to recognise the inadequate nature of the intake. As described above, prevention of clinical symptoms only indicates that this severe situation has not developed, but the overall adequacy of the provision cannot be deduced.

Optimal substrate utilisation

Maintenance of normal growth and development in children

One of the most sensitive markers of adequacy of provision of certain nutrients is a normal rate of growth. These nutrients have been classified as type 1 nutrients (Golden, 1989). Such nutrients tend to be fundamental to nutrition and metabolism e.g. amino acids, energy substrates, phosphorus, potassium. Of the micronutrients, only zinc probably falls into this category. In the rapidly growing infant, limitation of zinc supply despite an adequate protein energy intake, has been shown to reduce growth rate (Golden & Golden, 1981). All other micronutrients can be classified as type 2, where deficiency is more likely to lead to localised signs and symptoms of deficiency, rather than disturbance of growth.

Of even more fundamental importance is the requirement for micronutrients in normal development. It is now clear that an adequate intake of folate during the early months of pregnancy, is essential for prevention of neural-tube defects (Czeizel & Dudas, 1992). Although folate has long been recognised to play a key role in nucleic acid metabolism and especially in red blood cell haemopoiesis, this recent finding demonstrates the wide-ranging effects of micronutrients at different stages of growth and development.

Maintenance of anabolism in adults

A comparable feature to growth in children would be tissue repair and healing in adults. Given the above classification of micronutrients in children (type 1/type 2), it might be expected that only zinc, of the micronutrients, would have a major effect on substrate utilisation and anabolism in adults. This has indeed proved to be the case. Optimisation of major nutrients of amino acids, energy, potassium, and phosphorus have been shown to improve significantly the nitrogen balance (Rudman et al., 1975). However, optimisation of zinc supply improves nitrogen balance only in a proportion of cases, probably because of the relative importance of other factors in sick patients (Wolman et al., 1979).

There have been various studies of healing in the post-operative period, as a model for tissue repair in adults. Zinc deficiency has been shown to reduce collagen synthesis *in vivo* (Prasad et al., 1978) – hence zinc deficiency would be expected to lead to impaired wound healing. The results of clinical trials of zinc supplementation in otherwise healthy individuals have, however, been contradictory and zinc supplements may be of value only in patients with severe zinc deficiency (Solomons, 1989).

Optimal biochemical and physiological function

Given the concern regarding sub-clinical effects of micronutrients, the best markers for adequacy of provision should be sensitive markers of tissue or organ function, which would detect potential inadequacy at an early stage. Such markers could be biochemical or physiological.

Biochemical markers of micronutrient adequacy

Free radicals A controversial area in biochemical assessment is whether evidence of free radical damage, and of the adequacy of micro-nutrients to limit such damage, could be used diagnostically or thera-peutically. Enthusiasts for the use of Vitamin E or selenium additives point to changes in membrane fatty acid content, or in malondialdehyde production, as evidence for free radical damage, which should be pre-vented. It is unlikely that such markers will gain wide acceptance until the role of free radicals in the aetiology of disease is more fully understood.

Maintenance of enzyme activity Many micronutrients are required for enzyme activity, either as coenzymes or as part of metalloenzymes, and hence measurement of that enzyme activity may be used to optimise provision. Thus, the intracellular concentration of thiamine can be assessed by transketolase activation within red cells (a high activation indicating poor thiamine status), intracellular Vitamin B_2 (by glutathione reductase activation, intracellular B_6 by transaminase activation), or whole body selenium status by red blood cell glutathione peroxidase activity.

For some micronutrients, although the enzyme itself may be difficult to measure, metabolites are available to assess enzyme activity, e.g. sulphite or hypoxanthine in molybdenum deficiency, or organic acids in biotin deficiency. Unfortunately, specific examples do not exist for most micronutrients and hence such tests have only limited application.

Maintenance of plasma concentration The most widely used test of micronutrient adequacy is the plasma concentration, mainly because the sample is so readily available. The relationship of plasma concentration to intracellular concentration is poor for most micronutrients, this being especially the case during illness. Thus, measurement of plasma concen-tration is of only limited value in assessing the intracellular content and function of a micronutrient.

It is widely recognised that illness causes a redistribution of trace elements and vitamins. Surgery or infection lead to a reduction in serum zinc and iron, and an increase in serum copper, due to the induction in the liver of metallothionein, of ferritin, and of caeruloplasmin respectively. It seems likely that the process is mediated by cytokines, especially IL-1 and TNF, which subsequently induce IL-6 production, which in turn leads to the synthesis of the acute phase proteins (Shenkin, 1993).

Similarly, the plasma concentration of Vitamin C falls during an acute phase response. The mechanism of this is not clear, although it does appear as though this is a redistribution of Vitamin C, rather than a demonstration of increased need (Gaby & Singh, 1991*a*).

Thus, interpreting the plasma concentration of most micronutrients can be attempted only if the state of the acute phase response is also known. Trends in the magnitude of the acute phase response (e.g. by assessing changes in plasma C-reactive protein concentration), are therefore helpful in interpreting changes in plasma concentration of micronutrients.

Physiological markers of micronutrient adequacy

Perhaps the most difficult aspect is to quantify the effects which micro-nutrients have on organ and tissue function. Unlike the biochemical consequences, where altering supply may cause a rapid change in biochemical activity of an enzyme or in the products of metabolism, the physiological changes are slow and hence are also less specific, since other factors are involved in bringing about similar effects. The evidence for the influence of micronutrients on tissue function is, however, compelling, and examples are summarised below. The major results have been:

(i) A reduced level of intake of a particular micronutrient is associ-ated with some tissue dysfunction, ultimately associated with disease, or:

(ii) Provision of extra amounts of micronutrients leads to an improve-ment in tissue function or to a reduction in the incidence or severity of disease.

This topic has been reviewed extensively (e.g. Benedich and Butterworth (1991); Gaby *et al.*, 1991*a*, *b*), and only some general examples will be given here:

Immune function Most micronutrients have been shown to have some immunostimulatory activity in *in vitro* systems. However, con-trolled evidence of efficacy *in vivo* has been limited. Chandra (1992) has demonstrated that supplements of a mixture of vitamins and trace elements led to a marked reduction in infection episodes, in apparently healthy elderly individuals. This was found to be related to an increase in T4 cell numbers, improved lymphocyte responsiveness to phyto-haemagglutinin (PHA), and an increase in Natural Killer (NK) cells. Only a small proportion of individuals were shown to have definite evidence of micronutrient deficiency at the start of the trial.

A recent meta analysis of 20 trials of Vitamin A supplementation in infectious diseases, has demonstrated that Vitamin A supplements to children in developing countries have anti-infective properties. There was a significant reduction in specific mortality from diarrhoeal disease in community studies, and in respiratory disease in children with measles (Glasziou& and Mackerras, 1983).

There are few other studies which have shown such a clear overall effect. Some studies have suggested a beneficial effect of Vitamin C in treatment of the 'common cold', but this has not, as yet, been proven (Gaby & Singh, 1991a).

A recent interesting study in burn patients has demonstrated that provision of a fairly large parenteral intake of zinc, copper, and selenium, appears to lead to a reduced incidence of infection (Berger *et al.*, 1992c).

Neoplastic disease A low intake and low serum concentration of various micronutrients has been associated with neoplastic disease. Of special current interest is the role of carotenoids in lung cancer. Large numbers of studies have now been performed which, with few exceptions, have demonstrated that individuals with high intakes of fruit and vegetables rich in β carotene, or having the highest blood concentration of β carotene, have approximately one half the risk of developing lung cancer, compared to the groups with the lowest β carotene intake or serum β carotene concentrations (Gaby & Singh, 1991b). The effect of β carotene appears to be independent of Vitamin A intake. It is also noteworthy that smokers with the same intake of β carotene as non-smokers, have lower serum concentrations of β carotene, suggesting some increase in its metabolism in smokers. Smokers may therefore have a requirement for a greater intake (Stryker *et al.*, 1988).

There is also highly suggestive evidence that a higher β carotene intake may be associated with lower incidence of other cancers, such as breast, oesophageal and gastric. Most of these studies depend upon an association between low serum β carotene and subsequent detection of cancer – such studies are limited by the possible effect which an undiagnosed neoplasm might have upon β carotene metabolism. Nonetheless, taken overall, the evidence is fairly compelling for some beneficial effect from β carotene (Gaby & Singh, 1991b). Whether the mechanism for this is through its free radical scavenging activity and whether oral β carotene supplements within an otherwise complete diet are effective in reducing the incidence or severity of neoplastic disease, remains to be established.

There have been long running controversies regarding the role of other micronutrients associated with free radical scavenging activity, i.e. Vitamin C, Vitamin E, and selenium, as to whether supplementation with these micronutrients reduces the incidence of various cancers. The variation in results in different studies makes this conclusion less likely, and further studies are indicated.

Cognition There are now a number of studies which purport to show that vitamin and trace element supplements may increase intelligence quotient (IQ). Although performance in certain types of tests has been significantly improved, major questions have been raised regarding the validity of the studies and the statistical analysis (Schoenthaler *et al.*, 1991; Peto, 1991).

None of these studies has, to date, provided evidence that vitamin status was poorest in those individuals whose performance was found to improve most following supplementation. Although grave doubts have been raised as to whether intelligence itself can be influenced by such supplements, it may be that at least some of the effects observed are due to an improvement in concentration power rather than intelligence (Benton, 1991). This would be consistent with some of the sub-clinical effects, such as fatigue and apathy often found in malnutrition. There can be little doubt that the overall role of nutritional effects within psychological functioning is small, but nonetheless further studies are required to determine the precise effect of vitamin and trace element supplements on cognitive skills, especially in individuals with varying extents of micronutrient depletion.

Recommended intake of vitamins and trace elements

Recommended oral intakes for vitamins and trace elements in health have been published in the most recent version of the Dietary Recommended Values for Food Energy and Nutrients in the United Kingdom Panel on Dietary Reference Values (1991). In these recommendations, the reference nutrient intake (RNI) is the amount which meets the requirements of 97.5% of the population in health. As has been described above, many individuals will have a greater requirement than this, especially if they are seriously ill or are in hospital. The intake present in most enteral feeds or in parenteral supplements generally provides 1–2 times the RNI and

Table 4.1. *Requirements, provision and toxicity of essential trace elements*

		Oral RNI[a]	Amount in 2000 Kcal tube feed[d]	I V reqts[b]	Toxic[c] oral intake
Zinc	mg	4.0–9.5	13–36	3.2–6.5	>100
	μmol	60–145		50–100	
Copper	mg	1.2	2–3.4	0.3–1.3	>35
	μmol	19		5–20	
Selenium	μg	40–75	30–130	30–60	>200
	nmol	500–900		400–800	
Manganese	mg	>1.4	2.4–8	0.3	>700
	μmol	26		5	
Chromium	μg	>25	30–200	10–20	Not known
	nmol	500		200–400	
Molybdenum	μg	50–400	>4–240	19	10–15 mg
	μmol	0.5–4		0.4	
Iron	mg	4.7–14.8	18–27	1.2	100–200
	μmol	80–260		20	

[a] From Panel on Dietary Reference Values, 1991. Not differentiated into male/female requirements.
[b] From Shenkin (1988); AMA 1979a, b, 1984.
[c] From Hathcock (1991).
[d] Values obtained from some representative enteral diets available in the UK.

hence should meet the requirements in most illnesses. However, in patients with special losses, or who start seriously depleted, greater amounts may be required. Table 4.1 and Table 4.2 summarise the recommended intakes and supply by oral and intravenous routes.

Toxicity of vitamin and mineral supplements

All essential micronutrients, with the possible exception of some of the water soluble vitamins, are toxic at high levels of intake (Hathcock, 1991). For some, the level required to achieve toxic effects would be outwith the amounts ever likely to be taken except in acute overdosage. However, for some of the fat soluble vitamins, such as Vitamin A and Vitamin D, and for minerals such as iron, selenium, zinc, and copper, chronic toxicity is a real concern, and care must be taken to match the dose of any supplement to the actual needs of the patient. Tables 4.1 and 4.2 also

Table 4.2. *Requirements, provision and toxicity of vitamins*

		Oral RNI[a]	Amount in 2000 Kcal tube feed[d]	I V reqts[b]	Toxic[c] oral intake
Vitamins					
A	µg	250–700	1000–2160	1000	7500
D	µg	0–10	8.5–14.6	5	50
E	µg	>4[c]	20–64	10	Not known
K	µg	1 µg/kg	100–200	150	Not known
B$_1$	mg	0.4 mg/1000 kcal	1.4–3.4	3.0	50 mg/kg
B$_2$	mg	1.3	2–6	3.6	Not known
B$_6$	mg	15 µg/g protein	2–13.8	4.0	50–500 mg
B$_{12}$	µg	5	3–15	5.0	Not known
Niacin	mg	6.6 mg/1000 kcal	18–45	40	3–6 g
Folate	µg	200	390–880	400	Not known
Biotin	µg	10–200	100–600	60	Not known
Ascorbic acid	mg	40	100–300	100	Uncertain

[a] From Panel on Dietary Reference Values, 1991. Not differentiated into Male/Female requirements.
[b] From Shenkin (1988); AMA 1979a, b.
[c] Depends upon intake of polyunsaturated fatty acids.
[d] Values obtained from some representative enteral diets in the UK.

summarises the relationship between the reference nutrient intake and the dose required to be taken on a chronic basis to achieve toxic effects. Given the potential for toxicity, it remains axiomatic that patients should not take nutrient supplements unless they are clinically indicated.

Summary

It is now clear that provision of adequate amounts of vitamins and trace elements involves more than just preventing clinical deficiency states. Micronutrients are required in all aspects of metabolism and inadequate supply may lead to sub-clinical, yet nonetheless important, effects which may have long-lasting consequences e.g. free radical damage or failure of tissue repair. Adequate intakes are therefore necessary both in 'at risk' groups in a general population, as well as in patients in hospital with increased requirements for protein-energy nutrition. It remains to be established whether provision of greater amounts of micronutrients will improve outcome, to a greater extent than the overall provision of an adequate amount of a well-balanced diet. Better tests of micronutrient status in disease states are required to optimise intake in the seriously ill patient.

References

Aggett, P. J. (1991). Severe zinc deficiency. In *Zinc in Human Biology*, ed. C. F. Mills. pp. 259–79, Springer-Verlag.

American Medical Association. (1979*a*). Guidelines for essential trace element preparations for parenteral use. *Journal of the American Medical Association*, **241**, 2051–4.

American Medical Association. (1979*b*). Multivitamin preparations for parenteral use: a statement by the Nutrition Advisory Group. *Journal of Parenteral and Enteral Nutrition*, **3**, 258–65.

American Medical Association. (1984). Working conference on parenteral trace elements. *Bulletin of the New York Academy of Medicine*, **60**, 115–212.

Benedich, A. & Butterworth, C. E. (1991). *Micronutrients in Health and in Disease Prevention*. Marcel Dekker, New York.

Benton, D. (1991). Vitamin and mineral intake and cognitive functioning. In *Micronutrients in Health and in Disease Prevention*, eds A. Bendich and C. E. Butterworth. pp. 219–32, Marcel Dekker, New York.

Berger, M. M., Cavadini, C., Bart, A. *et al.* (1992*a*). Selenium losses in 10 burned patients. *Clinical Nutrition*, **11**, 75–82.

Berger, M. M., Cavadini, C., Bart, A. *et al.* (1992*b*). Cutaneous copper and zinc losses in burns. *Burns*, **18**, 373–80.

Berger, M. M., Cavadini, C., Guinchard, S., Krupp, S. & Dirren, H. (1992*c*). Effect of increased Cu, Zn, and Se on leucocytes in burns. *Clinical Nutrition* **11**, Suppl., 111.

Chandra, R. K. (1992). Effect of vitamin and trace element supplementation on immune response and infection in elderly subjects. *Lancet*, **340**, 1124–7.

Cruickshank, A. M., Telfer, A. B. M. & Shenkin, A. (1988). Thiamine deficiency in the critically ill. *Intensive Care Medicine*, **14**, 384–7.

Czeizel, A. E. & Dudas, I. (1992). Prevention of the first occurrence of neural-tube defects by periconceptional vitamin supplementation. *New England Journal of Medicine*, **327**, 1832–5.

Dreosti, I. E. (1991). *Trace Elements, Micronutrients and Free Radicals*. Humana Press, New Jersey.

Fidanza, F. (1991). *Nutritional Status Assessment*. Chapman & Hall, London.

Gaby, S. K., Benedich, A., Singh, V. N. & Machlin, L. J. (1991). *Vitamin Intake and Health – a scientific review*. pp. 1–217, Marcel Dekker, New York.

Gaby, S. K. & Singh, V. N. (1991*a*). Vitamin C. In *Vitamin Intake and Health – a scientific review*. eds S. K. Gaby, A. Benedich, V. N. Singh and L. J. Machlin. pp. 103–61, Marcel Dekker, New York.

Gaby, S. K. & Singh, V. N. (1991*b*). β-carotene. In *Vitamin Intake and Health – a scientific review*. eds S. K. Gaby, A. Benedich, V. N. Singh and L. J. Machlin. pp. 29–57, Marcel Dekker, New York.

Glasziou, P. P. & Mackerras, D. E. M. (1983). Vitamin A supplementation in infectious diseases; a meta-analysis. *British Medical Journal*, **306**, 366–70.

Golden, M. H. N. (1989). The diagnosis of zinc deficiency. In *Zinc in Human Biology*, ed. C. F. Mills, pp. 32–33, Springer-Verlag.

Golden, M. H. C. & Golden, B. E. (1981). Effects of zinc supplementation on the dietary intake, rate of weight gain and energy cost of tissue deposition in children recovering from malnutrition. *American Journal of Clinical Nutrition*, **34**, 900–8.

Hathcock, J. N. (1991). Safety of vitamin and mineral supplements. In *Micronutrients in Health and in Disease Prevention*, ed. A. Bendich and C. E. Butterworth. pp. 439–50, Marcel Dekker, New York.

Kopple, J. D. (1988). Nutrition. Diet and the kidney. In *Modern Nutrition in Health and Disease*, ed. M. E. Shils and V. R. Young. 7th Ed. pp. 1230–68, Lea and Febiger, Philadelphia.

O'Dell, B. L. (1984). Bioavailability of trace elements. *Nutrition Reviews*, **42**, 301–8.

Panel on Dietary Reference Values, Department of Health. (1991). *Dietary Reference Values for Food Energy and Nutrients for the United Kingdom*. HMSO, London.

Peto, R. (1991). Vitamins and IQ. *British Medical Journal*, **302**, 906.

Prasad, A. S., Rabbani, P., Abbasi, A., Bowersox, E., Fox, M. R. S. (1978). Experimental zinc deficiency in humans. *Annals of Internal Medicine*, **89**, 483–90.

Rudman, D., Millikan, W. J., Richardson, T. J. *et al.* (1975). Elemental balances during intravenous hyperalimentation of underweight adult subjects. *Journal of Clinical Investigations*, **55**, 94–104.

Schoenthaler, S. J., Amios, S. P., Eysenck, H. J., Peritz, E. & Yudkin, J. (1991). Controlled trial of vitamin – mineral supplementation: effects on intelligence and performance. *Personality and Individual Differences*, **12**, 351–62.

Shenkin, S. D., Cruickshank, A. M. & Shenkin, A. (1989). Subclinical riboflavin deficiency is associated with outcome of seriously ill patients. *Clinical Nutrition*, **8**, 269–71.

Shenkin, A. (1988). Clinical aspects of vitamin and trace element metabolism. *Ballières Clinical Gastroenterology*, **2**, 765–98.

Shenkin, A. (1993). Trace elements and acute illness. *Care in the Critically Ill*, **9**, 60–3.

Solomons, N. W. (1989). Putative therapeutic roles of zinc. *Zinc in Human Biology*, ed. C. F. Mills. pp. 297–321, Springer-Verlag.

Stryker, W. S., Kaplan, L. A., Stein, E. A. *et al.* (1988). The relation of diet, cigarette smoking, and alcohol consumption to plasma β carotene and α-tocopherol levels. *American Journal of Epidemiology*, **127**, 283–96.

Tasman-Jones, C., Kay, R. G. and Lee, S. P. (1978). Zinc and copper deficiency with particular reference to parenteral nutrition. In *Surgery Annual*, ed. L. M. Nybus. pp. 23–52, Appleton, New York.

Wolman, S. L., Anderson, G. H., Marliss, E. B. & Jeejeebhoy, K. N. (1979). Zinc in total parenteral nutrition: requirements and metabolic effects. *Gastroenterology*, **76**, 458–67.

5

Nutritional immunology

A. ANIMASHAUN AND R. V. HEATLEY

Immunological studies in people with nutritional deficiencies have revealed a wide spectrum of complex dysfunction depending on the degree of malnutrition. This can range from mild deficiencies involving individual nutrients or excess in people with apparently normal nutritional status to those with severe forms of protein-energy malnutrition (PEM). PEM was initially described in children in non-industrialised nations although it is now clear that this condition in varying degrees is commonly found among ill and hospitalised patients throughout the world (Puri & Chandra, 1985).

It has been suggested that malnutrition is the commonest cause of secondary immunodeficiency (Puri & Chandra, 1985). However, the relationship between the two is complex and it is difficult to separate the effect of an illness *per se* from any observed immune dysfunction. A vicious cycle ensues in some individuals in which malnutrition impairs immune function, thus reducing antimicrobial protection and the resulting infection causes further nutritional deficiency.

Overview of immunology

The immune system has developed principally against infective pathogenic agents. This defence is performed bilaterally through the innate and adaptive systems. The innate system acts non-specifically against foreign or non-self material and inhibits the infective process; simultaneously, the adaptive system stimulates a specific response to an infective agent (Roitt, Brostoff & Male, 1985).

The key cells involved in immune reactions are lymphocytes, which can be subdivided into T cells (which mature and differentiate in the thymus); B cells (which mature in the spleen and lymph nodes) and null cells which do not express classical T- or B-cell markers and include natural killer (NK) and killer (K) cells (Roitt *et al.*, 1985). Using monoclonal antibodies it is possible to characterise and identify these T cells and the cluster of differentiation (CD) nomenclature is now used (McMichael, 1987):

(a) CD3+ cells: comprise 95% of all circulating T cells and contain an approximate ratio of 2:1 of CD4+:CD8+ cells (Janossy & Prentice, 1982).
(b) CD4+ cells: consist of helper/inducer (or 'helper') cells and are required for both cellular and humoral immunity (Gansbacher & Levinson, 1986).
(c) CD8+ cells: consist of cells with suppressor functions that may inhibit or downgrade the inflammatory response (Janossy & Prentice, 1982).
(d) CD16+ cells: natural killer cells.

Other cells involved in the immune reactions are mononuclear phagocytes (monocytes (CD11+ cells) and macrophages) and polymorphonuclear phagocytes. Soluble factors include lysozyme, complement and interleukins (Roitt *et al.*, 1985).

Immune responses may be subdivided into cellular and humoral reactions.

Cellular immunity

This involves the interaction between T lymphocytes and antigen.

Immune responses to any antigen involve the modification of the antigen by cells known as antigen-presenting or accessory cells, usually monocytes or macrophages (Grey & Chestnut, 1985). T cell division occurs and clones of antigen-specific cells are formed: soluble lymphokines are released from the T cells and the antigen destroyed, with the aid of other cells such as macrophages.

Functional assays for T lymphocytes include the proliferative response to recall antigens such as the purified protein derivative Bacillus Calmette-Guérin (BCG) where only sensitised individuals respond to skin testing (delayed cutaneous hypersensitivity) *in vivo* and the *in vitro* proliferative response to lectin mitogens. Certain lectins such as phytohaemagglutinin (PHA) and pokeweed mitogen (PWM) can substitute for antigen in the accessory cell signal and preferentially stimulate certain T cell subsets. PHA stimulation leads to proliferation predominantly of CD4+ cells and to a lesser extent CD8+ cells (Reinherz & Schlossman, 1982). PWM preferentially stimulates CD4 + cells to generate helper cells which in turn stimulate B cells to secrete immunoglobulin (Janossy & Prentice, 1982). Monocytes also play a pivotal role in PWM-driven lymphocyte stimulation (Stevenson *et al.*, 1983).

Another commonly used mitogen, concanavalin A (Con A) stimulates CD8 + cells preferentially to generate suppressor cells.

Clinically, impaired cell-mediated immunity increases susceptibility to bacterial, viral, fungal and parasitic disease.

Humoral responses

These result in the production of antibodies (immunoglobulins), following contact with a specific antigen, which stimulate the B cell to divide into antibody-secreting plasma cells. This response involves not only accessory cells but also CD4 + lymphocytes (Hood, Weissman & Ward, 1978). Clinically, B lymphocyte deficiency increases susceptibility to bacterial and viral infections.

Natural killer cells are a third lineage of lymphocytes (Legros, Herbert & Watson, 1984; Baines, 1986) with high spontaneous cytotoxic activity whose activity is promoted by lymphokines such as interleukin-2 and interferon. Accessory cells can release soluble factors which may non-specifically alter cells. Interleukin-1, the lymphocyte activating factor can also stimulate the release of interleukin-2 (IL-2) (Robb, 1984). IL-2 is secreted by activated CD4 + cells (Kahan, 1981) and promotes CD4 + cell proliferation. IL-2 also induces interferon secretion and increases NK cell proliferation, as well as stimulating B cells to secrete antibody (Robb, 1984; Christou, 1990).

Antigen non-specific immune mechanisms include phagocytosis, involving circulating cells such as monocytes and granulocytes, or fixed cell macrophages. Both monocytes and macrophages may act as accessory cells. The process of phagocytosis depends on a complex interaction that includes opsonins, antibody production and complement, all of which lead to intracellular killing. Complement also mediates some aspects of inflammation.

Single nutrient deficiencies and immune function

The effects of deficiencies of individual nutrients can have devastating consequences on the immune system. Almost all micronutrients have been implicated in normal cellular and humoral function but certain nutrients are of particular importance.

Zinc

This trace element is an essential micronutrient required for many physiological functions. Its vital importance is reflected by the hereditary zinc deficiency state, acrodermatitis enteropathica, which leads to a variety of defects which can be reversed by the reintroduction of zinc (Prasad, 1985). Zinc plays a central role in cell mediated immunity, with brief episodes of total deprivation leading to thymic hypoplasia, and premature splenic and lymph node involution (Fraker, Haas & Luecke, 1977; Chandra, 1980; Ronnlund & Suskind, 1983; McClain, Kasarkis & Allen, 1985). Low levels of circulating thymic factors (Blaszek & Mathé, 1984) and increased numbers of immature T cells and lymphopaenia may result (Malave, Claverie-Benureau & Benaim, 1983).

Animal studies have demonstrated that zinc deficiency may reduce the following: CD4+ cell activity (Fraker, Haas & Luecke, 1977); mitogen responsiveness (Gross *et al.*, 1979; Zanzonico, Fernandes & Good, 1981); delayed cutaneous hypersensitivity (Fraker, Zwickl & Luecke, 1982), long-term memory of T lymphocytes (de Pasquale-Jardieu & Fraker, 1984), natural killer cell activity (Fernandes *et al.*, 1979; Allen *et al.* 1983) and monocyte cytotoxicity (Allen *et al.*, 1983). Some of these changes may be completely reversed by the re-introduction of zinc (Fraker *et al.*, 1978).

Zinc deficiency probably compromises the immune response through its role as a co-factor in the enzymes required for cell replication and protein synthesis (Blaszek & Mathé, 1984). *In vitro*, zinc appears to have a variable mitogenic response on lymphocytes, similar to PHA (Kirchner & Rühl, 1970; Berger & Skinner, 1974) though other studies have shown exogenous zinc *in vitro* has an inhibitory effect on lymphocyte transformation (Gaworski & Sharma, 1978; Rao, Schwartz & Good, 1979). The effect of zinc on other immunocytes is less well defined. T cells appear to be less sensitive than B cells to zinc deprivation (Ronnlund & Suskind, 1983).

Several diseases are associated with altered zinc metabolism including acrodermatitis enteropathica (Moynahan, 1974). Lesser degrees of disturbed metabolism occur in other conditions including PEM, Crohn's disease, alcoholic liver disease, Down's syndrome and chronic renal failure. Although immune defects are well recognised in these disorders the relationship between mild to moderate zinc depletion and altered immune function is not clear cut.

The potential use of zinc as an immunostimulant has been explored. Supplemental zinc has been given in a number of conditions in an attempt to improve immune function, with variable results even in the same disease. In Down's syndrome, individuals with low zinc levels were shown to improve skin reactivity, mitogen transformation and phagocytic function with zinc supplementation (Björksten *et al.*, 1980). Similarly patients with chronic renal failure given additional zinc improved their skin reactivity while untreated patients did not (Antoniou, Shalhoub & Schechter, 1981).

Studies in healthy people given supplemental zinc have also shown variable results. An enhanced mitogenic response has been found after a month of extra zinc, and since the patients were not initially plasma zinc depleted, the improvement was not attributed to zinc depletion (Duchateau, Delespesse & Verseecke, 1981*a*). However plasma zinc levels do not always accurately reflect zinc nutrition (Solomons, 1979; Keeling *et al.*, 1980). In other studies oral zinc has been shown to have an enhancing effect on selected immune functions in healthy old people (Duchateau *et al.*, 1981*b*; Wagner *et al.*, 1983; Chandra, 1992). Conversely, excessive intakes may lead to a reduction in immune function in healthy individuals (Chandra, 1984). In the studies discussed the doses of elemental zinc used were well in excess of the recommended daily allowance of 15 mg and it is therefore possible that the immune responses were due to the correction of a substantial deficiency or to a non-nutritional, pharmacological effect of zinc.

Other trace elements

Iron deficiency, ubiquitous and commonly associated with paediatric PEM, may increase susceptibility to infection and depress cellular and humoral immunity (Gross & Newberne, 1980; Rogers & Newberne, 1987; Strauss, 1978), but the results are highly variable suggesting a differential effect on lymphoid populations. Phagocytic function may also be reduced (Dowd & Heatley, 1984). Magnesium appears to be necessary for activation of the complement cascade but deficiency has not been shown to affect cellular immune function in humans. Cobalt, selenium and manganese may have immunostimulatory properties (Hui, Berebitsky & Harmony, 1979; Mulhern *et al.*, 1981; Heatley, 1992).

Vitamin C

Vitamin C is a vital element in wound healing and may have a role in immunological surveillance. The relationship between Vitamin C and lymphocyte function is, however, complex. Animal studies suggest that ascorbic acid deficiency is associated with decreased mitogen-induced T cell blastogenesis (Mueller & Kies, 1962; Thomas & Holt, 1978) with reversal by Vitamin C repletion (Anthony, Kurahara & Taylor, 1979) and an increase in both Con A mitogenesis (Siegel & Morton, 1977) and interferon production (Siegel & Morton, 1977).

In humans, total T cell numbers and subsets do not seem to be influenced by administration or withdrawal of Vitamin C (Kay *et al.*, 1982; Kennes *et al.*, 1983). Supplementation has been variously shown to enhance mitogen transformation to PHA, PWM and Con A (Anderson *et al.*, 1980; Panush *et al.*, 1982; Kennes *et al.*, 1983). Conversely other studies have failed to demonstrate an effect on mitogen transformation using large doses of Vitamin C *in vivo* (Panush, 1982; Goodwin & Garry, 1983) or *in vitro* (Anderson, Oosthuizen & Gatner, 1979) or on the percentage of CD4+ or CD8+ T cells in humans with experimentally induced scurvy before or during the ascorbutic period (Kay *et al.*, 1982). Both *in vitro* stimulatory (Manzella & Roberts, 1979; Panush & Delafuente, 1979) and inhibitory (Munster *et al.*, 1977; Ramirez *et al.*, 1980) mitogen transformation effects have been reported. Neutrophil (Thomas & Holt, 1978) and monocyte (Sandler, Gallin & Vaughan, 1975) functions are increased by exogenous Vitamin C supplementation *in vivo* and *in vitro*. The reported effects of Vitamin C on humoral immunity are conflicting (Prinz *et al.*, 1979; Anderson *et al.*, 1980; Kennes *et al.*, 1983).

The potential role of Vitamin C as a modulator of the immune system is therefore somewhat contentious. Most studies have used doses considerably in excess of the recommended daily allowance of 30 mg and at high doses Vitamin C may be acting as a pharmacological agent rather than a nutrient. Reports of harmful (Editorial, 1979; Thomas & Holt, 1978) and other (Hanck, 1982) effects of megadose therapy have been documented.

Other vitamins

Vitamins A and E are dietary antioxidants which scavenge free radicals thus protecting cell membranes from oxidative damage. They play a vital role therefore in immunodefence. Deficiencies of either or both vitamins may predispose towards infections by reducing the cellular integrity of epithelial and mucosal surfaces. High concentrations of Vitamin E appear to correlate with a reduced risk of infection in people over the age of 60;

similarly Vitamin A deficiency seems to increase the incidence of spontaneous infection (Kelleher, 1991).

The majority of studies have been undertaken in animal models but it has been shown that both CD3+ and CD4+ numbers and mitogen responsiveness can be improved by supplementation in elderly people (Penn et al., 1991). Conversely, megadose therapy with Vitamin E may have an inhibitory effect on cellular immune function (Goodwin & Garry, 1983). Patients with Vitamin B_{12} and folic acid deficiencies show impaired mitogen transformation responses (Gross et al., 1981) and neutrophil dysfunction (Youinou et al., 1982). Pyridoxine deficiency may have profound effects on both humoral and cellular immunity (Axelrod & Trakatellis, 1964).

Lipids and amino acids

The administration of enteral and intravenous lipids may affect immune functions in various ways. Deficiencies of polyunsaturated and essential fatty acids may depress humoral immunity (de Wille, Fraker & Romsos, 1979) and have different effects on cell-mediated immunity (Krause, Williams & Broitman, 1980). Immunosuppression may result from the excessive administration of polyunsaturated fatty acids (Uldall et al., 1975: McHugh et al., 1977).

Although it is clear that normal immune function depends on an adequate protein intake, it is not clear whether single amino acids play an individual role in maintaining immunocompetence. Animal studies suggest that deficiencies of branched-chain or sulphur-containing amino acids lead to reduced cellular immunity secondary to atrophy of lymphoid tissue (Gross & Newberne, 1980). These changes appear to reflect the change seen in paediatric protein-energy malnutrition (Jose & Good, 1973). Concurrent infectious illness may be responsible for the normal or high immunoglobulin levels seen in these children (Wannemacher et al., 1971).

Clinical situations associated with altered immunity

The assessment of undernutrition may be made on clinical evaluation and anthropometric indices. Haematological and biochemical measurements are also important, especially of serum albumin, transferrin and zinc (Puri & Chandra, 1985). Concurrent functional immunological indices will give in vivo and in vitro information which may be valuable in predicting outcome. Moderately severe undernutrition of different aetiologies has detrimental effects on cellular immune functions in particular.

Immune responses in protein-energy malnutrition in children and adults

The majority of studies relating to protein-energy malnutrition and immunity have been undertaken in malnourished children in developing countries (Chandra & Newberne, 1977). In severe malnutrition, pronounced involution of the thymus occurs as well as a reduction in the weight of the tonsils, lymph nodes and spleen, indicating an inhibitory effect of PEM on the lymphoid system (Christou, 1990). Cell-mediated immunity especially is affected leading to reduced numbers of circulating (CD3+, CD4+ and CD8+ cells) T lymphocytes (Puri & Chandra, 1985), poor primary recall and delayed cutaneous hypersensitivity response (Neumann *et al.*, 1975; McMurray *et al.*, 1981), and decreased proliferation to PHA (Neumann *et al.*, 1975; McMurray *et al.*, 1981). Some other studies in severe PEM, however, have shown normal PHA transformation (Dourov, 1986).

Although B cell numbers and serum immunoglobulin concentrations may be normal (Kahan, 1981) or even increased, suggesting decreased CD8+ activity (Christou, 1990), functional studies indicate a variable quality of response to PWM (Kahan, 1981). Natural killer cell numbers may be increased (Kahan, 1981) though activity may be reduced in children with marasmus and/or kwashiorkor (Salimonu *et al.*, 1983) with normal NK activity in nutritionally recovered children (Salimonu *et al.*, 1983). Other abnormalities include reduced monocyte phagocytic activity (Kahan, 1981), depressed complement activity (Puri & Chandra, 1985), decreased interferon production (Salimonu *et al.*, 1983) and normal or reduced polymorphonuclear function (Chandra, Chandra & Ghai, 1976). In paediatric populations which are undernourished as opposed to malnourished, it appears that under-nutrition affects the cellular immune response less severely (Greenwood *et al.*, 1986).

Many of the abnormalities documented above can be partly or completely restored by nutritional repletion (Neumann *et al.*, 1975; Salimonu *et al.*, 1983). It has unfortunately not proved possible to titrate the body's cellular immune response to malnutrition in order to determine the minimum level necessary for prevention of infection. Although both the *in vivo* and *in vitro* tests described are related to antimicrobial function in cellular immunity they do not directly examine the ability of the malnourished individual to protect him or herself against infectious disease.

Between 25% of moderately ill and 50% of severely ill hospital patients have been estimated to be suffering from malnutrition (Bollett & Owens, 1973; Dowd *et al.*, 1986). Chronic organ failures such as that observed with renal, hepatic and cardiac impairment are commonly associated with malnutrition. Adult kwashiorkor may ensue when a rapid reduction in serum albumin level occurs in the presence of an only moderate carbohydrate and low protein diet while severe catabolism is occurring. It is identical to the picture commonly associated with paediatric malnutrition in developing countries. Adult marasmus results from insufficient dietary intake without severe catabolism; this is cachexia and is characterised by markedly reduced anthropometric measurements with normal albumin and transferrin concentrations (Bistrian *et al.*, 1976; Bistrian, 1977).

Patients may be denied access to high quality nutrition for prolonged periods because of post-operative states, gastrointestinal or neurological dysfunction secondary to conditions that preclude oral feeding (Law, Dudrick & Abdou, 1973). To compound the problem, other factors operating in a nosocomial environment also have deleterious effects on the immune system such as drugs, anaesthesia, infection, septic shock, cancer, trauma and burns (McIrvine & Mannick, 1983). Frequently, nutritional deficiency, infection and reduced immunocompetence coexist in the same person and it may be impossible to elucidate the primary problem.

Even relatively short periods of nutritional deprivation can result in immunodysfunction, particularly cellular. Studies in adult marasmus/kwashiorkor undertaken in acutely and chronically ill hospitalised patients have demonstrated reduced skin reactivity (Law *et al.*, 1973; Bistrian, 1977; Chandra, Baker & Kumar, 1985), impaired B lymphocyte function (Law *et al.*, 1973) and depressed (Law *et al.*, 1973) or normal (Bistrian, 1977) mitogen transformation to phytohaemagglutinin, pokeweed mitogen and concanavalin A. Chronically malnourished individuals produce less IL-1 than controls (Keenan *et al.*, 1982; Kauffman, Jones & Kluger, 1986) which may explain the poor febrile response often noted. Re-feeding increases IL-1 levels, the rate of rise being proportional to the amount of protein and carbohydrate ingested (Keenan *et al.*, 1982) and intravenous hyperalimentation improves the depressed cellular immunity seen in other malnourished patients (Law *et al.*, 1973; Bistrian, 1977).

In general, apart from some specific conditions which will be discussed later such as alcoholic liver disease, Crohn's disease and cancer, there does not appear to be a clear-cut correlation between nutritional deprivation and cellular immunocompetence.

Immunocompetence in specific clinical conditions

Immunocompetence in patients with cancer

In patients with cancer, defects in cell-mediated immunity occur which outweigh those found in the humoral and phagocytic systems. A reduction in immunocompetence may be secondary to the type of tumour, its size and staging, to anaesthesia and operative treatment, radiotherapy, chemotherapy and malnutrition (Daly, Dudrick & Copeland, 1980). Sepsis is the commonest cause of death in patients with cancer (Inagaki, Rodriguez & Bodey, 1974) and the enhanced susceptibility to infection may be related to the patient's nutritional status. This may have a predictive role in relation to immune function in patients with neoplasia and both factors may be of prognostic importance.

Cutaneous anergy (Daly, Dudrick & Copeland, 1980) and reduced *in vitro* cellular immunity (Haffejee *et al.*, 1978) are commonly seen and in those who are malnourished there is greater post-operative morbidity and mortality (Daly *et al.*, 1980). Reduced natural killer activity may occur in malnourished but not well-nourished patients with cancer, unrelated to tumour size, age of patient or body weight reduction (Villa *et al.*, 1991). Interleukin-2 levels may also be decreased (Villa *et al.*, 1991). The role of tumour necrosis factor (TNF), an important cytokine with various antitumour and antiviral effects which may stimulate weight loss in malignancy, is unclear (Vaisman, Schattner & Hahn, 1989).

The majority of refeeding trials undertaken have been done in patients with cancer. It has been shown conclusively that enteral or parenteral nutrition can improve the cellular immune response in various neoplastic lesions, for example increase CD3 + cell numbers and complement levels (Bozzetti, 1989), increase NK activity (Villa *et al.*, 1991), increase mitogen responsiveness (Haffejee *et al.*, 1978) and restore cutaneous reactivity (Daly *et al.*, 1980). Although nutritional replenishment may not change the ultimate outcome, it has been associated with a more favourable response to operative therapy and fewer post-operative complications (Daly *et al.*, 1980) and may have a role in patients who would otherwise be unsuitable for chemotherapy because of their cachectic state (Bozzetti, 1989). The demonstration that parenteral or enteral nutrition can restore some immune activities to normal indicates a central role of malnutrition in the genesis of immunodysfunction.

Immunocompetence in ageing individuals

The incidence and severity of infections is increased in elderly populations and although it is impossible to assess the contribution of age-related immunodeficiency to this process, it is clear that immune function does decline with increasing age. However, it may be impossible to separate the effect of age *per se* on the immune system from the considerable contribution of extraneous factors such as concurrent disease, nutritional status, stress and environmental exposure to pathogens.

Humoral immunity may be decreased (Kishimoto *et al.*, 1980) and a decline in cellular immunity is commonly reported (Gillis *et al.*, 1981; Lokhorst *et al.*, 1983; Chandra, 1990; Penn *et al.*, 1991) though may not be universal (Saltzman & Peterson, 1987). Among the factors responsible are thymic involution, an increase in the number of immature CD3 + cells and a qualitative change in T lymphocytes including alterations in cell surface receptors with the development of a new membrane 'senescent cell' antigen (Saltzman & Peterson, 1987; Chandra, 1990). Mitogen responses vary, possibly reflecting that only some T lymphocytes are affected by ageing. IL-2 levels may be reduced (Saltzman & Peterson, 1987) although IL-1 and TNF levels in chronically malnourished, elderly individuals are not reduced when compared to well-nourished age-matched controls (Bradley *et al.*, 1990). Of considerable interest and concern is the effect that ageing, with its inherent effects on T cell function, will have on the increasingly large number of people infected with the human immunodeficiency virus (HIV). Although apparently in good health now, as cellular immune function declines with age, a large number of asymptomatic HIV-antibody positive people may develop the acquired immunodeficiency syndrome.

Nutritional advice and supplementation both in healthy old people without signs of systemic disease (Chandra, 1990) and elderly long-stay patients given vitamins A, C, E (Penn *et al.*, 1991) can reduce cutaneous anergy and improve CD3 + cell numbers and mitogen responsiveness. Multivitamin and trace element supplementation given in physiological doses to healthy elderly people improved numbers of certain T cell subsets and NK cells; NK activity, mitogen responsiveness and IL-2 production were also enhanced. The incidence of infectious disease in the supplemented group was also reduced (Chandra, 1992). The relative contribution of single micronutrient deficiency is unknown. Investigations have documented evidence of cellular zinc depletion in hospitalised but not in healthy elderly subjects (Goode *et al.*, 1991), and it has been shown that

Vitamin C depletion is associated with an increased risk of bedsores (Goode, Burns & Walker, 1992). Supplementation with zinc (Duchateau *et al.*, 1981*b*) and Vitamin C (Kennes *et al.*, 1983) has been shown to improve cellular immune function both *in vivo* and *in vitro*. Refeeding poorly nourished elderly patients with fractured femurs has been shown to improve anthropometric measures as well as clinical outcome (Bastow, Rawlings & Allison, 1983; Delmi, 1990). Presumably the latter benefit was as a result of improved immune function which in turn may have increased the host's response to infection, thus aiding recovery. It has been suggested that nutritional deficiency is the common link between response to infection and immune dysfunction in the elderly (Makinodan *et al.*, 1984).

Immunocompetence in Crohn's disease

Immune dysfunction frequently accompanies Crohn's disease, although whether this is a primary phenomenon or occurs secondarily to mucosal inflammation, immunosuppressant drug treatment or the nutritional disturbances that commonly occur is unknown. Many of the clinical signs seen such as poor wound healing, fistulae, muscle wasting, hypo-proteinaemia, weight loss and immunodysfunction are commonly seen in other conditions where malnutrition coexists. Similarly, many mucosal and peripheral blood immunocyte abnormalities found in Crohn's disease such as colonic autoantibodies (Strickland & Jewell, 1983), lymphocyte cytotoxicity against colonic epithelial cells (Hodgson & Jewell, 1987) and periphera T cell immune defects (Brandtzaeg, 1985) are not specific for the condition.

Several studies of cellular immunity have yielded conflicting results, for example the number of T lymphocytes and their subsets has been found to be normal (Thayer, Charland & Field, 1976; Victorino & Hodgson, 1980; Roche, Watkins & Cook, 1982; Goronzy, Weyand & Waase, 1985; Pallone *et al.*, 1985), increased (Pallone *et al.*, 1983; Selby & Jewell, 1983) or decreased (Meyers *et al.*, 1976; Panush & Delafuente, 1979; Selby & Jewell, 1983). However, although these results are at variance with each other, reported differences are small and there do not appear to be substantial quantitative changes in the absolute number of lymphocyte subsets. Studies of cellular immunity have also yielded conflicting results with variable lymphocyte responses to PHA (Bird & Britton, 1974; Lyanga, Davis & Thomson, 1979; Victorino & Hodgson, 1980; Watanabe *et al.*, 1984); PWM (Victorino & Hodgson, 1980; Danis & Heatley, 1983;

Fujita, Okabe & Yao, 1985) and Con A (Lyanga, Davis & Thomson, 1979; Victorino & Hodgson, 1980; Fujita, Okabe & Yao, 1985). NK cell activity may be reduced (Auer, Ziemer & Sommer, 1980; Gibson & Jewell, 1986) with normal peripheral blood numbers. IL-1 activity may be increased (Satsangi *et al.*, 1987); IL-2 activity is variable (Ebert *et al.*, 1984; Ming *et al.*, 1987). Monocyte function appears normal although turnover may be increased (Thayer, Charland & Field, 1976; Auer *et al.*, 1978). B cell function appears variable (Auer *et al.*, 1979; Pfreundschüh *et al.*, 1981). The explanation for such results may lie in the clinical, therapeutic and pathological differences between patients as well as methodological variation.

Nutritional therapeutic approaches have been used in Crohn's disease ranging from elemental (O'Morain, Segal & Levi, 1980; O'Morain, Segal & Levi, 1984) to parenteral (Heatley, 1984) and support with mineral and vitamin supplementation (Animashaun *et al.*, 1990). A documented improvement in immune function with improved CD3 + lymphocyte numbers, immunoglobulin production and monocyte function along with enhanced anthropometric measurements occurred when malnourished Crohn's disease patients were given an enteral polymeric food supplement (Harries, Danis & Heatley, 1984), suggesting that malnutrition was a prime factor leading to the original immunodysfunction. Oral Vitamin C supplements have also been shown to improve PHA transformation in well-nourished Crohn's disease patients, although no change was noted in the normal T lymphocyte subsets, monocyte function or humoral immunity. It is possible that Vitamin C had an immunostimulatory effect on CD4 + cells. Oral zinc supplementation did not alter immune function (Animashaun, 1988; Animashaun *et al.*, 1990).

Immunocompetence in alcoholic liver disease

Genetic, nutritional and immune mechanisms (Neuberger & Williams, 1987) all contribute to an individual's susceptibility to the development of alcoholic liver disease. Malnutrition frequently coexists with alcoholic liver disease (World, Ryle & Thomson, 1985) and severe marasmus and kwashiorkor is not uncommon (Mendenhall *et al.*, 1984).

A number of immune abnormalities are documented although it is difficult to separate those which are primarily pathogenic from those secondary to ethanol ingestion, hepatocyte dysfunction or associated with malnutrition. Peripheral B lymphocyte counts are normal (Bernstein *et al.* 1974; MacSween & Anthony, 1985) although polyclonal hypergammaglobulinaemia is common (Zetterman & Sorrell, 1981). Peripheral blood subpopulations of lymphocytes and subsets have been found to be increased (McKeever *et al.*, 1983), or decreased (Couzigou *et al.*, 1984; Perrin *et al.*, 1984). Functional studies are again conflicting, reflecting differing populations with decreased (Lundy *et al.*, 1975; Chelazzi *et al.*, 1985) or normal (Hsu & Leevy, 1971; Lundy *et al.*, 1975; Ericsson *et al.*, 1980) mitogen responsiveness. These abnormalities may be reversed on alcohol withdrawal. NK cells numbers are variable (Ericsson *et al.*, 1980) although function may be reduced (Charpentier *et al.*, 1984). Reduced skin test reactivity can occur (Björkholm, 1980) which may be secondary to malnutrition (Bagasra *et al.*, 1986).

Zinc (Sullivan & Heaney, 1970; Walker *et al.*, 1973) and Vitamin C (Baines, 1982) deficiencies have been documented in alcoholic liver disease, and in one study delayed cutaneous hypersensitivity was improved by zinc supplementation (Labadie *et al.*, 1986). It is therefore possible that depletion of these nutrients affects immune function in this condition. In another study involving well-nourished patients with alcoholic liver disease, reduced lymphocyte transformation to PWM was shown which was responsive to neither zinc nor ascorbic acid supplementation (Animashaun, 1988).

Conclusion

Globally, malnutrition remains one of the greatest challenges to mankind. Nutrition is an essential determining factor in immune function. There can be no doubt of the severe effects of nutritional deprivation on the immune system. From individual depletions through to deficiencies of several essential dietary constituents, immunocompetence may be seriously challenged. The position is complicated by the observation that many poorly nourished individuals have concurrent diseases that may themselves enhance the degree of nutritional deficiency and immunodysfunction, thereby increasing the risk of sepsis. It has been shown that supplementation with selected nutrients or refeeding may improve certain immune functions. Further scientific studies need to be undertaken, particularly supplementation trials, to fully explore the complex relationship between nutrition and immunity.

References

Allen, J. I., Perri, R. T., McClain, C. J. & Kay, N. E. (1983). Alterations in human natural killer cell activity and monocyte cytotoxicity induced by zinc deficiency. *Journal of Laboratory and Clinical Medicine*, **102**, 577–89.

Anderson, R., Oosthuizen, R. & Gatner, E. M. S. (1979). Effects of ascorbate and calcium and sodium ascorbate on certain functions of human blood lymphocytes *in vitro. South African Medical Journal*, **56**, 511–15.

Anderson, R., Oosthuizen, R., Maritz, R., Theron, A. & van Rensburg, A. J. (1980). The effects of increasing weekly doses of ascorbate on certain cellular and humoral immune functions in normal volunteers. *American Journal of Clinical Nutrition*, **33**, 71–6.

Animashaun, J. A. (1988). *The Influence of Nutrition on Immune Function in Crohn's Disease and Alcoholic Liver Disease*, MD Thesis, University of Leeds.

Animashaun, A., Kelleher, J., Heatley, R. V., Trejdosiewicz, L. K. & Losowsky, M. S. (1990). The effect of zinc and vitamin C supplementaion on the immune status of patients with Crohn's disease. *Clinical Nutrition*, **9**, 137–46.

Anthony, L. E., Kurahara, C. G. & Taylor, K. B. (1979). Cell-mediated cytotoxicity and humoral immune response in ascorbic acid-deficient guinea pigs, *American Journal of Clinical Nutrition*, **32**, 1691–8.

Antoniou, L. D., Shalhoub, R. J. & Schechter, G. P. (1981). The effect of zinc on cellular immunity in chronic uraemia. *American Journal of Clinical Nutrition*, **34**, 1912–17.

Auer, I. O., Weschler, W., Ziemer, E., Malchow, H. & Sommer, H. (1978). Immune status in Crohn's disease: 1. Leucocyte and lymphocyte subpopulations in peripheral blood. *Scandinavian Journal of Gastroenterology*, **13**, 561–71.

Auer, I. O., Götz, S., Ziemer, E., Malchow, H. & Ehms, H. (1979). Immune Status in Crohn's disease: 3. Peripheral blood B lymphocytes, enumerated by means of F (ab)$_2$ antibody fragments, null cells and T lymphocytes. *Gut*, **20**, 261–8.

Auer, I. O., Ziemer, E. & Sommer, H. (1980). Immune status in Crohn's disease: 5. Decreased *in vitro* natural killer cell activity in peripheral blood. *Clinical & Experimental Immunology*, **42**, 41–9.

Axelrod, A. E. & Trakatellis, A. C. (1964). Relationship of pyridoxine to immunological phenomena. *Vitamin & Hormones*, **22**, 591–607.

Bagasra, O., Howeedy, A., Dorio, R. & Kajdacsy-Balla, A. (1986). Functional analysis of T-cell subsets in chronic experimental alcoholism. *Immunology*, **61**, 63–9.

Baines, M. (1982). Vitamin C and exposure to alcohol. *International Journal of Vitamin and Nutrition Research*, **23**, 287–93.

Baines, M. G. (1986). Natural killer cells. *Immunology Today*, **7**, 22–3.

Bastow, M. D., Rawlings, J. & Allison, S. P. (1983). Benefits of supplementary tube feeding after fractured neck of femur: a randomised controlled trial. *British Medical Journal*, **287**, 1589–92.

Berger, N. A. & Skinner, A. M. (1974). Characterization of lymphocyte transformation induced by zinc ions. *Journal of Cell Biology*, **61**, 45–55.

Bernstein, I. M., Webster, H., Williams, R. C. & Strickland, R. G. (1974). Reduction in circulating T-lymphocytes in alcoholic liver disease. *Lancet*, **ii**, 488–90.

Bird, A. G. & Britton, S. (1974). No evidence for decreased lymphocyte reactivity in Crohn's disease. *Gastroenterology*, **67**, 926–32.

Bistrian, B. R., Blackburn, G. L., Vitale, J., Cochran, D. & Naylor, J. (1976). Prevalence of malnutrition in general medical patients. *Journal of the American Medical Association*, **235**, 1567–70.

Bistrian, B. R. (1977). Cellular immunity in adult marasmus. *Archives of Internal Medicine*, **137**, 1408–11.

Björkholm, M. (1980). Immunological and haematological abnormalities in chronic alcoholism. *Acta Medica Scandinavica*, **207**, 197–200.

Björksten, B., Back, O., Gustavson, K. H., Hallmans, G., Hagglorf, B. & Tarnvik, A. (1980). Zinc and immune function in Down's syndrome. *Acta Paediatrica Scandinavica*, **69**, 183–7.

Blazsek, I. & Mathé, G. (1984). Zinc and immunity. *Biomedicine and Pharmacotherapy*, **38**, 187–93.

Bollett, A. J. & Owens, S. (1973). Evaluation of nutritional status of selected hospitalized patients. *American Journal of Clinical Nutrition*, **26**, 931–8.

Bozzetti, F. (1989). Effects of artificial nutrition on the nutritional status of cancer patients. *Journal of Parenteral and Enteral Nutrition*, **13**, 406–20.

Bradley, S. F., Vibhagool, A., Fabrick, S., Terpenning, M. S. & Kauffman, C. A. (1990). Monokine production by malnourished nursing home patients. *Gerontology*, **36**, 165–70.

Brandtzaeg, P. (1985). Immunopathology of Crohn's disease. *Annals of Gastroenterology and Hepatology*, **21**, 201–20.

Chandra, R. K., Chandra, S. & Ghai, O. P. (1976). Chemotaxis, random motility and mobilization of polymorphonuclear leucocytes in malnutrition. *Journal of Clinical Pathology*, **29**, 224–7.

Chandra, R. K. & Newberne, P. M. (1977). *Nutrition, Immunity and Infection: Mechanisms of Interactions*, New York, Plenum.

Chandra, R. K. (1980). Single nutrient deficiency and cell-mediated immune responses. *American Journal of Clinical Nutrition*, **33**, 736–8.

Chandra, R. K. (1984). Excessive intake of zinc impairs immune responses. *Journal of the American Medical Association*, **252**, 1443–6.

Chandra, R. K., Baker, M. & Kumar, V. (1985). Body composition, albumin levels and delayed cutaneous cell-mediated immunity. *Nutrition Research*, **5**, 679–84.

Chandra, R. K. (1990). The relation between immunology, nutrition and disease in elderly people. *Age & Ageing*, **19**, S25–31.

Chandra, R. K. (1992). Effect of vitamin and trace-element supplementation on immune responses and infection in elderly subjects. *Lancet*, **340**, 1124–7.

Charpentier, B., Franco, D., Paci, L. *et al.* (1984). Deficient natural killer cell activity in alcoholic cirrhosis. *Clinical & Experimental Immunology*, **58**, 107–15.

Chelazzi, G., Piccinelli, O., Senaldi, G., Rossi, D. & Brugo, M. A. (1985). Cellular immunity in alcohol-induced liver disease. *Acta Gastroenterologica Belgica*, **48**, 111–17.

Christou, N. (1990). Perioperative Nutritional Support: Immunologic Defects. *Journal of Parenteral and Enteral Nutrition*, **14**, 186S–96S.

Couzigou, P., Vinchendeau, P., Fleury, B. *et al.* (1984). Etude des modifications des sous-populations lymphocytaires circulantes au cours des hepatopathies alcooliques. Rôle respectif de l'alcool, de l'insuffisance hépato-cellulaire et de la nutrition. *Gastroenterologica Clinica Biologica*, **8**, 915–19.

Daly, J. M., Dudrick, S. J. & Copeland, E. M. (1980). Intravenous hyperalimentation: effects on delayed cutaneous hypersensitivity in cancer patients. *Annals of Surgery*, **192**, 587–92.

Danis, V. A. & Heatley, R. V. (1983). Pokeweed mitogen-stimulated immunoglobulin production by peripheral blood lymphocytes *in vitro*: evidence for disordered immunoregulation in patients with ulcerative colitis and Crohn's disease. *Clinical & Experimental Immunology*, **54**, 739–46.

Delmi, M., Rapin, C-H., Bengoa, J-M., Delmas, P. D., Vasey, H. & Bonjour, J-P. (1990). Dietary supplementation in elderly patients with fractured neck of the femur. *Lancet*, **335**, 1013–16.

De Pasquale-Jardieu, P. & Fraker, P. J. (1984). Interference in the development of a secondary immune response in mice by zinc deprivation: persistence of effects. *Journal of Nutrition*, **114**, 1762–9.

De Wille, J. W., Fraker, P. J. & Romsos, D. R. (1979). Effects of essential fatty acid deficiency and various levels of dietary polyunsaturated fatty acids, on humoral immunity in mice. *Journal of Nutrition*, **109**, 1018–27.

Dourov, N. (1986). Thymic atrophy and immune deficiency in malnutrition. In *The Human Thymus: Histopathology and Pathology*, ed. H. K. Miller-Hermalink. p. 127, Springer-Verlag, Berlin.

Dowd, P. S. & Heatley, R. V. (1984). The influence of undernutrition on immunity. *Clinical Science*, **66**, 241–8.

Dowd, P. S., Kelleher, J., Walker, B. E. & Guillou, P. J. (1986). Nutrition and cellular immunity in hospital patients. *British Journal of Nutrition*, **55**, 515–27.

Duchateau, J., Delespesse, F. & Vereecke, P. (1981*a*). Influence of oral zinc supplementation on the lymphocyte response to mitogens of normal subjects. *American Journal of Clinical Nutrition*, **34**, 88–93.

Duchateau, J., Delespesse, F., Vrijens, R. & Collet, H. (1981*b*). Beneficial effects of oral zinc supplementation on the immune response of old people. *American Journal of Medicine*, **70**, 1001–4.

Ebert, E. C., Wright, S. H., Lipshutz, W. H. & Hauptman, S. P. (1984). T-cell abnormalities in inflammatory bowel disease are mediated by interleukin-2. *Clinical Immunology and Immunopathology*, **33**, 232–44.

Editorial. (1979). Ascorbic acid: immunological effects and hazards. *Lancet*, **i**, 308.

Ericsson, C. D., Kohl, S., Pickering, L. K., Davis, J., Glass, G. S. & Faillace, L. A. (1980). Mechanisms of host defence in well-nourished patients with chronic alcoholism. *Alcoholism: Clinical and Experimental Research*, **4**, 261–5.

Fernandes, G., Nair, M., Onge, K., Tanaka, T., Floyd, R. & Good, R. (1979). Impairment of cell-mediated immunity functions by dietary zinc deficiency in mice. *Proceedings of the National Academy of Science*, **76**, 457–61.

Fraker, P. J., Haas, S. M. & Luecke, R. W. (1977). Effect of zinc deficiency on the immune response of the young adult A/J mouse. *Journal of Nutrition*, **107**, 1889–95.

Fraker, P. J., De Pasquale-Jardieu, P., Zwickl, C. M. & Luecke, R. W. (1978). Regeneration of T-cell helper function in zinc deficient adult mice. *Proceedings of the National Academy of Science*, **73**, 5660–5.

Fraker, P. J., Zwickl, C. M. & Luecke, R. W. (1982). Delayed type hypersensitivity in zinc-deficient adult mice: impairment and restoration of responsibity to dinitrofluorobenzene. *Journal of Nutrition*, 112, 309–13.

Fujita, K., Okabe & Yao, T. (1985). Immunological studies in Crohn's disease: 2. Lack of evidence for humoral and cellular dysfunctions. *Journal of Clinical and Laboratory Immunology*, **16**, 155–61.

Gansbacher, B. & Levinson, A. I. (1986). Effects of PHA-activated T-cells on B-cell differentiation. *Immunology*, **58**, 191–6.

Gaworski, C. L. & Sharma, R. P. (1978). The effect of heavy metals on [^{3}H]-thymidine uptake in lymphocytes. *Toxicology and Applied Physiology*, **46**, 305–13.

Gibson, P. R. & Jewell, D. P. (1986). Local immune mechanisms in inflammatory bowel disease and colorectal cancer. *Gastroenterology*, **90**, 12–19.

Gillis, S., Kozak, R., Durante, M. & Weksler, M. E. (1981). Immunological studies of ageing: decreased production of and response to T cell growth factor by lymphocytes from aged humans. *Journal of Clinical Investigation*, **67**, 937–42.

Goode, H. F., Penn, N. D., Kelleher, J. & Walker, B. E. (1991). Evidence of cellular zinc depletion in hospitalised but not healthy elderly subjects. *Age and Ageing*, **20**, 345–8.

Goode, H. F., Burns, E. & Walker, B. E. (1992). Vitamin C depletion and pressure sores in elderly patients with femoral neck fracture. *British Medical Journal*, **305**, 925–7.

Goodwin, J. S. & Garry, P. J. (1983). Relationship between megadose vitamin supplements and immunological function in a healthy elderly population. *Clinical & Experimental Immunology*, **51**, 647–53.

Goronzy, J., Weyand, C. M. & Waase, I. (1985). T-cell subpopulations in inflammatory bowel disease: evidence for a defective induction of T8 + suppressor/cytotoxic T lymphocytes. *Clinical & Experimental Immunology*, **61**, 593–600.

Greenwood, B. M., Bradley-Moore, A. M., Bradley, A. K., Kirkwood, B. R. & Gilles, H. M. (1986). The immune response to vaccination in undernourished and well-nourished Nigerian children. *Annals of Tropical Medicine & Parasitology*, **80**, 537–44.

Grey, H. M. & Chestnut, R. (1985). Antigen processing and presentation to T cells. *Immunology Today*, **6**, 101–6.

Gross, R. L., Osdin, N., Fong, L. & Newberne, P. M. (1979). Depressed immunological function in zinc-deprived rats as measured by mitogen response of spleen, thymus and peripheral blood. *American Journal of Clinical Nutrition*, **32**, 1260–5.

Gross, R. L., Reid, J. V. O., Newberne, P. M., Burgess, Marston, R. & Hift, W. (1981). Depressed cell-mediated immunity in megaloblastic anaemia due to folic acid deficiency. *American Journal of Clinical Nutrition*, **28**, 225–32.

Gross, R. L. & Newberne, P. M. (1980). Role of nutrition in immunologic function. *Physiology Review*, 188–302.

Haffejee, A. A., Angorn, I. B., Brain, P. B., Duursma, J. & Baker, L. W. (1978). Diminished cellular immunity due to impaired nutrition in oesophageal carcinoma. *British Journal of Surgery*, **65**, 480–2.

Hanck, A. (1982). Tolerance and effects of high doses of ascorbic acid. *International Journal of Vitamin A & Nutritional Research*, **23**, 221–38.

Harries, A. D., Danis, V. A. & Heatley, R. V. (1984). Influence of nutritional status on immune functions in patients with Crohn's disease. *Gut*, **25**, 465–72.

Heatley, R. V. (1984). Nutritional implications of inflammatory bowel disease. *Scandinavian Journal of Gastroenterology*, **19**, 995–8.

Heatley, R. V. (1994). Immune Systems and Nutritional Support. In *Artificial Nutrition Support in Clinical Practice*, ed. J. Payne-James, G. Grimble and D. Silk (in press). Edward Arnold, Sevenoaks, Kent.

Hodgson, H. J. F. & Jewell, D. P. (1987). Immunology of inflammatory bowel disease. *Ballière's Clinical Gastroenterology*, **1**, 531–45.

Hood, L., Weissman, I. L. & Ward, W. B. (1978). *Immunology*, ed. J. Hall. Benjamin Cummings Publishing Company, California, London, Sydney.

Hsu, C. C. S. & Leevy, C. M. (1971). Inhibition of PHA-stimulated lymphocyte transformation by plasma from patients with advanced alcoholic cirrhosis. *Clinical & Experimental Immunology*, **8**, 749–60.

Hui, D. Y., Berebitsky, G. L. & Harmony, J. A. K. (1979). Mitogen-stimulated calcium ion accumulation by lymphocytes. Influence of plasma lipoproteins. *Journal of Biology & Chemistry*, **254**, 4666–73.

Inagaki, J., Rodriguez, V. & Bodey, G. P. (1974). Causes of death in cancer patients. *Cancer*, **33**, 568–73.

Janossy, G. & Prentice, H. G. (1982). T-cell subpopulations, monoclonal antibodies and their therapeutic applications. *Clinics in Haematology*, **11**, 631–60.

Jose, D. G. & Good, R. A. (1973). Quantitative effects of nutritional essential amino acid deficiency upon immune responses to tumors in mice. *Journal of Experimental Medicine*, **137**, 1–9.

Kahan, B. D. (1981). Nutrition and host defence mechanisms. *Surgical Clinics of North America*, **61**, 557–70.

Kauffman, C. A., Jones, P. G. & Kluger, M. J. (1986). Fever and malnutrition: endogenous pyrogen/interleukin-1 in malnourished patients. *American Journal of Clinical Nutrition*, **4**, 449–52.

Kay, N. E., Holloway, D. E., Hutton, S. W., Bone, N. D. & Duane, W. C. (1982). Human T-cell function in experimental ascorbic acid deficiency and spontaneous scurvy. *American Journal of Clinical Nutrition*, **36**, 127–30.

Keeling, P. W. N., Jones, R. B., Hilton, P. J. & Thompson, R. P. H. (1980). Reduced leucocyte zinc in liver disease, *Gut*, **21**, 561–4.

Keenan, R. A., Moidawer, L. L., Yang, R. D., Kawamura, I., Blackburn, G. L. & Bistrian, B. R. (1982). An altered response by peripheral leucocytes to synthesis or release leucocyte endogenous mediator in critically ill, protein-malnourished patients. *Journal of Laboratory and Clinical Medicine*, **100**, 844–57.

Kelleher, J. (1991). Vitamin E and the immune response. *Proceedings of the Nutrition Society*, **50**, 245–9.

Kennes, B., Dumont, I., Brohee, D., Hubert, C. & Neve, P. (1983). Effect of Vitamin C supplements on cell-mediated immunity in old people. *Gerontology*, **29**, 305–10.

Kirchner, H. & Rühl, H. (1970). Stimulation of human peripheral lymphocytes by zinc^{2+} *in vitro*. *Experimental & Cellular Research*, **61**, 229–30.

Kishimoto, S., Tomino, S., Mitsuya, H., Fujiwara, H. & Tsuda, H. (1980). Age-related decline in the *in vitro* and *in vivo* synthesis of anti-tetanus toxoid antibody in humans. *Journal of Immunology*, **5**, 2347–52.

Krause, L., Williams, M. & Broitman, S. A. (1980). Relationship of diet high in lipid and cholesterol on immune function in rats given 1,2 dimethyl hydrazine (DMH). *American Journal of Clinical Nutrition*, **33**, 937.

Labadie, H., Verneau, A., Trinchet, J. G. & Beaugrand, N. (1986). L'apport oral de zinc amélior-t-il l'immunité cellulaire des malades atteints de cirrhose alcoolique? *Gastraoenterologica Clinica Biologica*, **10**, 799–803.

Law, D. K., Dudrick, S. J. & Abdou, N. I. (1973). Immunocompetence of patients with protein-calorie malnutrition: the effects of nutritional repletion. *Annals of Internal Medicine*, **79**, 545–50.

Legros, G. S., Herbert, A. G. & Watson, J. D. (1984). *In vitro* modulation of thymus-derived lymphocytes with monoclonal antibodies in mice. 2. Separation of natural killer cells and cytotoxic T cells. *Immunology*, **51**, 103–13.

Lokhorst, H. M., Van Linden, J. A., Schuurman, J. J., Gmelig Meyling, F. H. J., Bast, E. J. E. G. & De Gast, T. (1983). Immune function during ageing in man: relationship between serological abnormalities and cellular immune states. *European Journal of Clinical Research*, **13**, 209–14.

Lundy, J., Raaf, J. H., Deekin, S. *et al.* (1975). The acute and chronic effects of alcohol on the human immune system. *Surgery, Gynaecology & Obstetrics*, **141**, 212–18.

Lyanga, J. J., Davis, P. & Thomson, A. B. R. (1979). *In vitro* testing of immunoresponsiveness in patients with inflammatory bowel disease: prevalence and relationship to disease activity (immunoresponsiveness in inflammatory bowel disease). *Clinical & Experimental Immunology*, **37**, 120–5.

MacSween, R. M. N. & Anthony, R. S. (1985). Immune mechanisms in alcoholic liver disease. In *Alcoholic Liver Disease – Pathobiology, Epidemiology & Clinical Aspects*, ed. P. Hall, pp. 69–89, Edward Arnold Ltd.

McClain, C. J., Kasarkis, E. J. & Allen, J. J. (1985). Functional consequences of zinc deficiency. *Progress in Food and Nutrition Science*, **9**, 185–226.

McHugh, M. I., Wilkinson, R., Elliot, R. W. *et al.* (1977). Immunosuppression with polyunsaturated fatty acids in renal transplantation. *Transplantation*, **24**, 263–7.

McIrvine, A. J. & Mannick, J. A. (1983). Lymphocyte function in the critically ill surgical patient. *Surgical Clinics of North America*, **63**, 295–361.

McKeever, U., O'Mahoney, C., Lawler, E., Kinsella, A., Weir, D. G. & Feighery, C. F. (1983). Monocytosis: a feature of alcoholic liver disease. *Lancet*, **ii**, 1492.

McMichael, A. J. (1987). *Leucocyte Typing III: White Cell Differentiation Antigens*, Oxford University Press, Oxford.

McMurray, D. N., Loomis, S. A., Casazza, L. J., Rey, H. & Miranda, R. (1981). Development of impaired cell-mediated immunity in mild and moderate malnutrition. *American Journal of Clinical Nutrition*, **34**, 68–77.

Makinodan, T., James, S. J., Inamizu, T. & Chang, M. (1984). Immunologic basis for susceptibility to infection in the aged. *Gerontology*, **30**, 279–89.

Malave, I., Claverie-Benureau, B. & Benaim, I. R. (1983). Modulation by zinc of the *in vitro* antibody response to T-dependent and T-independent antigens. *Immunological Communications*, **12**, 397–406.

Manzella, J. P. & Roberts, N. J. (1979). Human macrophage and lymphocyte responses to mitogen stimulation after exposure to influenza virus, ascorbic acid and hyperthermia. *Journal of Immunology*, **123**, 1940–4.

Mendenhall, C. L., Anderson, S., Weesner, R. E., Goldberg, S. J. & Crolic, K. A. (1984). Protein-calorie malnutrition associated with alcoholic hepatitis. *American Journal of Medicine*, **76**, 211–22.

Meyers, S., Sachar, D. B., Taub, R. N. & Janowitz, H. D. (1976). Anergy to dinitrochlorobenzene and depression of T-lymphocytes in Crohn's disease and ulcerative colitis. *Gut*, **17**, 911–15.

Ming, R. H., Atluru, D., Spellman, C. W., Imir, T., Goodwin, J. S. & Strickland, R. G. (1987). Peripheral blood mononuclear cell interleukin-2 production, receptor generation and lymphokine-activated cytotoxicity in inflammatory bowel disease. *Journal of Clinical Immunology*, **7**, 59–63.

Moynahan, E. J. (1974). Acrodermatitis enteropathica: a lethal inherited human zinc deficiency disorder, *Lancet*, **ii**, 399–400.

Mueller, P. S. & Kies, M. W. (1962). Suppression of tuberculin reaction in the scorbutic guinea pig. *Nature*, **195**, 813.

Mulhern, S. A., Morris, V. C., Vessey, A. R. & Levander, O. A. (1981). Influence of selenium and chow diets on immune function in first and second generation mice. *Federal Proceedings*, **40**, 935.

Munster, A. M., Loadholdt, C. B., Leary, A. G. & Barnes, M. A. (1977). The effect of antibiotics on cell-mediated immunity. *Surgery*, **81**, 692–5.

Neuberger, J. & Williams, R. (1987). Immunology of drug and alcohol induced liver disease. *Ballière's Clinical Gastroenterology*, **1**, 707–22.

Neumann, C. G., Lawlor, G. J., Stiehm, E. R. *et al.* (1975). Immunological responses in malnourished children. *American Journal of Clinical Nutrition*, **28**, 89–104.

O'Morain, C., Segal, A. W. & Levi, A. J. (1980). Elemental diets in treatment of acute Crohn's disease. *British Medical Journal*, **281**, 1173–5.

O'Morain, C., Segal, A. W. & Levi, A. J. (1984). Elemental diet as primary treatment of acute Crohn's disease: a controlled trial. *British Medical Journal*, **288**, 1859–62.

Pallone, F., Montano, S., Fais, S., Boirivant, M., Signore, A. & Pozzilli, P. (1983). Studies of peripheral blood lymphocytes in Crohn's disease. *Scandinavian Journal of Gastroenterology*, **18**, 1003–8.

Pallone, F., Squarcia, O., Fais, S., Boirivant, M., Biancone, C. & Tonietti, G. (1985). T-cell differentiation antigens expressed by peripheral blood lymphocytes in Crohn's disease. *Boll. Ist. Sieroter Milan*, **64**, 394–9.

Panush, R. S. & Delafuente, J. C. (1979). Modulation of certain immunologic responses by Vitamin C. *International Journal of Vitamin & Nutrition Research*, **19**, 179–99.

Panush, R. S., Delafuente, J. C., Katz, P. & Johnson, J. (1982). Modulation of certain immunological responses by Vitamin C. 3. Potentiation of *in vitro* and *in vivo* lymphocyte responses. *International Journal of Vitamin & Nutrition Research*, **23**, 35–47.

Penn, N. D., Purkins, L., Kelleher, J., Heatley, R. V., Mascie-Taylor, B. H. & Belfield, P. W. (1991). The effect of dietary supplementation with Vitamins A, C and E on cell-mediated immune function in elderly long-stay patients: a randomized controlled trial. *Age & Ageing*, **20**, 169–74.

Perrin, D., Bignon, J.-D., Beaujard, E., Cheneau, M.-L. (1984). Populations de lymphocyte T circulants chez les patients atteints de cirrhose alcoolique. *Gastroenterologica Clinica Biologica*, **8**, 907–10.

Pfreundschüh, M., Feurle, G. E., Springer, A., Gouse, A. & Beck, J. (1981). T Lymphocyte subpopulations in the peripheral blood of patients with Crohn's disease. *Scandinavian Journal of Gastroenterology*, **16**, 845–51.

Prasad, A. S. (1985). Clinical manifestations of zinc deficiency. *Annual Review of Nutrition*, **5**, 341–63.

Prinz, W., Bortz, R., Hersch, M. & Gilich, G. (1979). Vitamin C and the humoral immune response. *International Journal of Vitamin Nutritional Research*, **19**, 25–34.

Puri, S. & Chandra, R. K. (1985). Nutritional regulation of host resistance and predictive value of immunological tests in assessment of outcome. *Paediatric Clinics of North America*, **32**, 499–416.

Ramirez, I., Richie, E., Wang, Y.-M. & Van Eys, J. (1980). Effect of ascorbic acid *in vitro* on lymphocyte reactivity to mitogens. *Journal of Nutrition*, **110**, 2207–15.

Rao, K. M. M., Schwartz, S. A. & Good, R. A. (1979). Age-dependent effects of zinc on the transformation response of human lymphocytes to mitogens. *Cellular Immunology*, **42**, 270–8.

Reinherz, E. & Schlossman, S. F. (1982). The characterization and function of human immunoregulatory T Lymphocyte subsets. *Pharmacological Review*, **34**, 17–22.

Robb, R. J. (1984). Interleukin-2: the molecule and its function. *Immunology Today*, **5**, 203–9.

Roche, J. H., Watkins, M. H. & Cook, S. L. (1982). Inflammatory bowel disease: prevalence and level of activation of circulating T-lymphocyte subpopulations mediating suppressor/cytotoxic and helper function as defined by monoclonal antibodies. *Clinical Immunology & Immunopathology*, **25**, 362–73.

Rogers, A. E. & Newberne, P. M. (1987). Nutrition and immunological responses. *Cancer Detection and Prevention Supplement*, **1**, 1–14.

Roitt, I., Brostoff, J. & Male, D. (1985). *Immunology*, Churchill Livingstone, Edinburgh.

Ronnlund, R. D. & Suskind, R. N. (1983). Iron, zinc and other trace elements' effect on the immune response. *Journal of Paediatric Gastroenterology & Nutrition*, **2**, S172–80.

Salimonu, L. S., Ojo-Amaize, E., Johnson, A. O. K., Laditan, A. A. O., Akinwolere, A. O. A. & Wigzell, H. (1983). Depressed natural killer cell activity in children with protein-calorie malnutrition. *Cellular Immunology*, **82**, 210–15.

Saltzman, R. L. & Peterson, P. K. (1987). Immunodeficiency of the elderly. *Reviews of Infectious Diseases*, **9**, 1127–39.

Sandler, J. A., Gallin, J. I. & Vaughan, M. (1975). Effects of serotonin carbamylcholine and ascorbic acid on leucocyte cyclic G.M.P. and chemotaxis. *Journal of Cellular Biology*, **67**, 480–4.

Satsangi, J., Wolstencroft, R. A., Cason, J., Ainley, C. C., Dumonde, D. C. & Thompson, R. P. H. (1987). Interleukin-1 in Crohn's disease. *Clinical and Experimental Immunology*, **67**, 594–605.

Selby, W. S. & Jewell, D. P. (1983). T lymphocyte subsets in inflammatory bowel disease. *Gut*, **24**, 99–105.

Siegel, B. V. & Morton, J. I. (1977). Vitamin C and the immune response. *Experientia*, **33**, 393–7.

Solomons, N. W. (1979). On the assessment of zinc and copper nutriture in man. *American Journal of Clinical Nutrition*, **32**, 856–71.

Stevenson, H. C., Miller, P. J., Waxdal, M. J., Haynes, B. F., Thomas, C. A. & Fauci, A. S. (1983). Interaction of pokeweed mitogen with monocytes in the activation of human lymphocytes. *Immunology*, **49**, 633–40.

Strauss, R. G. (1978). Iron deficiency, infections and immune function: a reassessment. *American Journal of Clinical Nutrition*, **31**, 660–6.

Strickland, R. G. & Jewell, D. P. (1983). Immunoregulatory mechanisms in non-specific inflammatory bowel disease. *Annual Review of Medicine*, **34**, 195–204.

Sullivan, J. F. & Heaney, R. P. (1970). Zinc metabolism in alcoholic liver disease. *American Journal of Clinical Nutrition*, **23** (2), 170–7.

Thayer, W. R., Charland, C. & Field, C. (1976). The subpopulations of circulating white blood cells in inflammatory bowel disease. *Gastroenterology*, **71**, 379–84.

Thomas, W. R. & Holt, P. G. (1978). Vitamin C and immunity: an assessment of the evidence. *Clinical & Experimental Immunology*, **32**, 370–9.

Uldall, P. R., Wilkinson, R., McHugh, M. I. *et al.* (1975). Linoleic acid and transplantation. *Lancet*, **ii**, 128–9.

Vaisman, N., Schattner, A. & Hahn, T. (1989). Tumour necrosis factor production during starvation. *American Journal of Medicine*, **87**, 115.

Victorino, R. M. M. & Hodgson, H. J. F. (1980). Alterations to T-lymphocyte subpopulations in inflammatory bowel disease. *Clinical & Experimental Immunology*, **41**, 156–65.

Villa, M. L., Ferrario, E., Bergamasco, E. *et al.* (1991). Reduced natural killer cell activity and IL-2 production in malnourished cancer patients. *British Journal of Cancer*, **63**, 1010–14.

Wagner, P. A., Jernigan, J. A., Bailey, L. B., Nickens, C. & Brazzi, G. A. (1983). Zinc nutriture and cell-mediated immunity in the aged. *International Journal of Vitamin & Nutrition Research*, **53**, 94–101.

Walker, B. E., Dawson, J. B., Kelleher, J. & Losowsky, M. S. (1973). Plasma and urinary zinc in patients with malabsorption syndromes or hepatic cirrhosis. *Gut*, **14**, 943–8.

Wannemacher, R. W., Powanda, M. C., Pekarek, R. S. & Beisel, W. R. (1971). Tissue amino acid flux after exposure of rats to Diplococcus pneumoniae. *Infection & Immunology*, **4**, 556–62.

Watanabe, M., Tsuru, S., Aiso, S. *et al.* (1984). Induction of impaired activation of lymphocyte by suppressive factor in Crohn's disease patients. *Journal of Clinical & Laboratory Immunology*, **14**, 29–34.

World, M. J., Ryle, P. R. & Thomson, A. D. (1985). Alcoholic malnutrition and the small intestine. *Alcohol & Alcoholism*, **20**, 89–124.

Youinou, P. Y., Garre, M. A., Menez, J. F. *et al.* (1982). Folic acid deficiency and neutrophil dysfunction. *American Journal of Medicine*, **73**, 652–7.

Zanzonico, P., Fernandes, G. & Good, R. A. (1981). The differential sensitivity of T-cell and B-cell mitogenesis to *in vitro* zinc deficiency. *Cellular Immunology*, **60**, 203–11.

Zetterman, R. K. & Sorrell, M. F. (1981). Immunological aspects of alcoholic liver disease. *Gastroenterology*, **81**, 616–24.

6

Physiology of nutrient absorption: a decade of advance in formulation of enteral diets

G. K. GRIMBLE

Introduction

The successful growth of enteral nutrition owes a great deal to the work of the scientific and clinical innovators who prepared a diet comprising 18 free *L*-amino acids, glucose, salts, fat soluble vitamins and ethyl linoleate (Randall, 1984). It was refined as a result of extensive studies in animals and further investigations (sponsored by NASA) into its suitability for astronauts during prolonged space flight, revealed no nutritional abnormalities through 2500 man-days of diet feeding of earth-bound volunteers (Winitz *et al.*, 1970; Winitz, Seedman & Graff, 1970). As a consequence 'chemically defined' elemental diets became known as 'space diets', although they were never actually fed to astronauts.

This diet was designed for patients with 'severely impaired gastro-intestinal function', of digestive or absorptive origin. The composition of this diet should be judged against the views of intestinal physiology which were current in the 1950s and 1960s, since each macronutrient was included in the form thought to be most easily assimilated (Table 6.1).

For a decade or more, 'elemental diets' found widespread application and apart from the specific clinical indication, Crohn's disease (Bowling *et al.*, 1993), they are generally prescribed to patients with 'severely impaired gastrointestinal function'. With advances in our understanding of nutrient absorption physiology, this definition requires revision. The discovery of the obvious, that the gastrointestinal tract has a huge reserve capacity, has led to development of polymeric diets. In addition, the *degrees* of clinical impairment of absorptive function have been more precisely defined in specific patient groups in whom growth impairment results from malabsorption, e.g. cystic fibrosis, or neonatal prematurity (Durie & Pencharz, 1992). 'Elemental' diets no longer comprise the monomeric absorptive elements of food. *L*-amino acids have been replaced

Table 6.1. *The physiological rationale for the composition of elemental diets*

Macronutrient	Form	Reason
Protein	L-amino acids	No digestion required Rapidly absorbed by L-amino acid transporters on brush-border membrane of enterocyte
Carbohydrate	Glucose/sucrose	Glucose absorbed directly Little digestion required by sucrase/isomaltase at brush-border membrane of enterocyte
Fat	Small amount of triglyceride	To prevent EFA deficiency

by partial enzymic hydrolysates of protein; most contain small amounts of emulsified lipid and free glucose has been replaced by partial enzymic hydrolysates of corn starch and some sucrose. In some respects they are similar to the latest generation of protein-hydrolysate based enteral diets.

The distinction between diets for patients with normal and abnormal gastrointestinal function has thus become blurred. Indeed, with the wisdom of hindsight it is hard to understand why it was ever considered that significant malabsorption of nutrients from nasoenterally-infused polymeric diets would occur. There is now a greater understanding of how to define the degree of impairment of any aspect of nutrient assimilation and of how simple dietetic and clinical manoeuvres can overcome slight impairment of any of these steps, without reducing the amount of nutrient administered each day.

Definition of malabsorption of nutrients

Reserve capacity or the 'safety margin' of the gastrointestinal tract

The term 'rate limiting' is borrowed from enzymology and implies that any of the steps of intestinal nutrient assimilation becomes so severely impaired as to cause malabsorption. In clinical terms, this may present as vitamin malabsorption and deficiency or as loose watery stools consequent on malabsorption of macronutrients and their fermentation by the colonic luminal microflora (Hammer *et al.*, 1990).

Although gastrointestinal pathology can affect nutrient assimilation, it is important to remember that the functional absorptive capacity of the human gastrointestinal tract for most nutrients is large. Indeed, malabsorption of some nutrients occurs only if 90% impairment of organ function has occurred, e.g. exocrine pancreatic disease (Crane, 1964). Because of the overlap between luminal and brush-border phases of digestion, the degree of impairment has to be profound before clinically significant malabsorption will occur.

The 'reserve capacity' or 'safey-margin' of total nutrient absorptive capacity of the small-intestine is better understood and in man, nasoduodenal intakes of up to 6000 kcal/day are efficiently assimilated (Raimundo *et al.*, 1988). Animal studies have demonstrated that the total absorptive area of intestine suits the *metabolic mass* of each species. Comparison of two species of similar size, habitat and diet but different *metabolic mass*, e.g. desert wood rat and iguana, shows them to have intestines of similar size but with markedly different surface area. The difference can be accounted for by the amplification of surface area by villi and microvilli, 1280-fold in the desert rat, much less in the iguana (Ferraris, Lee & Diamond, 1989). In one ingenious study of mice, hyperphagia consequent on transfer to a 6°C environment did not alter digestion efficiency, but a slight intestinal adaptation to a higher nutrient load resulted in reduction of the 'safety margin' from 220–300% to 60–90% (Toloza, Lam & Diamond, 1991). In man, this would correspond to a safety margin of about 4500–7000 kcal/day.

This should be borne in mind when considering studies which show impairment of absorptive function, e.g. reduced pancreatic secretions, brush-border membrane hydrolases of kinetics of substrate uptake, in different disease states. Few of these studies have addressed the question as to whether such changes give rise to *clinically* significant impairment of nutrient uptake. Thus, in a recent double-blind, prospective controlled crossover trial of a polymeric and a predigested chemically defined formula diet, we observed no difference in any nutritional parameter, even though the attending physicians had diagnosed moderately impaired gastrointestinal function (Rees *et al.*, 1992). This would support the concept that the general use of predigested chemically defined formula diets should be confined to patients with severely (rather than moderately) impaired gastrointestinal function.

The concept of nutrient 'load'

Malabsorption may occur if digestive and absorptive systems are overwhelmed by too high a luminal nutrient concentration. Load can thus be defined as the product of the rate of administration of a nutrient and the resulting luminal concentration, *in relation to mouth-to-caecum transit time*. In this equation, the constant k, defines the complex interaction between nasogastric infusion of a hypothetical nutrient, gastric emptying and pancreatobiliary secretions in producing the final luminal concentration:

$$\text{Load (mmoles/h)} \times k = \text{Infusion rate } (l/h)$$
$$\times \text{ luminal concentration (mmol/l)}$$

Lactose and its hydrogenated derivative lactitol provide a good example of this concept, because lactitol is not absorbed to any appreciable extent in the human small intestine. Regardless of the oral load of lactitol given, it will traverse the small intestine intact (accompanied by water) to be rapidly fermented by luminal microflora (Grimble, Patil & Silk, 1988) and at a high enough dose will elicit a laxative effect (Patil, Grimble & Silk, 1987). Lactose can be hydrolysed by β-galactosidase to galactose and glucose which are absorbed, but in lactase-deficient patients, a bolus of lactose will cause diarrhoea (O'Keefe *et al.*, 1984), whereas 24-hour nasogastric infusions of lactose-containing enteral diets do not (Keohane *et al.*, 1983). The difference can be explained by the fact that in alactasic patients, brush-border β-galactosidase is never entirely absent but is insufficient to hydrolyse a lactose bolus (high 'load') within the orocaecal transit time. During continuous infusion, load is low and residual β-galactoside activity is not saturated by the rate of delivery.

This concept can be applied to the patient who presents with gastrointestinal symptoms (which are not antibiotic related) on supplemental feeding. A slower nasoenteral nutrient infusion rate, over an extended period of the day may resolve the problem, without recourse to 'half-strength' regimes, which limit nutrient intake.

Protein absorption

Assimilation of dietary protein proceeds by two complementary phases. Luminal digestion produces small peptides and free L-amino acids which are then subject to further hydrolysis or absorption at the enterocyte brush border.

Gastric luminal protein digestion

Efficient hydrolysis of dietary protein in the stomach relies on acid denaturation which renders stable protein structures, susceptible to hydrolysis. The gastric pepsins have a functional pH optimum towards intact protein of *c*. pH 2.0 (lower than their optimal pH for soluble oligo-peptides) as a result of the combined effects of gastric-acid denaturation, dicarboxylic acid side-chain protonation and the catalytic properties of the enzymes themselves. This co-operative mechanism will convert dietary protein to large oligopeptides only (Foltmann, 1986). This soluble mixture is thus a susceptible substrate for luminal digestion by pancreatic endo- and exo-peptidases, for which the pH optimum is much higher. The peptide-bond specificities of the three endo- and two exo-peptidases are co-operative, and will release large amounts of free amino acids and small peptides (Desnuelle, 1986; Puigserver, Chapus & Kerfelec, 1986).

Poor solubilisation of protein in the stomach during enteral nutrition can cause adverse effects. Of all dietary proteins, casein is probably the worst culprit and retrograde reflux of gastric contents along the feeding-tube can lead to blockage (Marcuard & Perkins, 1988), or even oeso-phageal obstruction (Turner *et al.*, 1991). In one study (Viall *et al.*, 1990), casein-based diets led to a higher incidence of gastric residue and side-effects, than did a highly soluble soy-protein hydrolysate. Whole protein is more slowly cleared from the gastric lumen than protein hydrolysates (Ziegler *et al.*, 1990), although this has not been observed in all studies (Mowatt-Larssen *et al.*, 1992). Concurrent medication may also adversely affect intestinal assimilation. Thus, H2-receptor antagonists which are widely used to control stress-ulceration in ICU patients who are being fed by TPN (Grimble *et al.*, 1991) may inhibit efficient gastric protein digestion during enteral nutrition, by raising luminal pH above the optimum for gastric enzymes. It has been noted that cimetidine markedly inhibits brush-border disaccharidases and glucose and amino acid absorption in the small intestine of mice (Gill, Sanyal & Sareen, 1990).

Intestinal nitrogen assimilation

Dietary and endogenous protein

Assimilation of dietary protein occurs mainly in the proximal jejunum, as deduced from the rapidity of amino acids in blood after a protein meal (Craft *et al.*, 1968; Silk *et al.*, 1979; Chung *et al.*, 1979). The increasing gradient of all major brush-border peptidases towards the ileocaecal valve also suggests that the ileum has considerable digestive and absorptive capacity (Skovbjerg, 1981; Triadou, Bataille & Schmitz, 1983; Tarvid, 1992). The colon is a major site of assimilation of endogenously derived protein (intestinal secretions, secreted plasma proteins and desquamated cells) in view of evidence of stomatal protein losses in ileostomy patients (Chacko & Cumming, 1988). Indeed, the luminal microflora of the colon have considerable capacity for digesting endogenous and dietary proteins *in vitro* and *in vivo* (Mortensen, Rasmussen & Holtug, 1988; Mortensen *et al.*, 1990; MacFarlane, Cumming & Allison, 1986). There is a co-operative interaction between protein fermentation (producing short-chain fatty acids (SCFA), isomeric SCFA and copious amounts of NH_4^+) and carbohydrate fermentation which consumes NH_4^+ (Mortensen *et al.*, 1990). This synergism has been exploited for many years in treatment of chronic hepatic encephalopathy with non-absorbable disaccharides such as lactulose or lactitol (Morgan, 1991).

Other modes of nitrogen uptake

Two other sources of nitrogen (N) which are assimilated in the large intestine have often been overlooked. These are nitrogen derived from urea recycling and amino acids derived from non-dietary sources. The human large intestine has a significant capacity to utilise urea as a source of nitrogen for resynthesis of the α-NH_2 of amino acids. Ruminants are able to utilise urea efficiently, after hydrolysis by the ruminal microflora, as the liberated NH_4^+ can be absorbed and incorporated into amino acids via the transaminase reaction. In man, the same mechanism has been demonstrated by stable-isotope studies with ^{15}N-urea. Permeation of urea from blood into the colonic lumen occurs in significant amounts, approximately 2.6 g N/d (of which 1.4 g N/d is recycled into amino acids) in comparison to a daily urea production rate of 8.5 g N from 14 g N protein intake (Moran & Jackson, 1990a, b); Hibbert, Forrester & Jackson, 1992). This source of NH_4^+ is additional to that derived from metabolic consumption of glutamine by the gastrointestinal tract (Windemueller, 1981; Souba, 1993).

A second, minor pathway, is recycling of D-amino acids though the action of D-amino acid oxidase DAO, which converts D-amino acids to their keto-form which can be transaminated to the L-form. The capacity of this pathway is surprisingly high as shown by the ability of patients to utilise intravenous solutions comprising racemic mixtures of D/L-amino acids (Tweedie, Spivey & Johnston, 1973). Studies of a genetic strain of mice which lack DAO have confirmed that the origin of part of the urinary excretion of D-amino acids is colonic and sensitive to antibiotic treatment (Konno, Niwa & Yasamura, 1990). The remainder comes from racemisation of amino acid residues in long-lived tissue protein, such as those in the lens or associated with myelin (Shapira & Chou, 1987).

Free amino acid transport

There are four major, Na^+-dependent, group-specific, active transport systems in the mammalian enterocyte (Matthews, 1991): (1) monoamino, monocarboxylic (neutral amino acids), (2) glycine, proline, hydroxy-proline, (3) dibasic amino acids and cystine, (4) dicarboxylic (acidic) amino acids. Their definition is complicated by the presence of multiple transport systems within each group, and differing transport character-istics for the same amino acid, at the enterocyte brush border and basolateral membrane (see Semenza & Cortelli, 1986).

A good example of this complexity is shown by the dibasic amino acids, which include arginine, currently under active investigation as a nutritional immune modulator (Kirk & Barbul, 1990). The presence of an active transport system has been shown by studies on patients with the inborn error, cystinuria, caused by a lesion at the level of the intestinal/renal active transporter, who characteristically have high urinary excretion of all dibasic amino acids and cystine. Uptake of dibasic amino acids is never entirely abolished because a component of uptake is passive and non-saturable (Milliner, 1990). Amino acids which do not share the same transporter, e.g. leucine, or metabolically related compounds, e.g. poly-amines, α-ketoglutarate can also stimulate dibasic amino acid uptake via a countertransport mechanism (Cheeseman, 1992; Medina *et al.*, 1991; Payne-James *et al.*, 1989).

All dibasic amino acids stimulate net water secretion in the perfused jejunum, but the most potent, arginine has a local effect (Hegarty *et al.*, 1981). An explanation could be that arginine, absorbed from the intestinal lumen is stoichiometrically converted to ornithine and citrulline and urea during passage through the enterocyte (Rerat *et al.*, 1988). It would be tempting to speculate that this unique metabolic adaptation represents an adaptive response to excessive stimulation of local motility effects by the arginine metabolite, nitric oxide (Calignano *et al.*, 1992; Palmer, Ferrige & Moncada, 1987).

Peptide transport

The close connection between brush-border membrane hydrolysis of peptides and their uptake is consistent with a 'dual hypothesis' of peptide

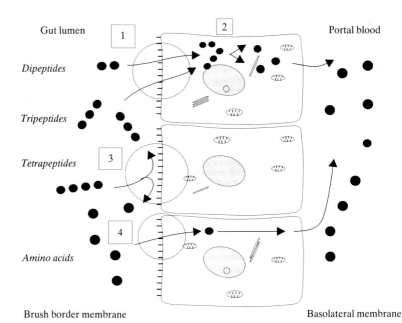

Fig. 6.1. Nitrogen assimilation in the small intestine. An idealised view of the intestinal wall is shown. Following luminal digestion by pancreatic proteases, di- and tri-peptides can be absorbed intact by a specific transporter 1 and are hydrolysed by intracellular peptidases 2. Tetra- and higher peptides are hydrolysed by brush-border peptidases 3. Free amino acids are absorbed by one of the specific active L-amino acid transporters 4.

assimilation (Grimble *et al.*, 1989; Matthews, 1991). In this scheme, a di- or tri-peptide can be absorbed intact by a system, distinct from any amino acid transporter, and will be hydrolysed intracellularly (Fig. 6.1). Alternatively, constituent amino acids or smaller peptide fragments may be absorbed after brush-border membrane hydrolysis of the peptide.

The transport characteristics of di- and tri-peptide uptake are unique. Uptake of dipeptides by brush-border membrane vesicles is pH sensitive and maximal if the external pH is less than intravesicular pH (Ganapthy & Leibach, 1985). This characteristic has been shown to be true for the brush-border membrane of the small-intestine and renal tubule (Ganapathy, Mendicino & Leibach, 1981) as well as the placental membrane (Ganapathy *et al.*, 1981) as well as the placental membrane (Ganapathy *et al.*, 1985). Proton-dependence, the hallmark of intact di- and tri-peptide uptake, has allowed the transporter protein to be characterised. Uptake of the cephalosporin antibiotics (containing a peptide bond) is active and competes for transport of dipeptides (Okano *et al.*, 1986). Kramer and colleagues, have therefore used H^3-labelled benzylpenicillin, or an azo-derivative of cephalexin, which, when treated with ultraviolet light, will covalently tag the transporter protein responsible for their uptake by brush-border membrane vesicles (Kramer, 1987; Kramer *et al.*, 1988). A protein of molecular weight 127000 daltons was identified and isolated and proved to have all of the characteristics of dipeptide transport when incorporated into synthetic liposomes. It is likely that this protein is either the peptide transporter system or a part of it. Investigation of uptake of over 60 model peptides by renal brush-border membrane vesicles has revealed the existence of two transport systems of low- and high-affinity (Daniel, Morse & Adibi, 1992), the latter having the following structural requirements for peptide uptake:

1. A free terminal α-NH_2 and COOH group.
2. α-configuration for both termini.
3. A *trans*- rather than *cis*-peptide bond.
4. *L*-amino acid isomers at both termini although hydrophobic D-amino acids are acceptable at the N-terminus.
5. Chain-length of two or three amino acids only.

These differences between L-amino acid and peptide transport are highly significant. Free L-amino acid transport often works 'uphill' against a transmembrane concentration gradient, whereas di- and tri-peptide uptake is 'downhill' because the high activity of intracellular peptidases rapidly removes them from the intracellular compartment. This would explain the inherent rapidity of di- and tri-peptide transport which may be exploited in feeding patients with severely impaired absorptive function. A second consideration is that stimulation of Na^+ and water uptake by dipeptides is less strong than by amino acids (Cook, 1972) because transport of the latter is generally Na^+-dependent. We have observed that hydrolysates containing $>70\%$ di- and tri-peptides had a rather weak effect on Na^+ (and water) uptake, in contrast to tetra- and penta-peptide preparation or free L-amino acids (Rees *et al.*, 1988a, b). Thus, the use of hydrolysates which are designed to promote maximum nitrogen absorption (di and tri-peptides) may not give optimal water and Na^+ uptake.

Quantitative aspects of dietary protein assimilation

Perfusion studies

Dipeptide transport predominates over free L-amino transport during early growth (Guadalini & Rubino, 1982; Miller *et al.*, 1984). It is less sensitive to the effects of starvation (Vasquez, Morse & Adibi, 1985), which upregulates brush-border peptidase activity (Vasquez *et al.*, 1985; Tarvid, 1992). This would imply that peptide assimilation in the small intestine is strongly conserved when dietary amino acid supply may be rate-limiting to growth. It would also suggest that, in the absence of protein intake, efficient assimilation of endogenous secretions is necessary. In addition, most human and animal intestinal-perfusion studies have shown that the rate of absorption of individual amino acid residues is faster and more even from partially hydrolysed protein than from its equivalent free amino acid mixture (Grimble *et al.*, 1986). These findings suggest that there may be an absorptive advantage in using protein hydrolysates rather than free amino acids in enteral diets.

Several factors affect uptake. The starter protein, the method of enzymic hydrolysis and the chain length of constituent peptides have all been shown to have profound effects on uptake of amino acid residues (Keohane *et al.*, 1985; Grimble *et al.*, 1986; Friedrich *et al.*, 1984). A small increase in the chain length of ovalbumin and casein hydrolysates from di- and tri-peptides to tetra- and penta-peptides (Table 6.2), markedly reduced N uptake from these preparations, at both high and low perfused concentrations (Grimble *et al.*, 1987; Rees *et al.*, 1988a, b). As in previous animal studies (Adibi & Morse, 1977), in the absence of luminal pancreatic enzymes, brush-border hydrolysis of tetra- and penta-peptides is rate-limiting to the uptake of constituent nitrogen.

It would clearly be profitable to investigate the effect of other hydrolysis variables in similar detail, as proposed before (Grimble *et al.*, 1989). For example, the sequence and hydrophobicity (Daniel, Morse & Adibi, 1992) of the constituent peptides of a protein hydrolysate will profoundly influence uptake. Thus, if two hydrolysates of identical chain-length profile were produced from the same protein by two groups of peptidases with different bond specificity, their absorption characteristics may be quite different. There may thus be scope for 'tailoring' hydrolysates for maximal amino acid absorption.

Table 6.2. *Effect of peptide chain-length on jejunal assimilation of protein hydrolysates*

Starter protein	Hydrolysate type	Peptide chain length ($\%$ by weight)				Nitrogen absorption ($\%$)	
		>5	4–5	2–3	Amino acids		
Whey	Short-chain	40	23	32	5	37.7	$p < 0.001$
	Long-chain	98	–	–	2	12.1	
Ovalbumin	Short-chain	Trace	16	75	9	33.6	$p < 0.05$
	Medium-chain	Trace	68	24	8	23.0	
Casein	Short-chain	Trace	22.5	69.5	8	32.0	$p < 0.05$
	Medium-chain	Trace	64	35	1	24.5	

Data from (Grimble *et al.*, 1986; Grimble *et al.*, 1987; Rees *et al.*, 1988*a, b*).
Determined by Cu(II)-Sephadex chromatography (Rothenbuhler, Waibel & Solms, 1979).

Animal feeding studies

The literature abounds with 'formula' trials comparing clinical benefit from enteral diets based on protein hydrolysates, free L-amino acids or whole proteins (e.g. see Viall *et al.*, 1990; Mowatt-Larssen *et al.*, 1992; Zaloga, Ward & Prielipp, 1991), in which the diets were not balanced in terms of energy or nitrogen intake. Indeed, in only two have the amino acid composition of the hydrolysate and protein been matched (Steinhardt *et al.*, 1989; Ziegler *et al.*, 1990). There is thus little clinical data on the relative nutritional efficacy of different forms of enteral nitrogen.

Diets based on casein or the identical amino acid mixture produce equal growth rates in young, healthy rats (Itoh, Kishi & Chibata, 1973). Similar, long-term comparisons in healthy volunteers showed that regardless of the degree of hydrolysis of lactalbumin, nitrogen balance remained the same (Moriarty *et al.*, 1985). In contrast, a whole-protein based diet elicited greater N retention, tissue weight and plasma protein levels in burned guinea-pigs than did the equivalent free amino acid diet (Trocki *et al.*, 1986). The basis of this difference may lie in methodology of balancing the amino acid content of diets, rather than any superiority of whole protein over free L-amino acids, or vice versa. The method of amino acid analysis, by HPLC after complete acid hydrolysis, results in the loss of the carboxamide groups of asparagine and glutamine from the protein (or partial hydrolysate) such that glutamine plus glutamate content is expressed as glutamate alone. This apparent 'loss' of nitrogen, is as much as 20% of total N (e.g. casein) and can be corrected only by adjusting the composition of an 'equivalent' amino acid diet, by addition of the dicarboxylic acids with their amides in the ratio found in the native protein by sequence analysis. Itoh and colleagues found that this correction made no difference to biological values of casein, its partial hydrolysate or *L*-amino acid mixture (Itoh *et al.*, 1973). In contrast, we found a whey hydrolysate or its 'equivalent' amino acid mixture equally effective in maintaining rat growth (Grimble *et al.*, 1989). The hydrolysate, however, caused marked caecal hypertrophy of the same magnitude as in pectin-supplemented rats (Koruda *et al.*, 1986). The reason for this is unclear but confirms that the form of dietary nitrogen affects distal intestinal growth. It would certainly suggest that a degree of caution should be exercised in considering clinical trials which claim metabolic advantages for enteral diets based on whole protein, hydrolysates, or free amino acids in stressed patients, if this simple correction has not been made (Trocki *et al.*, 1986).

In only one study has a metabolic advantage been claimed for hydrolysates vs. free amino acids (Monchi *et al.*, 1991). However, this mode of administration (two infusions of 10–15 minutes per day) probably influenced this result. The more rapid aminoacidaemia which follows an oral bolus of hydrolysates (Silk *et al.*, 1979; 1980) stimulates insulin secretion more, as proved to be the case (48.4 ± 11.2 vs. 20.0 ± 5.0 mIU/ml, hydrolysate vs. amino acids, Monchi *et al.*, 1991). During continuous 24-hour nasoenteral infusion, absorptive differences are likely to be minimal because the 'load' is modest. However, with increased use of 'cyclical' nasoenteral nutrition, these absorptive differences will be accentuated, as suggested by a recent trial in post-surgical patients (Ziegler *et al.*, 1990).

Feeding studies in man

Normal or moderately impaired gut function

Two studies have shown that there is no absorptive or metabolic advantage of whole-protein, protein hydrolysates, or the equivalent amino acid mixtures. The first was in normal subjects (Moriarty *et al.*, 1985), in the second we investigated patients with impaired gastrointestinal function judged by the attending physician to be moderate (Rees *et al.*, 1992). Similar results have been obtained in patients with only 60–150 cm of intestine remaining (McIntyre, Fitchen & Lennard-Jones, 1986).

Severely reduced absorptive area

When absorptive area was more severely reduced (50–80 cm jejunum), no difference was observed in N balance, N absorption of ^{13}C-leucine kinetics when patients received a whey–protein–hydrolysate-based or equivalent amino acid-based enteral diet (Rees *et al.*, 1988*a*, *b*). The whey protein hydrolysates used in both studies contained mainly tetra- and penta-peptides and it is possible that brush-border hydrolysis rate-limited their uptake.

Impaired pancreatic function

Crane observed that ^{15}N-labelled yeast protein was malabsorbed only if pancreatic enzyme secretion was impaired by more than 90% (Crane, 1964). This has been confirmed in patients with total pancreatectomy who absorbed 91% of nitrogen from a lactalbumin, hydrolysate-based diet, compared to only 61% from a similar diet based on intact lactalbumin. What is most remarkable about this study, is that over half the protein was assimilated in the absence of measurable luminal pancreatic enzymes (Steinhardt *et al.*, 1989). Although malabsorbed protein was partly utilised after fermentation in the large bowel, this study does point to the high capacity and versatility of the brush-border peptidases towards oligopeptides liberated during the gastric phase of digestion.

Non-nutritional, non-absorptive aspects of peptides for clinical nutrition

Formulation issues

Industrial processes for manufacture of hydrolysates for food and clinical use have to reconcile a number of conflicting requirements. A final product must be safe to use, of good nutritional value, stable and with reasonable taste properties and cost. There are many possible ways of achieving this as can be seen from the peptide chain-length profile of a number of hydrolysate-based enteral diets which are currently available (Table 6.3).

The use of pancreatic endopeptidases for industrial hydrolysis of food-grade proteins has several disadvantages. Their peptide-bond specificity results in release of large quantities of free tyrosine and phenylalanine whose low solubility may result in processing losses and reduced nutritional value, as shown with some of the earlier casein hydrolysates

Table 6.3. *Peptide chain-length profile of several protein hydrolysates used in enteral diets*

Diet	L-amino acids	Peptide chain-length (%)								
		2	3	4	5	6	7	8	9	10
Survimed[a]	18.0	5.0	5.0	1.0	1.0	24.0	10.0	2.0	17.0	17.0
Travasorb[b]	20.0	15.0	5.0	1.0	1.0	29.0	29.0	–	–	–
Amirige[c]	15.0	5.0	21.0	12.0	12.0	1.0	2.0	2.0	16.5	16.5
Pepti 2000[c]	17.0	11.0	16.0	14.0	14.0	13.0	15.0	–	–	–
Peptisorb[d]	28.0	11.0	17.0	11.0	12.0	1.0	10.0	10.0	–	–
Steraldiet[e]	25.0	1.0	28.0	18.0	17.0	11.0	–	–	–	–
Reabilan[f]	2.0	11.0	21.0	1.0	17.0	17.0	15.0	16.0	–	–
Tipeptid[g]	8.0	34.0	35.0	16.0	7.0	–	–	–	–	–
Tolerex[h]	100.0	–	–	–	–	–	–	–	–	–

Note: Peptide profile measured by Cu(II)-sephadex chromatography. Some of these diets are no longer available or may be marketed under other names in various countries.
[a] Fresenius, Bad Homburg, Germany.
[b] Clintec, Deerfield, Illinois, USA.
[c] Nutricia, Zoetermeer, Holland.
[d] E. Merck Pharmaceuticals, Alton, UK.
[e] Dubenard, Paris, France.
[f] Roussel, Puteaux, France.
[g] Laboratoires Roger Bellon, Neuilly-sur-Seine, France.
[h] Norwich Eaton, New York, USA.

used for parenteral nutrition (Table 6.4). Other plant-derived, fungal or bacterial proteases and peptidases have been used to reduce free amino acid release whilst maintaining a reasonable degree of hydrolysis (Adler-Nissen, 1986a; Andrews, 1987; Neurath, 1989). A second disadvantage of pancreatic enzymes is that hydrolysates with bitter or 'off-flavours' may be produced, which reduce palatability in oral products. This is a function of the presence of short hydrophobic peptides whose bitterness can be predicted by hydrophobicity scales (Ney, 1979; Adler-Nissen, 1986a). The value of theories of taste has been demonstrated for casein hydrolysates, especially in relation to the 'bitter' oligopeptide of casein (residues 53–79) which enclose β-casomorphin, a peptide with opioid-like activity which can stimulate small intestine water and electrolyte absorption (Hautefeuille et al., 1986; Teschemacher & Koch, 1991; Britton & Kastin, 1991). Although resistant to pancreatic proteases, it can be cleaved by plant or renal endopeptidases, thus reducing 'bitterness' markedly (Umetsu, Matsuoka & Ichishima, 1983).

Table 6.4. *Percentage recovery of amino acids in three casein hydrolysates*

Amino acid	Recovery (%) compared to casein		
	Aminosal[a]	Amigen[b]	New preparation[c]
Essential			
Ile	102.7	104.8	111.1
Leu	113.2	101.0	96.5
Lys	102.6	114.0	98.6
Met	99.2	89.2	100.0
Phe	109.4	61.8	95.1
Thr	82.5	102.1	101.8
Trp	133.3	100.0	N/A
Val	107.9	107.5	95.7
Semi-essential			
Arg	94.8	112.3	100.0
His	99.5	100.9	100.0
Non-essential			
Ala	95.0	118.7	105.0
Asp	99.9	104.6	106.1
Cys	213.5	N/A	100 (est)
Glu	111.5	107.9	93.3
Gly	114.6	128.9	96.7
Pro	111.4	121.4	97.6
Ser	63.6	99.4	94.4
Tyr	21.4	14.1	91.9

Adapted from [a](Wretlind, 1952), [b](Patel, Anderson & Jeejeebhoy, 1973), [c](Chataud *et al.*, 1986a, b).

The most difficult technological aspect of hydrolysate production is to allow hydrolysis to proceed to di- and tri-peptides, but at the same time to limit the amount of free L-amino acid released. This has been achieved in one process by use of several peptidases in a carefully controlled time sequence, or 'cascade hydrolysis' (Chataud, Desreumaux & Cartwright 1986a, b). Final ion-exchange purification yielded a desalted, apyrogenic casein hydrolysate comprising 78% di- and tri-peptides, or 95.5% di- to tetra-peptides (Chataud *et al.*, 1986a, b). This composition can doubtless be improved upon by use of other proteases and peptidases with differing bond-specificity. The choice of such enzymes is large (Adler-Nissen, 1986b; Neurath, 1989). In addition to their optimal jejunal absorption (Grimble *et al.*, 1987; Rees *et al.*, 1988a, b), these preparations may have use as a low

Casein hydrolysate (Wretlind, 1952)	**Casein hydrolysate** (Chataud, Desreumaux & Cartwright, 1986*a*, *b*)
Substrate	
Casein acid precipitation from milk washed with boiling ether	Casein
Enzyme source	
Trypsin glycerol fraction of acetone/ether extracted fresh pancreas Enterokinase extracted from fresh animal intestines (same method as for trypsin)	alkaline bacterial protease neutral bacterial protease trysin + chymotrypsin
Conditions	
Single temperature incubation	Sequential addition of enzymes pH control for each enzyme addition
Reaction time	
3–4 days	4.5 hours
Final treatments	
Cellophane membrane dialysis (×3) at 70°C–80°C. Vacuum drying resuspension in distilled water. Precipitation of tyrosine at 0°C. Sterile filtration	Ion-exchange purification, ultrafiltration

Fig. 6.2. Methods of preparation of protein hydrolysates for intravenous use.

osmolality small peptide source for intravenous nutrition (Grimble & Silk, 1989, 1990) (Fig. 6.2).

Carbohydrate absorption

The carbohydrate source of enteral diets usually comprises partially hydrolysed corn starch or 'maltodextrins', which are produced by the action of bacterial and fungal α-amylase, glucoamylase and pullulanase (Pedersen & Norman, 1987).

Digestion and absorption of dietary carbohydrate

Dietary carbohydrate is predominantly absorbed in the proximal small intestine, approximately 75% of absorption occurring in the first 70 cm

(Johansson, 1975). The luminal hydrolysis of starch is catalysed by two α-amylases (salivary and pancreatic) whose pH optimum of 7 corresponds to the luminal pH of the duodenum and upper jejunum (Meldrum *et al.*, 1972). Both α-amylases are endo-glycosidases with an absolute specificity for α-1,4 glucose linkages with two adjacent α-1,4-linkages, and will not hydrolyse lactose or sucrose. Thus, the end products of starch digestion are maltose, maltotriose and the α-limit dextrins, with no free glucose release. The α-limit dextrins are branched structures containing both α-1,4 and α-1,6 linkages; the smallest which can be produced by α-amylase attack is a pentasaccharide comprising maltotriose linked by an α-1,6 bond to maltose at the central glucose moiety (Gray, 1970). Further hydrolysis of this compound can only occur through the action of brush-border glucoamylase. The chain-length of the linear, α-1,4-linked dextrins in the lumen after a starch meal depends on the extent to which α-amylase digestion has gone to completion, but is probably in the range 5–10 glucose units, similar to the chain-length profile of maltodextrins used in enteral diets.

Membrane digestion and the brush-border oligosaccharidases

In man, the most significant mode of transmucosal passage of dietary carbohydrate is as monosaccharides. This is not to say that di- and oligo-saccharides cannot permeate the brush-border membrane (transcellular route) or pass through the tight-junction (paracellular route). Indeed, a small amount is translocated this way and can be exploited as a useful non-invasive marker for increased intestinal permeability to sugar probes, e.g. lactulose, lactitol, in inflammatory illness, such as Crohn's disease (Maxton *et al.*, 1986; Maxton, Catt & Menzies, 1990; Katz *et al.*, 1989). Quantitatively this route is small, less than 2% for lactitol (Grimble, Patil & Silk, 1988). Fragments of dietary starch digestion, the α-limit dextrins can also permeate the mucosal barrier and be excreted in urine. Their excretion rate is sensitive to high carbohydrate meals and episodes of acute pancreatitis, suggesting that part comes from liver glycogen degradation (Kumlien *et al.*, 1988, 1989).

The final stages of the digestion of dietary disaccharides and the products of luminal amylase digestion of starch involve the brush-border hydrolysis (by several saccharidases) to produce monosaccharides (Fig. 6.3). These enzymes are all inserted, as multisubunit structures, into the brush-border membrane via a hydrophobic domain, whilst the

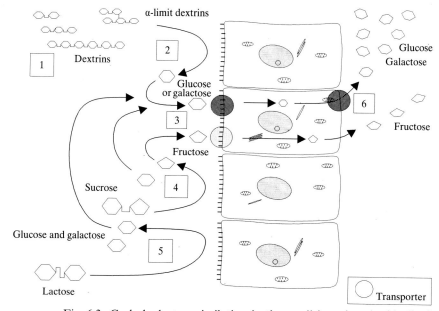

Fig. 6.3. Carbohydrate assimilation in the small intestine. An idealised view of the intestinal wall is shown. The products of luminal digestion by pancreatic α-amylase 1 (maltose, maltotriose, longer dextrins and α-limit dextrins) are hydrolysed by brush-border α-glucosidases to free glucose 2 which is absorbed by the Na^+-dependent glucose/galactose cotransporter 3. Sucrose is hydrolysed by brush-border sucrase 4 and the fructose absorbed by a specific transporter 3. Lactose is hydrolysed by brush-border β-galactosidase 5 to glucose and galactose which can both be absorbed via the Na^+-dependent glucose/galactose cotransporter. At the basolateral membrane, a specific glucose transporter controls efflux into the portal circulation 6.

hydrophilic domains contain the active site of the enzyme (Kenny & Maroux, 1982).

A classification of the maltases and sucrase is shown in Table 6.5. The maltases all hydrolyse external α-1,4-glycosidic linkages at the non-reducing end of maltose, maltotriose, amylose or amylopectin. Maltases Ib, II and perhaps III also have activity towards α-1,6 linkages, that is the branch points of the α-limit dextrins and in amylopectin (Noren *et al.*, 1986). Sucrase-isomaltase is a hybrid enzyme with two activities. The isomaltase moiety has the ability to split α-1,6 linked glucose oligomers, albeit at a slower rate than α-1,4 linkages. In contrast, the sucrase moiety has activity towards α-1,4 linkages, e.g. maltose in addition to that of

Table 6.5. *Membrane digestion of dietary starch*

Enzyme trivial name	Alternative name	Enzyme number	Substrate	Product
Sucrase	Maltase Ia	3.2.1.48	Sucrose	Glucose Fructose
Isomaltase	Maltase Ib	3.2.1.10	Maltose α-1,4/α-1,6-linked oligomers	Glucose
Glucoamylase	Maltase II	3.2.1.20	Starch α-1,4 $\gg$ α-1,6	Glucose
Maltase	Maltase III	3.2.1.20	Maltose α-1,4 linked oligomers	Glucose
Other membrane saccharidases				
Lactase	β-D-galactoside	3.2.1.23 3.2.1.62	Lactose	Glucose Galactose

sucrose (Noren *et al.*, 1986). Lactase/β-galactosidase exists as two forms in a dimeric structure, both of which can cleave lactose to glucose and galactose (Noren *et al.*, 1986).

Thus, hydrolysis of starch to glucose at the brush border utilises all of the 'maltases' of which sucrase-isomaltase is the most important, ca: 80% of total activity. The isomaltase moiety alone accounts for 50% of total activity, and Maltase II (glucoamylase) has considerable activity towards oligosaccharides (Gray, 1975). These considerations help explain why starch assimilation can proceed after total pancreatectomy.

Rate-limiting steps in carbohydrate assimilation

When normal human volunteers consumed 50 grams of glucose, maltose, a maltodextrin or starch, there were no differences in the shape or area under the curve of the plasma glucose response (Wahlqvist *et al.*, 1978). If the α-amylase inhibitor is used to completely inhibit luminal amylase, the degree of starch malabsorption is not total (Layer, Sinmeister & Di Magno, 1986). These data suggest that glucose polymer chain-length has no effect on assimilation, in the presence of normal pancreatic secretions and that brush-border saccharidase activity is high.

We were interested in defining the total assimilatory capacity of the small intestine in a series of studies in which loads of nutrient up to 6000 kcal/d were infused into the duodenum (Raimundo *et al.*, 1988). An alternative approach which did not rely on perfusion techniques of inhibitors of α-glucosidases, was to use a glucose polymer which was resistant to hydrolysis by α-amylase, but not by the brush-border α-glucosidases. Dextrans, which comprise linear polymers of α-1,6 linked glucose are completely resistant to α-amylase hydrolysis and were available in high molecular weight form (40 000 daltons). It has been shown that in rats, this material was malabsorbed (Edwards, Bruce & Ferguson, 1992) and we therefore fed this to healthy volunteers who were consuming an oral enteral diet (Grimble *et al.*, 1992). On the basis of gastrointestinal symptoms, and glycaemia, all of the dextran was assimilated in the small intestine in the presence of large competing amounts of maltodextrins. The brush-border glucosidases of the small intestine therefore have extremely high efficiency and activity and are unlikely to be rate limiting towards soluble maltodextrins, unless the absorptive area is markedly reduced.

Uptake of fructose is by what appear to be multiple carriers, since part can be inhibited by phlorizin, a specific inhibitor of the Na^+-glucose cotransporter (Milla *et al.*, 1977). A second component is by diffusion and is not inhibitable by phlorizin or by metabolic inhibitors (Crouzoulon & Korieh, 1991). The process of glucose uptake by membranes of different tissues has been described in much greater detail and two separate transport proteins identified. Immunochemical studies have confirmed the common identity of the Na^+-glucose cotransporter in brush-border membranes of intestine and renal tubules (Pajor, Hirayama & Wright, 1992). The kinetic and biochemical properties of this tetramer with 73 000 dalton subunits is reviewed elsewhere (Stevens, 1992). A second transporter is responsible for facilitated diffusion exit of glucose from the basolateral membrane of mucosal cells of the intestine and renal tubule, as well as uptake into liver cells (Thorens *et al.*, 1990). In addition, the density of this transporter on the basolateral membrane of intestinal cells is modulated by circulating glucose concentration, being upregulated in diabetes (Cheeseman, 1992). This may be a key control point for intracellular compartmentation of glucose and its uptake by the enterocyte, since only a small fraction of the glucose is metabolised during passage through the absorptive cell (Fernandez Lopez *et al.*, 1992).

Absorption of carbohydrates from enteral diets

We have expended considerable effort in defining the composition of the maltodextrins used in elemental diets, by developing chromatographic

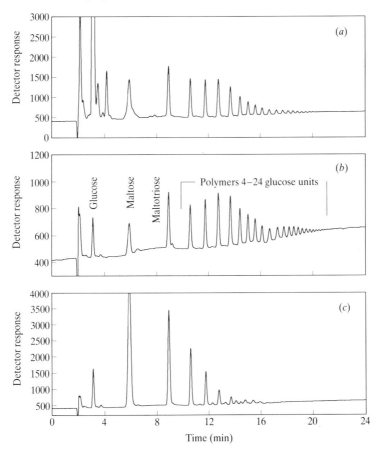

Fig. 6.4. HPLC analysis of maltodextrins commonly used in enteral diets. High-performance liquid chromatography of 'maltodextrins' commonly used in enteral diets. Depending on the enzymes used, and length of digestion, different chain-length material can be produced. (*a*) Caloreen; (*b*) Glucidex 6: short-digestion, long chain-length; (*c*) Glucidex 29: long-digestion, short chain-length.

methods of increasing power (Grimble, 1992). Although it is claimed that the composition is simple, we have found that most consist of a very heterogeneous mixture of glucose polymers as shown in Fig. 6.4. As a result, it is impossible to describe the material simply as 'maltodextrin' without referring to its absorptive characteristics.

In vitro rabbit jejunal preparations in an Using chamber transport less glucose from bathing media containing a short-chain maltodextrin

(4–9 glucose units) than from free glucose solutions (Heitlinger *et al.*, 1992). Although this suggests that brush-border hydrolysis is rate-limiting to uptake, cf. peptide transport above, we have not observed the same in the perfused human jejunum. Maltodextrins were fractionated into different size-ranges and two differed in having an average size-range of < 10 glucose units or > 10 glucose units. In the absence of luminal α-amylase, the lower MWt glucose polymers were assimilated more rapidly than higher MWt glucose polymers and seemed to be conferring a kinetic advantage on glucose uptake. An α-amylase hydrolysate of the low MWt glucose polymer fraction (< 10 glucose molecules) conferred the expected kinetic advantage on glucose transport, the high molecular weight fraction (osmolality $\frac{1}{5}$ of the starting material) was surprisingly well absorbed even in the absence of α-amylase. In addition, the low MWt polymer was as efficiently assimilated as maltose and maltotriose, more so than equivalent concentrations of free glucose (Jones *et al.*, 1981; Jones *et al.*, 1984; Jones, Higgins & Silk, 1987). Thus, the energy content of enteral diets can be *increased* and diet osmolality *reduced*, by substituting the (commonly used) heterogeneous starch hydrolysates with purified high molecular weight fractions. In one diet (Vivonex TEN, Norwich Pharmaceuticals Inc.) this concept has been utilised, with a subsequent lowering of osmolality from 830 to 630 mosmol/kg. Where digestive and absorptive functions are both severely impaired, a low molecular weight maltodextrin could be used.

Sucrose and enteral nutrition

In patients with a very short small intestine, the factors which may limit uptake of glucose from glucose polymer mixtures, would be the remaining capacity of the intraluminal and brush-border saccharidases and in a few instances, when these are not rate limiting, the capacity of the membrane carrier to mediate uptake of the released monosaccharide. Jejunal studies have shown that if glucose transport from glucose polymers is saturated, sugar absorption can be enhanced, if the disaccharide sucrose is added (Spiller, Jones & Silk, 1986). This is so, because although sucrose is hydrolysed by the sucrase moiety of the hybrid brush-border hydrolase, sucrase-isomaltase, absorption of fructose is by a carrier distinct from that of glucose/galactose. The linkage between brush-border hydrolysis of sucrose and absorption of the monosaccharides fructose and glucose absorption appears to confer a kinetic advantage of fructose uptake, since in one study 8/10 subjects malabsorbed 50 g of fructose, whereas none malabsorbed 100 g of sucrose (Rumessen & Gudmand Hoyer, 1986). Thus, the addition of sucrose to enteral diets can further enhance carbohydrate uptake, quite apart from its beneficial taste properties.

Fat absorption

The majority dietary fats are triglycerides, cholesterol and the fat soluble vitamins. Triglycerides (TG) are fatty acid triesters of glycerol, which may contain long chain fatty acids (C16–C18 – long chain triglycerides, LCT) or medium chain fatty acids (C6–C12 – medium chain triglycerides, MCT) and inclusion of either in the fat source of enteral diets is related to the physiology of fat digestion and absorption.

Triglycerides are insoluble in water and if absorption were solely on the basis of direct uptake of TG at the brush-border membrane, it should be severely limited by the droplet-size of the TG emulsion and by the limited permeability of fat droplets across the mucosal barrier and unstirred water layer. The efficiency of lipid assimilation is ensured by exogenous (bile acids) or endogenous (fatty acids, monoglycerides released *in situ*) chemical emulsificants, which produce an emulsion with high surface area/volume for efficient enzyme hydrolysis. The first phase in emulsification occurs in the stomach by mechanical action and lingual lipase partially hydrolyses some TG to free fatty acid and diglyceride (DG) (Hamosh *et al.*, 1975). Transfer of gastric contents, rich in fat, to the duodenum has two consequences:

- H^+ stimulated secretin stimulates pancreatic water and HCO^3- secretion into the duodenum, raising the pH to 6–7.
- Luminal free fatty acids in the duodenum stimulate cholecystokinin-pancreozymin (CCK-PZ) release by duodenal epithelial cells. This signals contraction of the gall bladder and release of bile acids into the intestinal lumen.

The higher pH of the duodenal contents aids in further emulsification and facilitates the action of pancreatic lipase. At pH 6–7, bile salts are soluble in water but above a certain concentration (Critical Micellar Concentration) will form pure bile salt micelles. Fatty acids, mono-glycerides and phospholipids interdigitate with this structure, forming mixed micelles with a hydrophobic core and hydrophilic outer surface. This has been reviewed in detail elsewhere (Gluckman, 1983; Stremmel, 1986; Hauton, 1986). Pancreatic colipase binds tightly to the surface of mixed micelles and acts as an electrostatic anchor for lipase which has considerable specificity for the 1,3 positions of TG.

In addition to lingual and pancreatic lipase, a third and distinct mucosal acid-active intestinal lipase has been partially characterised and found in the villus tips in the proximal intestine (Rao & Mansbach, 1990): that is the most mature population of enterocytes engaged in the absorption and transport of dietary lipid. Its binding to the brush border involves heparin (Bonner *et al.*, 1989), which allows fatty acids and monoglycerides (MG) to be generated in close proximity to the intestinal membrane prior to absorption.

Osmotic and other pressures generated within the micelle by extensive TG hydrolysis cause budding of smaller micelles from the surface of these structures. The resulting smaller micelles are then available for uptake of MG and fatty acids at the microvilli surface. Lipolysis products are absorbed in the proximal intestine, whereas bile salts are absorbed at the distal ileum, so mixed micelles must dissociate.

The acidic microenvironment adjacent to the brush-border membrane is important in promoting lipid absorption since protonation of fatty acids allows their diffusion through the membrane (Shiau, 1990). Within the enterocyte, the higher intracellular pH results in their ionisation, thus reducing the likelihood of back-diffusion. Notwithstanding this, mucosal uptake of long chain fatty acids is now known to occur as a result of binding to a specific intestinal membrane binding protein that is a member of a family of cytoplasmic hydrophobic ligand-binding proteins (Sacchettini, Gordon & Banaszak, 1989). This intestinal fatty acid binding protein is thought to participate in the uptake, intracellular targeting and metabolic processing of fatty acids within the intestinal epithelial cell.

Within the enterocyte, fatty acids are transferred by their specific cytoplasmic carrier proteins to the smooth endoplasmic reticulum for re-esterification to TG (Stremmel, 1986). These TG are transferred, along with cholesterol, phospholipids and fat soluble vitamins, to the Golgi apparatus where they combine with apolipoproteins to form chylomicrons and very low density lipoproteins. The Golgi apparatus is transferred to the enterocyte lateral membrane and fuses with it. Subsequent rupture of the fused vesicle by exocytosis results in the release of lipid into the lymphatic system.

Although probably not of any clinical significance, not all the neutral lipid absorbed from the lumen of the intestine is destined for packaging and transport via the lymphatics in chylomicrons (Mansbach, Arnold & Cox, 1985; Tipton, Frase & Mansbach, 1989). Experimental animal studies indicate that nearly half of neutral lipids may be transported out of the enterocytes via non-lymphatic pathways (presumably via the portal vein). These are postulated to require prior hydrolysis by a specific, non-pancreatic, alkaline-active lipase.

Medium chain triglycerides appear to 'short-circuit' some of these processes because they are more water soluble than LCT and may either be absorbed intact or undergo considerably more rapid lipase hydrolysis than LCT, with subsequent direct uptake of MG and fatty acid. There is no absolute requirement for mixed micelle formation with bile acids and, within the enterocyte, short and medium chain fatty acids are generally not re-esterified to TG and incorporated into chylomicrons but may be released directly into the portal circulation where they bind to albumin (Stremmel, 1986).

Perspectives

Protein assimilation

The past 20 years of research into nitrogen assimilation suggest that a significant proportion of dietary N is absorbed in the form of di- and tri-peptides. The most recent studies have identified the major component of the transport protein, and more importantly, its tissue distribution. Thus, assimilation of peptides in the small intestine mirrors the process by which filtered peptides are salvaged by the renal tubular brush-border membrane. The reason why there is apparent duplication of amino acid and peptide uptake is not entirely clear. For the kidney, it is not of primary nutritional importance because the filtered peptide load is never large, but may relate to the need to hydrolyse peptide fragments which would exert adverse physiological effects at high concentrations, when water is reabsorbed from the tubule. In the intestine, there may be several good reasons why peptide transport occurs. The first is that luminal protein digestion never proceeds to completion, i.e. free amino acids within the timescale of orocaecal transit time. In addition, pancreatic and other secretions produce luminal protein away from the major site of luminal hydrolysis, the duodenum and jejunum. These secretions are, by their nature, resistant to pancreatic proteolytic attack, and the coupling of peptide uptake to brush-border peptidases with different specificity may provide an efficient means for their salvage. A second reason for duplication is that peptide transport serves to relieve competition for transport between free amino acids, which share the same carrier. This may be especially true in cases where poor protein quality and malabsorption coexist with a high requirement for essential amino acid residues, e.g. rapid growth in infants.

Although dietary protein assimilation is a remarkably efficient process, there may be a need for highly purified protein hydrolysates containing a blend of free L-amino acids and di- and tri-peptides only, for use in patients with severely reduced absorptive area *and* pancreatic function. In this way, both nitrogen transport systems will be utilised. This is especially true if one considers that dietary protein assimilation is a jejunal event, whereas endogenous protein secretions are assimilated more distally. This is reflected in the increasing gradient of brush-border endo- and exo-peptidases towards the ileocaecal valve (Skovbjerg, 1981). Thus, adaptation which will occur in the remaining intestine after resection, has more limited scope for maintenance of protein assimilation (Curtis, Sleisenger & Kim, 1984; Bristol & Williamson, 1988).

Carbohydrate assimilation

As for the process of protein digestion, this has been helped by description of inborn errors of metabolism in which one or more of the brush-border disaccharidases is absent (Maxton, Catt & Menzies, 1990). There is now a clearer understanding of the molecular biology of the transport proteins responsible for monosaccharide translocation from apical to basolateral membranes of the enterocyte. In addition, the reserve capacity of the small intestine for carbohydrate assimilation has been defined by different experimental strategies. Current knowledge suggests that it is two to three times the maximum nutrient intake which is likely to be used in enteral feeding, and would comfortably exceed the necessary intake of a hyper-metabolic, severely burned patient.

Where absorptive function has been severely reduced by distal small bowel resection, remaining reserve capacity is often sufficient to allow complete assimilation of carbohydrate (Althausen, Uyeyama & Simpson, 1949; McIntyre, Fitchen & Lennard-Jones, 1986) as opposed to protein (Chacko & Cummings, 1988). The reason for this difference is that carbohydrate assimilation is primarily duodenal and jejunal, as shown by the longitudinal distribution gradient for the brush-border dissac-charidases and the Na^+-glucose cotransporter (Haase *et al.*, 1990; Skovbjerg, 1981).

Fat assimilation

Normal lipid digestion and absorption is dependent on a host of mechanisms, the most important of which appear to be adequate luminal levels of pancreatic lipase and bile salts, as well as sufficient absorptive area. In some patients, some or all of these factors may be limiting and diets containing excessive amounts of LCT should be avoided to prevent essential fatty acid and vitamin deficiency caused by competition for uptake by other long chain fatty acids (Dodge & Yarson, 1980). Such patients include those with severe exocrine pancreatic insufficiency (chronic pancreatitis and cystic fibrosis), severe abnormalities of intestinal mucosa (untreated coeliac disease), or extensive small bowel resection (Stremmel, 1986). Although MCT has been proposed as an efficiently absorbed fat source in these cases (Dodge, 1992; Durie & Pencharz, 1992) it does not contain linoleic acid and exclusive use of MCT may provoke essential fatty acid deficiency (Pettei, Daftary & Levine, 1991). Thus, for this group, (and especially in infants), it is preferable to use combination therapy of diets containing mixtures of MCT and LCT, as well as oral, enteric-coated pancreatic enzyme supplements which enhance utilisation of LCT and MCT and reduce steatorrhoea (Hamosh *et al.*, 1991; Bronstein *et al.*, 1992).

References

Adibi, S. A. & Morse, E. L. (1977). The number of glycine residues which limits intact absorption of glycine oligopeptides in human jejunum. *Journal of Clinical Investigation*, **60**, 1008–16.

Adler-Nissen, J. (1986*a*). Relationship of structure to taste of peptides and peptide mixtures. In *Protein Tailoring and Reagents for Food and Medical Uses*, pp. 97–122, ed. R. E. Feeney and J. R. Whitaker. Marcel Dekker Inc., New York.

Adler-Nissen, J. (1986*b*). *Enzymatic Hydrolysis of Food Proteins*. Elsevier Applied Science Publishers, London.

Althausen, T. L., Uyeyama, K. & Simpson, R. G. (1949). Digestion and absorption after massive resection of the small intestine. I. Utilisation of food from a 'natural' versus a 'synthetic' diet and a comparison of intestinal absorption tests with nutritional balance studies in a patient with only 45 cm of small intestine. *Gastroenterology*, **12**, 795–807.

Andrews, A. T. (1987). Enzymatic modification of dairy and other food proteins. In *Chemical Aspects of Food Enzymes*, pp. 230–58, ed. A. T. Andrews. Royal Society of Chemistry, London.

Bonner, M. S., Gulick, T., Riley, D. J. S., Spilburg, C. A. & Lange, L. G. (1989). Heparin-modulated binding and pancreatic lipase and uptake of hydrolysed triglycerides in the intestine. *Journal of Biological Chemistry*, **264**, 20261–4.

Bowling, T. E., Jameson, J. J., Grimble, G. K. & Silk, D. B. A. (1993). Enteral nutrition as a primary therapy in active Crohn's disease. *European Journal of Gastroenterology & Hepatology*, **5**, 1–7.

Bristol, J. B. & Williamson, R. C. N. (1988). Nutrition, operations, and intestinal adaptation. *Journal of Parenteral and Enteral Nutrition*, **12**, 299–309.

Britton, J. R. & Kastin, A. J. (1991). Biologically active polypeptides in milk. *American Journal of Medical Science*, **301**, 124–32.

Bronstein, M. N., Sokol, R. J., Abman, S. H., Chatfield, B. A., Hammond, K. B., Hambidge, K. M., Stall, C. D. & Accurso, F. J. (1992). Pancreatic insufficiency, growth, and nutrition in infants identified by newborn screening as having cystic fibrosis. *Journal of Pediatrics*, **120**, 533–40.

Calignano, A., Whittle, B. J. R., Di Rosa, M. & Moncada, S. (1992). Involvement of endogenous nitric oxide in the regulation of rat intestinal motility *in vivo*. *European Journal of Pharmacology*, **229**, 273–6.

Chacko, A. & Cummings, J. H. (1988). Nitrogen losses from the human small bowel: obligatory losses and the effect of physical form of food. *Gut*, **29**, 809–15.

Chataud, J., Desreumaux, S. & Cartwright, T. (1986*a*). Procéde de fabrication d'un hydrolysat enzymatique de proteines riche en di- et tri-peptides, utilisable notament en nutrition artificielle et en diètétique. French Patent 86 17516, 15th December.

Chataud, J., Desreumaux, S. & Cartwright, T. (1986*b*). Procède de preparation d'un melange peptidique, riche en di- et tri-peptides, utilisable notament en nutrition artificielle et en dietetique, melange ainsi obtenu, et utilisation de ce melange en nutrition artificielle et en diététique. French Patent 86 17515, 15th December.

Cheeseman, C. (1992). Role of intestinal basolateral membrane in absorption of nutrients. *American Journal of Physiology*, **263**, R482–8.

Chung, Y. C., Kim, Y. S., Shadchehr, A., Garrido, A., MacGregor, I. L. & Sleisenger, M. H. (1979). Protein digestion and absorption in human small intestine. *Gastroenterology*, **76**, 1415–21.

Cook, G. C. (1972). Comparison of intestinal absorption rates of glycine and glycylglycine in man and the effect of glucose in the perfusing fluid. *Clinical Science*, **43**, 443–53.

Craft, I. L., Geddes, D., Hyde, C. W., Wise, I. J. & Matthews, D. M. (1968). Absorption and malabsorption of glycine and glycine peptides in man. *Gut*, **9**, 425–37.

Crane, C. W. (1964). Studies on the absorption of ^{15}N labelled yeast in normal subjects and patients with malabsorption. In *The Role of the Gastrointestinal Tract in Protein Metabolism*, pp. 33–47, ed. H. N. Munro. F. A. Davis, Philadelphia.

Crouzoulon, G. & Korieh, A. (1991). Fructose transport by rat intestinal brush border membrane vesicles. Effect of high fructose diet followed by return to standard diet. *Comparative Biochemistry & Physiology A*, **100**, 175–82.

Curtis, JK. J., Sleisenger, M. H. & Kim, Y. S. (1984). Protein digestion and absorption after massive small bowel reaction. *Digestive Diseases & Science*, **29**, 834–40.

Daniel, H., Morse, E. L. & Adibi, S. A. (1992). Determinants of substrate affinity for the oligopeptide/H^+ symporter in the renal brush border membrane. *Journal of Biological Chemistry*, **267**, 9565–9573.

Desnuelle, P. (1986) Chemistry and enzymology of pancreatic endopeptidases. In *In Molecular and Cellular Basis of Digestion*, pp. 195–211 (ed. P. Desnuelle, H. Sjostrom and O. Noren. Elsevier, Amsterdam.

Dodge, J. A. (1992). Nutrition in cystic fibrosis: a historical overview. *Proceedings of the Nutrition Society*, **51**, 225–35.

Dodge, J. A. & Yarson, J. G. (1980). Essential fatty acid deficiency after prolonged treatment with elemental diet. *Lancet*, **ii**, 1256–7.

Durie, P. R. & Pencharz, P. B. (1992). Cystic fibrosis: nutrition. *British Medical Bulletin*, **48**, 823–46.

Edwards, C. A., Bruce, M. & Ferguson, A. (1992). The effect of supplementing elemental diet with dextran on colonic short-chain fatty acids and cellular proliferation. *Proceedings of the Nutrition Society*, **51**, 5A.

Fernandez Lopez, J. A., Casado, J., Argiles, J. M. & Alemany, M. (1992). Intestinal handling of a glucose gavage by the rat. *Molecular Cell Biochemistry*, **113**, 43–53.

Ferraris, R. P., Lee, P. P. & Diamond, J. M. (1989). Origin of regional and species differences in intestinal glucose uptake. *American Journal of Physiology*, **257**, G689–97.

Foltmann, B. (1986). Pepsin, chymosin and their zymogens. In *Molecular and Cellular Basis of Digestion*, pp. 491–505, ed. P. Desnuelle, H. Sjostrom and O. Noren. Elsevier Science Publishers B.V. (Biomedical Division), Amsterdam.

Friedrich, M., Noack, J., Proll, J. & Noack, R. (1984). Untersuchungen zur Absorption enzymatischer Proteinhydrolysate sowie aquimolarer Aminosauremischungen am perfundierten Dunndarm der Ratte. *Biomedica et Biochemica Acta*, **43**, 117–30.

Ganapathy, V., Mendicino, J. F. & Leibach, F. H. (1981). Transport of glycyl-L-proline into intestinal and renal brush border vesicles from rabbit. *Journal of Biological Chemistry*, **256**, 118–124.

Ganapathy, M. E., Mahesh, V. B., Devoe, L. D., Leibach, F. H. & Ganapathy, V. (1985). Dipeptide transport in brush-border membrane vesicles isolated from normal term human placenta. *American Journal of Obstetrics and Gynecology*, **153**, 83–6.

Ganapathy, V. & Leibach, F. K. (1985). Is intestinal transport energized by a proton gradient? *American Journal of Physiology*, **249**, G153–60.

Gill, M., Sanyal, S. & Sareen, M. L. (1990). Effect of cimetidine on intestinal absorption & digestive functions in mice. *Indian Journal of Medical Research*, **92**, 109–14.

Gluckman, R. M. (1983). Fat absorption and malabsorption. In *Clinics in Gastroenterology*, pp. 323–334, ed. M. H. Sleisenger. W. B. Saunders Co., London, Philadelphia, Toronto.

Gray, G. M. (1970). Carbohydrate digestion and absorption. *Gastroenterology*, **58**, 96–107.

Gray, G. M. (1975). Carbohydrate digestion and absorption. Role of the small intestine. *New England Journal of Medicine*, **292**, 1225–30.

Grimble, G. K. (1992). Ion chromatography in clinical research: a neglected technique? *Analytical Proceedings*, **29**, 468–70.

Grimble, G. K. & Silk, D. B. A. (1989). Peptides in human nutrition. *Nutrition Research Reviews*, **2**, 87–108.

Grimble, G. K. & Silk, D. B. A. (1990). Intravenous protein hydrolysates – time to turn the clock back? *Clinical Nutrition*, **9**, 39–41.

Grimble, G. K., Keohane, P., Higgins, B. E., Kaminski, M. V. & Silk, D. B. A. (1986). Effect of peptide chain-length on amino acid and nitrogen absorption from two lactalbumin hydrolysates in the normal human jejunum. *Clinical Science*, **71**, 65–9.

Grimble, G. K., Rees, R. G., Keohane, P. P., Cartwright, T., Desreumaux, M. & Silk, D. B. A. (1987). The effect of peptide chain-length on absorption of egg-protein hydrolysates in the normal human jejunum. *Gastroenterology*, **92**, 136–42.

Grimble, G. K., Patil, D. H. & Silk, D. B. (1988). Assimilation of lactitol, an 'unabsorbed' disaccharide in the normal human colon. *Gut*, **29**, 1666–71.

Grimble, G. K., Preedy, V., Garlick, P. & Silk, D. B. A. (1989). Trophic effects of dietary peptides on the rat intestinal tract. *Journal of Parenteral and Enteral Nutrition*, **13** (Supplement), 6S.

Grimble, G. K., Hunjan, M. K., Payne-James, J. J. & Silk, D. B. A. (1991). Long-term stability of ranitidine in total parenteral nutrition solutions: effects on lipid emulsion stability. *British Journal of Intensive Care*, **1**, 32–7.

Grimble, G. K., Mofokeng, E., Collins, S. & Silk, D. (1992). Is dextran 40KDa a soluble, low viscosity fibre suitable for use in enteral diets? *Journal of Parenteral and Enteral Nutrition*, **11** (Supplement), 107

Guandalini, S. & Rubino, A. (1982). Development of dipeptide transport in the intestinal mucosa of rabbits. *Pediatric Research*, **16**, 99–103.

Haase, W., Heitmann, K., Friese, W., Ollig, D. & Keopsell, H. (1990). Characterization and histochemical localization of the rat intestinal Na(+)-D-glucose cotransporter by monoclonal antibodies. *European Journal of Cell Biology*, **52**, 297–309.

Hammer, H. F., Fine, K. D., Santa Ana, C. A., Porter, J. L., Schiller, L. R. & Fordtran, J. S. (1990). Carbohydrate malabsorption. Its measurement and its contribution to diarrhea. *Journal of Clinical Investigation*, **86**, 1936–44.

Hamosh, M., Klaeveman, H. L., Wolf, R. D. & Scow, R. D. (1975). Pharyngeal lipase and digestion of dietary triglyceride in man. *Journal of Clinical Investigation*, **55**, 908–13.

Hamosh, M., Mehta, N. R., Fink, C. S., Coleman, J. & Hamosh, P. (1991). Fat absorption in premature infants: medium-chain triglycerides and long-chain triglycerides are absorbed from formula at similar rates. *Journal of Pediatric Gastroenterology & Nutrition*, **13**, 143–9.

Hautefeuille, M., Brantl, V., Dumontier, A. M. & Desjeux, J. F. (1986). In vitro effects of beta-casomorphins on ion transport in rabbit ileum. *American Journal of Physiology*, **250**, G92–7.

Hauton, J. C. (1986). A quantitative dynamic concept of the role of bile in fat digestion. In *Molecular and Cellular Basis of Digestion*, ed. P. Desnuelle, H. Sjostrom and O. Noren. Elsevier, Amsterdam.

Hegarty, J. E., Fairclough, P. D., Clark, M. L. & Dawson, A. M. (1981). Jejunal water and electrolyte secretion induced by L-arginine in man. *Gut*, **22**, 108–13.

Heitlinger, L. A., Sloan, H. R., DeVore, D. R., Lee, P-C., Lebenthal, E. & Duffry, M. E. (1992). Transport of glucose polymer–derived glucose by rabbit jejunum. *Gastroenterology*, **102**, 443–7.

Hibbert, J. M., Forrester, T. & Jackson, A. A. (1992). Urea kinetics: comparison of oral and intravenous dose regimens. *European Journal of Clinical Nutrition*, **46**, 405–9.

Itoh, H., Kishi, T. & Chibata, I. (1973). Comparative effects of casein and amino acid mixture simulating casein on growth and food intake in rats. *Journal of Nutrition*, **103**, 1709–15.

Johansson, C. (1975). Studies of gastrointestinal interactions: VII. Characteristics of the absorption pattern of sugar, fat and protein from composite meals in man: a quantitative study. *Scandinavian Journal of Gastroenterology*, **10**, 33–42.

Jones, B. J. M., Brown, B. E., Spiller, R. C. & Silk, D. B. A. (1981). Energy dense enteral feeds – the use of high molecular weight glucose polymers. *Journal of Parenteral and Enteral Nutrition*, **5**, 567.

Jones, B. J. M., Brown, B. E., Loran, J. S., Kennedy, J. F., Stead, J. A. & Silk,

D. B. A. (1984). Glucose absorption from starch hydrolysates in the human jejunum. *Gut*, **24**, 1152–60.

Jones, B. J. M., Higgins, B. E. & Silk, D. B. A. (1987). Glucose absorption from maltotriose and glucose oligomers in the human jejunum. *Clinical Science*, **72**, 409–14.

Katz, K. D., Hollander, D., Vadheim, C. M. *et al.* (1989). Intestinal permeability in patients with Crohn's disease and their healthy relatives. *Gastroenterology*, **97**, 927–31.

Kenny, A. J. & Maroux, S. (1982). Topology of microvillar membrane hydrolases of kidney and intestine. *Physiological Reviews*, **62**, 91–128.

Keohane, P. P., Attrill, H., Jones, B. J. M., Brown, B., Frost, P. & Silk, D. B. A. (1983). The roles of lactose and *Clostridium difficile* in the pathogenesis of enteral feeding associated diarrhoea. *Clinical Nutrition*, **1**, 259–64.

Keohane, P. P., Grimble, G. K., Brown, B., Spiller, R. C. & Silk, D. B. A. (1985). Influence of protein composition and hydrolysis method on intestinal absorption of protein in man. *Gut*, **26**, 907–13.

Kirk, S. J. & Barbul, A. (1990). Role of arginine in trauma, sepsis and immunity. *Journal of Parenteral and Enteral Nutrition*, **116**, 36–44.

Konno, R., Niwa, A. & Yasumura, Y. (1990). Intestinal bacterial origin of D-alanine in urine of mutant mice lacking D-amino-acid oxidase. *Biochemical Journal*, **268**, 263–5.

Koruda, M. J., Rolandelli, R. H., Settle, R. G., Saul, S. H. & Rombeau, J. L. (1986). The effect of a pectin-supplemented elemental diet on intestinal adaptation to massive small bowel resection. *Journal of Parenteral and Enteral Nutrition*, **10**, 343–50.

Kramer, W. (1987). Identification of identical binding polypeptides for cephalosporins and dipeptides in intestinal brush-border membrane vesicles by photoaffinity labeling. *Biochemica et Biophysica Acta*, **905**, 65–74.

Kramer, W., Girbig, F., Leipe, I. & Petzoldt, E. (1988). Direct photoaffinity labelling of binding proteins for beta-lactam antibiotics in rabbit intestinal brush border membranes with [^{3}H]benzylpenicillin. *Biochemical Pharmacology*, **37**, 2427–35.

Kumlien, J., Chester, M. A., Lindberg, B. S., Pizzo, P., Zopf, D. & Lundblad, A. (1988). Urinary excretion of a glucose-containing tetrasaccharide. A parameter for increased degradation of glycogen. *Clinica Chemica Acta*, **176**, 39–48.

Kumlien, J., Andren Sandberg, A., Zopf, D. & Lundblad, A. (1989). Determination of a glucose-containing tetrasaccharide in urine of patients with acute pancreatitis. *International Journal of Pancreatology*, **4**, 139–47.

Layer, P., Sinmeister, A. R. & DiMagno, E. P. (1986). Effect of decreasing intraluminal amylase activity on starch digestion and post-prandial gastrointestinal functions in humans. *Gastroenterology*, **91**, 41–8.

MacFarlane, G. T., Cummings, J. H. & Allison, C. (1986). Protein degradation by human intestinal bacteria. *Jourrnal of General Microbiology*, **132**, 1647–56.

Mansbach, C. M., II, Arnold, A. & Cox, M. A. (1985). Factors influencing triacylglycerol delivery into mesenteric lymph. *American Journal of Physiology*, **249**, G642–8.

Marcuard, S. P. & Perkins, A. M. (1988). Clogging of feeding tubes. *Journal of Parenteral and Enteral Nutrition*, **12**, 403–5.

Matthews, D. M. (1991). *Protein Absorption: Development and Present State of the Subject*. Wiley–Liss, New York.

Maxton, D. G., Bjarnason, I., Reynolds, A. P., Catt, S. D., Peters, T. J. &

Menzies, I. S. (1986). Lactulose, ^{51}Cr-labelled ethylenediaminetetra-acetate, L-rhamnose and polyethyleneglycol 400 [corrected] as probe markers for assessment *in vivo* of human intestinal permeability. *Clinical Science*, **71**, 71–80.

Maxton, D. G., Catt, S. D. & Menzies, I. S. (1990). Combined assessment of intestinal disaccharidases in congenital asucrasia by differential urinary disaccharide excretion. *Journal of Clinical Pathology*, **43**, 406–9.

McIntyre, P. B., Fitchen, M. & Lennard-Jones, J. E. (1986). Patients with a high ileostomy do not need a special diet. *Gastroenterology*, **91**, 25–33.

Medina, M. A., Urdiales, J. L., Nunez de Castro, I. & Sanchez Jimenez, F. (1991). Diamines interfere with the transport of L-ornithine in Ehrlich-cell plasma-membrane vesicles. *Biochemical Journal*, **280**, 825–7.

Meldrum, S. J., Watson, B. W., Riddle, H. C., Bown, R. L. & Sladen, G. E. (1972). pH profile of gut as measured by a radiotelemetry capsule. *British Medical Journal*, **2**, 104.

Milla, P. J., Oyesiku, J. E. J., Mullet, D. P. R. & Harries, J. T. (1977). Fructose absorption and the effects of other monosaccharides on its absorption in the rat jejunum *in vivo*. *Gut*, **18**, 425.

Miller, P. M., Burston, D., Brueton, M. J. & Matthews, D. M. (1984). Kinetics of uptake of L-leucine and glycylsarcosine into normal and protein malnourished young rat jejunum. *Pediatric Research*, **18**, 504–8.

Milliner, D. S. (1990). Cystinuria. *Endocrinology & Metabolism Clinics of North America*, **19**, 889–907.

Monchi, M., Vaugelade, P., Vaissade, P. & Rérat, A. (1991). Net protein utilisation after duodenal infusion of small peptides of free amino acids in growing rats. *Clinical Nutrition*, **10** (Supplement 2), 31. (Abstract)

Moran, B. J. & Jackson, A. A. (1990a). ^{15}N-urea metabolism in the functioning human colon: luminal hydrolysis and mucosal permeability. *Gut*, **31**, 454–7.

Moran, B. J. & Jackson, A. A. (1990b). Metabolism of ^{15}N-labelled urea in the functioning and defunctional human colon. *Clinical Science*, **79**, 253–8.

Morgan, M. Y. (1991). The treatment of chronic hepatic encephalopathy. *Hepatogastroenterology*, **38**, 377–387.

Moriarty, K. J., Hegarty, J. E., Fairclough, P. D., Kelly, M. J., Clark, M. L. & Dawson, A. M. (1985). Relative nutritional value of whole protein, hydrolysed protein and free amino acids in man. *Gut*, **26**, 694–9.

Mortensen, P. B., Rasmussen, H. S. & Holtug, K. (1988). Lactulose detoxifies *in vitro* short-chain fatty acid production in colonic contents induced by blood: implications for hepatic coma. *Gastroenterology*, **94**, 750–4.

Mortensen, P. B., Holtug, K., Bonnen, H. & Clausen, M. R. (1990). The degradation of amino acids, proteins, and blood to short-chain fatty acids in colon is prevented by lactulose. *Gastroenterology*, **98**, 353–60.

Mowatt-Larssen, C. A., Brown, R. O., Wojtysiak, S. L. & Kudsk, K. A. (1992). Comparison of tolerance and nutritional outcome between a peptide and a standard enteral formula in critically ill, hypoalbuminemic patients. *Journal of Parenteral and Enteral Nutrition*, **16**, 20–4.

Neurath, H. (1989). The diversity of proteolytic enzymes. In *Proteolytic Enzymes: A Practical Approach*, pp. 1–13, ed. R. J. Beynon and J. S. Bond. IRL Press, Oxford.

Ney, K. H. (1979). Bitterness of peptides: amino acid composition and chain length. In *In Food Taste Chemistry*, pp. 149–173, ed. J. C. Boudreau. American Chemical Society Symposium Series 115.

Noren, O., Sjostrom, H., Danielson, E. M., Cowell, G. M. & Skovbjerg, H.

(1986). The enzymes of the enterocyte plasma membrane. In *Molecular and Cellular Basis of Digestion*, pp. 335–65, ed. P. Desnuelle, H. Sjostrom and O. Noren. Elsevier Science Publishers BV, Amsterdam.

O'Keefe, S. J. D., Adam, J. K., Cakata, E. & Epstein, S. (1984). Nutritional support of malnourished lactose intolerant African patients. *Gut*, **25**, 942–7.

Okano, T., Inui, K. I., Takano, M. & Hori, R. (1986). H + gradient-dependent transport of aminocephalosporins in rat intestinal brush-border membrane vesicles. *Biochemical Pharmacology*, **35**, 1781–6.

Pajor, A. M., Hirayama, B. A. & Wright, E. M. (1992). Molecular biology approaches to comparative study of Na(+)-glucose cotransport. *American Journal of Physiology*, **263**, R489–95.

Palmer, R. M. J., Ferrige, A. G. & Moncada, S. (1987). Nitric oxide release accounts for the biological activity of endothelium-derived relaxing factor. *Nature*, **327**, 524–6.

Patel, D., Anderson, G. H. & Jeejeebhoy, K. N. (1973). Amino acid adequacy of parenteral casein hydrolysate and oral cottage cheese in patients with gastrointestinal disease as measured by nitrogen balance and blood aminogram. *Gastroenterology*, **65**, 427–37.

Patil, D. H., Grimble, G. K. & Silk, D. B. (1987). Lactitol, a new hydrogenated lactose derivative: intestinal absorption and laxative threshold in normal human subjects. *British Journal of Nutrition*, **57**, 195–9.

Payne-James, J., Grimble, G., Cahill, E. & Silk, D. B. A. (1989). Jejunal absorption of ornithine-oxoglutarate (OKGA) in man. *Journal of Parenteral and Enteral Nutrition*, **13** (Supplement), 22S.

Pedersen, S. & Norman, B. E. (1987). Enzymatic modification of food carbohydrates. In *Chemical Aspects of Food Enzymes*, pp. 156–87, ed. A. T. Andrews. Royal Society of Chemistry, London.

Pettei, M. J., Daftary, S. & Levine, J. J. (1991). Essential fatty acid deficiency associated with the use of a medium-chain triglyceride infant formula in pediatric hepatobiliary disease. *American Journal of Clinical Nutrition*, **53**, 1217–21.

Puigserver, A., Chapus, C. & Kerfelec, B. (1986). Pancreatic exopeptidases. In *Molecular and Cellular Basis of Digestion*, pp. 235–47, ed. P. Desnuelle, H. Sjostrom and O. Noren. Elsevier, Amsterdam.

Raimundo, A. H., Rogers, J., Grimble, G., Cahill, E. & Silk, D. B. A. (1988). Colonic in-flow and small bowel motility during intraduodenal enteral nutrition. *Gastroenterology*, **29**, A1469–70.

Randall, H. T. (1984). Enteral Nutrition: Tube feeding in acute and chronic illness. *Journal of Parenteral and Enteral Nutrition*, **8**, 113–36.

Rao, R. H. & Mansbach, C. M., II (1990). Acid lipase in rat intestinal mucosa: physiological parameters. *Biochimica et Biophysica Acta*, **1043**, 273–80.

Rees, R. G., Grimble, G. K., Halliday, D., Ford, C. & Silk, D. B. A. (1988a). Influence of orally administered amino acids and peptides on protein turnover kinetics in the short bowel syndrome. *Gut*, **28**, A1397.

Rees, R. G., Raimundo, A. H., Grimble, G. K., Hunjan, M. K. & Silk, D. B. A. (1988b). Peptide based nitrogen source of enteral diets: Studies with casein hydrolysates in man. *Journal of Parenteral and Enteral Nutrition*, **12**, 21S.

Rees, R. G. P., Hare, W. R., Grimble, G. K., Frost, P. G. & Silk, D. B. A. (1992). Do patients with moderately impaired gastrointestinal function requiring enteral nutrition need a predigested nitrogen source? A prospective crossover controlled clinical trial. *Gut*, **33**, 877–81.

Rerat, A., Simoes-Nunes, C., Mendy, F. & Roger, L. (1988). Amino acid absorption and production of pancreatic hormones in non-anaesthetised pigs after duodenal infusions of a milk enzymic hydrolysate or of free amino acids. *British Journal of Nutrition*, **60**, 121–36.

Rothenbuhler, E., Waibel, R. & Solms, J. (1979). An improved method for the separation of peptides and alpha-amino acids on copper sephadex. *Analytical Biochemistry*, **97**, 367–75.

Rumessen, J. J. & Gudmand Hoyer, E. (1986). Absorption capacity of fructose in healthy adults. Comparison with sucrose and its constituent monosaccharides. *Gut*, **27**, 1161–8.

Sacchettini, J. C., Gordon, J. I. & Banaszak, L. J. (1989). Refined apoprotein of rat intestinal fatty acid binding protein produced in *Escherichia coli*. *Proceedings of the National Academy of Science (USA)*, **86**, 7736–40.

Semenza, G. & Cortelli, A. (1986). The absorption of sugars and amino acids across the small intestine. In *Molecular and Cellular Basis of Digestion*, pp. 318–412, ed. P. Desnuelle, H. Sjostrom and O. Noren, Elsevier, Amsterdam.

Shapira, R. & Chou, C. H. (1987). Differential racemization of aspartate and serine in human myelin basic protein. *Biochemical & Biophysical Research Communications*, **146**, 1342–9.

Shiau, Y. (1990). Mechanism of intestinal fatty acid uptake in the rat: the role of an acidic environment. *Journal of Physiology*, **421**, 463–74.

Silk, D. B. A., Chung, Y. C., Berger, K. L. et al. (1979). Comparison of oral feeding of peptide and amino acid meals to normal human subjects. *Gut*, **20**, 291–9.

Silk, D. B. A., Fairclough, P. D., Clark, M. L. et al. (1980). Uses of a peptide rather than a free amino acid nitrogen source in chemically defined elemental diets. *Journal of Parenteral and Enteral Nutrition*, **4**, 548–53.

Skovbjerg, H. (1981). Immunoelectrophoretic studies on human small intestinal brush border proteins – the longitudinal distribution of peptidases and disaccharidases. *Clinica Chimica Acta*, **112**, 205–12.

Souba, W. W. (1993). Intestinal glutamine metabolism and nutrition. *Journal of Nutritional Biochemistry*, **4**, 2–9.

Spiller, R. C., Jones, B. J. M. & Silk, D. B. A. (1986). Jejunal water and electrolyte absorption from two proprietary enteral feeds in man: importance of sodium content. *Gut*, **28**, 681–7.

Steinhardt, H. J., Wolf, A., Jakober, B. et al. (1989). Nitrogen absorption in pancreatectomised patients: protein versus protein hydrolysate as substrate. *Journal of Laboratory Clinical Medicine*, **113**, 162–7.

Stevens, B. R. (1992). Vetebrate intestine apical membrane mechanisms of organic nutrient transport. *American Journal of Physiology*, **263**, R458–63.

Stremmel, W. (1986). Intestinal absorption of fat and fat-soluble vitamins. In *Clinical Nutrition and Metabolic Research*, pp. 118, ed. G. Dietze, A. Grunert and G. Wolfram. Karger, Basel, Munich.

Tarvid, I. (1992). Effect of early postnatal long-term fasting on the development of peptide hydrolysis in chicks. *Comparative Biochemistry & Physiology A*, **101**, 161–6.

Teschemacher, H. & Koch, G. (1991). Opioids in the milk. *Endocrine Regulation*, **25**, 147–50.

Thorens, B., Cheng, Z. Q., Brown, D. & Lodish, H. F. (1990). Liver glucose transporter: a basolateral protein in hepatocytes and intestine and kidney cells. *American Journal of Physiology*, **259**, C279–85.

Tipton, A. D., Frase, S. & Mansbach, C. M., II (1989). Isolation and characterisation of a mucosal triacylglycerol pool undergoing hydrolysis. *American Journal of Physiology*, **257**, G871–8.

Toloza, E. M., Lam, M. & Diamond, J. (1991). Nutrient extraction by cold-exposed mice: a test of digestive safety margins. *American Journal of Physiology*, **261**, G608–20.

Triadou, N., Bataille, J. & Schmitz, J. (1983). Longitudinal study of the human intestinal brush border membrane proteins: distribution of the main disaccharidases and peptidases. *Gastroenterology*, **85**, 1326–32.

Trocki, O., Mochizuki, H., Dominioni, L. & Alexander, J. W. (1986). Intact protein versus free amino acids in the nutritional support of thermally injured animals. *Journal of Parenteral and Enteral Nutrition*, **10**, 139–45.

Turner, J. S., Fyfe, A. R., Kaplan, D. K. & Wardlaw, A. J. (1991). Oesophageal obstruction during nasogastric feeding. *Intensive Care Medicine*, **17**, 302–3.

Tweedie, D. E. F., Spivey, J. & Johnston, I. D. A. (1973). Choice of intravenous amino acid solutions for use after surgical operation. *Metabolism*, **22**, 173–8.

Umetsu, H., Matsuoka, H. & Ichishima, E. (1983). Debittering mechanism of bitter peptides from milk casein by wheat carboxypeptidase. *Journal of Agricultural Food Chemistry*, **31**, 50–3.

Vasquez, J. A., Morse, E. L. & Adibi, S. A. (1985). Effect of starvation on amino acid and peptide transport and peptide hydrolysis in humans. *American Journal of Physiology*, **249**, G563–6.

Viall, C., Porcelli, K., Teran, J. C., Varma, R. N. & Steffee, W. P. (1990). A double-blind clinical trial comparing the gastrointestinal side effects of two enteral feeding formulas. *Journal of Parenteral and Enteral Nutrition*, **14**, 265–9.

Wahlqvist, M. L., Wilmshurst, E. G., Murton, C. R. & Richardson, E. N. (1978). The effect of chain length on glucose absorption and the related metabolic response. *American Journal of Clinical Nutrition*, **31**, 1998–2001.

Windemueller, H. G. (1982). Glutamine utilisation by the small intestine. *Advances in Enzymology*, **53**, 201–38.

Winitz, M., Adams, R. F., Seedman, D. A. et al. (1970). Studies in metabolic nutrition employing chemically defined diets II. Effects on gut microflora populations. *American Journal of Clinical Nutrition*, **23**, 546–59.

Winitz, M., Seedman, D. A. & Graff, J. (1970). Studies in metabolic nutrition employing chemically defined diets. I. Extended feeding of normal human adult males. *American Journal of Clinical Nutrition*, **23**, 525–45.

Wretlind, K. A. J. (1952). The amino acid content of a dialysed enzymatic casein hydrolysate. *Acta Physiologica Scandinavica*, **27**, 189–203.

Zaloga, G. P., Ward, K. A. & Prielipp, R. C. (1991). Effect of enteral diets on whole body and gut growth in unstressed rats. *Journal of Parenteral and Enteral Nutrition*, **15**, 42–7.

Ziegler, F., Ollivier, J. M., Cynober, L., Masini, J. P., Coudray Lucas, C., Levy, E. & Giboudeau, J. (1990). Efficiency of enteral nitrogen support in surgical patients: small peptides *v* non-degraded proteins. *Gut*, **31**, 1277–83.

7

Enteral and parenteral nutrition

C. R. PENNINGTON

The development of artificial nutritional support

The recognition that undernutrition was a common problem in hospital patients led to an appreciation of the associated morbidity which stimulated the development of techniques for artificial nutritional support. Artificial nutritional support, by enteral and parenteral nutrition, represents one of the more important yet least heralded advances in therapeutics. Nutritional support has a wide application in clinical practice, particularly in gastroenterology, general surgery and intensive care. There have been important improvements in the methods of nutrient delivery, notably percutaneous endoscopic gastronomy and peripheral parenteral nutrition. Now, attention is focussing on the possible therapeutic merit of supplementing nutrients with specific substrates such as glutamine, arginine, and the omega-3-fatty acids. This chapter summarises the current practice and recent developments in the supervision of artificial nutritional support.

Enteral nutrition

Indications

The indications and contraindications for enteral nutrition are summarised in Table 7.1. The reasons for enteral nutrition administered over a one year period in one health district (Wilcock *et al.*, 1991) are shown in Table 7.2.

The importance of anorexia in the genesis of malnutrition merits emphasis. Anorexia accompanies many diseases including renal failure, liver failure and alcoholic liver disease, Crohn's disease, cancer, and AIDS. Many anorexic patients can be managed with oral supplements, others benefit from enteral nutrition pending the treatment of their underlying disease. The use of enteral feeding in these circumstances can save much

Table 7.1. *Indications and contra-indications for enteral feeding*

Indications
  (a) Anorexia
       e.g. Crohn's disease, malignancy, alcoholic liver disease.
  (b) Inability to eat
       e.g. oropharyngeal neoplasia, cerebrovascular disease, motor neurone disease.
  (c) Supplemental feeding in intestinal failure
       e.g. malabsorption syndromes, Crohn's disease, short-bowel syndrome.
  (d) Protection and maintenance of intestinal integrity
       e.g. burns, intestinal adaptation following resection.

Contraindications
  (a) Intestinal obstruction.
  (b) Vomiting and severe diarrhoea.
  (c) High intestinal fistulae.

Table 7.2. *Enteral tube feeding in selected Cambridge Hospitals: diagnostic groups and duration of treatment*

Diagnostic group	Patient number	Treatment duration (days)
Neurological	144 (49%)	4428 (64%)
Malignancy	47 (16%)	1005 (14%)
Gastrointestinal	36 (12%)	577 (8%)
Respiratory	24 (8%)	216 (3%)
Miscellaneous	40 (15%)	744 (11%)
Total	291	6970

Adapted from Wilcock *et al.*, 1991.

nursing time and relieve the patient of unnecessary stress which accompanies the forced ingestion of unwanted meals.

Some patients are unable to eat for mechanical reasons. These include patients with oral or pharyngeal carcinoma, and patients with chronic neurological disorders such as cerebrovascular disease and motor neurone disease. Patients who have impaired intestinal function can sometimes maintain energy, nitrogen and electrolyte balance when nutrients are infused over prolonged periods, including overnight, to supplement their oral diet. Those with intestinal failure due to Crohn's disease or radiation enteritis fall into this category.

Recent interest has focussed on the possible advantages of enteral nutrition in intensive care when the use of special formulae may help reduce bacterial translocation from the gut, and sepsis (Mclave, Lowen & Snider, 1992). Such patients often have gastric stasis and simultaneous gastric decompression will be needed.

Enteral nutrition is contraindicated in patients with intestinal obstruction, high entero-cutaneous fistulae and those suffering from severe diarrhoea or vomiting. The absence of bowel sounds or gastric stasis in the post operative patient does not preclude enteral feeding. Under these circumstances jejunal infusion may be combined with gastric aspiration.

Nutrient solutions

Enteral diets may be considered in three categories: polymeric diets, chemically defined diets, and special formulations. Some examples of enteral feeds are given in Table 7.3. The majority of these solutions provide 1 kcal per ml, and are designed to meet average requirements of nitrogen, energy, minerals, vitamins and trace elements in two litres.

Polymeric diets

Polymeric diets contain a whole protein nitrogen source for use in patients who do not have severe impairment of intestinal function. The protein source is usually milk, casein and lactalbumin, with or without soya protein. Fat is supplied from vegetable oils and carbohydrate from corn starch and maltodextrin. These feeds do not contain gluten or significant amounts of lactose.

Some preparations provide fat in the form of medium chain triglycerides, for example, Triosorbon, which may be beneficial in patients with steatorrhoea and limited intestinal function. Solutions are also available with a low sodium content for patients with cirrhosis or cardiac failure, e.g. Fortison Low Sodium. Some feeds have increased energy density, these products are used in patients with burns or trauma and when fluid restriction is required. Examples include Ensure plus and Fortison plus which provide 1.5 kcal per ml.

Patients who need prolonged and particularly total enteral nutrition, including those with cerebrovascular disease and motor neurone disease, may benefit from the use of polymeric feeds which contain fibre. Enrich includes 5 g of carbohydrate as dietary fibre in a 250 ml can, Fresubin Plus F solutions provide 3–5 g in 500 ml.

Table 7.3. *Some examples of enteral feeds. Not all of the disease-specific products are available in the UK*

(a) Polymeric feeds
  Clinifeed
  Ensure
  Fortison
  Fresubin
  Isocal
  Liquisorbin
(b) Special formulations of polymeric feeds
  Enrich
  Ensure plus
  Fortison Energy Plus
  Fortison Low Sodium
  Fresubin Plus F
(c) Elemental feeds
  Elemental 028
  Flexical
  Fresubin OPD
  Peptamen
  Pepditre 2 Plus
  Reabilan
(d) Formulations for specific disease states
  Alitrac
  Dialamine
  Generaid
  Hepaticaid
  Nephranutril
  Perative
  Pulmocare

Chemically defined diets

These diets contain predigested nutrients with nitrogen in the form of amino acids, and most have low fat content. They were originally marketed for patients with severe impairment of digestion and absorption. Vivonex and Elemental 028 both provide only 40 g of protein in 2 litres, Elemental 028 provides 1600 kcal in this volume. The recently introduced Elemental 028 Extra provides more energy and nitrogen. Vivonex HN contains twice as much nitrogen, but the osmolality is very high. Vivonex is no longer available in the UK.

The use of these products has been extended to include the management and investigation of patients with alleged food allergy or intolerance, as well as the treatment of Crohn's disease (O'Morain, Segal & Levi, 1984). Studies have shown that elemental diets are as effective as corticosteroid therapy for the induction of remission. Debate continues, however, about the relative merits of polymeric diets for this purpose.

The recognition that small peptides are preferentially absorbed (Zeigler *et al.*, 1990) led to the introduction of peptide feeds; these have a similar nutrient profile. They may be preferred in patients with severely impaired intestinal function, although most patients with intestinal disease can be managed satisfactorily with the cheaper polymeric products.

Special formulations

Many specialised diets have been designed for the management of children with inborn errors of metabolism but these will not be considered in this chapter. Recently, enteral feeds have been designed to meet perceived requirements in specific disease states. Thus, Pulmocare has a reduced ratio of carbohydrate to fat to reduce respiratory demands in patients with respiratory failure (Weiner *et al.*, 1987). Formulations enriched with essential amino acids are available for patients with chronic renal failure (Nephranutril and Dialamine). Other solutions have an increased content of branch chain amino acids and minimum methionine content for the treatment of patients with chronic liver disease and portal systemic encephalopathy (Hepato-Nutril, Hepaticaid and Hepatomine). These solutions also have a reduced sodium content. Feeds designed for hypercatabolic stress are also enriched with branch chain amino acids.

There is increasing interest in the use of nutrient substrates for the modification of the immunological and inflammatory response (Katz, Kvefan & Askanazi, 1990). Long chain fatty acids such as the polyunsaturated fatty acids of the omega 6 variety derived from linoleic acid, are given in the form of Intralipid in parenteral nutrition and are also found in enteral products. By stimulating the synthesis of thromboxane A2 and prostaglandin E2 they can encourage thrombosis and suppress complement synthesis, respectively, and impair delayed cell mediated hypersensitivity reactions. These effects are less marked with omega-3-fats derived from linolenic acid which lead to the formation of less potent metabolites. Arginine has been shown to have a significant immunostimulatory effect (Barbul *et al.*, 1983). It can prevent the thymic atrophy which follows injury, and it leads to the increased release of interleukin 2. RNA has also been shown to stimulate the immune response, and, in

Table 7.4. *The relative merits of naso-gastric and percutaneous endoscopic gastric (PEG) tubes*

	N–G tube	PEG tube
Advantages	Easily passed	Better tolerated
		More reliable nutrient delivery
Disadvantages	Inappropriate removal	Invasive procedure
	Loss of prescribed nutrients	Complications of placement
	Tracheal intubation	
	Cosmetic	

the animal model, glutamine protects the integrity of the intestinal epithelium reducing microbial translocation. These observations have been utilised in the formulation of some enteral feeds.

Perative is a recently introduced product which contains partially hydrolysed proteins, arginine, beta-carotene and omega-3-fatty acids. Impact is an enteral product fortified with nucleotides and arginine. The use of this preparation has been shown to reduce the incidence of infections in burn patients (McDonald, Sharp & Deitch, 1992). Immuno-nutril is enriched with arginine and glutamine, and it contains omega-3-fats. Alitrac is enriched with glutamine and marketed for the stressed patient. Studies are needed to define the clinical advantage of these more expensive products. Work with burn patients already suggests that they may have an important role.

Methods

Enteral feeding may be achieved by naso-gastric tube, percutaneous endoscopic gastrostomy, naso-jejunal tube or jejunostomy. The relative merits of these routes of administration are summarised in Table 7.4.

Nasogastric feeding

This route is preferred in patients with temporary impairment of oral nutrition or who need short-term supplemental feeding. Final-bore PVC or polyurethane nasogastric tubes are used. The stiff, wide-bore Ryles tubes are not appropriate for enteral feeding because of patient discomfort and the risk of oesophageal damage. The Silk Corpak tube is made of polyurethane and designed with a bullet end and anticlog ports, through

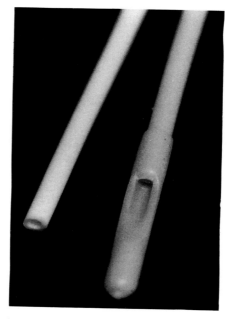

Fig. 7.1. The Silk Corpak naso-gastric tube showing the bullet end and anticlog port.

which the guide wire will not protrude (Fig. 7.1). The end of the tube is lubricated with water and passed via the nose with the patient in the sitting position. The patient is told to swallow when he is aware of the tube at the back of the throat. With repeated swallows, the tube is passed into the stomach, correct placement is best checked by the aspiration of gastric fluid, which is recognised by the use of litmus paper. This type of tube may remain *in situ* for many months, although percutaneous endoscopic gastrostomy tubes are now increasingly used for patients who need long-term treatment. The more mobile patients who require overnight feeding, may prefer to remove the tube after each feed. Endoscopic placement of the tube can be useful in the unconscious patient, and when intubation of the jejunum is required, for example, in patients with gastric stasis.

The tube is flushed with 20–50 ml of water with a 50 ml syringe before and after the feed, or 6 hourly in patients who need prolonged feeding periods. Flushing should also occur before and immediately after the administration of liquid medication.

Percutaneous endoscopic gastrostomy (PEG)

This is a major advance, which is particularly useful for the management of patients who need prolonged nutritional support and who are unable to eat or swallow (Steigmann *et al.*, 1990). Examples include patients with nasopharyngeal tumors, cerebrovascular disease and motor neurone disease.

The tube is inserted endoscopically under antibiotic cover (Fig. 7.2). The endoscope is passed in the normal manner and the patient is then rolled onto the back. The site of insertion between the umbilicus and the xiphisternum is identified by transillumination and or gastric identation seen through the endoscope, when an assistant presses the abdominal wall. Failure to transilluminate or indent the stomach may mean that other structures are interposed between the abdominal wall and the stomach and the procedure must be abandoned. The chosen site is then infiltrated with local anaesthetic and a small incision is made through the skin. The stomach is adequately inflated and a cannula inserted through the incision. The needle is seen to pierce the anterior gastric wall by the endoscopist. Provided the position is satisfactory the needle is withdrawn and a guide wire is passed through the cannula into the stomach where it is grasped by an endoscopic snare. The endoscope is withdrawn pulling the snare and wire back through the mouth where the wire is attached to the gastrostomy tube. The tube is then pulled into the stomach by traction on the other end of the wire which emerges from the abdominal wall. The endoscope is again passed and follows the gastrostomy tube into position until it is satisfactorily placed against the wall of the stomach, avoiding blanching. Tubes are fitted with flanges or balloons to prevent displacement. Those with balloons which can be deflated by cutting the tube are easier to remove.

Provided the recommended procedure is observed PEG tube placement is relatively safe (Fig. 7.3). However, complications can occur. They include exit-site infection, peritonitis due to leakage if the stomach is not properly opposed, and damage to adjacent organs.

After a few months the gastrostomy tube can be removed and replaced with a button gastrostomy tube which lies flush with the abdominal wall. This is preferable for the mobile patient.

Jejunal tubes

Jejunal feeding may be achieved by jejunostomy in which a fine-bore feeding tube is placed into the jejunum at open operation. This usually

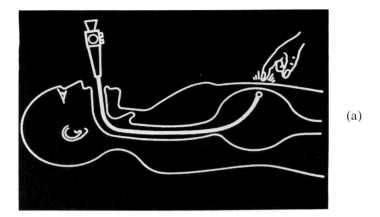

(a)

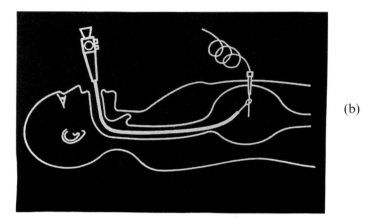

(b)

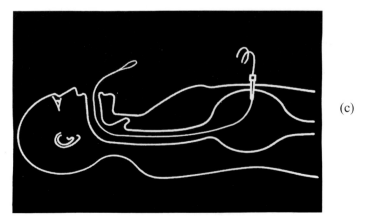

(c)

Fig. 7.2. (a)–(c) (*continued*)

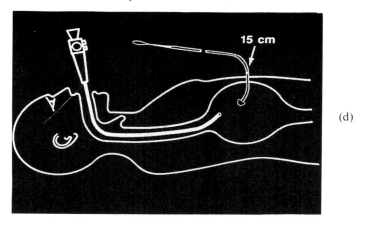

(d)

Fig. 7.2 (*continued*). The insertion of a percutaneous endoscopic gastrostomy tube: (a) The endoscope is passed and the insertion site is identified by transillumination or indentation. (b) Under local anaesthetic, a cannula is inserted through the abdominal wall into the inflated stomach, the needle is removed and the wire is passed through the cannula into the stomach where it is grasped by an endoscopic snare. (c) The endoscope with the snare and wire is withdrawn, the wire is attached to the gastrostomy tube, and the tube is drawn into the stomach by traction on the other end of the wire. (d) The gastroscope is reinserted to check that the tube is in a satisfactory position with the gastric wall. The abdominal attachments are placed to secure the gastrostomy tube.

coincides with planned surgery. Adequate fixation is important to prevent peritoneal leakage of nutrient or intestinal content. Alternatively, a per-nasal tube can be placed into the jejunum using an endoscope. A guide wire is passed through the endoscope into the jejunum. The endoscope is removed and the nasojejunal tube is then passed over the wire into the jejunum. The proximal end of the tube is routed through the nose by directing it through a naso-pharyngeal tube. This system may have advantages in the intensive care unit, where a multilumen tube designed to facilitate simultaneous gastric decompression is an advantage.

The relative merits of the different methods of nutrient delivery are summarised in Table 7.4. The advantage of the PEG tube in comparison with nasogastric administration for patients with chronic neurological disability is shown in Fig. 7.4. These patients had been fed by nasogastric tubes before the insertion of PEG tubes. They were malnourished because of the unreliable nutrient delivery by the nasogastric route. The reasons included repeated tube displacement with loss of the prescribed nutrient (Wicks *et al.*, 1992).

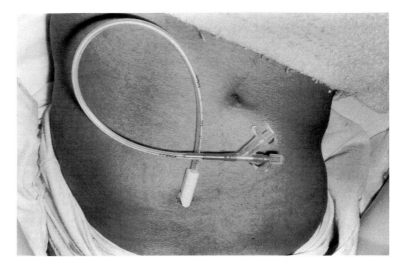

Fig. 7.3. A recently inserted PEG tube for nutritional access in a severely handicapped pateint.

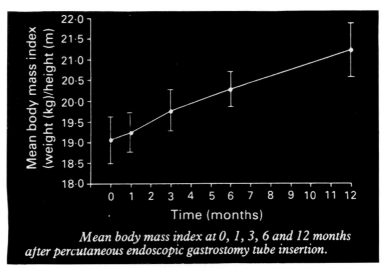

Mean body mass index at 0, 1, 3, 6 and 12 months after percutaneous endoscopic gastrostomy tube insertion.

Fig. 7.4. The improvement in the nutritional state following the insertion of PEG tubes in patients previously fed by nasogastric tube (Wicks *et al.*, 1992, reproduced with the permission of the editor of GUT).

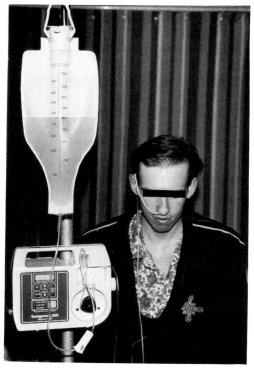

Fig. 7.5. A simple naso-gastric feeding system which is suitable for temporary use in the immobile patient, or for overnight supplemental feeding.

Regardless of the route of administration, patients require nutrient reservoirs, giving sets and infusion pumps (Fig. 7.5). Small portable pumps with rechargeable batteries are helpful for the mobile patient, who wears a strap which supports the pump and reservoir (Fig. 7.6). The giving set and reservoir are discarded after each feed, to avoid the risk of bacterial contamination and abnormal rates of infusion, due to the stretching of the tubing.

Nutrients are infused in a cyclical fashion in those patients who just require overnight supplemental feeding, and in those needing total enteral feeding who are able to take negligible oral diet. As with parenteral feeding there are significant advantages in cyclical as opposed to continuous feeding (Gayle *et al.*, 1985). Cyclical feeding leads to improved nitrogen retention with reduced fat deposition. It also has important psychological

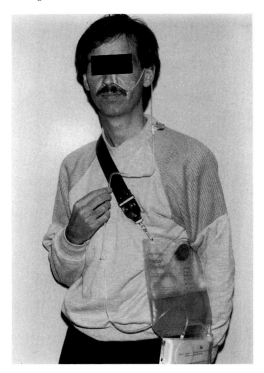

Fig. 7.6. A portable enteral feeding system.

advantages in liberating the patient from infusion for part of the day. Bolus feeding with the intermittent administration of large volumes of feed is discouraged because of the greater risk of complications. When overnight feeding is prescribed the patients are requested to sleep in a semi-upright position with three pillows, to minimise gastro-oesophageal reflux.

Complications

Complications of enteral feeding can be considered in three groups: complications of nutrient delivery, gastrointestinal complications, and nutritional and metabolic problems.

Complications of nutrient delivery

Nutrients may be delivered in the wrong place. Obvious examples include delivery into the lung leading to pneumonia when naso-gastric tubes are placed in the trachea or following gastric aspiration. Lung infection, with gram negative organisms, has also been attributed to continuous enteral feeding in intensive care patients. This is because the feeding increases the pH, permitting the proliferation of bacteria, which subsequently migrate on the external surface of the catheter to reach the trachea (Jacobs *et al.*, 1990). Aspiration may be minimised by jejunal feeding.

Peritonitis will follow the displacement of PEG and jejunostomy tubes. All feeding tubes may be blocked if they are not managed properly, particularly when they are used for the frequent administration of medication.

Gastrointestinal complications

Diarrhoea and vomiting have been attributed to enteral feeding. The rapid infusion of cold solutions may be an important factor. Osmolality within the range found in commercial feeds, is unlikely to be important. Patients with hypoalbuminaemia are particularly prone to diarrhoea, as are those patients who are receiving antibiotics. When diarrhoea occurs the cause should be investigated, the rate of infusion reduced, and the possible advantage of a different type of feed considered. This might include a peptide feed, or a product containing fat in the form of MCT, for patients with severe intestinal impairment.

Nutritional and metabolic problems

The nutrient solutions contain average recommended requirements of macronutrients, micronutrients, electrolytes, minerals and water in 2 litres of feed. Monitoring of nutritional state, electrolyte balance, and glucose homeostasis is essential. Patients with cirrhosis and cardiac failure may develop fluid overload with conventional feeds. Under these circumstances feeds with a reduced sodium content are preferred. Conversely, additional electrolytes and water may be needed in patients who have intestinal failure and diarrhoea. Hypomagnesaemia is a feature of Crohn's disease (Park *et al.*, 1990).

The refeeding syndrome complicates the initiation of nutritional support in severely malnourished patients, such as those with a history of ethanol abuse. The administration of nutrients can precipitate severe hypo phosphataemia, hypomagnesaemia, and thiamin deficiency. Careful monitoring is important.

Parenteral nutrition

Terminology

This treatment is frequently described as total parenteral nutrition (TPN). TPN implies that all the nutrition is being administered by the intravenous route. The majority of patients who require parenteral feeding are able to consume and absorb small amounts of nutrient via the oral route. In these patients parenteral nutrition is supplemental. Some oral diet should be encouraged wherever possible for social, psychological and economic reasons. Oral nutrition is important for the encouragement of intestinal adaptation and the prevention of hepatobiliary disease. Thus, the general term parenteral nutrition should be used. Total parenteral nutrition describes treatment in the limited number of patients who are unable to eat. Many patients who need short-term parenteral nutrition, particularly those on surgical wards, can receive their nutrient solution via a peripheral vein, thus avoiding the complications associated with central venous catheters. Conversely, patients who suffer from prolonged intestinal failure need central catheters with either an external segment (Broviak, Cuff-Cath) or subcutaneous port (Port-A-Cath). Catheter patency is maintained by a heparin lock when the patient is disconnected from the infusion fluid. Finally, wherever possible patients should be fed in a cyclical manner rather than by continuous infusion. This has metabolic advantages with reduced fluid retention and fat accumulation. Thus, parenteral nutrition (PN) may be total (TPN), supplemental (SPN), central (CPN), peripheral (PPN), continuous or cyclical; or combinations of these options!

Indications

Parenteral nutrition is indicated when intestinal function is unavailable or inadequate. The intestine may be unavailable in patients with intestinal obstruction and after intestinal surgery, although some of these patients have gastric ileus and can be fed enterally into the jejunum with con-comitant gastric aspiration. Inadequate intestinal function can occur in various intestinal disorders, summarised in Table 7.5. Common reasons for intestinal failure include Crohn's disease, radiation enteritis, motility dis-orders, and short-bowel syndrome, following resection for inflammatory or vascular disease. HIV infection is a recognised cause of intestinal failure in the absence of specific pathogens. Increasing numbers of AIDS patients are under treatment by home parenteral nutrition in the USA (Singer *et al.*, 1991). Controversy surrounds the use of parenteral nutrition in patients

Table 7.5. *Causes of intestinal failure*
which may require parenteral nutrition

Inflammatory disease
  e.g. Crohn's disease
    Radiation enteritis
Motility disorders
  e.g. Idiopathic intestinal pseudo obstruction
    Scleroderma
Short bowel syndrome
  e.g. Volvulus
    Crohn's disease
Miscellaneous
  e.g. AIDS
    Malignant disease

---

with AIDS and also inoperable malignant intestinal obstruction (August *et al.*, 1991). More work is required to define the role of parenteral nutrition in patients with AIDS.

Parenteral nutrition is contraindicated in patients whose nutritional needs can be met by the oral or enteral route. Cardiac failure, electrolyte imbalance, and the last stages of terminal disease should also preclude this treatment. When benefit may be expected, disorders of electrolyte balance must be corrected before this treatment is begun.

Nutrient solutions

The required nutrients are illustrated in Fig. 7.7. Nitrogen is provided in the form of amino acid solutions. There are many commercially available preparations which vary in nitrogen concentration and electrolyte provision (Table 7.6). These solutions provide essential amino acids. However, the insoluble amino acids arginine, glutamine and taurine which are considered non-essential are not included. Under some circumstances some of these amino acids may be beneficial. Glutamine may have an important role in the preservation of the integrity of the intestinal epithelium and along with arginine it may enhance immune function. Consequently, the use of peptide solutions which will facilitate the delivery of these amino acids is being explored.

Energy is delivered in the form of dextrose and lipid. The concomitant use of lipid to supply part of the energy requirements is recommended. Energy needs cannot be satisfied with dextrose in the stressed patient

Table 7.6. *Some examples
of amino acid solutions*

Solution	Nitrogen: g/l
Aminoplex	12, 24
Freamine	13, 15
Synthamin	9, 14, 17
Vamin	9, 14, 18

Note: The electrolyte content differs between the solutions. Electrolyte-free preparations are available for patients with renal failure.

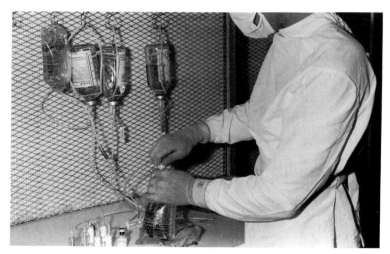

Fig. 7.7. The nutrients required for parenteral nutrition are compounded under sterile conditions in the pharmacy.

because of limited dextrose tolerance. Reliance on dextrose, increases sodium and water retention as well as the tendency to reactive hypoglycaemia at the end of infusion. Lipid solutions provide phosphate and serve as a carrier for the fat soluble vitamins. Furthermore, solutions containing lipid as a second energy source may be less prone to cause central vein thrombosis than concentrated dextrose solutions (Pithie & Pennington, 1987).

Commercially prepared micronutrient solutions of water-soluble vitamins, and trace element preparation, such as Additrace, make nutrient prescription much easier. The sodium, potassium, magnesium, calcium and phosphate content is adjusted to requirement. Most amino acid solutions contain some electrolytes. Electrolyte-free preparations are available for patients with renal failure. Finally, the different concentrations of amino acids and dextrose allow the volume and water content to be adjusted to the patients' needs. In exceptional circumstances, for example in patients with a high output fistula, the patient may need an electrolyte bag to supplement the electrolyte provision of the nutrition bag.

Methods

The need for supplemental or total, peripheral or central parenteral nutrition is assessed. When central feeding is needed, the relative merits of the subcutaneous and external catheter are discussed with the patient, and the chosen catheter is placed so that the tip lies at the junction of the superior vena cava and the right atrium. Our preferred external catheter is currently the Cuff Cath (Fig. 7.8). This is a strong polyurethane catheter with a Teflon cuff and an on–off switch, which removes the need for clamping and thus renders the extension set redundant. The switch can be replaced by unscrewing it from the end of the catheter. Extension sets are advisable when patients have a conventional silicon-type Broviak catheter, if prolonged treatment is envisaged. The extension set is attached to the end of the catheter between the catheter and spigot or giving set. It is used for routine clamping during setting-up and discontinuing the feed. Extension sets are changed at regular intervals and reduce the wear and tear on the catheter. Some patients prefer subcutaneous ports. The port can be changed when the membrane fails, but this requires a surgical procedure.

The nutrient solution is compounded in the pharmacy under aseptic conditions (Fig. 7.7). The shelf-life will depend upon the type of solution prescribed. Lipid containing mixes have a shorter shelf-life than conventional solutions. The solution is stored in the 'fridge until it is used and infusion must be completed before the expiry date.

Nutrient solutions are infused via a volumetric pump with a suitable air-in-line and occlusion alarm. Mobile patients may prefer portable pumps. Unfortunately the giving sets for these pumps are significantly more expensive. Cyclical infusion is preferred so that most patients infuse

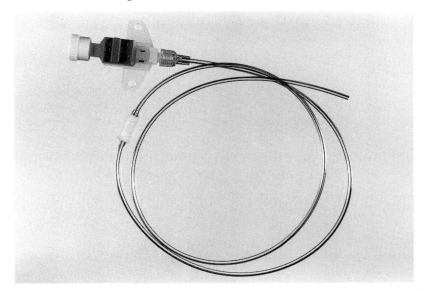

Fig. 7.8. Catheters for central venous access for prolonged parenteral nutrition: the Cuff Cath is a tough polyurethane catheter with a Teflon cuff and a very useful on–off switch.

overnight for 12–18 hours. This gives the patient 8–12 hours free from the encumbrance of the infusion and infusion equipment. The speed at which the solution can be infused will be determined by the volume, the electrolyte and nutrient content, and the cardiovascular status of the patient. The infusion rate is reduced before the giving set is disconnected, particularly in patients who are receiving concentrated dextrose solutions, to reduce the risk of reactive hypoglycaemia. Patients who receive solutions containing lipid are tested for lipid clearance by visual inspection of the serum after a test dose of the lipid solution has been infused through a peripheral vein.

All catheter procedures are conducted with an aseptic technique because catheter junctions are the commonest portal of entry for infecting microorganisms (Linares et al., 1985). Many centres prefer to keep the junction enclosed in a Betadine-impregnated swab. At the end of the infusion, this swab is removed, and the junction and adjacent ends of the catheter and giving set are wiped with antiseptic solution. The junction is encased in a clean Betadine-soaked swab which is left in place for three minutes. The pump is then switched off, the switch on the end of the catheter is also turned off. The giving set is removed from the catheter and a syringe containing a flushing solution is placed on the end of the catheter. This is usually saline, but a 20% ethanol solution may be preferred for patients receiving lipid-containing mixes (Johnston *et al.*, 1992). The flush is used not only to clear the line of nutrient solution, but also to gauge resistance in order to detect impending occlusion. Thereafter, a latex-ended spigot is attached to the end of the catheter, through which a heparin solution is injected to retain line patency until the next infusion. The junction may then be wrapped in a protective dressing. Patients with subcutaneous catheters require skin cleansing with antiseptic solution before the insertion of the Heubner needle, which is then secured in position.

Each unit should have a protocol for catheter care. Catheters are best managed by accredited nurses who must also be familiar with potential complications, their recognition and management. Patients who may benefit from home feeding should receive similar instructions backed up by explanatory literature. Before going home they must prove competent with catheter methods. Domiciliary visits by the nutrition nurses are helpful.

Complications

The complications of parenteral nutrition may be considered in three groups: nutritional complications, catheter-related complications, and the effect of parenteral nutrition on other organ systems (Table 7.7).

Nutritional complications

The common errors fall into two groups: the over-provision of macro-nutrients, and the underprovision of micronutrients.

The excessive administration of dextrose leads to lipogenesis with hepatic steatosis (Kaminski, Adams & Jellinek, 1980) and the increased production of carbon dioxide. The latter sometimes causes difficulty when patients are being weaned from a ventilator. Excessive amino-acid administration can cause cholestasis (Black, Suttle & Whittington, 1981), particularly in paediatric practice. It is also one of the factors which may be incriminated in the development of bone disease.

Commercial micronutrient solutions should ensure that trace element deficiency syndromes no longer occur. However, it must be remembered that the amounts of nutrients such as selenium are based upon estimated daily needs. Account should be taken of pre-existing deficiency. Many patients who require long-term parenteral nutrition do not need a

Table 7.7. *The complications of parenteral nutrition*

Nutritional complications
Overprovision of macronutrients
e.g. hepatic steatosis with dextrose
Cholestasis and amino acids
Underprovision of micronutrients
e.g. selenium deficiency
Catheter-related complications
Catheter sepsis
Catheter fracture
Catheter occlusion
Central vein thrombosis
Effect on other organ systems
Hepatic disease
e.g. steatosis
cholestasis
Biliary disease
e.g. biliary sludge
gallstones
Bone disease
e.g. osteoporosis
osteomyelitis
Cardiac disease
e.g. endocarditis
atrial thrombus

daily nutrient infusion, additional selenium supplements are required under these circumstances. Furthermore, there is evidence that some vitamins degrade rapidly during the infusion time. This particularly applies to vitamin C (Allwood *et al.*, 1992). Multilayer bags may prevent the oxidation of this vitamin but they are more expensive.

Catheter-related complications

There are four major catheter-related complications: infection, occlusion, central vein thrombosis, and fracture with or without air embolism.

Infection: Infection most commonly gains access through the catheter junctions. The exit-site, contamination of the nutrient solution and haematogenous seeding are other potential routes of contamination. Exit-site infection is recognised by erythema and exudation at the skin junction. There may be tenderness extending up the catheter tunnel. When catheter infection occurs, the patient becomes abruptly ill with a high temperature and tachycardia. Blood cultures should be obtained through the central catheter and peripheral vein. A heparin lock is applied, and antibiotic therapy is administered pending the culture results. The combination of vancomycin and netilmicin will cover the common catheter pathogens. If the blood cultures are sterile, catheter infection is unlikely and other reasons for the illness are sought. Conversely, positive cultures suggest catheter infection, or contamination from another source. Semi-quantitative central vein cultures have been proposed to identify catheter infection (Mosca *et al.*, 1987), which is probable if *Staph epidermidis* is cultured. When infection is confirmed the line is either removed or decontaminated with antibiotic locks (Messing *et al.*, 1990). This decision is influenced by the need for continuing central vein feeding, and the nature of the offending pathogen. For example, attempted eradication would seem unwise with pathogens such as *Staphylococcus aureus* and *Candida* sp. Finally, the risk of metastatic infection such as osteomyelitis and endocarditis must always be considered.

Occlusion: Catheter occlusion may be caused by fibrin, lipid-sludge, or amorphous debris. Lipid sludge (Fig. 7.9) is the probable cause with lipid-containing mixes when increasing resistance over a few days will culminate in complete blockage. Before total occlusion a 70% ethanol lock may free the line (Pennington & Pithie, 1987). Furthermore, the use of a 20% ethanol flush instead of saline when patients receive such nutrient mixes, may prevent this complication (Johnston *et al.*, 1992). Fibrin can form a sleeve around the distal end of the catheter. This can act as a flap preventing the withdrawal of blood. Occasionally it can encase the catheter so that the nutrient solution emerges at the exit site. Alternatively, the catheter lumen may be occluded. A urokinase lock will sometimes disperse the fibrin. When the catheter is completely blocked it may be worth attaching a syringe with a 10 ml solution of 10 000 units of urokinase to the hub for 24 hours. This will sometimes free the occlusion, presumably because the urokinase diffuses down the catheter lumen. Hydrochloric acid has been advocated for the clearance of amorphous debris.

Central vein thrombosis: This may present with clinical evidence of occlusion of the superior vena cava, pulmonary embolism, or pyrexia. The risk of thrombosis can be reduced by the avoidance of very concentrated dextrose solutions, placing the catheter in the right atrium rather than the superior vena cava (Pithie *et al.*, 1988), and the use of heparin. However the value of heparin in this context has only been demonstrated with doses of 3 units per ml of nutrient solution (Mughall, 1989). There is a theoretical risk of aggravating the tendency for parenterally fed patients to develop osteoporosis, and heparin cannot be mixed with lipid-containing nutrient solutions. Warfarin is an effective prophylactic agent, but it is not without risk of haemorrhage especially in the patient with inflammatory bowel disease. Solutions which contain

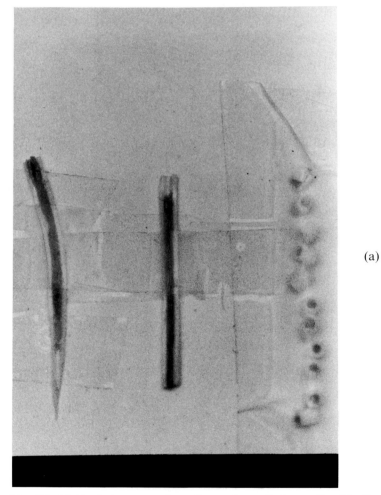

(a)

Fig. 7.9. Lipid sludge may deposit on the catheter wall with the prolonged use of lipid containing parenteral nutrition solutions. (a) Macroscopic appearance of occluded catheter. (*continued*).

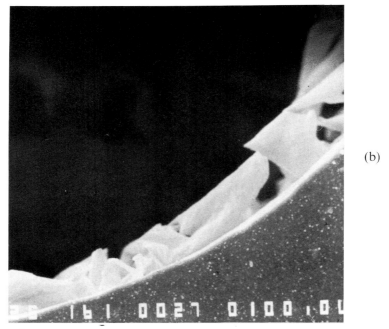

(b)

Fig. 7.9 (*continued*). (b) Microscopic examination of a catheter wall after one month's infusion of lipid mixes. This catheter was removed when parenteral nutrition was no longer required.

lipid also interact with oral anticoagulants. When central vein thrombosis occurs (Fig. 7.10) effective thrombolysis can be achieved with streptokinase (and tissue plasminogen activator).

Fracture of external catheters: This can be prevented by minimising catheter clamping through the use of extension sets, catheters with an on–off switch or the Groshong valve. In the event of fracture, patients should have ready access to clamps. Repair kits are available. The latex membrane of the subcutaneous catheter may also fail. This is heralded by soreness during infusion at the site of the port. Replacement of the port is then required.

Effect on other organs

Parenteral nutrition may adversely affect the hepatobiliary system, the intestine, the skeleton and the heart.

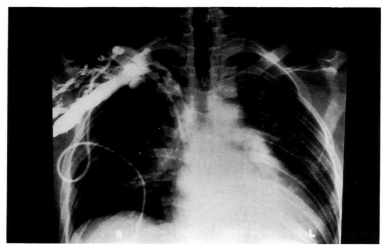

Fig. 7.10. Upper limb venogram showing venous thrombosis. This study was obtained after the patient woke with distension of the face and upper limbs.

Hepatobiliary complications: These may arise for three reasons; the failure to provide enteral nutrition, the provision of intravenous nutrients, and the omission of certain non-essential, insoluble amino acids from the nutrient solution. Lack of enteral stimulation will encourage stasis with accompanying biliary sludge, bacterial overgrowth, and the absorption of bacterial toxins. This may be facilitated by intestinal atrophy, which accompanies the absence of glutamine in the nutrient solution. Excess dextrose will lead to steatosis (Kaminski *et al.*, 1980). Cholestasis has been associated with the overprovision of amino acids in paediatric practice (Black *et al.*, 1981), and possibly also the absence of taurine. The risk of hepatic disease can be reduced by the encouragement of oral nutrition and the avoidance of excessive nutrient administration (Fisher, 1989).

Intestine: Intestinal atrophy leading to the translocation of microorganisms and bacterial products has been linked to the lack of glutamine in an animal model rather than in the clinical context. Nevertheless, peptide solutions which provide a more complete range of amino acid delivery are under trial.

Skeleton: Bone disease has occurred because of inadequate provision of vitamin D and calcium, and the contamination of older amino

Table 7.8. *Suggested monitoring protocol for patients who are receiving long-term parenteral nutrition*

		Frequency	
Category	Measurement	Acute/hospital	Chronic/home
Clinical	Pulse, BP temp, respiration	4 hourly	As clinically indicated
	Fluid balance	Daily	As clinically indicated
	Weight	Daily	Monthly
	Inspection of exit site	Daily	Weekly
	Catheter hub	Daily	Daily
Blood	Sodium, potassium, chloride, urea glucose, haemoglobin, WCC + lymphocyte count	Daily	Monthly or as clinically indicated
	Calcium, magnesium, phosphorus, zinc, albumin, transferrin, bilirubin, alk. phos., AST, yGT	Twice weekly	Monthly or as clinically indicated
	Trace elements Screen	Not needed in short-term unless malnourished	1–3 monthly
Urine	Glucose	Daily	As clinically indicated
	Volume	Daily	As indicated
	Urea	Daily	As indicated
	Electrolytes	As indicated	As indicated
Anthropometrics	Weight Skin fold thickness Mid-arm muscle Circumference	Weekly	Monthly

acid solutions with aluminium. In addition, patients who receive prolonged parenteral nutrition appear at risk from osteoporosis (Koo, 1992). This may reflect changes in acid balance.

The heart: This can be adversely affected by the underprovision of selenium and thiamine, spread of infection from the catheter to the endocardium, and lipomatous deposits in the inter-atrial septum which is of uncertain clinical significance (Beau *et al.*, 1991). Intracardiac thrombus formation is rare in adult practice.

Monitoring

Patients who receive artificial nutritional support need monitoring. During the early phase of treatment, attention must be given to measurements of blood glucose and electrolytes. The fluid balance, and the temperature chart should be reviewed. Subsequent attention should be given to the adequacy of nutritional replacement and the continuing need for such treatment, in addition to the state of the underlying disease. The development of complications must be sought and treated as required. The influence of the disease and its treatment on the psychological welfare of the patient and the family must not be overlooked, especially in patients who need prolonged nutritional support at home.

Monitoring is best undertaken by a team which should include a nutrition nurse specialist, a dietitian, and a clinician with experience in gastroenterology. A suggested monitoring protocol for patients receiving parenteral nutrition is outlined in Table 7.8. Less intensive monitoring is needed for most patients who receive enteral nutrition. The adequacy of nutritional support is measured in the usual way. This includes the height and bone age in children.

References

Allwood, M. C., Brown, P. B., Ghedini, C. & Hardy, G. (1992). The stability of ascorbic acid in total parenteral nutrition mixtures stored in a multilayer bag. *Clinical Nutrition*, **11**, 284–8.

August, D., Thorn, D., Fisher, R. L. & Welchek, C. M. (1991). Home parenteral nutrition for patients with inoperable malignant bowel obstruction. *Journal of Parenteral and Enteral Nutrition*, **15**, 323–7.

Barbul, A., Rettura, G., Levenson, S. M. & Seifter, E. (1983). Wound healing and thymotrophic effects of arginine: a pituitary mechanism of action. *American Journal of Clinical Nutrition*, **37**, 786–94.

Beau, B., Michel, P., Coisne, D. *et al.* (1991). Lipomatous hypertrophy of the cardiac intraatrial septum. An unusual complication of long term home parenteral nutrition in adult patients. *Journal of Parenteral and Enteral Nutrition*, **15**, 659–62.

Black, D. D., Suttle, E. A. & Whittington, P. F. (1981). The effect of short term parenteral nutrition on hepatic function in the human neonate. A prospective randomised study demonstrating alteration of hepatic canalicular function. *Journal of Pediatrics*, **99**, 445–9.

Fisher, R. L. (1989). Hepatobiliary abnormalities associated with total parenteral nutrition. *Gastroenterology Clinics of North America*, **18**, 645–67.

Gayle, D. Pinchcofsky-Devlin, R. D. & Kaminski, M. V. (1985). Visceral protein increase associated with interrupt versus continuous enteral hyperalimentation. *Journal of Parenteral and Enteral Nutrition*, **9**, 474–6.

Jacobs, S., Chong, R. W. S., Lee, B. *et al.* (1990). Continuous enteral feeding: A major cause of pneumonia among ventilated intensive care unit patients. *Journal of Parenteral and Enteral Nutrition*, **14**, 353–6.

Johnston, D., Walker, K., Richard, J. & Pennington, C. R. (1992). An ethanol flush for the prevention of catheter occlusion. *Clinical Nutrition*, **11** (in press).

Kaminski, D. I., Adams, A. & Jellirek, M. (1980). The effect of hyperalimentation on hepatic lipid content and lipogenic enzyme activity in rats and man. *Surgery*, **88**, 93–100.

Katz, D. P., Kvetan, V. & Askanazi, J. (1990). Enteral nutrition: potential role in regulating immune function. *Current Opinion in Gastroenterology*, **6**, 199–203.

Koo, W. W. K. (1992). Parenteral nutrition related bone disease. *Journal of Parenteral and Enteral Nutrition*, **16**, 386–94.

Linares, J., Sitges-Sera, A., Garaas, J. *et al.* (1985). Pathogenesis of catheter sepsis: a prospective study with quantitative and semi-quantitative culture of hub and segments. *Journal of Clinical Microbiology*, **21**, 357–60.

McDonald, W. S., Sharp, C. W. & Deitch, E. A. (1992). Immediate enteral feeding in burn patients is safe and effective. *Annals of Surgery*, **21**, 177–83.

Mclave, S. A., Lowen, C. & Snider, H. L. (1992). Immunonutrition and enteral hyperalimentation of critically ill patients. *Digestive Diseases and Sciences*, **37**, 1153–61.

Messing, B., Man, R., Coliman, R. *et al.* (1990). Antibiotic lock technique as an effective treatment of bacterial catheter related sepsis during parenteral nutrition. *Clinical Nutrition*, **9**, 220–5.

Mosca, R., Curtas, S., Forbes, B. & Meguid, M. M. (1987). The benefits of isolator cultures in the management of suspected catheter sepsis. *Surgery*, **102**, 718–23.

Mughall, M. M. (1989). Complications of intravenous feeding catheters. *British Journal of Surgery*, **76**, 15–21.

O'Morain, C., Segal, A. W. & Levi, A. J. (1984). Elemental diet as primary treatment of acute Crohn's disease. *British Medical Journal*, **288**, 1859–63.

Park, R. H. R., Galloway, A., Shenkin, A. *et al.* (1990). Magnesium deficiency in patients on home enteral nutrition. *Clinical Nutrition*, **9**, 147–9.

Pennington, C. R. & Pithie, A. D. (1987). Ethanol lock in the management of catheter occlusion. *Journal of Parenteral and Enteral Nutrition*, **8**, 507–8.

Pithie, A. D. & Pennington, C. R. (1987). The incidence, aetiology and management of central vein thrombosis during parenteral nutrition. *Clinical Nutrition*, **6**, 151–3.

Pithie, A. D., Soutar, J. S. & Pennington, C. R. (1988). Catheter tip position in central vein thrombosis. *Journal of Parenteral and Enteral Nutrition*, **12**, 613–14.

Singer, P., Rothkopf, M. M., Kvetan, V. *et al.* (1991). Risks and benefits of home parenteral nutrition in the acquired immunodeficiency syndrome. *Journal of Parenteral and Enteral Nutrition*, **15**, 75–9.

Steigmann, G., Goff, J. S., Silas, D. *et al.* (1990). Endoscopic versus operative gastronomy: final results of prospective randomised trial. *Gastrointestinal Endoscopy*, **36**, 1–5.

Weiner, M., Rothkopf, M. M., Rothkopf, G. *et al.* (1987). Fat metabolism in injury and stress. *Critical Care Clinics*, **3**, 25–56.

Wicks, C., Gimson, A., Vlavionos, P. *et al.* (1992). Assessment of percutaneous endoscopic gastrostomy tube feeding as part of an integrated approach to enteral nutrition. *Gut*, **33**, 613–16.

Wilcock, H., Armstrong, J., Cottee, S. *et al.* (1991). Artificial nutritional support for the patients in the Cambridge health district. *Health Trends*, **23**, 93–100.

Zeigler, F., Olliver, J. M., Cynober, L. *et al.* (1990). Efficacy of enteral nutritional support in surgical patients; small peptides versus non-degraded proteins. *Gut*, **31**, 1277–83.

8

Is nutritional support worthwhile?

R. L. KORETZ

'Worthwhile: Important or valuable enough to repay time or effort
spent; of true value'

Webster's New World Dictionary
Second College Edition (1986)

Worthwhileness, like beauty, is in the eye of the beholder. For example, a young group of rock musicians may find it very important to spend hours practising, using a high-decibel sound system. If they do this in your backyard, you may not find these efforts very valuable at all. For purposes of this chapter, I am going to look at nutritional support (NS) from the perspective of a patient. The question to be asked is whether NS is of true value to that patient.

Hiram Studley noted, in 1936, that patients who died in the immediate postoperative period had 'regularly lost preoperatively a considerable portion of their weight' (Studley, 1936). He concluded that 'there is reason to believe that more patients will be saved provided efforts are concentrated on the preoperative preparation of those who have lost a good deal of weight, regardless of other appearances of the individual.' Over the next 30 years, investigators attempted to develop techniques to provide nutrition to individuals who could not, or would not, eat, and who had lost weight. The early attempts were frustrated by the volume and/or osmolality of the requisite infusates. These obstacles were overcome with the use of central vein catheters and superior vena caval infusions.

Since the 1960s, NS has grown into a multi-billion dollar (American) a year industry, spurred by the assumption that such an intervention would improve patient outcome. Therapeutic enthusiasts have made very optimistic claims; for example, Dudrick and Ruberg stated in 1971: '... the provision of adequate calories and nutrients given intravenously can significantly decrease the morbidity and mortality associated with a wide variety of disease processes' (Dudrick & Ruberg, 1971).

The basis for this wide acceptance of NS (parenteral NS (PNS) originally, but subsequently enteral NS (ENS) as well) rests on four lines

158

of 'evidence':

1. Any living organism, when deprived of nutrient intake for a long enough period, will die.
2. An individual with a given disease who is also malnourished has a poorer prognosis than does one with the same disease who is not malnourished (Studley's observation).
3. NS improves measured parameters of malnutrition (especially such things as body weight or nitrogen balance).
4. Retrospective or prospective (with or without non-randomized control groups) reports allegedly demonstrate therapeutic efficacy.

In consideration of these rationales for using NS as adjunctive treatment for various diseases, it would seem inherently obvious that any organism, if deprived of nutrients for a long enough period, will perish. Prisoners' of war experiences have, however, suggested that it was only when weight loss was excessive ($>40\%$), that mortality increased (Keys, 1962). Patients who suffer from underlying illnesses which then produce malnutrition ('secondary malnutrition') may not be comparable to healthy people who are starved ('primary malnutrition'); it is unknown if the degree of malnutrition which *causes* morbidity or mortality is less, the same, or even more.

The second rationale assumes that a causative association exists between nutritional and clinical parameters, that is, the malnutrition is responsible for the increased morbidity or mortality. However, the presence of an association between two factors does not prove a causative relationship. While malnutrition may cause the poor clinical outcome, it is also possible that malnourished patients have more severe disease, and that this more severe disease produces adverse nutritional and clinical consequences. In this latter case, the malnutrition is only a marker (a messenger) telling the clinician that severe disease exists. Killing the messenger would not alter the content of the message.

As we will see, the provision of NS has been shown to make certain nutritional parameters (tests) better. If our ultimate goal is to improve a test (which may be of value to the physician), these observations are quite important. However, if the objective is to make the quality and quantity of the patient's life better, we need to know that improving these tests improves clinical outcome.

A large number of opinions and/or uncontrolled (or poorly controlled) reports have been published attesting to the efficacy of NS. However, a more convincing test of efficacy would be the demonstration of an improved clinical outcome in a prospective randomised controlled trial (PRCT) comparing NS to a control group receiving no NS. This chapter will focus on the results of such PRCTs and look at the impact of either PNS or ENS on a variety of disease states. Separately, consideration will be given as to how NS affected clinical outcomes and how this therapy impacted on nutritional status. This latter analysis will more directly assess the issue of whether improving nutritional status improves clinical outcome.

Methodologic considerations

Through an ongoing review of the medical literature, as well as reviews of selected scientific medical meetings, 120 PRCTs (see Appendix) have been identified before early 1992. In these NS was compared to a control group receiving no more nutrition than the provision of standard foodstuffs and/or no more than 5% dextrose solutions intravenously. Recipients of PNS received at least intravenous nitrogen (in the form of amino acids or protein hydrolysates). Recipients of ENS participated in an organized effort to provide enteral nutrition through intensive nutritional counselling, additional commercial formula supplements, or enteral tube feedings. In all 120 studies, at least one clinical outcome (mortality, morbidity, or duration and/or cost of hospitalisation) was assessed. In 90 of them, at least one of the following 'nutritional outcomes' was also measured: body weight, triceps skinfold thickness, nitrogen balance, serum albumin.

In some of these reports (Reilly *et al.*, 1990; Hyde & Floch, 1984; Bonau *et al.*, 1984; Simms, Oliver & Smith, 1980; Hansell *et al.*, 1989; Muller *et al.*, 1986; Calvey, Davis & Williams, 1985; Evans *et al.*, 1987), two different NS regimens were compared to one control group. For the purposes of this analysis, each regimen was separately compared to the control group and thus considered a single trial. Two of the ENS reports (Harries *et al.*, 1983; Eriksson, Persson & Wahren, 1982) were randomised crossover trials.

Since the issue was the efficacy of NS, other studies in which the control groups received some form of non-nutritional therapy which was not available to the NS recipients, were excluded from the primary analysis, although they will be briefly considered later. An example of such a trial would be a comparison of elemental diets to steroid therapy in Crohn's disease.

Many of these PRCTs evaluated relatively small numbers of patients, and the possibility of a type 2 error (missing a difference which truly existed) was large. The data were thus considered not only from the perspective of statistical significance (in which the treated group had a 'statistically better' (SB) or 'statistically worse' (SW) outcome), but also from that of possible arithmetic trends. Any absolute difference in incidence between the two groups which was $> 5\%$ but not statistically significant, was considered to be 'better' (B) or 'worse' (W), depending on whether the differences favoured the treated or control group. If data were presented as absolute numbers, rather than incidences, B or W referred to the following differences: median survival > 1 month different (if there was < 1 year average survival in each group); mean albumin differences $\geqslant 0.3$ g%; mean hospital duration differences $\geqslant 3$ days; differences in frequency of analgesic usage $> 1/\text{day}$.

Effect of nutritional support on clinical outcome

The effects of NS on the mortality and morbidity associated with a wide variety of disease states are summarised in Tables 8.1 and 8.2. There was no obvious impact of either PNS or ENS on survival in any of the diseases studied. In only five PRCTs were any statistically significant differences seen. In three studies (Solassol, Joyeux & Dubois, 1979; Serrou *et al.*, 1981; Muller *et al.*, 1982), the PNS recipients fared better. In two others (Nixon *et al.*, 1981; Jordan *et al.*, 1981), the patients in the control groups survived longer.

The apparent beneficial effect of PNS on the morbidity of liver disease was mostly related to an improvement in the serum bilirubin. In four of the trials (Nasrallah & Galambos, 1980; Naveau *et al.*, 1986; Achord, 1987; Simon & Galambos, 1988), the elevated serum bilirubin did fall faster in the PNS recipients. However, in two of these reports (Naveau *et al.*, 1986; Simon & Galambos, 1988) the control groups had at least arithmetically better outcomes with regard to ascites, infection rates, and/or hepatic encephalopathy. Hence, these studies were considered to show no difference with regard to morbidity.

Several trials examined the role of parenteral branched-chained amino acids (BCAAs) in treating hepatic encephalopathy. In all of the studies, the recipients of the BCAAs had improvement in their encephalopathy (Koretz, 1986). This was also the conclusion of a meta-analysis (Naylor *et al.*, 1989). What cannot be determined from the design of these trials is whether this is due to nutritional supplementation or to a pharmacologic effect of the BCAAs. Even if the latter, this will be a very expensive way to treat encephalopathy (Koretz, 1986).

Table 8.1 *Summary of PRCTs of NS: effect on mortality*[a]

Route of NS	Disease state	Mortality B (SB)	No difference	W (SW)
PNS	Liver disease	4 (0)	2	1 (0)
	Inflammatory bowel disease	0	1	0
	Cancer therapy	3 (2[b])	9	7 (2)
	Pancreatitis	0	1	0
	Low birth weight infants	1 (0)	1	4 (0)
	Peri-operative	7 (1)	23	1 (0)
ENS	Liver disease	2 (0)	1	1 (0)
	Cancer therapy	4 (0)	3	1 (0)
	Peri-operative	2 (0)	4	1 (0)
	Hip fracture	1 (0)	1	0

PRCTs = Prospective randomised controlled trials.
NS = Nutritional support; PNS = Parenteral NS; ENS = Enteral NS.
B/W = Outcome in treated group better/worse than in control group (as defined in text).
SB/SW = Outcome in treated group statistically significantly better/worse than in control group.
[a] Numbers equal the number of PRCTs.
[b] Includes one study of terminal patients who received no radiation or chemotherapy.

Most of these latter trials of BCAAs were not included in this analysis because the control group received some type of NS (usually high-calorie infusions of glucose with or without lipid and with or without standard amino acid formulations). In the meta-analysis (Naylor *et al.*, 1989), it was suggested that there may have been a survival advantage in the recipients of BCAA-based PNS given with glucose as the sole calorie source. However, since the control groups received similar amounts of glucose without amino acids, and since BCAAs stimulate insulin release, it may have been a matter of having provided a survival disadvantage to the control group (i.e. giving glucose 'without insulin' to sick patients who tend to have glucose intolerance).

PNS appears to have a detrimental effect on cancer patients undergoing chemotherapy. In all of the trials in which data on infection rates were reported, the incidences were higher in the treated groups (Koretz, 1986). A meta-analysis of these studies led the American College of Physicians to release a position paper stating that 'the routine use of parenteral nutrition for patients undergoing chemotherapy should be strongly

Table 8.2. *Summary of PRCTs of NS: effect on morbidity*[a]

Route of NS	Disease state	Morbidity		
		B (SB)	No difference	W (SW)
PNS	Liver disease	5 (2)	2	0
	Inflammatory bowel disease	0	0	2 (0)
	Cancer therapy	5 (3)	1	11 (7)
	Pancreatitis	2 (0)	1	0
	Low birth weight infants	0	1	2 (2)
	Peri-operative	13 (3)	8[b]	11 (3)
ENS	Liver disease	3 (2)	2	1 (1)
	Inflammatory bowel disease	1 (0)	0	1 (1)
	Cancer therapy	9 (4)	2	2 (0)
	Peri-operative	9 (2)	3	3 (1)
	Chronic lung disease	2 (1)	0	0
	Hip fracture	2 (2)	0	0
	Colon preparation	1 (1)	1	0
	Amytrophic lateral sclerosis	1 (1)	0	0
	Allergic conditions	1 (1)	0	1 (0)

[a] Abbreviations all the same as in Table 8.1.
[b] Studies in which data only reported as 'no significant difference' assumed to show no difference at all.

discouraged' because 'the evidence suggests that parenteral nutritional support was associated with net harm, and no condition could be defined in which such treatment appeared to be of benefit' (American College of Physicians, 1989).

The clinical situation most often studied has been the perioperative one. The data in Table 8.2 would seem to suggest that the studies have shown no particular trend toward any benefit. A number of PRCTs evaluated the use of amino acids alone or given with only a small amount of glucose (Garden *et al.*, 1983; Hogbin, Smith & Craven, 1984; Hensle, 1978; Culebras-Fernandez *et al.*, 1987; Figueras *et al.*, 1988; Hansell *et al.*, 1989; Gys, Peeters & Hubens, 1990; Neuvonen *et al.*, 1986), a programme which might be considered to be inadequate 'nutritional support'. However, even if these trials are deleted from the analysis, the numbers of studies falling in the B (SB) column was about the same as those in the W (SW) column (10 (3) vs 9 (2)).

It is thus of interest to note that two meta-analyses of the surgical studies (Klein, Simes & Blackburn, 1986; Detsky *et al.*, 1987) both described at least trends towards improved morbidity in the recipients of the PNS.

A major problem in the 'scoreboard approach' employed is the inherent assumption that all PRCTs are created equal. This is not true, and thus one has to exercise a certain amount of caution in interpreting such data displays. PRCTs of higher quality should obviously be given more weight.

One of the 'quality' issues in any PRCT is the size of the trial, since one containing a small number of patients may not yield a statistically significant result (the classic 'type II' or 'beta' error). Attempts to get around this issue have been made by looking for the presence of arithmetic differences, since, if the therapy offers a less than dramatic benefit, the recipients of it should have an 'edge' and should tend to have at least arithmetically better outcomes. However, other quality issues may be obscuring the analysis. Meta-analysis is a mathematical way of assessing and weighing the overall quality of a trial and may be a more appropriate way to assess these data.

In one of the meta-analyses of the surgical studies (Detsky *et al.*, 1987), there was a trend ($p = 0.21$) for the PNS recipient to have an absolute reduction in the post-operative complication rate of 5%. In the other meta-analysis (Klein, Simes & Blackburn 1986), it was claimed that PNS would halve the incidence of major complications, although the absolute rate was not stated. Both of these meta-analyses were done prior to the publication of a number of other trials, including the largest PRCT in the NS literature, the Veterans Affairs study. In this study, more than 400 patients were randomised (Veterans Affairs Total Parenteral Nutrition Cooperative Study Group, 1991). In that trial, the recipients of the PNS had an arithmetically higher mortality rate (13% vs 11%), an arithmetically lower post-operative non-infectious complication rate (17% vs 22%), and a statistically significantly higher post-operative infectious complication rates (14% vs 6%). When Dr Klein included these later trials, he found that the use of PNS may be associated with an absolute reduction in the major complication rate of 5% (S. Klein, personal communication).

If the assumption is that PNS will provide a 5% benefit, if a patient needs seven to ten days of pre-operative PNS, at $800 (American) per day (Twomey & Patching, 1985), it will cost $112–160 000 to treat the 20 patients needed to prevent one complication. This limited benefit may be too expensive, a fact alluded to by others (Heatley, Williams & Lewis, 1979).

A discussion of the effect of PNS on morbidity would not be complete without considering one more issue. It has already been noted that there were higher infection rates (not just contaminations of the central venous line) in the recipients of PNS who were receiving cancer chemotherapy. A similar phenomenon was also seen in the Veterans Affairs peri-operative study, in which the recipients of pre-operative PNS had more post-operative infections. A recent meta-analysis of mostly unpublished trials comparing ENS to PNS in critically ill patients also found higher infection rates in the recipients of PNS (Moore *et al.*, 1992). Does PNS, in some way, pre-dispose patients to having more infections? If it does, then any clinical advantage it can provide will have to overcome this disadvantage.

The data regarding the impact of ENS on morbidity are more promising. A variety of particular disease states have been studied.

At least one significant difference in morbidity (always favouring the treated group) was seen in four (out of 11) PRCTs evaluating ENS in cancer patients undergoing radiation and/or chemotherapy. In three trials (Bounous *et al.*, 1975; Foster *et al.*, 1980; Lipschitz & Mitchell, 1980) there was better preservation of the leucocyte count. In one trial there was less diarrhoea (Bounous *et al.*, 1975) and, in another, less mucositis (Tandon *et al*, 1984). In other trials, there were arithmetical trends showing improved haematological parameters (Elkort *et al.*, 1981), less gastro-intestinal toxicity (Bounous, Gentile & Hugon, 1971; Nayel, El-Ghoneimy & El-Haddad, 1992; Cousineau *et al.*, 1973), better performance status (Tandon *et al.*, 1984; Nayel, El-Ghoneimy & El-Haddad, 1992) and better tumour response (Tandon *et al.*, 1984). However, beneficial arithmetical trends were not uniformly found. ENS recipients in other studies had arithmetically more severe gastrointestinal toxicity (Evans *et al.*, 1987 (one colorectal subgroup); Elkort *et al.*, 1981) and poorer tumour response (Bounous, Gentile & Hugon, 1971; Moloney, Moriarty & Daly, 1983). Since other studies showed no apparent differences (Evans *et al.*, 1987 (other sub-groups)), we cannot conclude that ENS is of benefit. However, the general trend for the results to have been better in the treatment groups should give impetus to conducting larger cooperative trials in various types of cancer, in an attempt to establish efficacy. There was no apparent increase in infectious complications in the recipients of ENS, as there was in those given PNS.

Most of the perioperative trials evaluated the utility of post-operative small intestinal feeding, and there were no apparent effects attributable to that intervention. A few of these studies examined the role of pre-operative ENS, and these will be examined in more detail.

Shukla *et al.* (1984) described a dramatic reduction in the incidence of post-operative wound infections in the treated group (10%, vs 37% in controls). Unfortunately, this study may have had a major breakdown in randomisation, as there was a significantly higher prevalence of cancer in the control group. Foschi *et al.* (1986) also reported an ENS-associated significant reduction in post-operative complications in patients with obstructive jaundice. Four patients were deleted from the ENS group because of metastatic disease or pre-operative biliary drainage complications. If these four also had post-operative complications, the differences would no longer be significant (intent-to-treat analysis). Two trials found arithmetically fewer post-operative complications in the ENS recipients (Flynn & Leightty, 1987; Meijerink *et al.*, 1992), although another one (Gurry & Ellis-Pegler, 1976) did not make this observation. These promising data should serve as the basis for developing a large PRCT to evaluate pre-operative enteral feedings. Because of the flaws in the two studies which claimed to show significant differences, it is premature to conclude that pre-operative ENS has been proven to be effective.

In an unblinded trial of enteral supplementation, patients with chronic lung disease had significant improvements in a series of subjective or effort-dependent parameters (Efthimiou *et al.*, 1988). In a small double-blinded study, there was a less impressive arithmetic improvement in subjective well-being (Otte *et al.*, 1989). This is yet another area where a large PRCT is needed.

Two trials have examined the role of nutritional supplements in elderly patients with hip fractures (Bastow, Rawlings & Allison, 1983; Delmi *et al.*, 1990). Both trials showed significant improvements in various aspects of healing. This is one area where ENS has proven efficacy.

Nine trials have compared elemental diets to steroids as primary therapy for Crohn's disease (Lochs *et al.*, 1991; Koretz, 1990). These studies are not included in the primary analysis because NS was not being compared to an untreated control group. The original reports contained relatively small numbers of patients and no significant differences in response rates were noted, leading the authors to conclude that both forms of therapy were equally efficacious. However, some of the trials excluded patients who could not tolerate the elemental diets. By intent-to-treat analysis, the steroid recipients had better outcomes. Indeed, in two larger studies, the groups randomised to elemental diets had significantly poorer response rates. Because of differences in the types of diets used, the relative efficacy of elemental diets containing only amino acids or very small peptides (theoretically containing no protein allergens) has not yet been established or refuted.

There are more limited data available concerning the impact of NS on the duration and cost of hospitalisation. These are available in the Appendix; no overall effect is apparent.

Up until now we have been considering the effect of NS on other diseases. A small number of patients have primary gastrointestinal tract inadequacy, that is, they are unable to assimilate enough nutrients to survive. If that state persists long enough, such patients will die of 'starvation'. When this condition is permanent, the only available therapy is long-term PNS, and performing a PRCT to establish efficacy is inappropriate. What is less clear is how long such a temporary state can exist before primary malnutrition becomes an important factor. It is likely that any patient can survive a few days and that most patients cannot survive a few months. For purposes of making clinical decisions as to how long to wait before beginning NS (usually PNS) to prevent the added problem of primary malnutrition, a period of three weeks has been chosen for my practice. This arbitrary decision was based on the observation that some PRCTs evaluated NS for periods of time of two weeks and failed to show any improvement in clinical outcome.

Effect of nutritional support on nutritional outcome

The effects of NS on body weight, triceps skinfold thickness, nitrogen balance, and serum albumin are summarised in Tables 8.3–8.6. As is obvious, NS appears to have much more profound effects on these parameters than on those of clinical outcome.

In 40 of 60 (67%) studies in which body weight information was available, weight was better preserved in the recipients of NS. Most of these differences were statistically significant.

The impact of NS on triceps skinfold thickness is also apparent. The recipients of NS had better measurements in 16 of the 26 (63%) PRCTs; again, most of the trials in which such differences were seen demonstrated statistical significance in the change.

Perhaps the most dramatic impact on NS on any parameter was its effect on nitrogen balance. All but one of the 33 trials (97%) demonstrated an improvement, and these differences were again usually statistically significant.

Another observation should be noted concerning the effect of NS on these three parameters. In no study was the outcome better (even arithmetically so) in the control group. In fact, it was only the serum albumin for which any trials were identified in which the control group fared better (Naveau *et al.*, 1986; Nixon *et al.*, 1981; Clamon *et al.*, 1985;

Table 8.3. *Summary of PRCTs of NS: effect on body weight*[a]

Route of NS	Disease state	Body weight		
		B (SB)	No difference	W (SW)
PNS	Liver disease	0	1	0
	Inflammatory bowel disease	0	1	0
	Cancer therapy	16 (12)	2	0
	Low birth weight infants	5 (5)	0	0
	Peri-operative	6 (6)	4	0
ENS	Liver disease	1 (1)	1	0
	Inflammatory bowel disease	1 (1)	0	0
	Cancer therapy	4 (4)	7	0
	Peri-operative	4 (4)	4	0
	Chronic lung disease	2 (2)	0	0
	Hip fracture	1 (1)	0	0

[a] Abbreviations all the same as in Table 8.1.

Table 8.4. *Summary of PRCTs of NS: effect on triceps skinfold thickness*[a]

Route of NS	Disease state	Tricep skinfold thickness		
		B (SB)	No difference	W (SW)
PNS	Liver disease	1 (0)	2[b]	0
	Cancer therapy	6 (4)	2	0
	Low birth weight infants	0	2	0
	Peri-operative	1 (1)	0	0
ENS	Liver disease	2 (1)	2[b]	0
	Inflammatory bowel disease	1 (1)	0	0
	Cancer therapy	1 (1)	2	0
	Peri-operative	1 (1)	0	0
	Chronic lung disease	2 (2)	0	0
	Hip fracture	1 (1)	0	0

[a] Abbreviations all the same as in Table 8.1.
[b] 'No significant difference' assumed to be no difference at all (as in Table 8.2).

Simko, 1983). Two of these four studies evaluated patients with liver disease, in whom serum albumin levels may have reflected underlying synthetic dysfunction rather than limited nitrogen availability. In fact, one might wonder how closely the serum albumin reflects nutrient deficiency

Table 8.5. *Summary of PRCTs of NS: effect on nitrogen balance*[a]

Route of NS	Disease state	Nitrogen balance		
		B (SB)	No difference	W (SW)
PNS	Liver disease	3 (2)	0	0
	Cancer therapy	2 (2)	0	0
	Pancreatitis	3 (3)	0	0
	Peri-operative	19 (14)	0	0
ENS	Liver disease	2 (1)	1	0
	Peri-operative	3 (3)	0	0

[a] Abbreviations all the same as in Table 8.1.

Table 8.6. *Summary of PRCTs of NS: effect on serum albumin*[a]

Route of NS	Disease state	Morbidity		
		B (SB)	No difference	W (SW)
PNS	Liver disease	3 (3)	1	1 (1)
	Cancer therapy	3 (1)	4	2 (2)
	Pancreatitis	0	2	0
	Low birth weight infants	2 (1)	0	0
	Peri-operative	4 (3)	10[b]	0
ENS	Liver disease	1 (1)	1	1 (1)
	Inflammatory bowel disease	1 (1)	0	0
	Cancer therapy	3 (2)	2	0
	Peri-operative	1 (1)	2	0
	Chronic lung disease	2 (2)	0	0
	Hip fracture	1 (1)	0	0

[a] Abbreviations all the same as in Table 8.1.
[b] 'No significant difference' assumed to be no difference at all.

in general. In patients with underlying inflammatory or malignant disease, various mediators (e.g. cytokines) may inhibit albumin synthesis even in the presence of adequate amino acid stores (Merritt *et al.*, 1985). Although many of the trials (21/47, 45%) did demonstrate that NS had a beneficial effect on serum albumin, this observation was less universal than it was for the other three nutritional parameters.

What should be obvious is that there is much more available evidence that NS can improve nutritional parameters than that showing it has a

Table 8.7. *Classification of studies by nutritional and clinical outcomes*

		Nutritional outcome		
		B (or SB)	No difference	W (or SW)
	B (or SB)	C	PD–CI	CD–CI
Clinical	No difference	PD–NI	C	PD–CI
Outcome	W (or SW)	CD–NI	PD–NI	C

B (SB) = Outcome better (statistically significantly better) in treatment group.
No difference = No difference (no statistically significant difference) in outcome.
W (SW) = Outcome worse (statistically significantly worse) in treated group.
C = Concordance; CI = Clinical improved; NI = Nutritional improved;
PD = Partial discordance [one outcome 0, the other B (SB) or W (SW)].
   PD–CI – Clinical outcome B (or SB), Nutritional outcome not different
           Clinical outcome not different, Nutritional outcome W (or SW).
   PD–NI – Nutritional outcome B (or SB), Clinical outcome not different
           Nutritional outcome not different, Clinical outcome W (or SW).
CD = Complete discordance.
   CD–CI – Clinical outcome B (or SB), Nutritional outcome W (or SW).
   CD–NI – Nutritional outcome B (or SB), Clinical outcome W (or SW).

favourable impact on clinical outcome. This, in turn, brings into question the nature of the relationship between malnutrition and a poor prognosis. If the association is causative, then improving the former should improve the latter. Since, in general, NS has been successful in doing the former, its relative failure in the latter suggests that the association is not causal.

This relationship can be investigated in more detail by considering the impact of NS on clinical and nutritional outcomes in individual studies. In the following analysis, only the 90 PRCTs which provided data on nutritional as well as clinical outcome were employed.

As discussed, if the association between malnutrition and outcome is causative, then NS would be expected to be effective only if it improved the nutritional parameters. In other words, a necessary condition to establish causality would be the demonstration of a concordance between nutritional and clinical outcomes. If the studies were to be arrayed as schematically demonstrated in Table 8.7, the large majority of them should line up in the spaces marked 'C' (for concordance). If the particular PRCT is located in one of the spaces labelled 'PD' (for partial discord-ance), then one of the outcomes was better or worse while the other was not. If the PRCT showed a B (or SB) outcome in either a nutritional

Table 8.8. *Nutritional outcome versus mortality*[a]

Nutritional outcome	Concordance	Partial discordance		Complete discordance		Per cent concordance
		CI	NI	CI	NI	
Body weight	14 (16)	3 (0)	14 (25)	0 (0)	11 (1)	33% (38%)
Nitrogen balance	6 (8)	0 (0)	17 (17)	0 (0)	2 (0)	24% (32%)
Triceps skinfold thickness	8 (12)	2 (0)	6 (7)	0 (0)	3 (0)	42% (63%)
Albumin	17 (21)	6 (3)	9 (11)	0 (0)	3 (0)	49% (60%)

CI = Clinical outcome better than nutritional one; NI = Nutritional outcome better then clinical one.
PRCT = Prospective randomised controlled trial.

$$\text{Per cent concordance} = \frac{\text{Number PRCTs concordant for that nutritional outcome}}{\text{Number PRCTs evaluating that nutritional outcome}}$$

[a] Numbers outside parentheses are numbers of studies when all arithmetical differences considered as better or worse. (Numbers in parentheses are the numbers when only statistically significant differences were considered.) As before, studies in which the data were reported as 'No significant difference' were assumed to show no difference at all.

Table 8.9. *Nutritional outcome versus morbidity*[a]

Nutritional outcome	Concordance	Partial discordance		Complete discordance		Per cent concordance
		CI	NI	CI	NI	
Body weight	20 (27)	10 (1)	9 (16)	0 (0)	14 (9)	38% (51%)
Nitrogen balance	13 (8)	0 (0)	9 (20)	0 (0)	9 (3)	42% (26%)
Triceps skinfold thickness	9 (9)	4 (4)	6 (8)	0 (0)	6 (4)	36% (36%)
Albumin	19 (26)	13 (7)	7 (7)	0 (0)	2 (1)	46% (63%)

CI, NI, PRCT and per cent concordance all as in Table 8.8.
Numbers outside and inside parentheses are the same as in Table 8.8.

or clinical parameter and a W (or SW) outcome in the other, complete discordance is present.

The data from analyses of these 90 trials are summarized in Tables 8.8 and 8.9, in which mortality and morbidity are separately compared to the four nutritional outcomes. All of the PRCTs are considered jointly, as there was no particular difference seen when individual disease states or route of NS were considered separately. There was substantial discordance (usually indicating that nutritional parameters fared better than clinical ones) regarding the impact of NS on clinical and nutritional outcomes, whether only statistically significant differences or all arithmetical ones were considered. This discordance was seen less frequently when serum albumin was used as the nutritional parameter, but even in this case over a third of the studies had this dissociation. These data suggest that a causal association is absent; they also again remind us that making nutritional status better will not guarantee that clinical improvement will ensue.

Conclusions

While the rationale(s) for NS may have a certain intuitive appeal, data from PRCTs have not been dramatically supportive. This is especially true for PNS, where evidence is beginning to emerge that the therapy may even have a previously unsuspected detrimental side effect.

It is clear from the above that several areas may exist where clinical benefit could be present, but data from large well-designed PRCTs are lacking. This is particularly true for ENS used as pre-operative preparation, in patients undergoing radiation and/or chemotherapy, and as support for advanced lung disease. The role of NS in liver disease is also not completely settled; we need large trials which will compare nutritional therapy (with and without the inclusion of BCAA-based formulations) to true control groups. There is a paucity of data comparing critically-ill nutritionally supported patients to non-nutritionally supported controls.

There are only two areas where we can consider NS as having established efficacy. One is the provision of supplements to older patients with hip fractures. The other is in the long-term management of patients with permanent gastro-intestinal tract inadequacy. While no PRCT has been done in the latter individuals, it would make no more sense to advocate that one be performed than it would be to call for a PRCT of chronic haemodialysis.

There are some patients who, while they do not have permanent 'short bowel syndrome', will be unable to eat for a period of weeks, e.g. patients with complicated intestinal fistulae or severe pancreatitis. We do not know how long is too long to go without 'eating'; perhaps insight into this question will emerge from future PRCTs, especially in those performed in the critically ill.

Future PRCTs must overcome the deficiencies of the past. Large enough numbers of patients must be included to ensure that less than dramatic but clinically meaningful differences are not being missed. Since previous trials have not found that NS has a dramatic effect, true control groups must be included, ones that receive no NS. It is not unethical to do so; NS is potentially dangerous, expensive, and without established efficacy. If it were a drug, it is unlikely that the United States Food and Drug Administration could find enough data to allow its use as 'therapy' in the wide variety of disease processes for which it has been proposed. The end points of these studies must be clinical, not nutritional, parameters. It has been established that improving body weight, anthropometrics, nitrogen balance, or even serum albumin (which may not even be a nutritional parameter) does not necessarily improve patient outcome.

Is NS worthwhile? It may be for physicians and other members of the health care team; they all obtain senses of fulfilment from providing a therapy which tests their skills, which produces 'beneficial' effects in some tests, and which even provides financial reward. It behooves us to make sure that this medical music will soothe our patients' ears.

References

Abel, R. M., Fischer, J. E., Buckley, M. J., Barnett, G. O. & Austen, W. G. (1976). Malnutrition in cardiac surgical patients. *Archives of Surgery*, **11**, 45–50.

Achord, J. (1987). A prospective randomized clinical trial of peripheral amino acid–glucose supplementation in acute alcoholic hepatitis. *American Journal of Gastroenterology*, **82**, 871–5.

American College of Physicians (1989). Parenteral nutrition in patients receiving cancer chemotherapy. *Annals of Internal Medicine*, **110**, 734–6.

Baker, F. S. (1978). Elemental diet and postoperative pain. *Diseases of the Colon and Rectum*, **21**, 535.

Bastow, M. D., Rawlings, J. & Allison, S. P. (1983). Benefits of supplementary tube feeding after fractured neck of femur: a randomised controlled trial. *British Medical Journal*, **287**, 1589–92.

Bellantone, R., Doglietto, G. B., Bossola, M. *et al.*, (1988). Preoperative parenteral nutrition in the high risk surgical patient. *Journal of Parenteral and Enteral Nutrition*, **12**, 195–7.

Bonau, R. A., Ang, S. D., Jeevanandam, M. & Daly, J. M. (1984). High-branched chain amino acid solutions: relationship of composition to efficacy. *Journal of Parenteral and Enteral Nutrition*, **8**, 622–7.

Bonkovsky, H. L., Fiellin, D. A., Smith, G. S. *et al.* (1991*a*). A randomized controlled trial of treatment of alcoholic hepatitis with parenteral nutrition and oxandrolone. I. Short-term effects on liver function. *American Journal of Gastroenterology*, **86**, 1200–8.

Bonkovsky, H. L., Singh, R. H., Jafri, I. H. *et al.* (1991*b*). A randomized controlled trial of treatment of alcoholic hepatitis with parenteral nutrition and oxandrolone. II. Short-term effects on nitrogen metabolism, metabolic balance, and nutrition. *American Journal of Gastroenterology*, **86**, 1208–18.

Bounous, G., Gentile, J. M. & Hugon, J. (1971). Elemental diet in the management of the intestinal lesion produced by 5-fluorouracil in man. *Canadian Journal of Surgery*, **14**, 312–24.

Bounous, G., LeBel, E., Shuster, J., Gold, P., Tahan, E. T. & Bastin, E. (1975). Dietary protection during radiation therapy. *Strahlentherapie*, **149**, 476–83.

Brans, Y. W., Summers, J. E., Dweck, H. S. & Cassady, G. (1974). Feeding the low birth weight infant: orally or parenterally? Preliminary results of a comparative study. *Pediatrics*, **54**, 15–23.

Cabre, E., Gonzalez-Huix, F., Abad-Lacruz, A. *et al.* (1990). Effect of total enteral nutrition in the short-term outcome of severely malnourished cirrhotics. *Gastroenterology*, **98**, 715–20.

Calvey, H., Davis, M. & Williams, R. (1985). Controlled trial of nutritional supplementation, with and without branched chain amino acid enrichment, in treatment of acute alcoholic hepatitis. *Journal of Hepatology*, **1**, 141–51.

Clamon, G. H., Feld, R., Evans, W. K. *et al.* (1985). Effect of adjuvant central i.v. hyperalimentation on the survival and response to treatment of patients with small lung cancer: a randomized trial. *Cancer Treatment Reports*, **69**, 169–77.

Coquin, J. Y., Maraninchi, D., Gastaut, J. A. & Carcassone, Y. (1981). Influence of parenteral nutrition (PN) on chemotherapy and survival of acute leukemias (AL); preliminary results of a randomized trial. (Abstract). *Journal of Parenteral and Enteral Nutrition*, **5**, 357.

Cousineau, L., Bounous, G., Rochon, M., Shuster, J., Gold, P. & Tahan, W. (1973). The use of an elemental diet during treatment with anticancer agents (Abstract). *Clinical Research*, **21**, 1067.

Cromack, D., Moley, J., Pass, H. *et al.* (1988). Prospective randomized trial of parenteral nutrition (TPN) compared to ad lib oral nutrition (ON) in patients with upper GI cancer and weight loss undergoing surgical treatment (Abstract). *Program of the 22nd Annual Meeting of the Association for Academic Surgery*, Salt Lake City, Utah, November 1988, p. 86.

Crossland, S. G., Geelhoed, G. W. & Guy, D. G. (1981). Evaluation of benefits of different nutritional pre- and postoperative management of hemor-rhoidectomy patients. *American Journal of Proctology, Gastroenterology and Colon and Rectal Surgery*, **32**(5), 8–14.

Culebras-Fernandez, J. M., de la Hoz Riesco, M., Garcia, C. V., Fernando-Llamazares, G. H. & Villalba, A. A. (1987). Improvement of the nutritional condition with hypocaloric peripheral parenteral nutrition (HPPN) in the immediate postoperative period of elective abdominal surgery. *Infusionstherapie*, **14**, 202–8.

Delmi, M., Rapin, C., Bengoa, J., Delmas, P. D., Vasey, H. & Bonjour, J. (1990). Dietary supplementation in elderly patients with fractured neck of the femur. *Lancet*, **335**, 1013–6.

Detsky, A. S., Baker, J. P., O'Rourke, K. & Goel, V. (1987). Perioperative parenteral nutrition: a meta-analysis. *Annals of Internal Medicine*, **107**, 195–203.

Dickinson, R. J., Ashton, M. G., Axon, A. T. R., Smith, R. C., Yeung, C. K. & Hill, G. L. (1980). Controlled trial of intravenous hyperalimentation and total bowel rest as an adjunct to the routine therapy of acute colitis. *Gastroenterology*, **79**, 1199–204.

Donaldson, S. S., Wesley, M. N., Ghavimi, F., Shils, M. E., Suskind, R. M. & DeWys, W. D. (1982). A prospective randomized clinical trial of total parenteral nutrition in children with cancer. *Medical and Pediatric Oncology*, **10**, 129–39.

Douglas, H. O., Milliron, S., Nava, H. *et al.* (1978). Elemental diet as an adjuvant for patients with locally advanced gastrointestinal cancer receiving radiation therapy: a prospectively randomized study. *Journal of Parenteral and Enteral Nutrition*, **2**, 682–6.

Drott, C., Unsgaard, B., Schersten, T. & Lundholm, K. (1988). Total parenteral nutrition as an adjuvant to patients undergoing chemotherapy for testicular carcinoma: protection of body composition – a randomized, prospective study. *Surgery*, **103**, 499–506.

Dudrick, S. J. & Ruberg, R. L. (1971). Principles and practices of parenteral nutrition. *Gastroenterology*, **61**, 901–10.

Efthimiou, J., Fleming, J., Gomes, C. & Spiro, S. G. (1988). The effect of supplementary oral nutrition in poorly nourished patients with chronic obstructive pulmonary disease. *American Review of Respiratory Disease*, **137**, 1075–82.

Elkort, R. J., Baker, F. L., Vitale, J. J. & Cordano, A. (1981). Long-term nutritional support as an adjunct to chemotherapy for breast cancer. *Journal of Parenteral and Enteral Nutrition*, **5**, 385–90.

Elmore, M. F., Gallagher, S. C., Jones, J. G., Koons, K. K., Schmalhausen, A. W. & Strange, P. S. (1989). Esophagogastric decompression and enteral feeding following cholecystectomy: a controlled, randomized prospective trial. *Journal of Parenteral and Enteral Nutrition*, **13**, 377–81.

Eriksson, L. S., Persson, A. & Wahren, J. (1982). Branched-chain amino acids in the treatment of chronic encephalopathy. *Gut*, **23**, 801–6.

Evans, W. K., Nixon, D. W., Daly, J. M. *et al.*, (1987). A randomized study of oral nutritional support versus *ad lib* nutritional intake during chemotherapy for advanced colorectal and non-small-cell lung cancer. *Journal of Clinical Oncology*, **5**, 113–24.

Figueras, J., Puig, P., Rafecas, A. *et al.* (1988). Postoperative hypocaloric parenteral nutrition. *Acta Chirurgica Scandinavica*, **154**. 435–8.

Fletcher, J. P. & Little, J. M. (1986). A comparison of parenteral nutrition and early postoperative enteral feeding on the nitrogen balance after major surgery. *Surgery*, **100**, 21–4.

Flynn, M. B. & Leightty, F. F. (1987). Preoperative outpatient nutritional support of patients with squamous cancer of the upper aerodigestive tract. *American Journal of Surgery*, **154**, 359–62.

Foschi, D., Cavagna, G., Callioni, F., Morandi, E. & Rovati, V. (1986). Hyperalimentation of jaundiced patients on percutaneous transhepatic biliary drainage. *British Journal of Surgery*, **73**, 716–19.

Foster, K. J., Brown, M. S., Alberti, G. M. M. *et al.* (1980). The metabolic effects of abdominal irradiation in man with and without dietary therapy with an elemental diet. *Clinical Radiology*, **31**, 13–17.

Frankel, A. M. & Horowitz, G. D. (1989). Nasoduodenal tubes in short-stay cholecystectomy. *Surgery, Gynecology, and Obstetrics*, **168**, 433–6.

Garden, O. J., Smith, A., Harris, N. W. S., Shenkin, A., Sim, A. J. W. & Carter, D. C. (1983). The effect of isotonic amino acid infusion on serum proteins and muscle breakdown following surgery. *British Journal of Surgery*, **70**, 79–82.

Ghavimi, F., Shils, M. E., Scott, B. F., Brown, M. & Tamaroff, M. (1982). Comparison of morbidity in children requiring abdominal radiation and chemotherapy, with and without total parenteral nutrition. *Journal of Pediatrics*, **101**, 530–7.

Gurry, J. F. & Ellis-Pegler, R. B. (1976). An elemental diet as preoperative preparation of the colon. *British Journal of Surgery*, **63**, 969–72.

Gutwein, I., Baer, J. & Holt, P. R. (1981). The effect of a formula diet in preparation of the colon for barium enema examination. *Archives of Internal Medicine*, **141**, 993–6.

Gys, T., Peeters, R. & Hubens, A. (1990). The value of short-term peripheral parenteral nutrition after colorectal surgery: a comparative study with conventional postoperative intravenous fluid. *Acta Chirurgica Belgica*, **90**, 234–9.

Hansell, D. T., Davies, J. W. L., Shenkin, A., Garden, O. J., Burns, H. J. G. & Carter, D. (1989). The effects of an anabolic steroid and peripherally administered intravenous nutrition in the early postoperative period. *Journal of Parenteral and Enteral Nutrition*, **13**, 349–58.

Harries, A. D., Jones, J. A., Danis, V. *et al.* (1983). Controlled trial of supplemented oral nutrition in Crohn's disease. *Lancet*, **i**, 887–90.

Hays, D. M., Merritt, R. J., White, L., Ashley, J. & Siegel, S. E. (1983). Effect of total parenteral nutrition on marrow recovery during induction therapy for acute nonlymphocytic leukemia in childhood. *Medical and Pediatric Oncology*, **11**, 134–40.

Heatley, R. V., Williams, R. H. P. & Lewis, M. H. (1979). Preoperative intravenous feeding – a controlled trial. *Postgraduate Medical Journal*, **55**, 541–5.

Hensle, T. W. (1978). Protein-sparing in cystectomy patients. *Journal of Urology*, **119**, 355–8.

Hogbin, B. M., Smith, A. M. & Craven, A. H. (1984). An evaluation of peripheral essential amino acid infusion following major surgery. *Journal of Parenteral and Enteral Nutrition*, **8**, 511–14.

Hoj, L., Osterballe, O., Bundgaard, A., Weeke, B. & Weiss, M. (1981). A double-blind controlled trial of elemental diet in severe, perennial asthma. *Allergy*, **36**, 257–62.

Holter, A. R. & Fischer, J. E. (1977). The effects of perioperative hyperalimentation on complications in patients with carcinoma and weight loss. *Journal of Surgical Research*, **23**, 31–4.

Hoover, H. C., Ryan, J. A., Anderson, E. J. & Fischer, J. E. (1980). Nutritional benefits of immediate postoperative jejunal feeding of an elemental diet. *American Journal of Surgery*, **139**, 153–9.

Hyde, D. & Floch, M. H. (1984). The effect of peripheral nutritional support and nitrogen balance in acute pancreatitis (Abstract). *Gastroenterology*, **86**, 1119.

Imes, S., Pinchbeck, B., Dinwoodie, A., Walker, K. & Thomson, A. B. R. (1986). Effect of Ensure®, a defined formula diet, in patients with Crohn's disease. *Digestion*, **35**, 158–69.

Issell, B. F., Valdivieso, M. D., Zaren, H. A. *et al.* (1978). Protection against chemotherapy toxicity by i.v. hyperalimentation. *Cancer Treatment Reports*, **62**, 1139–43.

Jensen, S. (1982). Parenteral nutrition and cancer surgery (Abstract). *Journal of Parenteral and Enteral Nutrition*, **6**, 335.

Jensen, S. (1985). Clinical effects of enteral and parenteral nutrition preceding cancer surgery. *Medical Oncology and Tumor Pharmacotherapy*, **2**, 225–9.

Jordan, W. M., Valdivieso, M., Frankmann, C. *et al.*, (1981). Treatment of advanced adenocarcinoma of the lung with ftoratur, doxorubicin, cyclophosphamide, and cisplatin (FACP) and intensive i.v. hyperalimentation. *Cancer Treatment Reports*, **65**, 197–205.

Kearns, P. J., Young, H., Garcia, G. *et al.* (1992). Accelerated improvement of alcoholic liver disease with enteral nutrition. *Gastroenterology*, **102**, 200–5.

Keys, A. (1962). Caloric deficiency and starvation. In *Clinical Nutrition*, ed. N. Joliffe, 2nd edn., pp. 122–36, Harper and Brothers, New York.

Kinsella, J. J., Malcolm, A. W., Bothe, A., Valerio, D. & Blackburn, G. L. (1981). Prospective study of nutritional support during pelvic irradiation. *International Journal of Radiation Oncology and Biological Physics*, 7, 543–8.

Klein, S., Simes, J. & Blackburn, G. (1986). Total parenteral nutrition and cancer clinical trials. *Cancer*, 58, 1378–86.

Koretz, R. L. (1986). Nutritional support: how much for how much. *Gut*, 27 (Suppl. 1), 85–95.

Koretz, R. L. (1990). Predigested diets: should we mash the meat when we mash the potatoes? *Nutrition in Clinical Practice*, 5, 241–6.

Lanzotti, V., Copeland, E., Bhuchar, V., Wesley, M., Correira, J. & Dudrick, S. (1980). A randomized trial of total parenteral nutrition (TPN) with chemotherapy for non-oat cell lung cancer (NOCLC). (Abstract). *Proceedings of the American Association for Cancer Research and the American Society of Clinical Oncology*, 21, 377.

Lipschitz, D. A. & Mitchell, C. O. (1980). Enteral hyperalimentation and hematopoietic toxicity caused by chemotherapy of small cell lung cancer (Abstract). *Journal of Parenteral and Enteral Nutrition*, 4, 593.

Lochs, H., Steinhardt, H. J., Klaus-Wents, B. *et al.* (1991). Comparison of enteral nutrition and drug treatment in active Crohn's disease. *Gastroenterology*, 101, 881–8.

McIntyre, P. B., Powell-Tuck, J., Wood, S. R. *et al.* (1986). Controlled trial of bowel rest in the treatment of severe acute colitis. *Gut*, 27, 481–5.

Meijerink, W. J. H. J., Von Meyenfeldt, M. F., Rouflart, M. M. J. & Soeters, P. B. (1992). Efficacy of perioperative nutritional support (Letter). *Lancet*, 340, 187–8.

Merritt, R. J., Kalsch, M., Roux, L. D., Ashley-Mills, J. & Siegel, S. S. (1985). Significance of hypoalbuminemia in pediatric oncology patients – malnutrition or infection? *Journal of Parenteral and Enteral Nutrition*, 9, 303–6.

Moghissi, K., Hornshaw, J., Teasdale, P. R. & Dawes, E. A. (1977). Parenteral nutrition in carcinoma of the esophagus treated by surgery: nitrogen balance and clinical studies. *British Journal of Surgery*, 64, 125–8.

Moloney, M., Moriarty, M. & Daly, L. (1983). Controlled studies of nutritional intake in patients with malignant disease undergoing treatment. *Human Nutrition: Applied Nutrition*, 37A, 30–5.

Moore, F. A., Feliciano, D. V., Andrassy, R. J. *et al.* (1992). Early enteral feeding, compared with parenteral, reduces postoperative septic complications. *Annals of Surgery*, 216, 172–83.

Muller, J. M., Brenner, U., Dienst, C. & Pichlmaier, H. (1982). Preoperative parenteral feeding in patients with gastrointestinal carcinoma. *Lancet*, i, 68–72.

Muller, J. M., Keller, H. W., Brenner, U., Walter, M. & Holzmuller, W. (1986). Indications and effects of preoperative parenteral nutrition. *World Journal of Surgery*, 10, 53–63.

Munkvad, M., Danielsen, L., Hoj, L. *et al.* (1984). Antigen-free diet in adult patients with atopic dermatitis. *Acta Dermatologica Venereologica*, 64, 524–8.

Nasrallah, S. M. & Galambos, J. T. (1980). Aminoacid therapy of alcoholic hepatitis. *Lancet*, ii, 1276–7.

Naveau, S., Pelletier, G., Poynard, T. *et al.* (1986). A randomized clinical trial of supplementary parenteral nutrition in jaundiced alcoholic cirrhotic patients. *Hepatology*, 6, 270–4.

Nayel, H., El-Ghoneimy, E. & El-Haddad, S. (1992). Impact of nutritional supplementation on treatment delay and morbidity in patients with head and neck tumors treated with irradiation. *Nutrition*, **8**, 13–18.

Naylor, C. D., O'Rourke, K., Detsky, A. S. & Baker, J. P. (1989). Parenteral nutrition with branched-chain amino acids in hepatic encephalopathy. *Gastroenterology*, **97**, 1033–42.

Neuvonen, P., Salo, M., Perttila, J. & Havia, T. (1986). Lack of modulation of postoperative immunosuppression by isotonic amino acid infusion. *Journal of Parenteral and Enteral Nutrition*, **10**, 160–5.

Nixon, D. W., Moffitt, S., Lawson, D. H. et al. (1981). Total parenteral nutrition as an adjunct to chemotherapy of metastatic colorectal cancer. *Cancer Treatment Reports* **65** (Suppl. 5), 121–8.

O'Mahoney, J. B., McIrvine, A. J., Palder, S. B. et al. (1984). The effect of short term postoperative intravenous feeding upon cell-mediated immunity and serum suppressive activity in well nourished patients. *Surgery, Gynecology, and Obstetrics*, **159**, 27–32.

Otte, K. E., Ahlburg, P., D'Amore, F. & Stellfield, M. (1989). Nutritional repletion in malnourished patients with emphysema. *Journal of Parenteral and Enteral Nutrition*, 13, 152–6.

Pildes, R. S., Ramamurthy, R. S., Cordero, G. V. & Wong, P. W. K. (1973). Intravenous supplementation of L-amino acids and dextrose in low-birth-weight infants. *Journal of Pediatrics*, **82**, 945–50.

Plaitakis, A., Smith, J., Mandeli, J. & Yahr, M. D. (1988). Pilot trials of branched-chain amino acids in amyotrophic lateral sclerosis. *Lancet* i, 1015–18.

Popp, M. B., Fisher, R. I., Simon, R. M. & Brennan, M. F., (1981a). A prospective randomized study of adjuvant parenteral nutrition in the treatment of diffuse lymphoma: effect on drug tolerance. *Cancer Treatment Reports*, **65** (Suppl. 5), 129–35.

Popp, M. B., Fisher, R. I., Wesley, R., Aamodt, R. & Brennan, M. F. (1981b). A prospective randomized study of adjuvant parenteral nutrition in the treatment of advanced diffuse lymphoma: influence on survival. *Surgery*, **90**, 195–203.

Preshaw, R. M., Attisha, R. P., Hollingsworth, W. J. & Todd, J. D. (1979). Randomized sequential trial of parenteral nutrition in healing of colonic anastomoses in man. *Canadian Journal of Surgery*, **122**, 437–9.

Reilly, J., Mehta, R., Teperman, L. et al., (1990). Nutritional support after liver transplantation: a randomized prospective study. *Journal of Parenteral and Enteral Nutrition*, **14**, 386–91.

Ryan, J. A., Page, C. P. & Babcock, L. (1981). Early postoperative jejunal feeding of elemental diet in gastrointestinal surgery. *American Surgeon*, **47**, 393–403.

Sagar, S., Harland, P. & Shields, R. (1979). Early postoperative feeding with elemental diet. *British Medical Journal*, **1**, 293–5.

Samuels, M. L., Selig, D. E., Ogden, S., Grant, C. & Brown, B. (1981). IV hyperalimentation and chemotherapy for stage III testicular cancer: a randomized study. *Cancer Treatment Reports*, **65**, 615–27.

Sax, H. C., Warner, B. W., Talamini, M. A. et al. (1987). Early total parenteral nutrition in acute pancreatitis: lack of beneficial effects. *American Journal of Surgery*, **153**, 117–24.

Scheurich, J. W., Wierman, M. E., Brown, B. G., Ferro, P. S. & Graham, D. Y. (1985). Preparation for barium enema. *Southern Medical Journal*, **78**, 838–40.

Schroeder, D., Gillanders, L., Mahr, K. & Hill, G. L. (1991). Effects of immediate postoperative enteral nutrition on body composition, muscle function, and wound healing. *Journal of Parenteral and Enteral Nutrition*, **15**, 376–83.

Sclafani, L., Shike, M., Quesada, E., Posner, M. & Brennan, M. (1991). A randomized prospective trial of TPN following major pancreatic resection or radioactive implant for pancreatic cancer (Abstract). *Program of the 22th Annual Cancer Symposium of the Society of Surgical Oncology*, Orlando, Florida, March 1991, pp. 96–7.

Serrou, B., Cupissol, D., Favier, F. & Michel, F. B. (1981). Opposite results in two randomized trials evaluating the adjunct value of peripheral intravenous nutrition in lung cancer patients. In *Adjunctive Therapy of Cancer III*, ed. S. E. Salmon & S. E. Johes, pp. 255–63, Grune and Stratton, New York.

Serrou, B., Cupissol, D., Plagne, R. *et al.* (1982). Follow-up of a randomized trial for oat cell carcinoma evaluating the efficacy of peripheral intravenous nutrition (PIVN) as adjunct therapy. *Recent Results in Cancer Research*, **80**, 246–53.

Shambarger, R. C., Brennan, M. F., Goodgame, J. T. *et al.* (1984). A prospective, randomized study of adjuvant parenteral nutrition in the treatment of sarcomas: results of metabolic and survival studies. *Surgery*, **96**, 1–12.

Shike, N., Feld, R., Evans, W. K., Shepherd, F. A., Harrison, J. E. & Jeejeebhoy, K. N. (1981). Long-term effect of TPN on body composition of patients with lung carcinoma. (Abstract). *Journal of Parenteral and Enteral Nutrition*, **5**, 564.

Shukla, H. S., Rao, R. R., Banu, N., Gupta, R. M. & Yadav, R. C. (1984). Enteral hyperalimentation in malnourished surgical patients. *Indian Journal of Medical Research*, **80**, 339–46.

Simko, V. (1983). Long-term tolerance of a special amino acid oral formula in patients with advanced liver disease. *Nutrition Reports International*, **27**, 765–73.

Simms, J. M., Oliver, E. & Smith, J. A. R. (1980). A study of total parenteral nutrition (TPN) in major gastric and esophageal resection for neoplasia (Abstract). *Journal of Parenteral and Enteral Nutrition*, **4**, 422.

Simms, J. H. & Smith, J. A. R. (1981). Intravenous feeding after total cystectomy – a controlled trial (Abstract). *Journal of Parenteral and Enteral Nutrition*, **5**, 357.

Simon, D. & Galambos, J. T. (1988). A randomized controlled study of peripheral parenteral nutrition in moderate and severe alcoholic hepatitis. *Journal of Hepatology*, **7**, 200–7.

Smith, R. C. & Hartemink, R. (1988). Improvement of nutritional measures during preoperative parenteral nutrition in patients selected by the prognostic nutritional index: a randomized controlled trial. *Journal of Parenteral and Enteral Nutrition*, **12**, 587–91.

Smith, R. C., Hartemink, R. J., Hollinshead, J. W. & Gillett, D. J. (1985). Fine bore jejunostomy feeding following major abdominal surgery: a controlled randomized clinical trial. *British Journal of Surgery*, **72**, 458–61.

Solassol, C., Joyeux, H. & Dubois, J. (1979). Total parenteral nutrition (TPN) with complete nutritive mixtures: an artificial gut in cancer patients. *Nutrition and Cancer*, **1**, 13–18.

Studley, H. O. (1936). Percentage of weight loss. *Journal of the American Medical Association*, 106, 458–60.

Tandon, S. P., Gupta, S. C., Sinha, S. N. & Naithani, Y. P. (1984). Nutritional support as an adjunct therapy of advanced cancer patients. *Indian Journal of Medical Research*, **80**, 180–8.

Thompson, B. R., Julian, T. B. & Stremple, J. F. (1981). Perioperative total parenteral nutrition in patients with gastrointestinal cancer. *Journal of Surgical Research*, **30**, 497–500.

Tomlinson, R. J. R., Newman, B. M. & Schofield, P. F. (1976). Is colostomy closure a hazardous procedure? A comparison of elemental diet and routine bowel preparation. *British Journal of Surgery*, **63**, 799–800.

Twomey, P. L. & Patching, S. C. (1985). Cost-effectiveness of nutritional support. *Journal of Parenteral and Enteral Nutrition*, **9**, 3–10.

Valdivieso, M., Frankmann, C., Murphy, W. K. *et al.*, (1987). Long-term effects of intravenous hyperalimentation administered during intensive chemotherapy for small cell bronchogenic carcinoma. *Cancer*, **59**, 362–9.

Van Eys, J., Copeland, E. M., Congir, A. *et al.* (1980). A clinical trial of hyperalimentation in children with metastatic malignancies. *Medical and Pediatric Oncology*, **8**, 63–73.

Veterans Affairs Total Parenteral Nutrition Cooperative Study Group (1991). Perioperative total parenteral nutrition in surgical patients. *New England Journal of Medicine*, **325**, 525–32.

Weiner, R. S., Kramer, B. S., Clamon, G. H. *et al.* (1985). Effects of intravenous hyperalimentation during treatment in patients with small-cell lung cancer. *Journal of Clinical Oncology*, **3**, 949–57.

Woolfson, A. M. J. & Smith, J. A. R. (1989). Elective nutritional support after major surgery: a prospective randomised trial. *Clinical Nutrition*, **8**, 15–21.

Yamada, M., Koyama, H., Hioki, K., Yamada, T. & Yamamoto, M. (1983). Effect of postoperative total parenteral nutrition (TPN) as an adjunct to gastrectomy for advanced gastric carcinoma. *British Journal of Surgery*, **70**, 267–74.

Yu, V. Y. H., James, B., Hendry, P. & MacMahon, R. A. (1979). Total parenteral nutrition in very low birthweight infants: a controlled trial. *Archives of Disease in Childhood*, **54**, 653–61.

Appendix: Summary of PRCTs

Disease	Reference (No. of Pts.)	Clinical outcome				Nutritional outcome			
		Mortality	Morbidity	Dur'n Hosp	Cost Hosp	Weight	TSF	N Balance	Albumin
	PNS studies								
Liver disease	Nasrallah & Galambos, 1980 (35)	B	SB				'NSD'		SB
	Naveau et al., 1986 (40)	0	0				B		SW
	Achord, 1987 (28)	B	SB						SB
	Bonkovsky et al., 1991a, b (21)	0	B			0	'NSD'	B	SB
	Reilly et al., 1990 (18)	B	B	SB	B			SB	
	Reilly et al., 1990 (20)	B	B	SB	B			SB	
	Simon & Galambos, 1988 (34)	W	0						0
IBD	Dickinson et al., 1980 (36)		W			0			

Cont.

Appendix – *Cont.*

Disease	Reference (No. of Pts.)	Clinical outcome				Nutritional outcome			
		Mortality	Morbidity	Dur'n Hosp	Cost Hosp	Weight	TSF	N Balance	Albumin
Oncotherapy	McIntyre et al., 1986 (47)	0	W						
	Popp et al., 1981 (41)	0				SB	0		B
	Nixon et al., 1981a,b (45)	SW	W			SB	B		SW
	Samuels et al., 1981 (30)	W	SW			SB	0		0
	Shambarger et al., 1984 (32)	W	SW			B		SB	0
	Van Eys et al., 1980 (20)	0	SW			0			
	Hays et al., 1983 (10)	W	W			SB	B		B
	Jordan et al., 1981 (43)	SW	W			B			
	Issell et al., 1978 (26)		SB			SB	0		
	Serrou et al., 1982 (31)	0	B			B			

Reference							
Valdivieso et al., 1987 (65)	0	SW			SB	SB	
Shike et al., 1981 (31)	W				SB	SB	SW
Clamon et al., 1985; Weiner et al., 1985 (119)	W	SW			SB		
Drott et al., 1988 (23)	0	0			B	SB	0
Solassol, Joyeux & Dubois 1979 (81)	0	SB			SB	SB	SB
Kinsella et al., 1981 (32)	0	B			0		0
Ghavimi et al., 1982 (25)	0	SW			SB	SB	
Donaldson et al., 1982 (25)	0	SW			SB	SB	
Solassol et al., 1979 (40)	SB	SW			SB		
Coquin et al., 1981 (23)	B	SB					
Lanzotti et al., 1980 (27)	0	W					
Serrou et al., 1981 (70)	SB						
Pancreatitis							
Sax et al., 1987 (55)	0	0	SW	SW		SB	0
Hyde & Floch 1984 (16)	B	B	B		SB	SB	0

Cont.

Appendix – *Cont.*

Disease	Reference (No. of Pts.)	Clinical outcome				Nutritional outcome			
		Mortality	Morbidity	Dur'n Hosp	Cost Hosp	Weight	TSF	N Balance	Albumin
	Hyde & Floch, 1984 (15)		B	B				SB	0
Low birth weight infants	Pildes *et al.*, 1973 (20)	W		B		SB			SB
	Pildes *et al.*, 1973 (19)	W		SB		SB			B
	Brans *et al.*, 1974 (15)	0	SW	B		SB	0		
	Brans *et al.*, 1974 (13)	W	SW	W		SB	0		
	Yu *et al.*, 1979 (34)	W	0	'NSD'		SB			
	Pildes *et al.*, 1973 (15)	B							
Peri-operative	Holter & Fischer, 1977 (56)	0	B			SB			SB
	Abel *et al.*, 1976 (44)	W	SW		SW			B	SB
	Preshaw *et al.*, 1979 (47)	0	W			0		B	0

Cont.

Reference						
Heatley, Williams & Lewis 1979 (74)	B	SB				0
Thompson, Julian & Stremple 1981 (21)	0	W				0
O'Mahony et al., 1984 (34)	0	0		SB		0
Garden et al., 1983 (20)	B	0	B	0	B	SB
Hogbin, Smith & Craven 1984 (43)	0	W	B		SB	
Yamada et al., 1983 (34)	B	B		SB		B
Bonau et al., 1984 (13)	0	0			SB	
Bonau et al., 1984 (10)	0	0			SB	
Fletcher & Little, 1986 (19)	0				SB	
Muller et al., 1982 (125)	SB	SB				0
Hensle, 1978 (44)	0	B	B		B	
Simms & Smith 1981 (?)		SB			SB	'NSD'
Culebras-Fernandez et al., 1987 (31)	0				SB	0
Jensen, 1985						
Jensen, 1982 (20)	B	B	SB	SB	SB	

Appendix – *Cont.*

Disease	Reference (No. of Pts.)	Clinical outcome				Nutritional outcome			
		Mortality	Morbidity	Dur'n Hosp	Cost Hosp	Weight	TSF	N Balance	Albumin
	Woolfson & Smith 1989 (122)	0	B	0				SB	
	Simms, Oliver & Smith 1980 (20)	0	'NSD'					B	SB
	Simms, Oliver & Smith 1980 (20)	B	W					SB	
	Moghissi et al., 1977 (15)	0	B			SB		SB	
	Figueras et al., 1988 (49)		B	0		0		SB	0
	Smith & Hartemink 1988 (34)	B	B	W		SB	SB		0
	Hansell et al., 1989 (20)	0	W	B				SB	
	Hansell et al., 1989 (20)	0	W	0				SB	
	Gys, Peeters & Hubens, 1990 (20)	0	SW			0		SB	
	Bellantone et al., 1988 (100)	0	B						'NSD'

Study						
Muller et al., 1986 (105)	–	0				
Muller et al., 1986 (113)	B	SB				
Neuvonen et al., 1986 (22)	0	0	0			
VA Group, 1991 (459)	0	SW				
Cromack et al., 1988 (26)	0	W	W			
Meijerink et al., 1992 (101)	0	W				
Sclafani et al., 1991 (51)	0	B				

ENS Studies

Study						
Liver disease						
Calvey, Davis & Williams, 1985 (43)	W	SW	SW		'NSD'	
Calvey et al., 1985 (42)	0	0		'NSD'	B	0
Cabre et al., 1990 (35)	B	SB	SB	B		SB
Kearns et al., 1992 (31)	B	SB	0	SB	0	SB
Simko, 1983 (15)	B	0	SB	0	SW	SW

Cont.

Appendix – *Cont.*

Disease	Reference (No. of Pts.)	Clinical outcome				Nutritional outcome			
		Mortality	Morbidity	Dur'n Hosp	Cost Hosp	Weight	TSF	N Balance	Albumin
IBD	Erikkson, Persson & Wahren 1982 (7-c)		B						
	Harries *et al.*, 1983 (28-c)		SW			SB	SB		SB
	Imes *et al.*, 1986 (125)		B						
Oncotherapy	Douglas *et al.*, 1978 (30)	B				0			B
	Foster *et al.*, 1980 (32)		SB			0			SB
	Elkort *et al.*, 1981 (47)	0	0			0	0		0
	Bounous *et al.*, 1975 (18)		SB			SB			SB
	Bounous, Gentile & Hugon 1971 (21)		0			SB			
	Evans *et al.*, 1987 (66)	B	B			0			
	Evans *et al.*, 1987 (66)	0	B			0			

Study						
Evans et al., 1987 (54)	W	W		0		0
Evans et al., 1987 (63)	B	B		0		
Tandon et al., 1984 (70)	B	SB		SB	0	0
Nayel, El-Ghoneimy-El-Haddad 1992 (23)		B		SB	SB	
Lipschitz & Mitchell 1980 (14)		SB				
Cousineau et al., 1973 (8)		B				
Moloney, Moriarty & Daly 1983 (84)	0	W				
Tomlinson, Newman & Schofield 1976 (26)		B	0	0		0
Peri-operative						
Fletcher & Little, 1986 (18)	0			SB		
Shukla et al., 1984 (110)	B	SB	B	SB	SB	SB
Sagar, Harland & Shields, 1979 (30)		B	SB	SB	SB	
Hoover et al., 1980 (48)		SW		SB	SB	
Ryan, Page & Babcock, 1981 (16)		B		0		

Cont.

189

Appendix – *Cont.*

Disease	Reference (No. of Pts.)	Clinical outcome				Nutritional outcome			
		Mortality	Morbidity	Dur'n Hosp	Cost Hosp	Weight	TSF	N Balance	Albumin
	Smith *et al.*, 1985 (50)	W	W	SW		0			0
	Schroeder *et al.*, 1991 (32)		B			0			
	Meijerink *et al.*, 1992 (100)	0	B						
	Foschi *et al.*, 1986 (60)	B	SB						
	Flynn & Leightty, 1987 (36)		B	B					
	Frankel & Horowitz, 1989 (50)	0	W	0					
	Elmore *et al.*, 1989 (50)		B	0					
	Crossland, Geelhoed & Guy 1981 (30)		0						
	Baker, 1978 (86)		0						
	Gurry & Ellis-Pegler, 1976 (51)	0	0	0					
Pulmonary	Otte *et al.*, 1989 (28)		B			SB	SB		SB

Hip Fracture	Efthimiou et al., 1988 (14)	SB			SB	SB
	Bastow, Rawlings & Allison 1983 (122)	0	SB		SB	SB
	Delmi et al., 1990 (59)	B	SB	SB		SB
Colon preparation	Scheurich et al., 1985 (61)	0				
	Gutwein, Baer & Holt, 1981 (98)	SB				
Amyotrophic lateral sclerosis	Plaitakis et al., 1988 (22)	SB				
Asthma	Hoj et al., 1981 (37)	SB				
Atopic dermatitis	Munkvad et al., 1984 (25)	W				

9

Enteral feeding and food intolerance in paediatrics

A. MacDONALD

Two areas in paediatrics which have received much attention are enteral feeding and food intolerance. Enteral tube feeds and diets for food intolerance were uncommonly used for children 10 years ago. Both areas require paediatric dietetic expertise to ensure that the nutritional requirements are met in order to achieve optimal growth in a way that is both practical and acceptable to the child and family.

Enteral feeding in paediatrics

History

Although some of the earliest reports of enteral feeding go back as far as ancient Egyptian times, one of the first reports of a child being fed by naso-gastric tube appeared in 1876 by Duke. A typical feeding regimen in young children consisted of 6 oz of milk with 1 oz brandy with digitalis every 6 hours (Randall, 1990). The first report of a child being successfully fed by gastrostomy was in 1880, when an 8-year-old boy with an oesophageal lye stricture was successfully fed for 15 years by masticating his food and then forcing it into the gastrostomy tube (Randall, 1990).

Indications for enteral feeding in paediatrics

Infants and children have fewer body reserves of all nutrients, particularly energy, than adults and enteral feeding is quickly resorted to if oral food intake fails to meet nutritional needs. It is estimated that the number of days before there is a total depletion of energy stores in a small pre-term infant is 5 days, in a term infant 32 days and in an adult as much as 90 days (Heird, 1977).

192

There are four broad categories for using enteral nutrition in paediatrics.

Inadequate energy and nutrient intake

This may be due to anorexia associated with a disease state, breathlessness associated with respiratory and cardiac disorders, structural and functional abnormalities of the gastrointestinal tract, neurological impairment of sucking, chewing and swallowing mechanisms.

Increased nutritional reqiuirements

Many infants and children with chronic or severe illnesses have a need for extra nutrients, particularly energy, but due to the anorexia associated with their disease, are unable to meet their nutritional requirements by normal eating. Examples of such disease states include liver disease, cystic fibrosis and congenital heart disease.

Metabolic disease

In some metabolic disorders, the body is unable to cope with long periods of fasting and continuous enteral feeds need to be given overnight to avoid hypoglycaemia.

Gastro-intestinal disease

Infants and children with a very short bowel may absorb nutrients more efficiently if their nutrition is given as a continuous enteral feed rather than as intermittent bolus feeds. Elemental feeds, used in the management of Crohn's disease are frequently administered via a tube as a result of their unpalatability.

Specific clinical indications for enteral feeding in paediatrics

Congenital heart disease

Failure to thrive (FTT) is a common problem in infants with congenital heart disease (CHD). The severity of FTT varies with the anatomic lesion and infants at particular risk are those with cyanotic CHD, left to right shunts, pulmonary hypertension and right sided cardiac failure (Poskitt, 1993). The cause of FTT is multifactorial. Reasons include: inadequate nutrient intake due to breathlessness associated with feeding and anorexia;

peripheral anoxia and acidosis leading to inefficient utilisation of nutrients (Menon & Poskitt, 1985); sodium depletion following diuretic therapy (Salmon *et al.*, 1989); increased resting energy expenditure in some children (Menon & Poskitt, 1985) and malabsorption (Carlin *et al.*, 1990) are also probably important. Increased stool fat and protein losses have been noted in CHD infants over 20 weeks of age (Sondheimer & Hamilton, 1978), although this has not been confirmed by all workers (Menon & Poskitt, 1985).

Enteral feeding should be considered in cases of poor oral intake and inadequate weight gain, inability to co-ordinate sucking, swallowing and respiration or breathlessness and exhaustion with feeding (Carlin *et al.*, 1990). Enteral feeding is usually provided in infancy either by continuous nasogastric feeds or overnight continuous feeds combined with intermittent small bottle feeds and 'top-up' bolus feeds during the day. Many infants with CHD who are failing to thrive appear to require as much energy as 150–200 kcal/kg. Bougle and co-workers gave 13 infants a continuous enteral feed providing 137 kcal/kg for 40 days and achieved good weight gain (Bougle *et al.*, 1986). More recently, Jackson and Poskitt gave 138 kcal/kg to 14 infants with CHD and improved their mean weight gain from 1.3 g/kg/day to 5.8 g/kg/day (Jackson & Poskitt, 1991). Energy supplementation of normal infant formula or breast milk with glucose polymers with or without fat supplements or concentrating the strength of normal infant formula, is the enteral feed of choice for infants in many cardiology units. It has been suggested that glucose polymers are preferable to a fat supplement as a source of additional energy, because shifting cardiac metabolism from β-oxidation of fatty acids to carbohydrate utilisation has beneficial effects (Menon & Poskitt, 1985). Care should be exhibited when concentrating normal infant formula, as this will increase renal solute load and electrolyte concentration of the feed.

Cerebral palsy

Nutritional problems and growth retardation (both low weight for age and low height for age) have been reported in children with cerebral palsy (CP) and have been related to the type of CP and degree of oral–motor dysfunction (Shapiro *et al.*, 1986). Rempel and co-workers described the growth characteristics of 57 children with severe CP and more than 90% of the patients were less than the fifth centile for both height and weight (Rempel, Colwell & Nelson, 1988). Krick and Van Duyn (1984) demonstrated that 12 CP children with oral motor impairment had decreased weight for age and height for age and this was significantly worse than children without oral–motor impairment with CP.

The poor nutrition of these children can easily be explained. Mechanical feeding problems such as weak or absent suck reflex, poor lip closure, hyperactive gag reflex, tongue thrust and chewing incoordination affect all stages of feeding and swallowing (Thommessen *et al.*, 1991; Jones, 1989). During mealtime there may be numerous episodes of food spillage, coughing, choking, regurgitation and spitting. Children with CP may lose up to 50% of their food through spillage. Other reasons for poor nutrition include prolonged length of time needed for oral feeding, since CP children may take 2–12 times longer to swallow a standard amount of pureed food (Gisel & Patrick, 1988). Low calorie density of pureed foods offered for children with mechanical feeding problems, lack of appetite, food aversion (Thommessen *et al.*, 1991), poor dentition (Shapiro *et al.*, 1986), lack of communication between carer and child (Dietz, 1987), gastro-oesophageal reflux and aspiration pneumonia (Gadol, Joshi & Young Lee, 1987) are further problems. There is some evidence that the energy expenditure may be increased in children both with athetoid and spastic CP (Dietz, 1987).

Nutritional support has been shown to improve weight (Shapiro *et al.*, 1986, Rempel, Colwell & Nelson, 1988, Patrick *et al.*, 1986) and achieve some improvement in height although less commonly (Shapiro *et al.*, 1986; Rempel, Colwell & Nelson, 1988). It may also improve oral–motor movements (Gisel & Patrick, 1988), heal persistent pressure sores, correct cold and cyanotic extremities (Patrick *et al.*, 1986), reduce irritability and induce improvement in behaviour (Gisel, 1991) and 'well-being' (Patrick *et al.*, 1986). Enteral feeding also allows therapists to focus on oral movements and coordination required for easy and efficient feeding, while the child's nutritional status is not in jeopardy (Gisel & Patrick, 1988). Some evidence would suggest that enteral feeding for the more severely affected CP children is more successful before two years of age than in older children when severe malnutrition is established. On the negative side, enteral feeding may cause obesity (Rempel *et al.*, 1988), and increase the incidence of reflux and mortality following gastrostomy insertion (Gisel & Patrick, 1988).

It is difficult to give precise recommendations for the nutritional requirements of CP children. However, if the child is very small and under the third centile for height, it is appropriate to base nutritional requirements on height age rather than actual age and initially provide an additional 20% more energy to permit catch-up weight gain and growth, i.e. 120% of the estimated average requirements (EAR) for height. Vitamin, mineral requirements and protein requirements should also be calculated according to height age.

Cystic fibrosis

Chronic malnutrition is particularly common in cystic fibrosis (CF) adolescents and it has been shown that up to 30% of patients are malnourished (Gaskin et al., 1990). This is mainly due to malabsorption, increased resting energy expenditure and poor energy intake. As a result many CF centres are resorting to overnight enteral feeding and so far the following benefits have been observed: increase in body fat, height, lean body mass and muscle mass, increased total body nitrogen, improved strength and development of secondary sexual characteristics (Ramsey et al., 1992; Levy et al., 1985; Boland et al., 1986).

It has been indicated that enteral feeding should begin if there is no weight gain over a 3-month period, or if the patient's weight/height ratio is less than 85% of ideal (Ramsey et al., 1992). Short-term overnight enteral feeding will usually produce immediate weight gain, but as soon as feeding has stopped weight loss may quickly result (Daniels et al., 1989). Long-term enteral feeding studies, where patients have been fed for up to 3 years, have demonstrated that patients have gained weight and grown satisfactorily. There is even some evidence to demonstrate that pulmonary function may decline at a slower rate (Gaskin et al., 1990; Levy et al., 1985; Boland et al., 1986).

The energy requirements of CF patients with severe chronic lung disease may be increased by at least 20%–50%. Patients who require enteral feeding usually have poor appetites and it may be necessary to give at least 40%–50% via the overnight enteral feed. A number of types of feed preparation have been used for enteral feeding including elemental, semi-elemental, polymeric and high fat feeds. Little work has been performed comparing the efficacy of feed preparation, although one study comparing an elemental with a polymeric feed demonstrated no clear benefits from the elemental formula (Kane, Hobbs & Black, 1990). The role of high fat feeds in CF has been unclear, although Kane and Hobbs demonstrated that Pulmocare (Abbot), a high fat enteral feed, resulted in lower CO_2 production and respiratory quotient in CF patients with moderate to severe pulmonary disease, when compared with a high carbohydrate feed (Kane & Hobbs, 1991). Hyperglycaemia requiring insulin therapy, has been reported as a complication of overnight feeds in CF and it is recommended that blood sugars are regularly monitored (Kane & Black, 1989).

Childhood cancer

The prevalence of malnutrition in childhood cancer has been correlated with diagnosis, extent of disease, age and treatment (Jaffe, 1987). Smith, Stevens and Booth (1990) demonstrated that 27% of newly diagnosed children with malignant solid tumours were malnourished and during therapy this increased to 46%. Children at high risk of developing nutritional problems, include those with a diagnosis of neuroblastoma, Ewing's sarcoma and metastic Wilms tumour (Jaffe, 1987). Although weight for height is commonly used as the main index of nutritional status, it is unreliable in patients with large tumour masses. Mid-upper arm circumference has been shown to be a better indicator of nutritional status in cancer children. Smith and co-workers demonstrated in a group of 48 children with malignant solid tumours, that height for age and weight for height did not differ from controls but mid-upper arm circumference was significantly lower (Smith, Stevens & Booth, 1990).

The cause of malnutrition is multi-factorial and includes the side effects of treatment e.g. vomiting, nausea, anorexia, dysphagia, diarrhoea and malabsorption, learned food aversions associated with vomiting, changes in taste perception, tumour-related anorexia (Jaffe, 1987) and behavioural feeding problems. There is evidence that improving nutritional status may reduce surgical morbidity, improve tolerance to chemotherapy and improve quality of life (Smith *et al.*, 1990).

Enteral feeding has been shown to be successful in a study feeding a small group of children with newly diagnosed malignancy (Smith *et al.*, 1992). It improved nutritional status as measured by mid-upper arm circumference, was well tolerated and produced apparent increase in child play-scale scores.

The energy requirements of these children do not appear to exceed normal EAR for actual age. Large volumes of feed are not well tolerated in children with malignancy and the use of a high energy density feed (1.5 kcal/ml) may be advisable (Smith *et al.*, 1992). In a child who has been vomiting, feeds should be cautiously introduced. Enteral feeding is usually short term, although most children will require overnight enteral feeding at home for a few months.

Nutritional requirements

There are few guidelines which give specific information about the nutritional needs of sick infants and children. The Dietary Reference Values (DRVs) for food and energy, published by the Department of Health, are for healthy people in the United Kingdom (Department of Health, 1991). DRVs for nutrients and EARs for energy, are meant to be applied to population groups and not individuals. DRVs and EARs for infants are based on the breast milk intake of normal infants. Few data are available on nutritional requirements for many of the nutrients for toddlers, school age children and adolescents. Thus, some of the DRVs and EARs are extrapolated from infant and adult data and do not take into account the effect of disease and growth failure. Energy and nutrient requirements for children with different clinical needs are given in Table 9.1. These are based on personal hospital practice and although there are few data to support these figures, they should at least provide a useful guideline.

Choice of feed

The type of feed is dependent upon the age, weight and clinical condition of the child. The common feeds used can be divided into three categories, i.e. polymeric, protein hydrolysate and elemental, and modular feeds.

Polymeric feeds for infants and children with a normal gut

0–12 months

Term infants less than 4 months of age can be given either expressed breast milk or an infant formula milk via a tube at a rate of between 150 ml and 200 ml/kg.

If infants are failing to thrive while taking maximum quantities of infant formula feed or are over the age of 4 months, additional energy supplementments need to be added to either feed. These are usually added in the form of glucose polymers or a fat emulsion, or a combination of both. The first stage is usually a gradual introduction of glucose polymers such as Maxijul (SHS), Polycal (Cow & Gate) or Caloreen (Roussel) in 1 g/100 ml increments to a maximum total carbohydrate feed concentration of 12 g/100 ml. (Normal infant milk carbohydrate concentration is 7.0 g/100 ml.) An extra 5 g/100 ml of added carbohydrate will provide an additional 19 kcal/100 ml. Higher carbohydrate concentrations may cause osmotic diarrhoea. If further energy supplementation is required, a fat emulsion may also be added in 1.0 g/100 ml increments, to a maximum total feed fat concentration of 5 g/100 ml. (Normal infant milk fat concentration is 3.5 g/100 ml). If 1.5 g/100 ml of fat is added it will provide 14 kcal/100 ml. A 50% long chain fat emulsion (LCT), i.e. Calogen (Scientific Hospital Supplies) is used in preference to a medium-chain triglyceride (MCT) emulsion (MacDonald & Booth, 1990).

Some centres prefer to increase the concentration of infant formula not only to improve the energy content of the feed, but also to increase the overall nutrient profile. This method should be cautiously used, as the protein and electrolyte content and renal solute load at high feed volumes, may be high.

1–5 years (8–20 kg)

There are two paediatric enteral feeds providing 1 kcal/ml, i.e. Nutrison Paediatric (Cow & Gate) and Paediasure (Abbot), whose formula is specifically developed for this age group.

Care should be exercised when using adult feeds providing 1 kcal/ml and 1.5 kcal/ml, as the electrolyte and protein contents are high. The vitamin and mineral profile is inappropriate for the needs of small children.

Over 5 years

Any commercially available standard formula providing 1 kcal/ml is suitable, given at appropriate volumes. If 1.5 kcal/ml feeds are used overnight for this age group of children, it is important to monitor overall protein intake to ensure this is not excessive. The intake from oral diet should be taken into account. 2.0 kcal/ml adult polymeric feeds are generally too high in protein for paediatric use.

Protein hydrolysate formula and elemental feeds

The majority of patients between 0 and 2 years with protracted diarrhoea, short-bowel-syndrome or cows' milk protein enteropathy who need a tube feed, can usually tolerate a commercially available standard protein-hydrolysate feed such as Nutramigen, Pregestimil (Mead Johnson), Peptijunior (Cow & Gate) or Pepdite 0–2 (SHS) (see section on food intolerance).

Elemental diets are used in paediatrics for Crohn's disease, multiple food intolerance, short gut syndrome and other malabsorption syndromes.

Table 9.1. *Nutrient requirements of paediatric patients with chronic disease*

	Normal	Failure to thrive/ poor growth	Cystic fibrosis	Cerebral palsy
Infants 0–1 year				
Energy	115 kcal/kg 0–3 months 100 kcal/kg 3–12 months	150–200 kcal/kg	If thriving as per normal infant If not thriving as per FTT	If thriving as per normal infant If not thriving as per FTT
Protein	2.0 g/kg 0–3 months 1.6 g/kg 4–12 months 1.5 g/kg 10–12 months	2.0 ± 0.5 g/kg		
Vitamins/minerals	As per DRV	As per DRV	8000 iu Vitamin A 800 iu in Vitamin E 50 mg Vitamin E Rest as for DRV	
Children 1–10 years				
Energy	As per EAR	EAR + 20% for height age	EAR + 20% actual age	EAR + 20% for height age
Protein	As per DRV	2.0 g/kg	2.0 g/kg	2.0 g/kg
Vitamins/minerals	As per DRV	As per DRV for height age	As per DRV for actual age + additional fat soluble vitamins A, D, E	As per DRV for height age
Children 11–15 years				
Energy	As per EAR	EAR + 20% for height age	EAR + 20% for actual age	EAR + 20% for height age
Protein	As per DRV	2.0 g/kg	2.0 g/kg	2.0 g/kg
Vitamins/minerals	As per DRV	As per DRV for height age	As per DRV for actual age + additional fat soluble vitamins A, D, E	As per DRV for height age

	Malignancy	Chronic liver disease	Cardiology	Short gut syndrome
Infants 0–1 year				
Energy	If thriving as per normal infant If not thriving as per FTT	150–200 kcal/kg	As per FTT infant if not thriving	150–200 kcal/kg
Protein		3.0 g/kg		2.5 g–3.0 g/kg
Vitamins/minerals		Sodium may be restricted Additional fat soluble vitamins Rest as per DRV		As per DRV Extra sodium and potassium may be needed
Children 1–10 years				
Energy	EAR	EAR + 20%	EAR	EAR + 20%
Protein	2.0 g/kg	2.0 g/kg–3.0 g/kg	2.0 g/kg	2.0 g–3.0 g/kg
Vitamins/minerals	As per DRV for actual age	Sodium may be restricted As per DRV for actual age + additional fat soluble vitamins	DRV	DRV. Extra sodiumn + potassium may be needed
Children 11–15 years				
Energy	EAR	EAR	EAR	EAR + 20%
Protein	1.5 g–2.0 g	1.5 g–2.0 g/kg	1.5 g–2.0 g/kg	2.0 g/kg
Vitamins/minerals	As DRV for actual age	Sodium may be restricted As per DRV for actual age + additional fat soluble vitamins	DRV	DRV. Extra sodium + potassium

EAR—estimated average requirements.
DRV—dietary reference values.
FTT—failure to thrive.

With the exception of one infant preparation, i.e. Neocate (SHS), elemental preparations that are available have been formulated for the adult and are generally high in protein and all contain variable amounts of electrolytes, vitamins and minerals. The elemental and semi-elemental feeds such as Pepdite 2+, Elemental 028 (SHS) and Flexical (Mead Johnson), contain less protein than the other similar feeds and have acceptable electrolyte, vitamin and mineral profiles, but these need to be matched to the specific nutritional requirements of the individual child. Elemental 028 has a very high osmolality and would need careful introduction into a child's diet. These preparations are not palatable and usually need to be given via a nasogastric tube (MacDonald, 1994).

Modular feeds

A modular feed is one which is based on separate protein, fat, carbohydrate, vitamin and mineral components, so that the individual ingredients and the quantities used can be adapted to meet the specific needs and tolerances of an infant or child. Modular feeds may be used in paediatrics, if nutritionally complete protein hydrolysate formulas or elemental feeds are not tolerated, e.g. in short gut syndrome or cows' milk intolerance, or if the fluid and nutrient requirements vary according to the clinical needs of the patient and this cannot be met by a nutritionally complete formula, e.g. in renal or liver disease. Examples of the ingredients used for the different types of modular feeds are given in Table 9.2.

The chief advantage of modular feeds is their flexibility: the ingredients can be adjusted from day to day according to the needs. However, they are complex, require time consuming calculations if not computerised and mistakes can easily be made during their preparation. It is important that these feeds are only calculated by qualified dietitians who have a thorough understanding of composition of the individual feed components and nutritional requirements of children.

Choice of route

In paediatrics, the choice of route partly depends upon the clinical condition, duration of feeding, age of the child and the preference of parent and child. Both nasogastric and gastrostomy feeding is commonly used in paediatric practice in the UK. Gastrostomy and nasogastric feeding is contraindicated for delayed gastric emptying, severe gastro-oesophageal reflux, intractable vomiting and impaired or absent gag reflex (Warman,

Table 9.2. *Examples of ingredients used in modular feeds*

	Modular feeds used in short gut syndrome and cows' milk intolerance	Modular feeds used in liver disease
Protein source	(a) Comminuted chicken (comminuted chicken in water)	(a) Whey protein
	(b) Hydrolysed whey	(b) Whey protein enriched with branch chain amino acids
Carbohydrate source	Glucose polymer ± Sucrose ± Glucose	Glucose polymer
Fat source	Long chain fat emulsion ± medium chain fat	Medium chain fat emulsion Long chain fat emulsion
Vitamins/minerals	*Comminuted chicken* Ketovite tablets and liquid + Aminogram mineral mixture *Hydrolysed whey protein* Paediatric Seravit	Paediatric Seravit (SHS)
Electrolytes	*Hydrolysed whey protein* Sodium Potassium ± Sodium (depending on profile of hydrolysed whey)	Potassium Sodium (to provide minimal requirements)
Feed thickener	*Comminuted chicken* 0.5% Nestargel (Nestlés) to ensure chicken fibres do not disperse out of solution to be given via a continuous tube	

1990). Although nasogastric tubes have been shown to be well tolerated in children, they can easily be dislodged by a toddler or forceful coughing, may cause nasal, oesophageal or tracheal irritation, can restrict mobility and are unpleasant to insert. Parent givers must be well trained and should demonstrate they are competent and safe before administering this form of nutritional support at home. Although gastrostomy tubes and buttons may allow greater mobility and may be more acceptable to some children requiring long-term feeding, they also have some disadvantages. They require a surgical procedure for placement, may result in increased gastro-oesophageal reflux, there may be leakage, skin irritation and infection around the insertion site, and feeding tubes may become clogged or blocked if inadequately cared for. Jejunostomy tubes are technically difficult to insert and in UK paediatric practice, jejunostomy feeding is resorted to only when nasogastric and gastrostomy feeding is contra-indicated. Nasojejunal feeding has some drawbacks as it is difficult to keep a tube in place for long periods in some children and considerable time is lost passing the tube through the pylorus (Sanderson & Walker-Smith, 1991).

Feeds are usually administered continuously but may be given inter-mittently by bolus for patients with neurological impairment. In children with intestinal disease on continuous feeds, nitrogen balance is more positive and output less (Parker, Stroop & Greene, 1981).

Complications of enteral feeding in paediatrics

A number of problems may be experienced with enteral feeding in children. Holden and co-workers demonstrated that sleep disturbance was common with overnight feeds. Fifty-nine parents and 35 out of 70 children reported sleep disturbance. Parents felt they had to check the feeding system overnight whilst the children's sleep problems were related to nocturia, the need to defaecate and abdominal pain (Holden *et al.*, 1991). However, Holden, and others, reported no major complications such as aspiration, hypoglycaemica after interruption of feed or entanglement in the tubing. Other problems associated with tube feeding include pulling out of tubes, by infants and children, when first inserted, gastro-oesophageal reflux, abdominal distension, vomiting, constipation, obesity and feed contamination, both in hospital and at home. Children with nasogastric tubes may be teased by their peers at school and may feel self-conscious about going out. Paediatric enteral feeding pumps are not all light-weight for portability, as well as being reliable and childproof and this may cause inconvenience. Parents may also have difficulty finding suitable baby sitters willing to supervise enteral feeding, as well as the child.

Reluctance to feed orally when enteral feeding has been discontinued is a further complication (Booth, 1991). For children who have never eaten by mouth or have had limited experience with oral feeding, an oral–motor stimulation programme is an important adjunct to tube feeding (Warman, 1990).

Food allergy and intolerance

It is common for parents to suspect that many of their children's problems may be related to food. Food additives, food allergy, E numbers and milk intolerance now appear to be everyday terms used by the general public. Even so, because there are inadequate diagnostic techniques, many doctors fail to take a 'middle of the road' approach when considering the possibility of food allergy and intolerance. They either choose to recognise it only when the cause and symptoms are obvious, or alternatively investigate every child they see for the possibility of food allergy and intolerance.

Definitions

During the past decade scientists have made serious attempts to reach a consensus on the use of terminology. The definitions given are those of the Royal College of Physicians/British Nutrition Foundation and Pearson (Lessoff, 1984; Pearson, 1987).

Food intolerance is any reproducible adverse reaction to a specific food or food ingredient which is not psychologically based. It is an umbrella term covering all organic reactions to food, including allergies, idio-syncratic, metabolic and pharmacologic reactions. Food allergy is an abnormal immunologic reaction to food. This term is often used indiscriminately to describe any food reaction but true food allergy is relatively rare. Examples of possible effects of the immunological response are food-specific antibodies, the production of immune complexes, and mucosal T cell mediated reactions (David, 1993).

Incidence and natural history

Although the true incidence of food intolerance is unknown, it is generally agreed that food intolerance is most common in infants and young children and decreases with age. Preliminary results from a study from High Wycombe would indicate that 1.4%–1.9% of the population react to common food allergens such as milk wheat, eggs, fish and nuts (DH/MAFF, 1991). The majority of studies conclude that less than 2% of the population have cows' milk protein intolerance (Halpern *et al.*, 1973; Jakobsson & Lindberg, 1979) and it has been estimated that only 0.01%–0.23% of the population react to food additives (Young *et al.*, 1987). There is a big difference between perceived food intolerance and proven food intolerance. In a number of carefully controlled double-blind studies in both children and adults with suspected classic symptoms, food allergy was confirmed in only 25%–40% of cases. Food allergy and intolerance is usually temporary but the outcome is partly dependent upon the type of food, severity of symptoms and age of the patient. There are several studies which have clearly demonstrated that most children acquire tolerance to milk by the age of three years (Bock, 1987; Businco *et al.*, 1985; Kjellman *et al.*, 1988). Egg intolerance may be more persistent (Eggleston, 1987) and it is even less common for patients to outgrow sensitivity to fish (Aas, 1987) and peanuts. Bock demonstrated that a group of 32 children still reacted to peanuts 2 to 14 years after their original intolerance was demonstrated (Bock & Atkins, 1989). Young children are more likely than older people to outgrow their food intolerance. It has been estimated that the computed mean development of tolerance to foods is 71% after 3 years, 50% after 6 years and 28% after 9 years (Kjellman, 1991).

Symptoms

Food allergy and intolerance can cause a diverse variety of symptoms in paediatrics, but these appear most commonly in the gastrointestinal tract or skin (Dannacus, 1987). Symptoms may be immediate and can occur within seconds, or up to two hours after eating a food, in the case of true IgE-mediated food allergy and may be life threatening. In the case of delayed food intolerance, reactions and symptoms may not occur for several hours or even days.

Gastro-intestinal

The oropharynx and the gastrointestinal tract are the first sites to be exposed to food allergens. Foods such as cows' milk, soya, egg, rice, chicken and fish have been clearly demonstrated to cause enteropathy of the small intestinal mucosa. It is a condition that usually affects only children under the age of three years, is temporary and is characterised by a combination of diarrhoea, vomiting, abdominal pain and failure to thrive (Ford & Walker-Smith, 1987). Unlike coeliac disease, there is a variably abnormal small intestinal mucosa which is patchy in distribution. Vomiting and diarrhoea are two of the commonest symptoms of cows' milk protein intolerance (CMPI) and infantile colitis resulting in chronic bloody loose stools or simple rectal bleeding in the first few weeks or months of life, has been clearly linked to milk (Hill & Milla, 1991, Harrison *et al.*, 1991). There are less objective data to demonstrate a link between food and other gastrointestinal symptoms such as colic, aphthous ulcers and constipation. There have been numerous studies that have suggested that cows' milk may be a possible cause of colic (Jakobsson & Lindberg, 1983; Lothe, Lindberg & Jakobsson, 1982; Iacono *et al.*, 1991) and one of the more convincing was a double-blind cross-over study by Lothe and Lindberg (1989) who gave a group of 24 infants, whose symptoms resolved on a casein hydrolysate formula, capsules containing either whey protein powder or a placebo powder. Of the 24 infants, 18 reacted to the whey protein powder (Lothe & Lindberg, 1989). In addition Clyne and Kulczycki (1991), demonstrated that bovine IgG is higher in breast milk of colicky infants and may be involved in the pathogenesis of colic. However, many workers have expressed doubt about some of these studies and it has been demonstrated that parental counselling is more effective at relieving crying, than elimination of cows' milk (Taubman, 1988). Food intolerance has been linked to recurrent mouth ulcers in a minority of cases and constipation in two anecdotal case reports (Chin, Tarlow & Allfree, 1983; McGrath, 1984), but in both conditions, it is an unlikely cause.

Skin

The most common symptoms affecting the skin are urticaria, angio-oedema and eczema. The role of food intolerance is considered to be more important in acute than in chronic urticaria. Common foods implicated with ordinary acute and contact urticaria are egg, cows' milk, fish, nuts, tomatoes and fruit (David, 1993). Yeasts have been implicated as a cause of chronic urticaria in adults and challenges with brewer's yeast have been shown to provoke urticaria (Atkins, 1991). Aspirin and food additives such as azo dyes, annatto, the antioxidants butylated hydroxy-anisole (BHA) and butylated hydroxytoluene (BHT) (Warin & Smith, 1976; Juhlin, 1985), have been implicated with chronic urticaria. Food is just one of the many triggers which can precipitate eczema and it is often difficult to distinguish between the effect of food and other triggers. Reactions to food tend to be delayed, rather than immediate. It has been estimated that only 10% of patients with eczema severe enough to warrant hospital attendance, will benefit from diet therapy (David, 1993). Many workers have used 'few food' diets with various degrees of success. Pike *et al.* found that only 18% of 66 children with severe atopic eczema responded to a 'few food' diet (Pike *et al.*, 1989). Armstrong and co-workers (1987) found that only 2 out of 12 patients improved on a 'few food' diet. The elemental diet has been shown to be successful. Devlin, David & Stanton (1991), reported an improvement in 27 out of 37 children with severe eczema using Vivonex and an antigen avoidance regimen, although some of this improvement may be due to a placebo effect. Parents have been reported to find diet therapy difficult in eczema (Hathaway & Warner, 1983) and many paediatricians consider that safe topical treatments should be tried before diet. However, if parents wish to try diet therapy it is important not to be too dismissive of this or else parents may seek the help of non-medical practitioners who may advocate restrictive and unsupervised diet therapy.

Respiratory

Although the incidence of food intolerance in asthma is disputed by some, it is generally thought to be small (Warner *et al.*, 1989). Novembre, Martino & Vierucci (1988) found that only 6% of 140 children with asthma had food reactions. In a study of 300 patients with asthma aged between seven months and eighty years, eleven patients were found to have reactions to foods following placebo-controlled double-blind challenges, but in five patients foods provoked symptoms other than asthma (Onorato *et al.*, 1986).

The chances of a child with asthma having food intolerance are much greater if the child has other atopic disorders (David, 1993). Foods reported to have triggered asthma include milk, eggs, nuts, cola, red wine and additives such as sulphur dioxide, tartrazine, sodium benzoate and salicylates (MacDonald, 1993*b*). In most cases of food-related asthma, symptoms occur within 30 minutes of ingestion and late reactions are unusual (David, 1993).

Neurological

The relationship between food allergy and intolerance and neurological symptoms such as hyperactivity, migraine and epilepsy is unclear. The idea that diet could affect behaviour and learning ability was proposed by Shannon in 1922 (Shannon, 1922). Although in 1973 Dr Feingold developed the widely publicised low additive- and salicylate-containing diet, objective evidence to support the effectiveness of this regimen is still lacking and probably food additives have an effect on only a minority of hyperactive children.

There is some evidence that hyperactive children may react to other foods in addition to food additives. Egger and co-workers studied 76 hyperactive children treated with 'few food' diet, of whom 62 improved, but only 28 of these completed a double-blind placebo-controlled challenge test. In total, 48 foods were incriminated. A high proportion of children had associated symptoms, e.g. headaches, fits and atopic symptoms such as asthma and eczema, which may not be typical of the average population of hyperactive children. The results of Egger's trial have been received with some scepticism and results from similar studies are awaited (Egger *et al.*, 1985).

Although there is evidence to suggest that foods may provoke migraine, the exact incidence and mechanism remains unknown. Egger *et al.* (1983) identified 55 foods causing migraine in 82 out of 88 children using a 'few food' diet. Using a similar diet, MacDonald, Forsyth & Wall (1989) found the incidence of food intolerance to be as little as 15% in a group of 60 children. Common foods implicated in migraine include milk, eggs, cheese, tea, coffee, red wine, chocolate, oranges, tomatoes and azo dyes.

There is a small amount of evidence to suggest that food intolerance may cause epilepsy and that anaphylaxis may occasionally provoke a seizure (David, 1993). Egger *et al.* (1989) could not demonstrate an improvement in 18 children with epilepsy alone using the 'few food' diet, but seizures did improve in 37 of 45 children with a combination of epilepsy, recurrent headaches, abdominal symptoms and hyperactivity. A further study using a similar 'few food' diet in 9 children demonstrated improvement in idiopathic epilepsy (Van Someren *et al.*, 1990).

Anaphylaxis

Systemic anaphylaxis is the most dangerous IgE medicated reaction and it usually occurs within minues after the ingestion of a food, but can still occur even after several hours. There is usually a clear-cut relationship to a food and foods such as fish, eggs, nuts, milk and certain grains are most frequently associated with anaphylaxis.

Food allergens

The definition of a food allergen is any food or its constituents able to produce an immune response in an individual. Most food allergens are acidic proteins or glycoproteins of a very specific configuration and size. Most are partially resistant to heat and to being broken down in the body by protein digesting enzymes. In British children, the most common food allergens include cows' milk, eggs, peanuts, fish, wheat and chocolate (Minford, MacDonald & Littlewood, 1982), although severe and even anaphylactic reactions have been reported to foods such as cabbage, white potatoes, chicory and mangoes (MacDonald, 1993*b*).

Diagnostic techniques

Although there are a number of laboratory diagnostic tests available they all have a limited ability to diagnose food intolerance.

Skin tests

A drop of allergen solution is placed on the skin which is either scratched to superficially penetrate the skin (scratch testing) or pricked with a hypodermic needle through the skin to a standard depth of 1 mm. The development of a wheal and flare response of greater than 3 mm to 4 mm within 20 minutes indicates a positive response. A positive reaction to an allergen demonstrates the presence of mast-cell fixed antibody (David, 1993). False positive and negative reactions are common with this test which rather limits its value. Factors affecting the results of skin tests include different potencies of allergen extracts, non-IgE mediated reactions and children and adults who have outgrown their food allergy may still retain positive skin tests (David, 1993).

RAST test

The radioallergosorbent test (RAST) is performed on serum to show the presence of IgE specific for the food antigen. In this test, solid phase-immobilised allergen is incubated with the patient's serum and after washing, the solid phase (usually a paper disc) is developed with radiolabelled anti-IgE (Freed, 1987). The RAST test is preferable to skin testing in patients with anaphylaxis and where the patient has widespread skin disease (David, 1993). However, there is poor correlation with skin test results (Adler *et al.*, 1991), and both false positive and negative results may occur.

Other tests

Basophil histamine release is a research diagnostic tool and is derived from the observation that peripheral blood leukocytes from allergic

Table 9.3. *Unorthodox diagnostic tests (David, 1993)*

Test	Explanation of test	Reliability of results
Pulse test	Increase in pulse rate following food challenge is likely to indicate food intolerance	Not validated No scientific basis
Cytotoxic test	In food-intolerant patients, white blood cells are reduced or leukocytes die in the presence of food allergen	Results unreliable
Hair analysis	Imbalance or lack of trace metals detected by hair analysis may cause food intolerance	Not validated No scientific basis
Radionics and dowsing	Forms of extra-sensory perception or radionic box. Usually pendulum is employed. A drop of saliva, urine, or sample of hair is placed under or inside the pendulum and the mode of oscillation indicates food intolerance	Not validated No scientific basis

individuals degranulate *in vitro* in the presence of antigen (Bjöksten, 1991). As it is dependent on allergen specific IgE, it is unlikely to be any more use than skin or RAST tests.

A number of unorthodox and unproved methods, comprehensively reviewed by David (1993) have been used both by non-medical and alternative practitioners to diagnose food allergy and intolerance and are summarised in Table 9.3.

Diet

Food withdrawal and symptom improvement followed by reappearance with a double-blind placebo-controlled food challenge, is seen as the best method of diagnosing food intolerance.

The type of diagnostic diet chosen will depend upon the patient's history, and severity of symptoms.

There are three main diagnostic diets in common use:

Exclusion diet

This is the commonest and simplest diagnostic diet and usually involves excluding one or two foods which appear from the history to be causing a reaction. It is usually recommended that this diet be continued for at least four weeks.

Empirical diet

An empirical diet involves excluding common food allergens associated with a specific condition but may not appear from the history to provoke symptoms. It should be continued for a period of approximately four weeks.

Few food diet or oligo-antigenic diet

This is a limited diet which should be used only when the symptoms are severe and the history is complex. It consists of a small number of basic foods (about 8–10), excluding all major food allergens, for a period of two to three weeks. The diet usually includes one meat, one cereal, two fruits and vegetables, a milk substitute and cooking oil or fat source. If there is an improvement in symptoms, omitted foods are systematically reintroduced into the diet at a frequency of one every seven days to identify which food(s) a patient is reacting to. The basic diet of 8–10 foods should not be attempted for longer than two or three weeks, any longer may result in poor compliance and nutritional deficiencies (MacDonald, 1993*b*).

Food reintroduction

With all three diagnostic diets, omitted foods should be reintroduced into the diet, usually in an open way initially, to see whether the original symptoms can be reproduced. Initially, foods should be introduced carefully, in minute quantities in case of anaphylactic reactions, but it is then important to gradually increase the dose to average portion sizes of the food. If there is any suggestion that a patient may react severely to a food, this should be conducted in hospital. If more than one food has to be reintroduced, it is important to leave a time interval of at least one week, in case of delayed reactions.

Double-blind placebo-controlled challenge tests

Experts in food intolerance would advocate a double-blind challenge test to refute or confirm the diagnosis of food intolerance beyond doubt. In this test, either the test food or a placebo is given in a hidden food and neither the patient nor the subject knows which substance has been given. This test is often labelled as the 'gold standard', but it has several limitations and is difficult to perform in routine practice. Suspected food allergens can either be disguised in another food, added to opaque capsules or given in a liquid medium via a nasogastric tube. It is difficult to mask the smell, texture and flavour of certain foods if disguised in another medium; capsules can contain only a limited quantity of food and if the food is given in another format or small quantities, it may not provoke a reaction. Subjects may require different quantities of allergen in order to provoke a response. Hill, Ball & Hoskins (1988), demonstrated that 8–10 g of cows' milk powder caused a reaction in some patients, whereas others required up to 10 times this volume of milk before symptoms developed. A negative reaction to the allergen in a blind challenge, does not always signify that food intolerance does not exist, as the quantity of food or length of challenge may have been inadequate, or the food itself administered in a less allergenic format. Anaphylaxis is always a danger of blind challenges and these should be reserved in routine clinical practice for food intolerance cases where the diagnosis is doubtful.

Specific diet therapies

Milk, wheat and eggs are the commonest components eliminated from the diet.

Milk free diets

Milk is one of the commonest foods to be eliminated from a young child's diet even though it is a cheap and valuable source of nutrition. 500 ml of cows' milk will provide 26% of the estimated average requirements for energy, 70% of the vitamin A and 100% of the calcium and riboflavin dietary reference values for a 1–3 year old boy (Department of Health, 1991).

In addition, many milk products such as cheese and yoghurt are convenient and milk derivatives such as lactose, whey and casein are used widely by the food industry and incorporated into a wide variety of manufactured foods as carriers or fillers, which makes it particularly difficult to exclude milk completely from the diet. Although a dietitian can teach parents how to interpret food labels and try and identify milk-containing components or provide lists identifying manufactured food free of milk, mistakes can still frequently occur. Manufacturers do not label all foods in e.g. home-baked cakes, chocolate and loose sweets and if an ingredient is added to another food ingredient (e.g. lactose added as a filler in monosodium glutamate, or milk is added to rusk in sausages), manufacturers need only identify the original ingredient, i.e. the additive or rusk. Many manufacturers produce substitutes for milk, products such as soya margarine, soya yoghurt, carob chocolate and soya-based cheese. However, sometimes milk derivatives are even added to these and death as a result of anaphylactic reaction has been reported in a 12-year-old boy, who was given a Tofu cheese which was thought to be milk free (David, 1993).

Milk substitutes

As milk is such a valuable food, it is important that children are provided with a nutritionally adequate, low allergenic formula. Unfortunately, probably no milk substitute is hypoallergenic and the main milk substitutes are summarised in Table 9.4. Hydrolysed protein formulas are popular in the treatment of CMPI, but it is now recognised that highly sensitive milk intolerant infants may react to these formulas. Although casein hydrolysates have been available for over 40 years, the first published case reports of reactions including anaphylaxis to them have appeared in the last few years (Bock, 1989; Saylor & Bahna, 1991; Rosenthal *et al.*, 1991; Sampson, James & Bernhisel-Broadbent, 1992). The two casein hydrolysate formulas available, i.e. Nutramigen and Pregestimil contain over 99% of peptides with a molecular weight of less than 1000 daltons. There are at least three reports of reactions to the more recently introduced whey hydrolysate formulae, including two reporting anaphylaxis (Heyman *et al.*, 1990; Businco *et al.*, 1989; Ellis, Short & Heiner, 1991). In clinical practice, there appears little difference between hydrolysed whey and casein formulas, although, one study comparing the two formulas in cows' milk sensitive enteropathy showed that small intestinal morphology was better with the whey hydrolysate (Walker-Smith, Digeon, Phillips, 1989).

If a young child refuses to take a milk substitute, it is probably advisable that a calcium supplement is given, even though the dietary reference value for healthy young children has been reduced to 350 mg per day (Kjellman *et al.*, 1988). Rickets has been reported in two children with a low calcium intake on a milk-free diet.

Egg free

All sources of egg need to be excluded from the diet including dried egg, egg white, egg yolk, egg albumen and egg lecithin. Examples of manufactured foods likely to contain egg include egg pasta, chewy sweets, sauces, salad cream, mayonnaise, cakes, biscuits, pastries and even malted milk drinks. It is possible to purchase egg substitutes based on potato starch, maize starch or tapioca flour, which can be used in cakes, biscuits, and sauces. Most people will eventually develop tolerance to egg. In the first instance they usually tolerate a small quantity of egg in cooking, as cooking helps to denature protein and render it less allergenic.

Wheat free

Wheat is one of many foods provoking food intolerance and a wheat-free diet should be distinguished from a gluten-free diet. A gluten-free diet omits wheat gluten, rye and usually oats and barley, but allows wheat starch, whereas a wheat-free diet excludes both wheat gluten and wheat starch. Sometimes there is a cross-reactivity between wheat and rye products. Unfortunately, some gluten-free special products such as gluten-free bread, flour and biscuits contain wheat starch and are therefore not suitable for wheat-free diets. A few special breads such as tapioca and rice bread are completely wheat-free and imaginative use should be made of non-wheat flours such as potato, sago, rice and buckwheat flour.

Nutritional adequacy of diet therapy

It is essential that all diet therapy is supervised by a qualified dietitian to ensure that the diet is nutritionally adequate. There have been several reports in the literature of poor growth and nutritional deficiencies and the diets have usually been self-selected or have been recommended and supervised by workers with little expertise in the field of nutrition (David, 1989). In a survey of children between 5 and 11 years, children who were perceived to have food intolerance and were avoiding three or more foods, were on average 4.2 cm shorter than children on a normal diet (Price, Rona & Chinn, 1988). David described a 10 month old child with eczema who had been diagnosed by a non-medical allergist as having an allergy to 57 foods. The child was placed on a diet comprising mashed potato, pure orange juice and pineapple juice only. Not only did the eczema fail to improve, but weight loss and failure to thrive occurred as a result of this inadequate diet (David, 1987).

Table 9.4. *Cows' milk substitutes*

Types	Examples	Nutritionally complete for infants	Advantages	Problems	Comments
Other animal milk	Goats' milk or sheep's milk	X Neither formula should be given to infants under 1 year Nutritionally incomplete	Cheap Readily available Palatable	• No microbiological standards in production. Pathogenic microorganisms may be found in goats' milk if unpasteurised • Strong immunological cross reactivity with cows' milk	Boil before use if comes from an unpasteurised source
Soya milk (a) Based on soya protein isolate	*Prescribable, nutritionally complete* Infasoy Isomil Prosobee Ostersoy Wysoy	✓ ✓ ✓ ✓	• Readily available • Palatable (relatively) • Cheap • Nutritionally complete	• Strong immunological cross reactivity with cows' milk Studies indicate 25–35% of infants reacting to cows' milk will react to soya	
Soya milk	Available from health stores, e.g. Plamil/Granose	X Not suitable for infants Low in calories, but some brands are now supplemented with calcium as well as other nutrients	• Readily available • Palatable (relatively) • Cheap	• Strong immunological cross reactivity with cows' milk Studies indicate 25–35% of infants reacting to cows' milk react to soya	Do no use for infants less than 1 year If used for young children, use a soya milk fortified with calcium

Types	Examples	Nutritionally complete for infants	Advantages	Disadvantages	Comments
Casein hydrolysates	Nutramigen Pregestimil	✓ ✓	• Low allergenicity • Nutritionally complete • Prescribable	• Expensive • Unpalatable • Case reports of reactions to casein hydrolysate are appearing	
Whey hydrolysates	Alfare Peptijunior	✓ ✓	• Low allergenicity • Nutritionally complete • Prescribable	• Expensive • Unpalatable • Case reports of reactions to whey hydrolysate are appearing	
Hydrolysed meat and soya	Prejomin Pepdite 0–2	✓ ✓	• Low allergenicity • Nutritionally complete • Prescribable	• Expensive • Unpalatable	• Little reported work evaluating these formulae
Amino acid	Neocate	✓	• Low allergenicity • Nutritionally complete • Prescribable	• Expensive • Unpalatable • Higher osmolality	• Little reported work evaluating amino acid formula

References

Aas, K. (1987). Fish allergy and the codfish allergens model. In *Food Allergy and Intolerance*, ed. J. Brostoff and S. J. Challacombe, pp. 356–6, Baillière-Tindall, London.

Adler, B. R., Assadullah, T., Warner, J. A. & Warner, J. O. (1991). Evaluation of a multiple food specific IgE antibody test compared to parental perception, allergy skin tests and RAST. *Clinical Experimental Dermatology*, **21**, 683–8.

Armstrong, D., Neild, V. S., Bailes, J. S. & Marsden, R. A. (1987). Exclusion diets in atopic eczema. In *Food Allergy*, ed. R. K. Chandra, pp. 262–72. Newfoundland Nutrition Research Education Foundation.

Atkins, F. M. (1991). Food-induced urticaria. In *Food Allergy. Adverse Reactions to Food and Food Additives*, ed. D. D. Metcalf, H. A. Sampson and R. A. Simon. Blackwell Scientific Publications, Oxford.

Bjöksten, B. (1991). *In vitro* diagnostic methods in the evaluation of food hypersensitivity. In *Food Allergy. Adverse Reactions to Food and Food Additives*, ed. D. D. Metcalf, H. A. Sampson and R. A. Simon. Blackwell Scientific Publications, Oxford.

Booth, I. W. (1991). Enteral nutrition in childhood. *British Journal of Hospital Medicine*, **46**, 111–13.

Bock, S. A. (1987). A prospective appraisal of complaints of adverse reactions to foods in children during the first three years of life. *Pediatrics*, **79**, 683–8.

Bock, S. A. (1989). Probable allergic reaction to casein hydrolysate formula. *Journal of Allergy and Clinical Immunology*, **84**, 272.

Bock, S. A., Atkins, F. M. (1989). The natural history of peanut allergy. *Journal of Allergy and Clinical Immunology*, **83** (5), 900–4.

Boland, M., Stoski, D. S., MacDonald, N. E., Scucy, P. & Patrick, J. (1986). Chronic jejunostomy feeding with a non-elemental formula in undernourished patients with cystic fibrosis. *Lancet*, **i**, 232–4.

Bougel, D., Iselin, M., Kahyat, A. & Duhamel, J.-F. (1986). Nutritional treatment of congenital heart disease. *Archives of Disease in Childhood*, **61**, 799–801.

Businco, L., Benincori, N., Cantari, A., Tacconi, L. & Picarazzi, A. (1985). Chronic diarrhoea due to cows' milk allergy. A 4 to 10 year follow-up study. *Annals of Allergy*, **53**, 844–7.

Businco, L., Cantani, A., Longhi, M. A. & Giampietr, P. G. (1989). Anaphylactic reactions to a cows' milk whey hydrolysate (Alfare, Nestlés) in infants with cows' milk allergy. *Annals of Allergy*, **62**, 333–5.

Carlin, A. C., Boatright Collier, S., Hendricks, K. M., Stoker, T. W. & Warman, K. Y. (1990). Paediatric disorders requiring specific nutrition management. In *Manual of Pediatric Nutrition*, ed. K. M. Hendricks and W. A. Walker, pp. 188–276. B. C. Decker, Toronto.

Chin, K. C., Tarlow, M. J. & Allfree, A. J. (1983). Allergy to cows' milk presenting as chronic constipation. *British Medical Journal*, **287**, 1593.

Clyne, P. S. & Kulczycki, A. (1991). Human breast milk contains bovine IgG. Relationship to infantile colic? Pediatrics, **87**, 439–44.

Dannaeus, A. (1987). Food allergy in infancy and children: state of the art. *Annals of Allergy*, **59**, Part II, 124–6.

Daniels, L., Davidson, G. P., Martin, A. J. & Pairas, T. (1989). Supplemental nasogastric feeding in cystic fibrosis patients during treatment for acute exacerbations of chest disease. *Australian Paediatric Journal*, **25**, 164–7.

David, T. J. (1987). Unhelpful recent developments in the diagnosis and treatment of allergy and food intolerance in children. In *Food Intolerance*, ed. J. Dobbing, pp. 185–214. Baillière Tindall, London.

David, T. J. (1989). Short stature in children with atopic eczema. *Acta Dermalogia Venerologia*, **114** (Suppl.), 41–4.

David, T. J. (1993). *Food and Food Additive Intolerance in Childhood*. Blackwell Scientific Publications, Oxford.

Department of Health (1991). *Dietary Reference Values for Food Energy and Nutrients for the United Kingdom*. London HMSO. Report on Health and Social Subjects 41.

DH/MAFF (1991). *Intolerance to Foods, Food Ingredients and Food Additives*. September.

Devlin, J., David, T. J. & Stanton, R. H. J. (1991). Elemental diet for refractory atopic eczema. *Archives of Disease in Childhood*, **66**, 93–9.

Dietz, W. H. (1987). Nutritional requirements and feeding of the handicapped child. In *Paediatric Nutrition Theory and Practice*, ed. R. J. Grand, J. L. Sutphen, and W. H. Dietz, pp. 387–92. Butterworth, Boston.

Egger, J., Carter, C. M., Graham, P. J., Gurnley, D. & Soothill, J. F. (1985). Controlled trial of oligoantigenic treatment in the hyperkinetic syndrome. *Lancet*, **i**, 540–4.

Egger, J., Carter, C. M., Wilson, J., Turner, M. W. & Soothill, J. F. (1983). Is migraine food allergy? A double-blind controlled trial of oligoantigenic diet treatment. *Lancet*, **ii**, 865–9.

Egger, J., Carter, C. M., Soothill, J. F. & Wilson, J. (1989). Oligoantigenic diet treatment of children with epilepsy and migraine. *Journal of Pediatrics*, **113**, 51–8.

Eggleston, P. A. (1987). Prospective studies in the natural history of food allergy. *Annals of Allergy*, **59**, Part II, 179–82.

Ellis, M. H., Short, J. A. & Heiner, D. C. (1991). Anaphylaxis after ingestion of a recently introduced hydrolysed whey protein formula. *Journal of Pediatrics*, **118**, 74–7.

Ford, R. P. K. & Walker-Smith, J. A. (1987). Paediatric gastrointestinal food allergic disease. In *Food Allergy and Intolerance*, ed. J. Brostoff and S. J. Challacombe, pp. 570–82. Baillière Tindall, London.

Freed, D. L. J. (1987). Laboratory diagnosis of food intolerance. In *Food Allergy and Intolerance*, ed. J. Brostoff and S. J. Challacombe, pp. 873–97. Baillière Tindall, London.

Gadol, C. L., Joshi, V. V. & Young Lee, E. (1987). Bronchiolar obstruction associated with repeated aspiration of vegetable material in two children with cerebral palsy. *Pediatric Pulmonology*, **3**, 437–9.

Gaskin, K. J., Waters, D. L., Baur, L. A., Soutter, V. L. & Gruca, M. A. (1990). Nutritional status, growth and development in children undergoing intensive treatment for cystic fibrosis. *Acta Paediatrica Scandinavica* (Suppl.), **366**, 106–10.

Gisel, E. G. (1991). Effect of food texture on the development of chewing of children between six months and two years of age. *Developmental Medicine and Child Neurology*, **33**, 69–79.

Gisel, E. G. & Patrick, J. (1988). Identification of children with cerebral palsy unable to maintain a normal nutritional state. *Lancet*, **i**, 283–7.

Halpern, S. R., Sellars, W. A., Johnson, R. B., Anderson, D. W., Saperstein, S. & Reisch, J. S. (1973). Development of childhood allergy in infants fed breast, soy or cows' milk. *Journal of Allergy and Clinical Immunology*, **51**, 139–51.

Harrison, C. J., Puntis, J. W. L., Durbin, G. M., Gornall, P. and Booth, I. W. (1991). Atypical allergic colitis in preterm infants. *Acta Paediatrica Scandinavica*, **80**, 1113–16.

Hathaway, M. J. & Warner, J. O. (1983). Compliance problems in the dietary management of eczema. *Arch. Dis. Child.*, **58**, 463–4.

Heird, W. E. (1977). Feeding the premature infant human milk or artificial formula. *American Journal of Disease of Childhood*, **131**, 468–9.

Heyman, M. B., Stoker, T. W., Rudolph, C. D. & Frick, O. L. (1990). Hypersensitivity reaction in an infant fed hydrolysed lactalbumin contained in a semi-elemental formula. *Journal of Pediatric and Gastroenterological Nutrition*, **10**, 253–6.

Hill, D. J., Ball, G. & Hoskins, C. S. (1988). Clinical manifestations of cows' milk allergy in childhood. Associations with *in-vitro* cellular immune responses. *Clinical Allergy*, **18**, 469–79.

Hill, S. M. & Milla, P. J. (1991). Infantile colitis. Allergy to food is the main non-infective cause and is easily treatable. *British Medical Journal*, **302**, 545–6.

Holden, C. E., Puntis, J. W. L., Charlton, C. P. L. & Booth, I. W. (1991). Nasogastric feeding at home: acceptability and safety. *Archives of Disease in Childhood*, **66**, 148–51.

Iacono, G., Garroccio, A., Montalto, G. *et al.* (1991). Severe infantile colic and intolerance. A long term prospective study. *Journal of Paediatric Gastroenterology and Nutrition*, **12**, 332–5.

Jackson, M. & Poskitt, E. M. E. (1991). The effects of high energy feeding on energy balance and growth in infants with congenital heart disease and failure to thrive. *British Journal of Nutrition*, **65**, 131–43.

Jaffe, N. (1987). Nutrition in cancer patients. In *Pediatric Nutrition Theory and Practice.* , ed. R. J. Grand, J. L. Sutphen & W. H. Dietz, pp. 571–8. Butterworth, Boston.

Jakobsson, I. & Lindberg, T. (1979). A prospective study of cows' milk protein intolerance in Swedish infants. *Acta Paediatrica Scandinavica*, **68**, 853–9.

Jakobsson, I. & Lindberg, T. (1983). Cows' milk proteins cause infantile colic in breast fed infants: a double-blind study. *Pediatrics*, **7**, 268–71.

Jones, P. M. (1989). Feeding disorders in children with multiple handicaps. *Developmental Medicine and Child Neurology*, **31**, 398–406.

Juhlin, L. (1985). Food additives in urticaria. In *The Urticarias*, ed. R. H. Champion, M. W. Greave, A. Kobza-Black and R. J. Pye, pp. 105–112.

Kane, R. E. & Black, P. (1989). Glucose intolerance with low-medium and high carbohydrate formulas during night time enteral feeding in cystic fibrosis patients. *Journal of Pediatric Gastroenterology and Nutrition*, **8**, 321–6.

Kane, R. E., Hobbs, P. J. & Black, P. (1990). Comparison of low, medium and high carbohydrate formulas for night time enteral feeding in cystic fibrosis patients. *Journal of Pediatric Enterology and Nutrition*, **14**, 47–52.

Kane, R. E. & Hobbs, P. J. (1991). Energy and respiratory metabolism in cystic fibrosis. The influence of carbohydrate content of nutritional supplements. *Journal of Pediatric Gastroenterology and Nutrition*, **12**, 217–23.

Kjellman, N. I. M. (1991). Natural history and prevention of food hypersensitivity. In *Food Allergy. Adverse Reactions to Food and Food Additives*, ed. D. D. Metcalf, H. A. Sampson and R. A. Simon. Blackwell Scientific Publications, Oxford.

Kjellman, N. I. M., Bjorksten, B., Hattevig, G. & Fath-Magnusson, K. (1988). Natural history of food allergy. *Annals of Allergy*, **61**, Part 2, 83–7.

Krick, J. & Van Duyn, M. A. S. (1984). The relationship between oral–motor involvement and growth: a pilot study in a paediatric population with cerebral palsy. *Journal of the American Dietetic Association,* **84**, 555–9.

Lessoff, M. H. (1984). Food intolerance and food aversion. A Joint Report of the Royal College of Physicians and the British Nutrition Foundation. *Journal of the Royal College of Physicians of London,* **18** (2), 83–123.

Levy, L. D., Durie, P. R., Pencharz, P. B. & Corey, M. L. (1985). Effects of long-term nutritional rehabilitation on body composition and clinical status in malnourished children and adolescents with cystic fibrosis. *Journal of Pediatrics,* **107**, 225–30.

Lothe, L., Lindberg, T. & Jakobsson, I. (1982). Cows' milk formula is a cause of infantile colic: a double-blind study. *Pediatrics,* **70**, 7–10.

Lothe, L. & Lindberg, T. (1989). Cow's milk whey protein elicits symptoms of infantile colic in colicky formula-fed infants: a double-blind crossover study. *Pediatrics,* **83**, 262–6.

MacDonald, A. (1994). Paediatric enteral nutrition. In *Manual of Dietetic Practice,* ed. B. Thomas. In press.

MacDonald, A. (1993b). *Food Allergy and Intolerance.* Profile Productions. In press.

MacDonald, A. & Booth, I. W. (1990). Nutrition. In *Paediatric Vade Mecum,* ed. J. A. Insley. Edward Arnold, London.

MacDonald, A., I. Forsyth & C. Wall (1989). Dietary treatment of migraine. In *Headache in Children and Adolescents,* ed. L. Lanzig, U. Balottin, and A. Cernibori. Elsevier Science Publishers BV (Biomedical Division).

McGrath, J. (1984). Allergy to cows' milk presenting as chronic constipation. *British Medical Journal,* **288**, 236.

Menon, G. & Poskitt, E. M. E. (1985). Why does congenital heart disease cause failure to thrive. *Archives of Disease in Childhood,* **60**, 1134–9.

Minford, A. M. B., MacDonald, A. & Littlewood, J. M. (1982). Food intolerance and food allergy in children: a review of 68 cases. *Archives of Disease in Childhood,* **57**, 742–7.

Novembre, E., Martino, M. & Vierucci, A. (1988). Foods and respiratory allergy. *Journal of Allergy and Clinical Immunology,* **81**, 1059–79.

Onorato, J., Merland, N., Terral, C. Y., Michel, F. B. & Bousquet, J. (1986). Placebo-controlled double-blind food challenge in asthma. *Journal of Allergy and Clinical Immunology.* **78** (6), 1139–46.

Parker, P., Stroop, S. & Green, H. L. (1981). A controlled comparison of continuous versus intermittent feeding in the treatment of infants with intestinal disease. *Journal of Pediatrics,* **99**, 360–4.

Patrick, J., Boland, M. P., Stoski, D. & Murray, G. E. (1986). Rapid correction of wasting in children with cerebral palsy. *Developmental Medicine Child Neurology,* **28**, 724–39.

Pearson, D. J. (1987). Problems with terminology and with study design in food sensitivity. In *Food Intolerance,* ed. J. Dobbing, pp. 1–13. Baillière-Tindall, London.

Pike, M. G., Carter, C. M., Boulton, P., Turner, M. W., Soothill, J. F. & Atherton, D. J. (1989). Few food diets in the treatment of atopic eczema. *Archives of Disease in Childhood,* **64**, 1691–8.

Poskitt, E. M. E. (1993). Failure to thrive in congenital heart disease. *Archives of Disease in Childhood,* **68**, 158–60.

Price, C. E., Rona, R. J. & Chinn, S. (1988). Height of primary school and parents' perceptions of food intolerance. *British Medical Journal,* **296**, 1696–9.

Ramsey, B. W., Farrell, P. M., Pencharz, P. and the Consensus Committee

(1992). Nutritional assessment and management in cystic fibrosis: a consensus report. *American Journal of Clinical Nutrition*, **55**, 108–16.

Randall, H. T. (1990). The history of enteral nutrition. In *Clinical Nutrition and Tube Feeding*, ed. J. L. Rombeau and M. D. Caldwell. W. B. Saunders, Philadelphia.

Rempel, G. R., Colwell, S. O. & Nelson, R. P. (1988). Growth in children with cerebral palsy fed via gastrostomy. *Pediatrics*, **82**, 857–61.

Rosenthal, E., Schlesinger, Y., Birnbaum, Y., Goldstein, R., Benderly, A. & Freier, S. (1991). Intolerance to casein hydrolysate formula. *Acta Paediatrica Scandinavica*, **80**, 958–60.

Salmon, A. P., Finkel, Y., Silove, E. D. *et al.* (1989). Sodium balance in infants with severe congestive heart failure. *Lancet*, **ii**, 875.

Sampson, H. A., James, J. M. & Bernhisel-Broadbent, J. (1992). Safety of an amino acid derived infant formula in children allergic to cows' milk. *Pediatrics*, **90**, 463–5.

Sanderson, I. R. & Walker Smith, J. A. (1991). Enteral feeding. In *Textbook of Paediatric Nutrition*, eds D. S. McLaren, D. Burman, N. R. Belton & A. F. Williams, pp. 321–336. Churchill Livingstone, Edinburgh.

Saylor, J. D. & Bahna, S. L. (1991). Anaphylaxis to casein hydrolysate formula. *Journal of Pediatrics*, **118**, 71–4.

Shannon, W. R. (1922). Neuropathic manifestations in infants and children as a result of anphylactic reaction to foods contained in their diet. *American Journal of Disease of Childhood*, **24**, 89–94.

Shapiro, B. K., Green, P., Krich, J., Allen, D. A. & Capute, A. J. (1986). Growth of severely impaired children: neurological versus nutritional factors. *Developmental Medicine and Child Neurology*, **28**, 729–33.

Smith, D. E., Handy, O., Holden, C. E., Stevens, M. C. G. & Booth, I. W. (1992). An investigation of supplementary naso-gastric feeding in malnourished children undergoing treatment for malignancy: results of a pilot study. *Journal of Human Nutrition and Dietetics*, **5**, 85–91.

Smith, D. E., Stevens, M. C. G. & Booth, I. W. (1990). Malnutrition in children with malignant solid tumours. *Journal of Human Nutrition and Dietetics*, **3**, 303–9.

Sondheimer, J. M. & Hamilton, J. R. (1978). Intestinal function in infants with severe congenital heart disease. *Journal of Pediatrics*, **92**, 572–8.

Taubman, B. (1988). Parental counselling compared with elimination of cows' milk or soya milk protein for the treatment of infantile colic syndrome. A randomised trial. *Pediatrics*, **81**, 756–61.

Thommessen, M., Heiberg, A., Kase, B. F., Larsen, S. & Riis, G. (1991). Feeding problems, height and weight in different groups of disabled children. *Acta Paediatrica Scandinavica*, **80**, 527–33.

Van Someren, V. V., Robinson, R. O., McCardle, B. & Sturgeon, N. (1990). Restricted diets for treatment of migraine. *Journal of Pediatrics*, **117**, 509–10.

Walker-Smith, J. A., Digeon, B. & Phillips, A. D. (1989). Evaluation of a casein and a whey hydrolysate for treatment of cows' milk sensitive enteropathy. *European Journal of Pediatrics*, **149**, 68–71.

Warin, R. P. & Smith, R. J. (1976). Challenge test battery in chronic urticaria. *British Journal of Dermatol.*, **94**, 401–6.

Warman, K. Y. (1990). Enteral nutrition: support of the paediatric patient. In *Manual of Pediatric Nutrition*, ed. K. M. Hendricks and W. A. Walker, pp. 72–109. B. C. Decker Inc., Toronto.

Warner, J. O., Gotz, M., Landau, L. I., Levison, H., Milner, A. D., Pedersen, S. & Silverman, M. (1989). Management of asthma; a consensus statement. *Archives of Disease in Childhood*, **64** (7), 1065–1079.

Young, E., Patel, S., Stoneham, M., Rona, R. & Wilkinson, J. D. (1987). The prevalence of reaction to food additives in a survey population. *Journal of the Royal College of Physicians of London*, **21** (4), 241–7.

10

Neonatal intravenous feeding

I. W. BOOTH

The nutritional vulnerability of the neonate

Together with better management of respiratory distress syndrome and intraventricular haemorrhage, the provision of parenteral nutrients to the very low birthweight (VLBW) neonate has played an important part in the improved survival of this high-risk group. Although most neonates who require parenteral nutrition need it for relatively short periods, about 2 weeks on average, this intervention comes at a time of immense nutritional vulnerability. Energy reserves are low and therefore early nutritional support is essential. It is also becoming clear that nutritional management may play a part in programming subsequent events, particularly neurodevelopment and the outcome of respiratory distress syndrome. However, considerable uncertainty remains about the precise indications for parenteral nutrition in the newborn.

Inability to withstand starvation

Studies of body composition at different ages have enabled the theoretical caloric reserve available for consumption during starvation to be estimated for different ages and sizes (Heird *et al.*, 1972). From these data, and a knowledge of resting energy expenditure at different ages, it is possible to estimate the length of time before death results from starvation. Thus, an adult, with nearly 2000 kcal/kilogram of caloric reserve is able to survive for 90 days. As subjects get smaller and younger, the maximum duration of starvation gets progressively less, so that a term infant can survive for about 30 days, a 2 kilogram pre-term baby for 2 weeks, and a 1 kilogram pre-term baby for only 4 days without nutrition. The need to provide nutritional support therefore becomes increasingly urgent, the smaller the patient.

Specific nutrient deficiencies also develop more readily in the newborn. For example, biochemical evidence of essential fatty acid deficiency can develop with a few days of birth (Gutcher & Farrell, 1992), and provides an important indication for the provision of parenteral lipid.

Nutrition and neuro-development

At birth, the brain accounts for approximately two-thirds of basal metabolic rate, and for about 50% at one year of age (Holliday *et al.*, 1972). Moreover, the human brain undergoes a growth spurt during the last trimester of pregnancy and for the first 2 years of life. The complexity of inter-neuronal connections also increases substantially during the first 2 years of life, and this process appears to be sensitive to undernutrition (Winick, Rosso & Waterlow, 1970).

It is perhaps not surprising therefore, that even modest energy deprivation during periods of rapid brain growth and differentiation may lead to an adverse neurodevelopmental outcome. Many studies have drawn attention to the delayed development seen in children suffering from primary protein-energy malnutrition. Under these circumstances, it seems that slowed development is related not only to undernutrition, but also to inadequate psycho-social stimulation (Grantham-McGregor, 1992). Hospital-based studies are few, but an intriguing series of observations by Georgieff *et al.* (1985) suggest that pre-term infants may be remarkably sensitive to even modest caloric deprivation. Infants were, as a result of intercurrent neonatal illness and despite the best efforts of the neonatologists, exposed to caloric deprivation (less than 85 kcal/kilogram/day) for increasing durations. Those infants who had been undernourished for between 4 to 6 weeks were significantly and substantially developmentally delayed at 12 months of age compared with the group of infants with only a few days' undernutrition. There also appeared to be a trend towards increasing deficit with an increased duration of undernutrition. Whilst these deficits may well correct in the long term, there is no evidence at present to suggest that they are rapidly reversible.

Early nutrition and long-term outcomes

Increasingly, we are becoming aware that nutritional experiences in early life may programme long-term outcomes. For example, pre-term babies who received mother's milk for the first few weeks of life had substantially improved IQ scores at 8 years of age compared with those who received

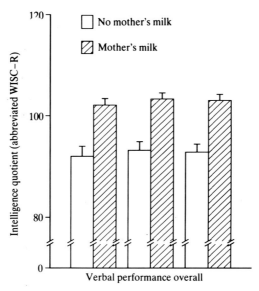

Fig. 10.1. IQ scores at 8 years of age in children who as pre-term infants received either mother's milk or formula (Lucas *et al.*, 1992).

formula (Fig. 10.1; Lucas *et al.*, 1992). It also seems that the adequacy of growth in utero and during the first 12 months of life may well affect outcome in adulthood with respect to ischaemic heart disease, hypertension and diabetes (Barker, 1992).

The infant brain and long chain polyunsaturated fatty acids

There is now mounting evidence that the neonate may be unable to elongate and desaturate the parent $n - 3$ or $n - 6$ fatty acids (Fig. 10.2). Brain growth is associated with an increase in the incorporation of the resulting long-chain polyunsaturated fatty acids (PUFA) into cerebral cortical phospholipids. Dietary manipulation in the experimental animals has suggested that the PUFA composition of the developing brain may be altered by extreme modifications of the essential fatty acids linoleic (C18:2$n - 6$) and α-linolenic (C18:3$n - 3$). Recent studies in man have shown a reduction in cerebral cortical phospholipid docosahexanoic acid in formula fed neonates compared with breast fed infants (Farquharson *et al.*, 1992). In contrast, supplementation of the diet of pre-term infants with long-chain PUFA $n - 3$ fatty acids improves retinal development (Uauy *et al.*, 1990). It therefore seems that provision of long-chain PUFA is

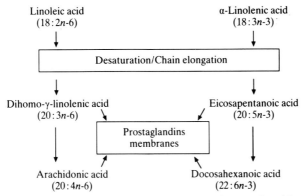

Fig. 10.2. Linoleic ($n - 6$) and alpha linolenic ($n - 3$) acids compete for the same enzyme system for desaturation and chain elongation to long-chain polyunsaturated fatty acids.

desirable, although evidence of functional deficit in association with biochemical deficiency is lacking. At present, parenteral lipids contain linoleic and linolenic acids, but do not contain the conditionally essential, longer chain, more unsaturated $n - 6$ and $n - 3$ fatty acids. Merely increasing the content of α-linolenic does not prevent a fall in red cell docosahexanoic acid content (Rhodes *et al.*, 1991).

Indications for parenteral nutrition (PN) (Table 10.1)

The criteria for using PN in the neonate remain poorly defined and its use is empirical, defined by over enthusiasm in some paediatricians, or by an irrational fear of side effects in others. As always, it is important to use the gut whenever possible. A number of recent studies have helped to define the place of enteral feeding in the VLBW infant.

Early feeding: enteral or parenteral?

The uncertainty about the optimal nutritional regimen for VLBW babies is reflected in a marked diversity of practice. In some neonatal units, enteral feeding is avoided for the first few weeks of life, whereas in others, the threshold for PN is much higher. Remarkably, this issue has not been convincingly addressed by clinical trials, nor do we really know whether or not PN does indeed reduce the risk of necrotising enterocolitis.

Three recent trials have clarified the role of enteral nutrition in VLBW

Table 10.1. *Indications for parenteral nutrition in the newborn*

Neonates	
Absolute indications	intestinal failure (short gut, functional immaturity, pseudo-obstruction)
	necrotising enterocolitis
Relative indications	hyaline membrane disease
	promotion of growth in pre-term infants
	possible prevention of necrotising entercolitis
Older infants and children	
Intestinal failure	short gut
	protracted diarrhoea
	chronic intestinal pseudo-obstruction
	post-operative abdominal or cardio-thoracic surgery
	radiation/cytotoxic therapy
Exclusion of luminal nutrient	Crohn's disease
Organ failure	acute renal failure
	acute liver failure
Hyper-catabolism	extensive burns
	severe trauma

neonates (Dunn *et al.*, 1988; Slagle & Gross, 1988; Meetze *et al.*, 1992). In each case babies were randomised to receive PN from birth, with or without the addition of small amounts of enteral nutrition. Those babies receiving early hypocaloric enteral feeds experienced less jaundice, required less phototherapy and had less metabolic bone disease (Dunn *et al.*, 1988) and subsequently had improved tolerance of enteral feeds (Slagle & Gross, 1988; Meetze *et al.*, 1992). It is well recognised in the experimental animal that total PN induces structural and functional atrophy in the gastro-intestinal tract, and these observations are consistent with a role for enteral nutrition in minimising these effects. Release of gastrointestinal peptides seems to be the most plausible mechanisms (Lucas, 1988).

Enteral nutrition and gastro-oesophageal reflux

Within the United Kingdom, anxiety about the risks of gastro-oesophageal reflux and pulmonary aspiration, particularly during mechanical ventilation, leads many neonatologists to avoid enteral nutrition during ventilation (Newell *et al.*, 1989). The effects of ventilation upon gastro-oesophageal reflux have now been investigated. Using a micro-antimony crystal intra-oesophageal pH electrode, Newell *et al.* (1989) demonstrated that ventilation actually reduces rather than promotes reflux, probably by increasing the anti-reflux pressure gradient across the gastro-oesophageal junction. There seems little justification for regarding mechanical ventilation as an indication for PN in this group of babies.

Enteral feeding and necrotising enterocolitis (NEC)

Along with hypoxia and mucosal injury, early enteral feeding has been thought to be a contributory factor in the pathogenesis of NEC. This has given rise to the practice of using PN prophylactically in the VLBW neonate in order to withhold enteral feeds (Eyal *et al.*, 1982). However, this practice has found little support in the more recent literature. The avoidance of early enteral feeding in three later studies failed to show a protective effect (LaGamma, Ostertag & Birenbaum, 1985; Unger *et al.*, 1986; Ostertag *et al.*, 1986). The situation is far from resolved. Meta-analysis of two of the studies examining the effect of early hypocaloric feeding (Dunn *et al.*, 1988; Slagle & Gross, 1988) has shown that NEC was more common in the early enteral feeding group (Heird, in press).

Macronutrient requirements

Energy

Reported resting energy expenditure in pre-term infants varies between 40 and 70 kcal/kg/day. The higher expenditures are usually seen in rapidly growing neonates in whom the energy cost of growth adds a substantial component (Heird, Jensen & Gomez, 1992). In the first few days of life, when growth is not an important consideration, the energy requirement is around 50 kcal/kg/day for parenterally delivered substrate. The parenteral nutrients required to meet this energy need are usually well tolerated. Most VLBW babies will assimilate the 40 kcal/kg provided by 5 g glucose, 1 g lipid and 2 g amino acid (all per kg/day). The next goal, that of matching *in utero* growth rate, is much more difficult and a consistent weight gain of 15 h/kg/day is rarely achieved. The required energy intake of around 90 kcal/kg/day is not usually tolerated because of hyperglycaemia or hypertriglyceridaemia.

Carbohydrate

Glucose is the preferred carbohydrate source and usually supplies 40–50% of total energy. There is no rationale for the use of fructose, which

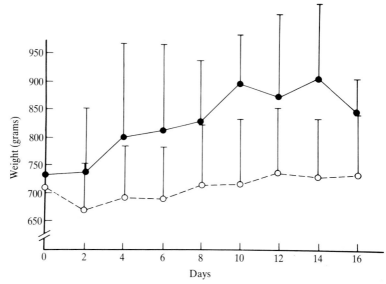

Fig. 10.3. Mean (SD) weight of insulin-treated (solid line) control (dashed line) infants. Weight was significantly greater in insulin-treated infants between days 4 and 15 (p, 0.05) (Collins *et al.*, 1991).

may precipitate death in patients with hereditary fructose intolerance, or lead to an accumulation of lactic acid (Collins, 1993).

Hyperglycaemia is common in the VLBW infant receiving parenteral glucose, even in the absence of recognised causes such as sepsis. Uncontrolled observations suggested that insulin may be helpful although initial improvements in glucose tolerance may not be sustained. Collins *et al.* (1991) have recently published the results of a trial in which VLBW neonates were randomised to receive either PN with a continuous insulin infusion or standard PN alone. Those infants receiving insulin tolerated higher glucose infusion rates, had greater non-protein energy intakes and better weight gain (Fig. 10.3). The addition of lipid emulsion to the regimen does not seem to impair efficiency (Kanarek, Santeiro & Malone, 1991). As the authors pointed out, glucose and insulin may just produce excess fat deposition, and an increased oxygen requirement. Although those infants receiving insulin did not require longer ventilation than controls, the effects of insulin on these, and additional factors such as linear growth and other growth factors, requires further study before routine insulin administration in this group of patients can be recommended. At present, it appears to be an effective, inexpensive and safe method of maintaining glucose homeostasis in VLBW infants who develop hyperglycaemia as a result of PN

Inositol

Inositol is a 6-carbon sugar alcohol which is an important component of membrane phospholipids and plays a crucial role in intracellular signal transduction. It is present in high concentration in breast milk, and administration to immature rabbits leads to increased pulmonary surfactant. The importance of inositol nutrition in early growth and development may have been understated. In a recent placebo-controlled study of parenteral inositol (80 mg/kg/d) during the first 5 days of life in ventilated neonates receiving total PN, supplementation was associated with reductions in the severity of respiratory distress syndrome (RDS), early mortality, retinopathy and bronchopulmonary dysplasia (Hallman *et al.*, 1992). If these striking results can be corroborated, there will be a strong argument for routine incorporation of inositol into PN regimens for VLBW infants with severe RDS.

Lipid

Parenteral lipid emulsions represent an important energy source, and are also a rich source of essential fatty acids; lipid oxidation also produces less carbon dioxide than an isocaloric amount of carbohydrate. Replacing 25% of parenteral glucose with the equivalent energy and lipid, leads to decreased energy expenditure in the newborn, and better growth (Van Aerde *et al.*, 1989). The differences between fat and carbohydrate in their nitrogen-sparing properties are not entirely clear, but are probably minimal in the very low birthweight infant (Pineault *et al.*, 1988).

The energy mix of PN does seem to influence the adaptive response of the small intestinal mucosa. In the newborn miniature pig, total PN with glucose as the sole energy source resulted in higher small intestinal sucrase and maltase activities, which were higher than in the group receiving 50:50 lipid carbohydrate mixture (Shulman & Burrin, 1991). Insulin may be the mediator of these differences.

A 20% lipid emulsion has a lower phospholipid/triglyceride ratio than a 10% emulsion. This probably explains the lower plasma cholesterol and triglyceride concentrations seen in infants receiving the 20% emulsion (Haumont *et al.*, 1984).

Medium chain triglycerides (MCT)

Parenteral MCT are currently under investigation as an alternative energy source to long chain triglycerides (LCT). Medium chain fatty acids are transported across the mitochondrial membrane independently of carnitine and are mainly oxidised, with a greater release of energy than from LCT. MCT emulsions lead to higher plasma free fatty acid concentrations, due to a higher availability to lipolytic enzymes, which in the jaundiced neonate could increase free bilirubin concentrations in plasma. In a comparative trial of an LCT emulsion with a 50:50 MCT/LCT mixture, the fraction of bilirubin unbound to albumin was significantly lower in the MCT/LCT group, supporting the idea that MCT-containing emulsions are safe energy sources in the pre-term infant (Rubin *et al.*, 1991).

Parenteral lipid and bronchopulmonary dysplasia

Parenteral lipid emulsions have a number of reported effects on pulmonary function in the neonate: decreased arterial oxygenation, deposition of lipid in alveolar macrophages and intravascularly, and increased pulmonary vascular tone. More recently, attention has focussed on lipid emulsions as a cause of bronchopulmonary dysplasia. A retrospective analysis from Liverpool suggested that a seven-fold increase in chronic lung disease was related to an increased use of early parenteral lipid emulsions in the ventilated VLBW infant (odds ratio 8:1) (Cooke, 1991). Furthermore, a small randomised study in which ventilated neonates were assigned to receive PN with or without lipid for the first five days, showed an adverse effect in the lipid group. Those infants who received early lipid, required more days ventilation and supplemental oxygen therapy, and had a high incidence of stage 3 bronchopulmonary dysplasia (5 out of 20 receiving lipid, compared with none of the 22 who did not receive early lipid) (Hammerman & Aramburo, 1988).

A further detailed study from London has failed to confirm these results. Early lipid infusion had no adverse effects on blood gases or a respiratory outcomes and the authors concluded that intravenous fat emulsions at rates not exceeding 0.15 g kg/h can be given safely to sick VLBW infants on the first day of life (Gilbertson *et al.*, 1991). The reasons for these conflicting results are unclear, but until more convincing evidence of a deleterious effect is produced, it seems wise not to withhold this valuable energy source from sick neonates.

Parenteral lipid and infection

Staphylococcus epidermidis is a common cause of bacteraemia in neonates receiving intensive care. Using a case-control methodology, Freeman *et al.* (1990) have shown that infants with this complication were 5.8 times more likely to have had a percutaneous central venous catheter. The authors suggest that heavy skin contamination with staphylococci, the growth promoting properties of lipid emulsion, the use of Teflon catheters and the suppressive effects of lipid emulsions on neutrophil and macrophage function, may be causative factors in this association. At present, the benefits of parenteral lipid in this nutritionally vulnerable group of infants, outweigh the risk of sepsis, although further study is needed to further define both pathogenesis and prevention.

Carnitine

L-carnitine is an essential in the transport of long-chain fatty acids across the mitochondrial membrane, which must take place before β-oxidation can occur. Deficiency may therefore impair lipid clearance from plasma, and reduce both ketogenesis and thermogenesis. PN solutions are carnitine-free and plasma carnitine deficiency has been documented in neonates receiving PN. However, studies of L-carnitine supplementation have yielded conflicting results (Schmidt-Sommerfeld & Penn, 1990). More recent studies have shown that L-carnitine supplementation (8–16 mg/kg/day) leads to modest increases in growth and nitrogen retention, with reduced triglyceride concentrations and free fatty acid/ketone body ratios (Helms *et al.*, 1990). However, higher dosage (48 mg/kg/day) is associated with increases in metabolic rate, fat oxidation and nitrogen excretion and impaired weight gain (Sulkers *et al.*, 1990). Although fat oxidation in the parenterally fed neonate may be limited by carnitine deficiency, it has yet to be established that this is of any clinical consequence, and it is difficult to support routine supplementation without further evidence.

Nitrogen

There is considerable uncertainty about how best to assess the most appropriate amino acid profile for neonatal solutions. It is unclear whether solutions should be designed to mimic the amino acid profile in the plasma of breast fed infants, cord blood, lean tissue, or the accretion rates for individual amino acids *in utero*. Synthetic crystalline L-amino acid solutions such as Vamin (Kabi Pharmaxia), which is based on the amino acid profile of egg protein, has been used as the nitrogen source of parenterally fed infants in the past, although these solutions were originally designed for adults. Compared with breast milk, this results in over-provision of certain amino acids such as phenylalanine, but under-provision of others such as taurine, which is now considered essential for patients on long-term PN. In addition, the most appropriate profile of amino acids administered to the neonate may not only be different but much less flexible. The need for growth means that the young infant requires relatively larger quantities of essential amino acids than an older child or adult. Moreover, immaturity of hepatic enzymes may reduce the synthesis and catabolism of certain amino acids. For example, liver cystathionase activity is low at full term, and endogenous synthesis of cystine from methionine is limited. In addition, histidine is required for normal growth in the newborn because of the increased demands for production of haemoglobin.

Plasma amino acid profiles in babies fed egg protein-based amino acid solutions have often shown increased concentrations of phenylalanine (Puntis *et al.*, 1986). Solutions designed to mimic the profile of amino acids seen in breast milk have been associated with lower plasma concentrations of phenylalanine and tyrosine, and plasma amino acid profiles closer to those found in breast fed infants (Puntis *et al.*, 1989). Such hyperphenylalaninaemia which does occur, does not seem to be associated with subsequent developmental delay (Lucas, Baker & Horley, 1993).

Taurine

Taurine is a sulphur-containing amino acid which is an end-product of methionine and cysteine metabolism. It is not incorporated into proteins. Bile acids are secreted in bile conjugated either to taurine or glycine, and taurine conjugates have superior detergent properties. Until recently this was felt to be the major physiological function of taurine. It is now clear that taurine is also important in the normal development of the brain and retina.

The activity of hepatic cysteinensulfinic acid decarboxylase, the rate-limiting enzyme in the biosynthesis of taurine from cysteine, is low in infancy. In contrast to infants receiving breast milk, in which taurine is abundant, formula-fed infants have biochemical taurine deficiency. Moreover, plasma taurine concentrations fall rapidly in pre-term infants receiving taurine-free PN solutions.

Children receiving long-term PN seem to be at particular risk of developing clinical taurine deficiency, and abnormal retinograms have been found in association with biochemical taurine deficiency. In three out of four children these became normal following taurine repletion (Geggel *et al.*, 1985). Taurine is therefore probably best regarded as a conditionally essential amino acid, and a taurine-containing amino acid solution is now available for use in infants (Vaminolac (Kabi Pharmacia); Thornton & Griffin, 1991).

Calcium and phosphate supplements

Limited solubilities often make meeting calcium and phosphate requirements of the rapidly growing neonate receiving PN difficult. In fact, conventional regimens can provide only about half the estimated requirements for an accretion rate which reflects intrauterine retention. Not surprisingly, metabolic bone disease is a common problem in infants receiving long-term PN. Organic phosphorus compounds (e.g. glycero- and glucose-phosphate) have been shown to be more compatible with calcium than conventionally used inorganic forms (Raupp *et al.*, 1991). Calcium glycerophosphate has now been shown to be effective in promoting mineral retention (Hanning *et al.*, 1991). It seems likely therefore, that organic phosphorus compounds represent an important vehicle for increasing the intake of calcium and phosphorus particularly in pre-term infants.

Venous access

A central venous catheter with the tip in the right atrium is the preferred route. Peripheral infusion leads almost inevitably to thrombophlebitis, requiring frequent line changes and loss of nutrient infusion. Patients are exposed to the risk of hypoglycaemia and hypothermia during the time when the infusion is not running or being resited.

For the neonate, a fine Silastic catheter inserted percutaneously is the most convenient method (Puntis, 1986). Peripheral veins should be reserved for the purpose in those neonates likely to require parenteral nutrition, and the catheter should be used exclusively for PN. The technique is carried out without anaesthesia with the infant in the incubator (Puntis, 1986).

Administration of PN through an umbilical arterial catheter is associated with infection, bleeding, limb ischaemia, embolism and hypertension. However, it provides easy vascular access and continues to be popular in some units. A recent study has suggested that the umbilical artery represents a reasonable alternative to a central venous catheter (Kanarek, Kuznicki & Blair, 1991), although most neonatologists would prefer to use a peripherally inserted percutaneous central venous catheter whenever possible.

References

Barker, D. J. P. (1992). Fetal and infant origins of adult disease. *British Medical Journal*, London.

Collins, J. W., Hoppe, M., Brown, K., Edidin, D. V., Padbury, J. & Ogata, E. D. (1991). A controlled trial of insulin infusion and parenteral nutrition in extremely low birthweight infants with glucose intolerance. *Journal of Pediatrics*, **11**, 921–7.

Collins, J. (1993). Time for fructose solutions to go. *Lancet*, **341**, 600.

Cooke, R. W. I. (1991). Factors associated with chronic lung disease in preterm infants. *Archives of Diseases of Childhood*, **66**, 26–8.

Dunn, L., Hulman, S., Weiner, J. & Kleigman, R. (1988). Beneficial effects of early hypocaloric enteral feeding on neonatal gastrointestinal function: preliminary report of a randomised trial. *Journal of Pediatrics*, 112, 622–9.

Eyal, F., Sagi, E., Arad, I. & Abital, A. (1982). Necrotising enterocolitis in the very low birth-weight infant: expressed breast milk feeding compared with parenteral feeding. *Archives of Diseases of Childhood*, **57**, 274–6.

Farquharson, J., Cockburn, F., Patrick, W. A., Jamieson, E. C. & Logan, R. W. (1992). Infant cerebral cortex phospholipid fatty-acid composition and diet. *Lancet*, 340, 810–13.

Freeman, J., Goldmann, D. A., Smith, N. E., Sidebottom, D. G., Epstein, M. F., & Platt, R. (1990). Association of intravenous lipid emulsion and coagulase-negative staphylococcal bacteremia in neonatal intensive care units. *New England Journal of Medicine*, 323, 301–8.

Geggel, H. S., Ament, M. E., Heckenlively, J. R., Martin, D. A. & Kopple, J. D. (1985). Nutritional requirement for taurine in patients receiving long-term parenteral nutrition. *New England Journal of Medicine*, **312**, 142–6.

Georgieff, M. K., Hoffman, J., Pereira, G. R. *et al.* (1985). Effect of neonatal caloric deprivation on head growth and one-year development status in pre-term infants. *Journal of Pediatrics*, **107**, 581–7.

Gilbertson, N., Kovar, I. Z., Cox, D. J., Crowe, L. & Palmer, N. T. (1991). Introduction of intravenous lipid administration on the first day of life in the very low birthweight neonate. *Journal of Pediatrics*, **119**, 615–23.

Grantham-McGregor, S. M. (1992). In *Protein-energy Malnutrition*, ed. J. C. Waterlow, pp. 344–60, Edward Arnold, London.

Gutcher, G. R. & Farrell, P. M. (1992). Intravenous infusion of lipid for the prevention of essential fatty acid deficiency in premature infants. *American Journal of Clinical Nutrition*, **54**, 1024–8.

Hallman, M., Bny, K., Hoppu, K., Lappi, M. & Pohjavvori, M. (1992). *New England Journal of Medicine*, **326**, 1233–9.

Hammerman, C. & Aramburo, M. J. (1988). Decreased lipid intake reduces morbidity in sick premature neonates. *Journal of Pediatrics*, **113**, 1093–8.

Hanning, R. M., Atkinson, S. A. & Whyte, R. K. (1991). Efficacy of calcium glycerophosphate vs conventional mineral salts for total parenteral nutrition in low-birth-weight infants: a randomised clinical trial. *American Journal of Clinical Nutrition*, **54**, 903–8.

Haumont, D., Deckelbaum, R. J., Richell, M. *et al.*, (1984). Plasma lipid and plasma lipoprotein concentrations in low birth-weight infants given parenteral nutrition with 20% compared to 10% Intralipid. *Journal of Pediatrics*, **115**, 787–93.

Heird, W. C., Driscoll, J. M., Schullinger, J. N. *et al.* (1972). Intravenous alimentation in paediatric patients. *Journal of Pediatrics*, **80**, 351–72.

Heird, W. C., Jensen, C. L. & Gomez, M. R. (1992). Practical aspects of achieving positive energy balance in low birth-weight infants. *Journal of Pediatrics*, **120**, S120–8.

Heird, W. C. (1992). Parenteral feeding. In *Effective Care of the Newborn Infant*. ed. J. C. Sinclair and J. F. Lucy, Oxford University Press, Oxford. (in press).

Helms, R. A., Mauer, E. C., Hay, W. W., Christensen, M. L. & Storm, M. C. (1990). Effect of intravenous L-carnitine on growth parameters and fat metabolism during parenteral nutrition in neonates. *Journal of Parenteral and Enteral Nutrition*, **14**, 448–53.

Holliday, M. A., Potter, D. *et al.* (1972). Metabolic rate and organ size during growth from infancy to maturity and during late gestation and early infancy. *Pediatrics*, **47**, 169–79.

Kanarek, K. S., Santeiro, M. L. & Malone, J. I. (1991). Continuous infusion of insulin in hyperglycemic low birth-weight infants receiving parenteral nutrition with and without lipid emulsion. *Journal of Parenteral and Enteral Nutrition*, 15, 417–20.

Kanarek, K. S., Kuznicki, M. B. & Blair, R. C. (1991). Infusion of total parenteral nutrition via the umbilical artery. *Journal of Parenteral and Enteral Nutrition*, **15**, 71–4.

LaGamma, E. F., Ostertag, S. G. & Birenbaum, H. (1985). Failure of delayed oral feeding to prevent necrotising enterocolitis. Results of a study in very low birth-weight neonates. *American Journal of Diseases of Children*, **139**, 385–9.

Lucas, A. (1988). Gut hormones and the adaptation to extrauterine nutrition. ed. P. J. Milla and D. P. R. Miller, pp. 302–17. Churchill Livingstone, Edinburgh.

Lucas, A., Morley, R., Lister, G. & Leeson-Payne, C. (1992). Breast milk and subsequent intelligence quotient in children born preterm. *Lancet*, **339**, 261–4.

Lucas, A., Baker, B. A. & Horley, R. M. (1993). Hyperphenylalaninaemia and outcome in the intravenously fed pre-term neonate. *Archives of Diseases of Childhood* (in press).

Meetze, W. H., Valentine, C., McGingan, J. E., Conlon, M., Sacks, N. & Neu, J. (1992). Gastrointestinal priming prior to full enteral nutrition in very low birth weight infants. *Journal of Paediatric and Gastroenterological Nutrition*, **15**, 163–70.

Newell, S. J., Booth, I. W., Morgan, M. E. I., Durbin, G. M. & McNeish, A. S. (1989). Gastro-oesophageal reflux in preterm infants. *Archives of Diseases of Childhood*, **64**, 780–6.

Ostertag, S. G., LaGamma, E. F., Reisen, C. E. & Ferrentino, F. L. (1986). Early enteral feeding does not affect the incidence of necrotising enterocolitis. *Pediatrics*, **77**, 275–80.

Pineault, M., Chexxex, P., Bisaillon, S. & Brisson, G. (1988). Total parenteral nutrition in the newborn: impact of the quality of infused energy on nitrogen metabolism. *American Journal of Nutrition*, **47**, 298–304.

Puntis, J. W. L., Edwards, M. A., Green, A., Morgan, M. E. I., Booth, I. W. & Ball, P. A. (1986). Hyperphenylalaninaemia in parenterally fed newborn babies. *Lancet*, **ii**, 1105–6.

Puntis, J. W. L., Ball, P. A., Preece, M. A., Green, A., Brown, G. A. & Booth, I. W. (1989). Egg and breast milk based nitrogen sources compared. *Archives of Diseases of Childhood*, **64**, 147–7.

Puntis, J. W. L. (1986). Percutaneous insertion of central venous feeding catheters. *Archives of Diseases of Childhood*, **61**, 1138–40.

Raupp, P., Kries, R., Pfahl, H. G. & Manz, F. (1991). Glycero- vs glucose-phosphate in parenteral nutrition of premature infants: a comparative *in vitro* evaluation of calcium/phosphorus compatibility. *Journal of Parenteral and Enteral Nutrition*, **15**, 469–73.

Rhodes, P. G., Reddy, N. S., Downing, G. & Carlson, S. E. (1991). The effects of different levels of intravenous alpha-linolenic acid and supplemental breast milk on red cell docosahexaneoic acid in very low birth-weight infants. *Journal of Pediatric and Gastroenterological Nutrition*, **13**, 67–71.

Rubin, M., Harell, D., Naor, N., Moser, A., Wielunsky, E., Merlob, P. & Lichtenberg, D. (1991). Lipid infusion with different triglycerine cores (long-chain vs medium-chain/long-chain triglycerides): effect on plasma lipids and bilirabin binding in premature infants. *Journal of Parenteral and Enteral Nutrition*, **15**, 469–73.

Schmidt-Sommerfeld, E. & Penn, D. (1990). Carnitine and total parenteral nutrition of the neonate. *Biology of the Neonate*, **58** (suppl. 1), 81–8.

Shulman, R. J. & Burrin, D. G. (1991). Total parenteral nutrition energy composition affects small intestinal disaccharidase activity in the newborn miniature pig. *Journal of Parenteral and Enteral Nutrition*, **15**, 560–3.

Slagle, T. A. & Gross, S. J. (1988). Effect of early low-volume enteral substrate on subsequent feeding intolerance in very low birthweight infants. *Journal of Pediatrics*, **113**, 526–31.

Sulkers, E. J., Lafeber, H. N., Degenhart, H. J., Przyrembel, H., Schlotzer, E. & Sauer, P. J. J. (1990). Effects of high carnitine supplementation on substrate utilisation in low-birthweight infants receiving total parenteral nutrition. *American Journal of Clinical Nutrition*, **52**, 889–94.

Thornton, L. & Griffin, E. (1991). Evaluation of a taurine containing amino acid solution in parenteral nutrition. *Archives of Diseases of Children*, **66**, 21–5.

Uauy, R. D., Birch, D. G., Birch, B. E., Tyson, J. E. & Hoffman, D. R. (1990). Effect of dietary N-3 fatty acids on retinal function of very low-birth weight neonates. *Pediatric Research*, **28**, 485–92.

Unger, A., Goetzman, B. W., Chan, C., Lyons, A. B. & Miller, M. F. (1986). Nutritional practices and outcome of extremely premature infants. *American Journal of Diseases in Children*, **140**, 1027–33.

Van Aerde, J. E. E., Sauer, P. J. J., Pencharz, P. B., Smith, J. M. & Swyer, P. R. (1989). Effect of replacing glucose with lipid on the energy metabolism of small infants. *Clinical Science*, **76**, 581–8.

Winick, M., Rosso, P. & Waterlow, J. C. (1970). Cellular growth of cerebrum, cerebellum and brain stem in normal and marasmic children. *Experimental Neurology*, **26**, 3939–4000.

11

Nutrition and the surgical patient

N. EVERITT and M. McMAHON

Introduction

Malnutrition amongst surgical patients is common, and mortality and morbidity are increased when malnourished patients undergo major surgical procedures (Warnold & Lundholm, 1984). Some studies have indicated that nutritional support can speed recovery from surgery with the reduction of mortality and morbidity, but others have not indicated benefit. It is now apparent that undernourishment may occur both as a consequence of reduced, or absent, food intake; and as a direct effect of underlying disease. The syndromes of multiple organ failure (MOF), and the septic state are associated with an altered pattern of metabolism, central to which is the futile cycling of substrates which is not suppressed by exogenous replacement. Nutritional support is frequently directed at the critically ill and it is only as the pathophysiology of MOF and the sepsis syndrome are understood, that treatment will be optimised. The lack of evidence of benefit from nutritional support may, in part, be because the metabolic burdens of surgical pathology, and of major operative procedures, are incompletely understood. In view of the complex nature of many diseases for which nutritional support appears logical, the lack of hard data to indicate a precise role for nutritional therapy, may reflect the difficulties encountered in the conduct of a strict clinical trial, rather than the value of nutritional support itself.

Prevalence of malnutrition amongst surgical patients

Malnutrition is common amongst surgical patients and is frequently overlooked. A survey, from the General Infirmary at Leeds, reported that 33% of patients on a general surgical ward displayed evidence of a nutritional disorder, when defined by two or more subnormal values for arm muscle circumference, weight loss and serum albumin (Hill *et al.*, 1977). When patients, who were more than seven days convalescent after surgery were considered as a separate group, the incidence of abnormally low values for two or more of the variables was 55%. In a study of 131 surgical patients on all wards in a North American hospital, in which nutritional status was assessed by arm muscle circumference, triceps skin-fold thickness and serum albumin, it was found that protein-calorie malnutrition was present in 55% of subjects and that severe malnutrition was more common in general surgical patients, than in patients from other surgical specialties (Bistrian *et al.*, 1974). It might be expected that there would be a higher incidence of malnutrition on surgical wards which serve communities in which poor nutrition is prevalent and on specialist units, which concentrate on surgery for gastrointestinal malignancy or inflam-matory bowel disease. Malnutrition was found to be present in over half of a group of long-stay patients with inflammatory bowel disease, who suffered complications after surgery (Hill *et al.*, 1977). Poor nutrition is not confined to general surgical patients; a British study indicated that approximately 20% of patients admitted to hospital with a fracture of the neck of the femur were undernourished, with skinfold thickness and arm muscle circumference more than two standard deviations below the mean values of an elderly reference population (Bastow, Rawlings & Allison, 1983).

Adverse effects of malnutrition in surgical patients

Poor nutritional status is associated with an increased risk of death and complication after major surgery; more than half a century ago, a correlation between pre-operative weight loss and mortality after gastrec-tomy in patients with peptic ulcer disease was recognised (Studley, 1936). Surgical incisions (Kobak *et al.*, 1947) and anastomoses are less likely to heal in the presence of malnutrition and therefore, wound dehiscence and anastomotic failure (Daly, Vars & Dudrick, 1972), are more likely. The immune response is impaired in the presence of malnutrition (Law, Dudrick & Abdou, 1973) and poorly nourished patients are more prone to develop major infective complications (Windsor & Hill, 1988*a*). Malnutrition affects the performance of skeletal muscles, including those which are concerned with breathing (Arora & Rochester, 1982), as well as cardiac muscle (Gottdiener *et al.*, 1978). Thus, pressure sores and venous thrombo-embolism (Holmes *et al.*, 1987), atelectasis and pneumonia (Windsor & Hill, 1988*b*), reduced cardiac output (Heymsfield *et al.*, 1978) and cardiac arrhythmias (Gottdiener *et al.* 1978), are associated with poor nutritional status. Malnutrition alters the normal respiratory response to hypoxaemia (Doeckel *et al.*, 1976) and it may be more difficult to wean the nutritionally depleted patient from mechanical ventilation (Benotti & Bistrian, 1989).

Causes of malnutrition amongst surgical patients

In surgical practice, malnutrition most frequently implies undernourishment and the usual pattern is protein-calorie deficit; deficiencies of vitamins and trace elements are less common and when they do occur, it is usually in the overall setting of protein-calorie malnutrition. Malnutrition may develop when nutritional intake is impaired, because gastrointestinal disease limits the absorption of nutrients, or because the patient's pathology imposes an 'obligatory' metabolic demand. In many instances, a combination of mechanisms is responsible for the nutritional deficit.

Malnutrition due to impaired intake

Intake may be impaired by psychological, socioeconomic, and physical limitations. The depressed, or apathetic patient is likely to neglect nutritional intake, both in respect of amount and content; and malnutrition may in turn affect mood and appetite adversely. Symptoms of anorexia and nausea, which are common to a wide variety of illnesses, will further reduce food intake. Once admitted to hospital, food is frequently found to be unfamiliar or unappetising. Moreover, extensive investigation may necessitate periods of starvation and absence from the ward at times when food is delivered. The management of certain conditions, for example acute pancreatitis, may require total abstinence from oral intake for a considerable period of time. Underlying pathology may interfere with the physical delivery of food, for example in individuals who suffer dysphagia, or patients for whom injury, rheumatological or neurological disease, limit function of the upper limb, jaw, or pharynx.

Malnutrition due to gastrointestinal disease

In surgical patients, malnutrition can occur either because there is malabsorption, or because of excess protein loss secondary to enteropathy.

Malabsorption may be due to altered gastrointestinal motility, reduced functional mucosal area, or digestive enzyme deficiency. Motility abnormalities include mechanical obstruction, ileus and pseudo-obstruction, and gastric stasis after head injury; whilst mucosal area is reduced by enteritis, resection, or fistulation. Digestive enzyme deficiency may occur as a consequence of pancreatic exocrine deficiency after pancreatitis or pancreatic resection. Pathology associated with excessive protein loss from the gastrointestinal tract includes Crohn's and Menetrier's diseases.

Malnutrition due to altered metabolic demand

Malnutrition can occur as a consequence of altered metabolic demand, when the patient may continue to lose lean body weight, fat, and micronutrients, despite the provision of sufficient nutrition to meet, or exceed, the requirements of oxidative metabolism. Altered metabolic demand may be due to malignant cachexia, or as part of the 'sepsis' response to infective, or inflammatory conditions (for example intraperitoneal abscess and inflammatory bowel disease). The most profound alterations in metabolism are seen when 'hypermetabolism' occurs as a component of the sepsis syndrome; when loss of body protein cannot be prevented despite adequate provision of energy (Streat, Beddoe & Hill, 1987). Improvement in nutritional status is unlikely to be achieved until the underlying pathology has been corrected; thus abscesses must be drained and necrotic tissue should be resected. However, it does not follow that nutritional support should not be provided in the interim, despite the lack of published evidence of benefit.

Sepsis, infection, and multiple organ failure

Improvements in intensive care, which include use of inotropes, ventilation and renal dialysis, have resulted in the survival of patients, often victims of trauma, who would previously have died. The increased survival has led to the recognition of the syndrome of MOF, in which there is a progressive failure of a variety of systems which, characteristically, were not involved in the original injury (Baue, 1975). Multiple organ failure is an host-dependent disease, caused by activation of endogenous humoral inflammatory mediators, which include cytokines, eicosanoids, complement, nitric oxide metabolites and free radicals (Cerra, 1991). The membranes are responsible for the altered microvascular circulation, increased cell membrane permeability, and intravascular thrombosis, seen in organs affected by MOF. Critically ill patients may have clinical episodes, manifest by pyrexia, a hyperdynamic circulation, and glucose intolerance, that suggest they may harbour an occult gram negative infection and yet in 30% of trauma patients who subsequently died of MOF no evidence of bacterial infection was found at post-morten examination (Goris *et al.*, 1985). Moreover, empirical treatment with broad spectrum antibiotics, has not been shown to reduce mortality from MOF. The terms 'sepsis' and 'septic syndrome' are used to describe the clinical situation in which the patient manifests a systemic response to an *apparent* infective focus, although in approximately 50% of 'septic' patients, bacteraemia cannot be demonstrated (Sprung, 1991). Much effort has been concentrated on the alteration of the effects of mediator activation, but it may be that intervention to prevent the initial release of inflammatory mediators is more appropriate. Stimuli thought to cause mediator release include necrotic tissue, unstable fractures, local hypo-tension, hypoxia and reperfusion injury. Evidence does exist which suggests that the gastrointestinal tract may have a central role in the development of MOF, for under physiological stress, the mucosa of the small intestine may become permeable either to lumenal bacteria (a process called translocation (Berg & Garlington, 1979)), or to bacterial endotoxin, which subsequently cause inflammatory mediator release.

Energy requirements in surgical patients

The energy expenditure, of surgical patients, is now recognised to be much less than was once thought. A study reported that few gastroenterological patients require more than 2000 kcal/day to achieve positive energy balance (MacFie, 1984), although requirements are increased in patients who have suffered multiple trauma and in the face of major sepsis (Streat *et al.*, 1987).

When nutritional support is required, energy can be provided either as carbohydrate or lipid. Glucose is a cheap carbohydrate, which is readily soluble in water and is an obligatory substrate for both erythrocytes and the brain. The use of glucose as the sole source of calories may, however, cause morbidity, particularly when the intravenous route of adminstration is used. Hyperglycaemia and hyperosmolar states may occur (Kirkpatrick, Dahn & Lewis, 1981), especially when there is glucose intolerance in sepsis, and there may be conversion of glucose to fat (MacFie *et al.*, 1983), with fatty infiltration of the liver (Sheldon, Petersen & Sanders, 1978). The respiratory quotient is increased, when glucose is the sole source of non-protein energy (MacFie *et al.*, 1983), to the extent that it may be more difficult to wean the ventilated patient on to spontaneous breathing (Askanazi, Nordenstrom & Rosenbaum, 1981). Lipid is more expensive than glucose and is not soluble in water, but it does not contribute to the osmolarity of the aqueous phase when in emulsion and thus the risk of plasma hyperosmolarity is reduced. Lower osmolarity is beneficial when intravenous nutrition (IVN) via a peripheral vein is considered, because the risk of thrombophlebitis, when a parenteral feed is infused via a peripheral vein (Gazitua *et al.*, 1979) is reduced, when feeds of lower tonicity are used. The amount of glucose necessary for nutritional support can be reduced, if lipid is used to provide approximately half of the non-protein energy requirements. Lipid can be oxidised by malnourished and surgically stressed patients (Nordenstrom *et al.*, 1982). Septic patients demonstrate an altered pattern of substrate utilisation, which favours the oxidation of lipid over glucose (Giovannini *et al.*, 1983), to the extent that endogenous lipid is oxidised, even when exogenous glucose is supplied in excess of total energy requirement (Askanazi *et al.*, 1980). Nitrogen is spared, when lipid is used to provide 50% of energy requirements (Jeejeebhoy *et al.*, 1976), but when greater proportions are used, oxidation of lipid is incomplete (Zeiderman *et al.*, 1984).

Plasma protein concentration in sepsis and nutritional repletion

Plasma proteins, especially albumin, are frequently and erroneously used as markers of nutritional status (O'Keefe & Dicker, 1988). Sepsis is associated with changes in cell membrane function, which cause increases in cellular and capillary permeability and redistribution of both body water and plasma proteins, which lead to expansion of the tissue fluid volume. As a consequence, plasma proteins are lost from the intravascular compartment to the interstitial compartment. Whilst total body albumin may alter little, the plasma concentration of albumin falls. Measurement of plasma protein does provide prognostic information related to the risks of an operation (O'Keefe & Dicker, 1988), but probably because it is related to the degree of abnormality of membrane function, rather than to a specific 'nutritional' risk. Expansion of the extracellular fluid volume in response to pre-operative nutritional support, has been associated with a poor outcome after surgery (Starker *et al.*, 1983) and patients who gained weight after pre-operative intravenous nutrition, but in whom plasma albumin levels fell, were found to be more prone to chest complications after major surgery (Fan *et al.*, 1989).

Indications for nutritional support in surgical patients

Nutritional support is not without risk, of injury from the insertion of enteral or intravenous catheters and of metabolic disturbances which are a consequence of a feed which is qualitatively or quantitatively unsuitable for the patient. The decision to provide nutritional support demands consideration of both the potential benefits and the possible complications which might occur.

Pre-operative nutritional support

Pre-operative patients may be divided into three groups. The first group, comprises the well nourished, who are at no added risk of post-operative morbidity secondary to nutritional status, whether they are to embark upon emergency or elective operation. The second group consists of patients who are malnourished and who require urgent elective or emergency surgery; and the final group consists of malnourished patients, for whom elective surgery is appropriate. Pre-operative nutritional support is not indicated for the first group: patients in the second group might benefit from nutritional intervention but the urgency of their disease renders the delay which would be necessary to restore lean body mass, undesirable. The second group would include a patient with dysphagia and weight loss secondary to a carcinoma of the oesophagus, for whom delayed surgery might allow progression of the tumour, which would prevent or contraindicate subsequent resection. However, patients in the third group may well benefit from nutritional support; a typical patient would present with multiple enterocutaneous fistulae secondary to Crohn's disease and time taken to improve nutritional status over several weeks, or months, could be expected to reduce the risk of post-operative complication.

Post-operative nutritional support

In the post-operative period, nutritional support is indicated, either when return to a full diet is expected to be delayed so that the risk of morbidity is increased or when post-operative complications occur which further impair nutritional status, for example gastrointestinal anastomotic leakage with intraperitoneal sepsis, or enterocutaneous fistulation.

Although impaired nutritional status is associated with an increased risk of post-operative morbidity, there is little scientific evidence to demonstrate that post-operative nutritional support improves outcome in the malnourished patient, nor that it is associated with outcome benefit in patients with post-operative complications that delay return to full diet. It is difficult to separate the relative influences of disease and nutritional status on patient outcome, especially in the critically ill. Ethical considerations prevent the conduct of studies in which patients in a control group would be denied nutritional support. However, overnight nasogastric supplementation of ward diet has been shown to significantly reduce the time taken to achieve independent mobility and the overall duration of hospital stay, for wasted patients after surgery for fractured neck of femur, compared to controls, who did not receive supplementation (Bastow *et al.*, 1983). Furthermore, provision of simple sip-feeds, in addition to ward food, was associated with reduced hospital stay and six month mortality and morbidity in patients who underwent hip surgery (Delmi *et al.*, 1990). The American Society of Parenteral and Enteral Nutrition have published guidelines (A.S.P.E.N. Board of Directors, 1986), for the use of intravenous nutrition in the post-operative period, which stress that nutritional support should be offered *in anticipation* of a delay in return to normal diet, rather than after a delay has occurred. Delay can be anticipated when surgery is likely to be associated with prolonged ileus, or when a gastrointestinal anastomosis requires enteral abstinence, for example after oesophagogastrectomy. The length of the anticipated delay depends upon the nutritional status of the patient. Thus, after major surgery, in a well-nourished patient, nutritional support would be considered when a delay of 7–10 days was anticipated, whilst in the severely malnourished, support would be started when a lesser delay was expected. IVN is required only when the gastrointestinal tract is unable to absorb sufficient nutrients. In many instances, post-operative enteral nutrition is possible, provided that the necessary access, for example a jejunostomy, has been provided at the time of surgery.

Route and timing of nutritional support

Influence on disease

The route by which nutritional support is provided appears to be of significance to the health of the small bowel mucosa and may have important consequences in the critically ill. In the mouse, severe injury (Maejima, Deitch & Berg, 1984) and protein calorie malnutrition (Deitch *et al.* 1987), have been shown to increase bacterial translocation from the lumen of the gut to mesenteric lymph nodes. Healthy mice deprived of enteral intake and maintained with complete IVN, undergo atrophy of the small bowel mucosa, whilst normal small bowel morphology is maintained in controls which receive an equivalent enteral diet (Levine *et at.*, 1974). Similarly rats maintained on IVN alone were found to have reduced secretion of secretory immunoglobulin A (Alverdy, Aoys & Moss, 1988) and were at increased risk of bacterial translocation (Alverdy, Chi & Sheldon, 1985), when compared to enterally fed controls.

No human study has demonstrated small bowel mucosal atrophy associated with restriction of enteral intake, IVN, or severe injury. However, a human volunteer study demonstrated increased small bowel mucosal permeability to lactulose, an exaggerated cytokine response, and augmented counter-regulatory hormone production in response to intravenous endotoxin, after 7 days of IVN (Fong, 1989). Intestinal mucosal permeability is increased in patients with severe burns (Deitch, 1990) and sepsis (Zeigler *et al.*, 1988). A study of severely injured patients who required nutritional support after laparotomy, demonstrated a decreased incidence of infective complications, when early enteral feeding was compared to IVN (Moore *et al.*, 1989). Supplementation of normal diet with whey protein was associated with improved opsonisation of bacteria, reduction in days of bacteraemia and improved outcome, in a study of children who had suffered greater than 60% surface area burns (Alexander *et al.*, 1980). All patients were able to take an enteral diet from admission and the protein-supplemented patients received less calories per gram of nitrogen than the control group. Thus, it has been suggested that in the critically ill patient, the optimal non-protein calorie ratio is lower than in less severely ill patients, while the protein requirement is higher (Deitch, 1992). Other studies have failed to demonstrate that enteral feeding is associated with a reduction in the incidence of MOF after sepsis, but it may be that the timing of nutritional support is crucial and that to prevent mediator activation, enteral nutrition should be started as soon after the initial insult as possible. In an animal study, enteral nutrition started immediately after 30% surface area burn, was associated with reduced jejunal mucosal atrophy, counter-regulatory hormone secretion, and resting metabolic expenditure, compared to delayed administration of the same enteral feed (Mochizuki *et al.*, 1984). A trial which compared immediate nasoduodenal feeding with nasoduodenal feeding delayed for 72 hours, in patients who had suffered greater than 30% body surface area burns, demonstrated reduced energy requirements in conjunction with early nutrition, and it was suggested that the hypermetabolic response to trauma was blunted (Jenken *et al.*, 1989)

Practical considerations

The enteral route is the first choice for administration of nutritional support for both pre-operative and post-operative surgical patients; it is cheaper, safer, and has potential therapeutic advantages. It is contra-indicated in the presence of gastro-intestinal failure, due either to inadequate functional mucosal surface for nutrient absorption, or abnormal gastrointestinal motility, when IVN is indicated. Oral and nasogastric feeding are inappropriate when there is oesophageal or gastroduodenal obstruction, or delayed gastric emptying after head injury but an enterostomy may allow the enteral route to be used provided small bowel motility is normal. Nasogastric feeding may be used safely when the stomach empties satisfactorily. Gastric emptying of liquid is primarily determined by volume and may be tested by bolus instillation of 5 ml/kg water, after which the nasogastric tube is spigotted for 1 hour; failure to aspirate gastric content after this period is taken as an indication to start nasogastric feeding (Columb *et al.*, 1992).

Specific nutrients

A number of nutrients, some of which have previously been ascribed little importance, now appear to have significant influence on mortality and morbidity in the critically ill. Some specific nutrients appear to exert control over metabolic pathways, whilst others seem to have pharmaceutical effects on a variety of organs, in particular the mucosa of the gastrointestinal tract.

Glutamine

Glutamine was traditionally considered a non-essential amino acid, but under conditions of physiological stress, the capacity of the body to synthesise sufficient to meet demands is exceeded and thus glutamine has been termed 'conditionally' essential (Meister, 1956). The gut is the principle organ of consumption of glutamine (Windmueller, 1982) and in man gastrointestinal consumption is increased by surgical stress (McAnena *et al.*, 1991). Depletion of glutamine in rats has been demonstrated to cause small bowel mucosal atrophy (Baskerville, Hambleton & Benbough, 1980) and glutamine is absent from commercial IVN for reasons of pharmaceutical stability and solubility. Standard IVN is associated with small bowel mucosal atrophy in healthy mice, but this did not occur when the intravenous feed contained glutamine, or in controls maintained with standard laboratory enteral feed (O'Dwyer *et al.*, 1989). Similarly, the impairment of secretory immune function and the risk of bacterial translocation, observed in parenterally fed rats, can be reduced by the inclusion of glutamine in the intravenous feed (Burke, 1989). Glutamine is a regulator of skeletal muscle protein synthesis (MacLennan, Brown & Rennie, 1987) and under conditions of physiological stress, glutamine is released by striated myocytes; studies performed in man have shown that parenteral administration of glutamine can improve nitrogen balance after surgery (Stehle *et al.*, 1989). No human studies have demonstrated changes in small bowel permeability associated with glutamine supplementation, but the subject remains one of much research interest and potential clinical importance. The blastogenic response of lymphocytes to mitogens is inhibited when glutamine is absent from cell culture media (Ardawi & Newsholme, 1983) and it may be that glutamine is required for normal lymphocyte function *in vivo*. Glutamine is also a precursor of glutathione, which is a natural anti-oxidant and thus it is possible that clearance of free radicals (*vide infra*) might be impaired in glutamine-depleted patients.

Arginine

Serum arginine concentrations are subnormal in septic patients (Freund, Ryan & Fischer, 1978) and are an indicator of poor prognosis (Freund *et al.*, 1979). Enteral supplementation of human volunteers with arginine, was associated with increased blastogenesis of peripheral blood monocytes in response to Concanavalin A (Barbul *et al.*, 1981) and similar results were observed when enteral arginine was given to patients after surgery for cancer (Daly *et al.*, 1988). Arginine is a precursor for nitric oxide production *in vivo* (Palmer, Rees & Ashton, 1988). Nitric oxide has been implicated as an endothelium-derived mediator of vascular relaxation and hence, arginine deficiency may contribute to the reduction of blood flow in the microcirculation and the subsequent tissue hypoxia, which is associated with the pathogenesis of MOF. Arginine supplementation can increase collagen synthesis at a site of injury (Barbul *et al.*, 1990) and increases pituitary release of growth hormone (Barbul, 1986) and it is postulated that arginine may be required for normal wound healing.

Alternative lipid substrates

Long-chain fatty acids and triglycerides are familiar sources of non- protein energy. Recently, interest has focussed on alternative lipid substrates, that include short-chain fatty acids (SCFA) and ω-3-polyunsaturated fatty acids, which appear to have roles other than those of simply energy sources. SCFA include acetate, propionate, and butyrate and are produced by fermentation of dietary fibre by commensal colonic bacteria. Butyrate is the preferred oxidative fuel source of colonocytes *in vitro*; intracolonic infusion of butyrate in the rat was associated with an increase in colonic mucosal weight and protein content, whilst intracolonic infusion of acetate, propionate and butyrate together, was associated with similar effects in the small intestine as well (Kripke *et al.*, 1989). Furthermore, intracolonic infusion of SCFA in rats, which had undergone colonic transection and anastomosis, was associated with an increase in colonic bursting pressure and a reduction in anastomotic leak, compared to animals which were infused with an electrolyte solution and to controls which were not infused (Rolandelli *et al.*, 1986). Small bowel mucosal atrophy was reduced in rats which received IVN supplemented with SCFA, compared to controls which received a non-supplemented intravenous feed (Koruda *et al.*, 1988).

The ω-3 PUFA, found in fish oils, are precursors for cell membrane eicosanoids that compete with arachidonic acid in the cyclo-oxygenase and lipo-oxygenase pathways, to form inflammatory mediators which are less potent. Dietary supplementation with ω-3 PUFA in the rat, was associated with reduced release of tumour necrosis factor, interleukin 1, prostaglandin and thromboxane from Kupffer cells in response to endotoxin (Billiar *et al.*, 1988).

Antioxidants

Free radicals are species which have an unpaired electron in the outer shell and are produced in response to a variety of factors which include cytokines, reperfusion injury, and ionising radiation. Free radicals cause indiscriminate damage by oxidation of various structures, which include the unsaturated fatty acid component of the cell membrane and protection may be offered by the use of antioxidants. Production of free radicals is reduced in the presence of zinc, and vitamins A, C, and B (Dormandy, 1983), while the propagation of free radicals is prevented by vitamins A, C, and E, which are more readily oxidised than the molecules in the target tissues. Vitamin E is found in high concentration in cell membranes (Fukuzawa *et al.*, 1982). Vitamins oxidised by free radicals may be regenerated by interaction with reduced glutathione, a reaction catalysed by glutathione reductase, the activity of which is reduced in selenium deficiency (Spallholtz, 1990). In stable patients, who receive a brief course of nutritional support, it may be unnecesary to supplement stores of fat-soluble vitamins and trace elements (MacFie, 1986), but in the presence of sepsis (Shanbhogue & Paterson, 1990) or MOF, depletion may occur much more rapidly and aggressive replacement may be necessary.

Summary

It is no longer sufficient to consider nutrition a supportive measure in the management of surgical disease; not only may nutritional status be altered by illness but nutritional therapy may alter the progression of disease. Early consideration of the role of nutritional intervention should be part of the management of all surgical patients.

References

Alexander, J. W., MacMillan, B. G., Stinnett, J. D. *et al.* (1980). Beneficial effects of aggressive protein feeding in severely burned children. *Annals of Surgery*, **192**, 505–17.

Alverdy, J. A., Chi, H. S. & Sheldon, G. S. (1985). The effect of parenteral nutrition on gastrointestinal immunity: the importance of enteral stimulation. *Annals of Surgery*, **202**, 681–4.

Alverdy, J. A., Aoys, E. & Moss, G. S. (1988). Total parenteral nutrition promotes bacterial translocation from the gut. *Surgery*, **104**, 185–90.

Ardawi, M. S. M. & Newsholme, E. A. (1983). Glutamine metabolism in lymphocytes of the rat. *Biochemistry Journal*, **212**, 835–42.

Arora, N. S. & Rochester, D. F. (1982). Respiratory muscle strength and maximal voluntary ventilation in undernourished patients. *American Review of Respiratory Disease*, **126**, 5–8.

Askanazi, J., Carpentier, Y. A., Elwyn, D. H. *et al.* (1980). Influence of total parenteral nutrition on fuel utilization in injury and sepsis. *Annals of Surgery*, **191**, 40–6.

Askanazi, J., Nordenstrom, J. & Rosenbaum, J. F. (1981). Nutrition for the patient with respiratory failure: glucose versus fat. *Anaesthesiology*, **54**, 373–7.

A.S.P.E.N. Board of Directors (1986). Guidelines for the use of total parenteral nutrition in the hospitalised adult patient. *Journal of Parenteral and Enteral Nutrition*, **10**, 441–5.

Barbul, A., Sisto, D. A., Wasserkrug, H. L. *et al.* (1981). Arginine stimulates lymphocyte immune response in healthy human beings. *Surgery*, **90**, 244–51.

Barbul, A. (1986). Arginine: biochemistry, physiology, therapeutic implications. *Journal of Parenteral and Enteral Nutrition*, **10**, 227–38.

Barbul, A., Lazarou, S. A., Efron, D. T. *et al.* (1990). Arginine enhances wound healing and lymphocyte immune response in humans. *Surgery*, **108**, 331–7.

Baskerville, A., Hambleton, P. & Benbough, J. E. (1980). Pathological features of glutaminase toxicity. *British Journal of Experimental Pathology*, **61**, 132–8.

Bastow, M. D., Rawlings, J. & Allison, S. P. (1983). Benefits of supplementary tube feeding after fractured neck of femur: a randomised controlled trial. *British Medical Journal*, **287**, 1589–92.

Baue, A. E. (1975). Multiple, progressive, or sequential systems failure. *Archives of Surgery*, **110**, 779–81.

Benotti, P. N. & Bistrian, B. (1989). Metabolic and nutritional aspects of weaning from mechanical ventilation. *Critical Care Medicine*, **17**, 181–5.

Berg, R. D. & Garlington, A. W. (1979). Translocation of certain indigenous bacteria from the gastrointestinal tract to the mesenteric lymph nodes and other organs in a gnotobiotic mouse model. *Infection and Immunity*, **23**, 403–11.

Billiar, T. R., Bankey, P. E., Svingen, B. A. *et al.* (1988). Fatty acid intake and Kupffer cell function: fish oil alters eicosanoid and monokine production to endotoxin stimulation. *Surgery*, **104**, 343–9.

Bistrian, B. R., Blackburn, G. L., Hallowell, E. & Heddle, R. (1974). Protein status of general surgical patients. *Journal of the American Medical Association*, **230**, 858–60.

Burke, D. J., Alverdy, J. C., Aoys, E. *et al.* (1989). Glutamine-supplemented total parenteral nutrition improves gut immune function. *Archives of Surgery*, **124**, 1396–9.

Cerra, F. B. (1991). Nutrient modulation of inflammatory and immune function. *American Journal of Surgery*, **161**, 230–4.

Columb, M. O., Shah, M. V., Sproat, L. J. *et al.* (1992). Assessment of gastric dysfunction. Current techniques for the measurement of gastric emptying. *British Journal of Intensive Care*, **2**, 75–80.

Daly, J. M., Vars, H. M. & Dudrick, S. J. (1972). Effects of protein depletion on strength of colonic anastomoses. *Surgery, Gynecology and Obstetrics*, **134**, 15–21.

Daly, J. M., Reynolds, J., Thom, A. *et al.* (1988). Immune and metabolic effects of arginine in the surgical patient. *Annals of Surgery*, 208, 512–23.

Deitch, E. A., Winterton, J., Li, M. *et al.* (1987). The gut as a portal of entry for bacteraemia. *Annals of Surgery*, **207**, 681–92.

Deitch, E. A. (1990). Intestinal permeability is increased in burn patients shortly after injury. *Surgery*, **107**, 411–16.

Deitch, E. A. (1992). Multiple organ failure. Pathophysiology and potential future therapy. *Annals of Surgery*, **216**. 117–34.

Delmi, M., Rapin, C.-H., Bengoa, J.-M. *et al.* (1990). Dietary supplementation in elderly patients with fractured neck of the femur. *Lancet*, **335**, 1013–16.

Doekel, R. C., Zwillich, C. W., Scoggin, C. H. *et al.* (1976). Clinical semi-starvation. Depression of hypoxic ventilatory response. *New England Journal of Medicine*, **295**, 358–61.

Dormandy, T. L. (1983). An approach to free radicals. *Lancet*, **ii**, 1010–14.

Fan, S. T., Lau, W. Y., Wong, K. K. *et al.* (1989). Pre-operative parenteral nutrition in patients with oesophageal cancer: a prospective randomised clinical trial. *Clinical Nutrition*, **8**, 23–7.

Fong, Y., Marano, M. A., Barber, A. *et al.* (1989). Total parenteral nutrition and bowel rest modify the metabolic response to endotoxin in humans. *Annals of Surgery*, **210**, 449–56.

Freund, H. R., Ryan, J. A. & Fischer, J. E. (1978). Amino acid derangements in patients with sepsis: treatment with branched chain amino acid rich infusions. *Annals of Surgery*, **188**, 423–30.

Freund, H., Atamian, S., Holroyde, J. *et al.* (1979). Plasma amino acids as predictors of the severity and outcome of sepsis. *Annals of Surgery*, **190**, 571–6.

Fukuzawa, K., Tokumura, A., Ouchi, S. *et al.* (1982). Antioxidant activities of tocopherols on Fe^{2+} ascorbate-induced lipid peroxidation in lecithin ribosomes. *Lipids*, **17**, 511–13.

Gazitua, R., Flatt, J. P., Bistrian, B. R. *et al.* (1979). Factors determining peripheral vein tolerance to amino acid infusions. *Archives of Surgery*, **114**, 897–900.

Goris, J. A., te Boekhurst, T. P. A., Nuytinck, J. K. S. *et al.* (1985). Multiple organ failure. Generalised autodestructive inflammation? *Archives of Surgery*, **120**, 1109–15.

Gottdiener, J. S., Gross, H. A., Henry, W. L. *et al.* (1978). Effects of self-induced starvation on cardiac size and function in anorexia nervosa. *Circulation*, **53**, 425–33.

Giovannini, I., Boldrini, G., Castagneto, M. *et al.* (1983). Respiratory quotient and patterns of substrate utilisation in human sepsis and trauma. *Journal of Parenteral and Enteral Nutrition*, **7**, 226–9.

Heymsfield, S. B., Bethel, R. A., Ansley, J. D. *et al.* (1978). Cardiac abnormalities in cachectic patients before and during repletion. *American Heart Journal*, **95**, 584–94.

Hill, G. L., Blackett, R. L., Pickford, I. *et al.*, (1977). Malnutrition in surgical patients: an unrecognised problem. *Lancet*, **i**, 689–92.

Holmes, R., MacChiano, K., Jhangiani, S. S. *et al.* (1987). Combating pressure sores – nutritionally. *American Journal of Nursing*, **87**, 1301–3.

Jeejeebhoy, K. N., Anderson, G. H., Nakhooda, A. F. *et al.* (1976). Metabolic studies in total parenteral nutrition with lipid in man: comparison with glucose. *Journal of Clinical Investigation*, **57**, 125–36.

Jenken, M., Gottschlich, M., Alexander, J. W. *et al.* (1989). Effect of immediate enteral feeding on the hypermetabolic response following severe burn injury. *Journal of Parenteral and Enteral Nutrition*, **13**, 12S.

Kobak, M. W., Benditt, E. P., Wissler, R. W. *et al.* (1947). The relation of protein deficiency to experimental wound healing. *Surgery, Gynecology, and Obstetrics*, **85**, 751–6.

Kirkpatrick, J. R., Dahn, M. & Lewis, L. (1981). Selective versus standard hyperalimentation. *American Journal of Surgery*, 141, 116–21.

Kripke, S. A., Fox, A. D., Berman, J. M. *et al.* (1989). Stimulation of intestinal mucosal growth with intracolonic infusion of short-chain fatty acids. *Journal of Parenteral and Enteral Nutrition*, **13**, 109–16.

Koruda, M. J., Rolandelli, R. H., Settle, R. G. *et al.* (1988). Effect of parenteral nutrition supplemented with short-chain fatty acids on adaptation to massive small bowel resection. *Gastroenterology*, **95**, 715–20.

Law, D. K., Dudrick, S. J. & Abdou, N. I. (1973). Immune competence of patients with protein-calorie malnutrition. The effects of nutritional repletion. *Annals of Internal Medicine*, **79**, 545–50.

Levine, G. M., Deren, J. J., Steiger, E. *et al.* (1974). Role of oral intake in maintenance of gut mass and disaccharide activity. *Gastroenterology*, **67**, 975–82.

McAnena, O. J., Moore, F. A., Moore, E. E. *et al.* (1991). Selective uptake of glutamine in the gastrointestinal tract: confirmation in a human study. *British Journal of Surgery*, **78**, 480–2.

MacFie, J., King, R. F. G. J., Holmfield, J. *et al.* (1983). Effect of the energy source on changes in energy expenditure and respiratory quotient during parenteral nutrition. *Journal of Parenteral and Enteral Nutrition*, **7**, 1–5.

MacFie, J. (1984). Energy requirements of surgical patients during intravenous nutrition. *Annals of the Royal College of Surgeons of England*, **66**, 39–42.

MacFie, J. (1986). Towards cheaper intravenous nutrition. *British Medical Journal*, **292**, 107–10.

MacLennan, P. A., Brown, R. A. & Rennie, M. J. (1987). A positive relationship between protein synthetic rate and intracellular glutamine concentration in perfused rat skeletal muscle. *FEBS Letters*, **215**, 187–91.

Maejima, K., Deitch, E. A. & Berg, R. (1984). Promotion by burn stress of the translocation of bacteria from the gastrointestinal tracts of mice. *Archives of Surgery*, **119**, 166–72.

Meister, A. (1956). Metabolism of glutamine. *Physiological Reviews*, **36**, 103–27.

Mochizuki, H., Trocki, O., Dominioni, L. *et al.* (1984). Mechanisms of prevention of post-burn hypermetabolism and catabolism by early enteral feeding. *Annals of Surgery*, **200**, 297–310.

Moore, F. A., Moore, E. E., Jones, T. N. *et al.* (1989). TEN vs TPN following major abdominal trauma-reduced septic mortality. *Journal of Trauma*, **29**, 916–23.

Nordenstrom, J., Carpentier, Y. A., Askanazi, J. *et al.* (1982). Metabolic utilization of intravenous fat emulsion during total parenteral nutrition. *Annals of Surgery*, **196**, 221–31.

O'Dwyer, S. T., Smith, R. J., Hwang, T. L. *et al.* (1989). Maintenance of small bowel mucosa with glutamine-enriched parenteral nutrition. *Journal of Parenteral and Enteral Nutrition*, **13**, 579–85.

O'Keefe, S. J. D. & Dicker, J. (1988). Is plasma albumin concentration the assessment of nutritional status of hospital patients? *European Journal of Clinical Nutrition*, **42**, 41–5.

Palmer, R. M. J., Rees, D. R. & Ashton, D. S. (1988). L-arginine is the physiological precursor for the formation of nitric oxide in endothelium-dependent relaxation. *Biochemical and Biophysical Research Communications*, **153**, 1251–6.

Rolandelli, R. H., Koruda, M. J., Settle, R. G. *et al.* (1986). Effects of intralumenal infusion of short-chain fatty acids on the healing of colonic anastomosis in the rat. *Surgery*, **100**, 198–203.

Shanbhogue, L. K. R. & Paterson, N. (1990). Effect of sepsis and surgery on trace minerals. *Journal of Parenteral and Enteral Nutrition*, **14**, 287–9.

Sheldon, G. F., Petersen, S. R. & Sanders, R. (1978). Hepatic dysfunction during hyperalimentation. *Archives of Surgery*, **113**, 504–8.

Spallholz, J. E. (1990). Selenium and glutathione peroxidase: essential nutrient and antioxidant component of the immune system. *Advances in Experimental Medicine Biology*, **262**, 145–58.

Sprung, C. L. (1991). Definitions of sepsis – have we reached a consensus? *Critical Care Medicine*, **19**, 849–51.

Starker, P. M., Lasala, P. A., Askanazi, J. *et al.* (1983). The response to TPN. A form of nutritional assessment. *Annals of Surgery*, **198**, 720–4.

Stehle, P., Zander, J., Mertes, E. *et al.* (1989). Effect of parenteral glutamine peptide supplements on muscle glutamine loss and nitrogen balance. *Lancet*, **i**, 231–3.

Streat, S. J., Beddoe, A. H. & Hill, G. L. (1987). Aggressive nutritional support does not prevent protein loss despite fat gain in septic intensive care patients. *Journal of Trauma*, **27**, 262–6.

Studley, H. O. (1936). Percentage of weight loss. A basic indicator of surgical risk in patients with chronic peptic ulcer. *Journal of the American Medical Association*, **106**, 458–60.

Warnold, I. & Lundholm, K. (1984). Clinical significance of preoperative nutritional status in 215 noncancer patients. *Annals of Surgery*, **199**, 299–305.

Windmueller, H. G. (1982). Glutamine utilization by the small intestine. *Advances in Enzymology*, **53**, 201–37.

Windsor, J. A. & Hill, G. A. (1988*a*). Weight loss with physiological impairment. A basic indicator of surgical risk. *Annals of Surgery*, **207**, 290–6.

Windsor, J. A. & Hill, G. L. (1988*b*). Risk factors for postoperative pneumonia. The importance of protein depletion. *Annals of Surgery*, **208**, 209–14.

Zeiderman, M. R., Karamatsu, J. R., King, R. F. G. J. *et al.* (1984). Does lipid induce thermogenesis in parenterally fed man? *British Journal of Surgery*, **71**, 908.

Zeigler, T. R., Smith, R. J., O'Dwyer, S. T. *et al.* (1988). Increased intestinal permeability associated with infection in burns patients. *Archives of Surgery*, **123**, 1313–19.

12

Peri-operative feeding

M. M. MEGUID and A. C. L. CAMPOS

Why feed a patient peri-operatively?

Starvation studies have shown that physical performance begins to deteriorate when more than 10% of body cell mass is lost (Daws *et al.*, 1972). This implies that the healthy adult can tolerate a net loss of 5% to 10% of body weight without functional disorder. The sequence of events precipitating clinically significant nutritional disorders is shown in Fig. 12.1. The determinants of the patient's nutritional reserve on admission to hospital include the length of antecedent illness with its associated degree of nutritional deprivation. Progressive nutrient deprivation during illness and its consequences on organ function and physical performance, are shown in Fig. 12.2. Whereas a patient's clinical course usually reflects the prognosis of the primary medical disorder, concomitant malnutrition greatly enhances the risk of serious complications, and deterioration of performance status which prejudices the ultimate survival.

As first reported in the early 1930s, patients with a pre-operative weight loss of more than 20% had a post-operative mortality of 33.3%. In contrast, in those with a lesser weight loss, post-operative mortality was only 3.5% (Studley, 1936). Within a decade, the sequelae of malnutrition came to be more fully understood. Hypoproteinaemia was shown to delay gastric emptying and to prolong ileus, increase the incidence of wound dehiscence, delay bone callus formation and increase the risk of infection. These early animal observations were extended to show that post-operative complications were more frequent in hypoproteinaemic surgical patients, that malnourished burned children had an increased risk of developing sepsis, and that haemorrhagic shock was not as well tolerated in a state of protein-depletion as in well-nourished controls. Thus, a variety of different physiological insults leads to similar results, from which it is concluded that complications are more like to occur in the

256

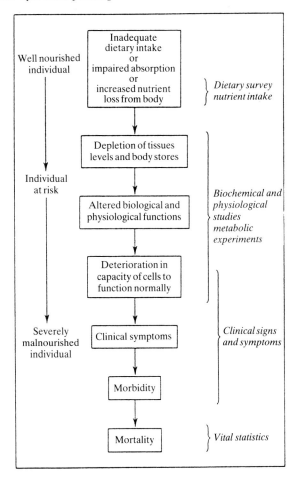

Fig. 12.1. Sequence of events leading to the precipitation of clinically significant nutritional disease and the methods used to assess nutritional status. (Reproduced with permission, from Beaton & Patwardhan (1976). *Nutr. Prev. Med., Geneva*, WHO, 445–81.)

poorly nourished. More recent studies have once again demonstrated this association in the post-operative clinical settings (Meguid *et al.*, 1988*a*).

The mechanisms by which malnourished patients are more prone to post-operative complications are often synergistic in producing their deleterious effects. In surgical patients, breaching the mechanical barriers of the skin and mucosa by surgical incisions and the subsequent

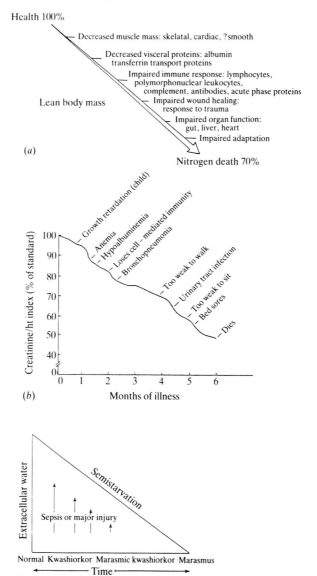

Fig. 12.2. (*a*) Sequence of clinical and laboratory events in the natural history of starvation. (Reproduced with permission, from Steffee, W. P. (1980). *JAMA*, **244**, 2630.) (*b*) Creatinine-height index is a measure of skeletal muscle mass. (Reproduced with permission, from Heymsfield *et*

manipulation of skin and deep tissues, leads to contamination by micro-organisms. Whereas in a well-nourished individual the host's defence mechanisms prevent septic complications, in the malnourished state impaired immunological function increases susceptibility to post-operative infections. Impaired immunological states include reduced cell-mediated immunity and inflammatory responses with decreases in humoral or antibody components (B-lymphocytes), cell-mediated components (T-lymphocytes), phagocytic components (polymorphonuclear neutrophils, macrophages, reticuloendothelial system) and direct or alternate complement pathways (Chandra, 1989).

Malnutrition leads to smooth muscle atrophy of the gastrointestinal tract. As shown in Table 12.1, relative to the well-nourished patient, a considerable delay occurs in the resumption of normal gastrointestinal tract function in the malnourished patients who undergo a similar operation and who do not experience a complication (Meguid *et al.*, 1988*b*). The occurrence of a complication significantly delays the resumption of oral intake and prolongs hospitalisation. Malnutrition also reduces skeletal muscle bulk and muscle metabolism, thereby affecting muscle function (Jeejeebhoy, 1986). This impairs not only gastrointestinal muscles but also respiratory muscle which leads to reduction of both the vital capacity and the resting minute ventilation, ultimately contributing to the occurrence of bronchopneumonia. Moderate starvation alone has been shown to cause a significantly impaired hypoxic ventilatory response. Cardiac mass and contractility is reduced compromising cardiovascular tone, and the malnutrition-related decrease in circulatory volume impairs renal function secondary to a fall in glomerular filtration. Fibroplasia is also reduced in malnourished patients, with resultant delayed wound healing. Starvation decreases the precursors for brain neurotransmitters, leading to a state of apathy with diminished sense of self motivation (Brozek, 1990; Larsson *et al*, 1993). Simply stated, malnutrition has a deleterious effect on every major system in the body. It is, therefore, not surprising that increases in morbidity and mortality occur following

Caption for Fig. 12.2 (*cont.*)
al. (1979). *Ann. Intern. Med.* **90**, 63.) (*c*) This scheme shows how semistarvation eventually leads to severe marasmus. Severe stress, from serious sepsis or major injury leads to rapid consumption of host tissues and expanded extracellular water (Kwashiorkor). Intermediate stages (Marasmic Kwashiorkor) are common. (Reproduced with permission. Hill, G. L. (1992). *Disorders of Nutrition and Metabolism in Clinical Surgery: Understanding and Management.* Churchill Livingstone.)

Table 12.1. *Relationships between resumption of normal oral intake in days, involved organ system, nutritional status, and complications in 464 surgical patients*

Involved organ system	Well-nourished patients		Malnourished patients	
	No compli-cation	Compli-cation	No compli-cation	Compli-cation
	Days	Days	Days	Days
Abdominal carcinomatosis	8	32	22	33
Oesophagus	7	18	30	40
Gastroduodenum	9	14	18	40
Pancreas	10	42*	15	29
Colorectum	8	12	19	19
Liver–gall bladder	5	13	11	62
Genitourinary/ gynaecological	6	16	8	20
Lymphoproliferative	6	45*	8	21
Other	13*	10	32	42

* Median duration of normal oral intake resumption is disproportionately prolonged by one or more extreme instances.
Reproduced with permission from Meguid *et al.* (1983). *Lancet*, **ii**, 230.

elective operation or accidental operative trauma, as well as following hospitalisation for medical conditions in malnourished patients (Campos & Meguid, 1992).

Unfortunately, a number of common medical/hospital-related routine practices increase the frequency and severity of malnutrition while in hospital. This includes the failure to weigh patients and the use of prolonged intravenous feeding with nutrient-deficient solutions. Thus, if a patient is admitted who is: (1) well-nourished and in whom a prolonged period of inadequate oral nutrient intake is anticipated (i.e. functional starvation >5 days), or (2) malnourished and a prolonged period of gastrointestinal dysfunction is inevitable, then early nutrient support to pre-empt the development of, or the further aggravation of, malnutrition, is clinically indicated and desirable. Not only is hospital-related malnutrition potentially avoidable, but it is very costly (Meguid, 1993).

How to meet the patient's nutrient requirements

The purpose of nutritional support is to achieve a positive nitrogen balance for the purpose of preserving or repleting the patient's lean body mass. It is important to determine the optimal quantity of nutrients to be given enterally or parenterally. Too little would not achieve this endpoint, while too much may lead to metabolic over-burden with its attendant potential metabolic complications (Askanazi *et al.*, 1980*a*; Meguid *et al.*, 1984*a,b*). Precise measurement of energy expenditure is not necessary in most clinical situations, but modifications of enteral or parenteral nutrient solutions are necessary in patients with diabetes, renal, hepatic and pulmonary disease. To determine nutrient requirements, a knowledge of the patient's (1) hydrational status, (2) nutritional reserve and status, and (3) the degree of metabolic stress is necessary. The aim of providing nutritional support is to provide sufficient energy to maintain or improve physiological function and to minimise further protein loss.

Baseline water requirements to meet obligatory fluid losses

Since water and electrolyte requirements are based on caloric expenditure, different schemas have been devised to calculate maintenance fluid needs based on surface area (1500 ml/m^2/24 h), body weight (20 ml/kg) or caloric expenditure (20 kcal/kg). Since 1 ml of water per 24 h is needed for each calorie expended, a system of calculating fluid requirements based on metabolic needs is useful. Thus, caloric and water maintance needs are 20 kcal/kg or 20 ml water/kg. Therefore, a 70 kg individual would need about 1400 ml of fluid per day. This amount of fluid replaces the daily obligatory losses from the kidney and insensible water losses. A number of factors can significantly increase water and energy needs including exposure to a cold environment, fever, sepsis, burns, trauma, cardiac or pulmonary disease and the rapid repletion after malnutrition. Thus, increased maintenance fluid requirements are needed for: a 1 °C rise in fever by 12%; hyperventilation by 10–60 ml/100 kcal; and sweating by 10–25 ml/100 kcal. For external gastrointestinal losses and in renal disease, fluid losses need to be monitored and analysed for major electrolyte content and fluid intake adjusted accordingly.

Electrolytes

Table 12.2 shows the normal daily needs of electrolytes during enteral or parenteral nutrition. Withdrawing sodium, potassium or phosphorus from

Table 12.2. *Typical electrolyte requirements during enteral or parenteral nutrition*

	Typical daily requirement	Forms used in TPN solutions
Sodium	70–100 meq/day	Chloride, acetate, phosphate
Potassium	70–100 meq/day	Chloride, acetate, phosphate
Magnesium	15–20 meq/day	Sulphate
Calcium	10–20 meq/day	Gluconate
Phosphate	20–30 mmol/day	Sodium, potassium

otherwise standard total parenteral nutrition (TPN) solution was shown by Rudman *et al.* (1975) to prevent retention of the remaining elements, including nitrogen. Thus, their addition is essential.

Energy needs

The energy derived from enteral or parenteral nutrients must include the caloric cost of: (1) resting energy requirements (5–10% greater than basal metabolic requirement), plus (2) the increased energy requirements due to the patient's illness (stress factor), plus (3) the energy expended on physical activity (activity factor).

In clinical practice, energy requirement to meet resting metabolic expenditure, is calculated using the Harris–Benedict equations. These predictive equations are based on height, weight, age and sex of normal adult men and women.

For men:
$$RME \text{ (kcal/d)} = 66.4730 + 13.7516 \text{ (W)} + 5.0033 \text{ (H)} - 6.7550 \text{ (A)}$$
For women:
$$RME \text{ (kcal/d)} = 655.095 + 9.563 \text{ (W)} + 1.8596 \text{ (H)} - 4.6756 \text{ (A)}$$

Where W = body weight in kg; H = height in cm; A = age in years. To calculate the patient's energy needs, the stress factor has to be considered, as outlined in Table 12.3. Activity decreased greatly on admission to hospital during critical illnesses and thus, this factor is necessarily always accounted for. Using this method, it should be recognised that, in some patients, caloric requirements are overestimated, while in others they are underestimated. In the malnourished patient, additional energy allowances are required for rapid repletion based on current weight and slow repletion based on ideal body weight. If a thermodilution pulmonary artery catheter

Table 12.3. *Adjustment of resting metabolic expenditure estimated by Harris–Benedict formula or kcal/kg method for changes imposed by various critical illnesses*

Patient	Stress factor	Reference
Well-nourished unstressed	1.0	Saffle *et al.*, 1985
		Van Lanschot *et al.*, 1986
Burned (prior to skin grafting)		Burke *et al.*, 1979
Normotensive		
0–20% BSA	1.2–1.5	
20–40% BSA	1.5–2.0	
>40% BSA	1.8–2.5	
'Burn shock'		
period of resuscitation	0.5	
Burned (after successful grafting)	1.0–1.3	
Septic (acute phase)		
Normotensive	1.2–1.7	
Hypotensive	0.5	Abraham *et al.*, 1984
		Giovannini *et al.*, 1983
Septic (recovery)	1.0	
Multiple trauma (acute phase)		
Normotensive	1.1–1.5	
Hypotensive	0.8–1.0	Shoemaker *et al.*, 1980
Multiple trauma (recovery)	1.0–1.2	

BSA: burn surface area.

is in place for close monitoring of cardiac responses to fluid resuscitation, it can be used to determine oxygen consumption, which is multiplied by the caloric value for oxygen (4.86 kcal/l at a nonprotein respiratory quotient of 0.85) (Liggett, St. John & Lefrak, 1987).

Maximum oxidation of the infused glucose is approximately 55%, while at higher infusion levels carbon dioxide production is increased and fat synthesis is stimulated. Excessive exogenous glucose infusions embarrass both respiratory and hepatic functions in severely stressed patients. The studies of Askanazi *et al.* (1980*b*) in which ventilatory oxygen and carbon dioxide exchange were measured, show that in injured and septic patients a high rate of endogenous fat oxidation occurs which is not suppressed to a normal extent by high concentration glucose infusion. Metabolic studies comparing the protein-sparing effect of exogenous glucose and fat calories, indicate that in injured and highly stressed patients, only glucose significantly suppresses gluconeogeneis (Long *et al.*, 1977). Thus, parenteral glucose should constitute the major caloric source in TPN with fat providing the rest of the caloric source. In most stressed patients, the enhanced oxidation of endogenous fat is not physiologically harmful, since fat stores tend to be present in generous amounts. In an occasional patient whose fat stores are markedly depleted, total caloric support is best provided by adding 10 to 15 kcal/kg/day as infused fat, because it circumvents the metabolic cost to the patient of converting glucose to fat. Furthermore, 2% of daily calories should be provided as intravenous fat to meet essential fatty acid requirements. A number of studies indicate that glucose and fat calories are interchangeable in patients who can achieve effective protein sparing and anabolism, with the addition of fat to glucose TPN (Jeejeebhoy *et al.*, 1976; Macfie, Smith & Hill, 1981).

Nitrogen

One gram of nitrogen is yielded by 6.25 g of protein (1 g of protein contains 16% nitrogen). Although the caloric density of protein is equal to 4 kcal/g, protein calories are usually not included in calculations of daily caloric intake. Protein requirements for intravenous feeding are the same as those for normal oral feeding (see Table 12.4). Amino acids or protein hydrolysates administered enterally have an effect similar to that observed when given parenterally. Based on these data, while it is recommended that 1.0–1.2 g/kg/day should be given for maintenance, 1.5–2.0 g/kg/day should be prescribed for repletion, and 2.0–2.5 g/kg/day in patients with excess losses.

Calorie to nitrogen ratio

Using a TPN formula with a calorie to nitrogen ratio of 1 to 150, which provided 1.75 times the Harris–Benedict estimation of caloric expenditure, Rutten *et al.* (1975) showed that optimal nitrogen balance was produced in a group of malnourished patients. Nitrogen balance studies (Peters & Fischer, 1980) and tracer kinetic studies (Sim *et al.*, 1979), have shown that, if a patient receives 35 to 40 kcal/kg/day and 0.2 to 0.3 g/kg/day of nitrogen, positive nitrogen balance is achieved in a wide spectrum of diseases. This represents a calorie:nitrogen ratio ranging from 200:1 to 130:1.

Vitamins and trace elements

The very few data on the vitamin and trace mineral requirements which exist for patients receiving TPN (AMA Department of Food and Nutrition,

Table 12.4. *Usual recommendations for TPN*

Maintenance	Moderate stress	Severe stress
	Elective surgery	Extensive burns
	Peritonitis	Multiple long fracture
	Soft tissue trauma	Closed head injury
	Malnutrition	Major sepsis
	Renal failure	Multiple trauma
	Respiratory failure	Multiple organ failure
	Pancreatitis	
	Dialysis	
Caloric requirements:		
25–30 kcal/kg/day	30–40 kcal/kd/day	40–45 kcal/kg/day
Protein requirements:		
1.0–1.2 g/kg/day	1.3–1.4 g/kg/day	1.5–2.0 g/kg/day
Protein restricted: 0.5–0.8 g/kg/day		
Non-protein calorie to nitrogen ratio: Protein (g) – 6.25 = Nitrogen (g)		
200–300:1	150:1	< 100:1

1975, 1979), indicate that parenteral requirements are at least as great as the oral requirement. This may reflect a number of factors: (1) loss of nutrient during storage and delivery from glass (Hartline & Zachman, 1976) and plastic (Howard *et al.*, 1980) containers and from administration sets; (2) loss because of systemic infusion with rapid renal excretion rather than via the normal portal circulation, which allows for more efficient nutrient storage and activation by the liver; and (3) interruption of the enterohepatic cycle in patients with extreme short bowel syndrome leading to loss of nutrients.

Clinical deficiency states do not usually single out a particular vitamin or trace element and the clinical syndromes initially observed with TPN, resulted from errors of omission. More commonly, combined deficiencies occur together with protein and energy malnutrition. Table 12.5 shows daily allowances for vitamins and trace elements. Recommended intravenous allowances are based on dietary allowances in healthy individuals. The influence of serious illness, sepsis and trauma on the requirements of vitamins and trace elements when these are given in conjunction with TPN or enteral formulae is not fully known.

Table 12.5. *Recommended daily maintenance dose for vitamins and trace elements*

Element	Oral[a]	Intravenous[b]
Thiamine (B_1)	1.4 mg	3 mg/day
Riboflavine (B_2)	1.6 mg	3.6 mg/day
Nicotinic acid (Niacin)	18 mg	40 mg/day
Pyridoxine (B_6)	2.2 mg	4 mg/day
Pantothenic acid	7 mg	15 mg/day
Folate	400 µg	400 µg/day
B_{12}	3 µg	5 mg/day
Ascorbic acid	60 mg	100 mg/day
Vitamin A	1000 µg RE[c]	2500 iu/day
D	5 µg	5 µg/day
E	10 mg	50 mg/day
K	NR[d]	10 mg/week
Iron	2 mg	2 mg
Zinc[e]	15 mg	4–10 mg[f]
Copper	2–3 mg	0.5 mg
Chromium	0.05–0.2 mg	10–15 µg
Iodine	150 µg	150 µg
Fluorine	1.5–4 mg	0.4 mg
Manganese	2.3 mg	0.15–0.8 mg
Molybdenum	100 mg	100–200 mg
Selenium	20–50 µg	40–120 µg

[a] Committee on Dietary Allowance, 1980.
[b] Nutrition Advisory Group, 1979.
[c] Retinal equivalents. 1 µg retinol equivalent = 1 µg retinol or 3.33 iu.
[d] NR = no recommendation.
[e] Patients with diarrhoea or ileostomies lose about 17 mg of zinc per litre of faeces, but for patients with a high small bowel fistula the losses are about 12 mg per litre of fistula discharge.
[f] Multiplied by 2.5 if given as zinc sulphate. Since only 20% of orally administered zinc is absorbed a further multiplication by 5 is required if given orally. Zinc levels in the blood reflect zinc ingestion rather than balance.

How to feed a patient

In any given clinical situation, optimal peri-operative feeding may be achieved by a combination of enteral and parenteral means. Each route will be discussed and their advantages and potential complications mentioned.

The enteral route

In the presence of a physiologically functional gastrointestinal tract, the use of the enteral route is desirable. Its advantages are: (1) maintenance of gastrointestinal tract mass and function (Thompson *et al.*, 1987); (2) maintenance of the patient's immune defence mechanisms (Border *et al.*, 1987); and (3) fewer metabolic complications and lower chances of systemic infection, than with parenteral nutrition. Lower cost may also be a factor which, however, varies from one geographic district to another (Twomey & Patching, 1985).

Nasogastric

Two feeding tubes are most commonly used: (1) large polyvinyl or a red rubber tube intended for gastrointestinal decompression but used instead for feeding; and (2) the softer small calibre tube designed specifically for tube feeding. The well-lubricated tube is inserted through the nostril and is advanced along the floor of the nasal cavity, being pushed steadily in a posterior direction. In the co-operative patient, the tube can be advanced while the patient drinks a sip of fluid which is then sucked out; in the comatose patient, flexion of the head closes the larynx and opens up the pharyngoesophageal tract.

Traditionally, the length of the tube to be inserted is equal to the sum of the distances from the tip of the nose to the tip of the ear lobe and from the earlobe to the xyphoid. Using this technique, the incidence of correct gastric placement is 72% (Hanson, 1979). Using the predictive equation: Patient's height (cm) $\times 0.2 + 17.1$, results in a 96% correct gastric tube placement. Nevertheless, the final position should be verified radiographically before using the tube.

The large stiff polyvinyl tubes are easier to insert. Infusion of nutrients is also easier due to less resistance. However, they are less well tolerated by the patient and carry a greater risk of injury. The small calibre tubes appear well tolerated and carry a lesser risk of injury but are more difficult to insert, tending to coil in the hypopharynx and are easily coughed up. The small bore tubes provide considerable resistance to flow of nutrients, necessitating either a low viscosity formula or the use of a pump.

The subjective distresses of nasogastric tube feeding in rank order are: (1) deprivation of the tasting, drinking and chewing of food; (2) soreness of the nose; (3) rhinitis, sinusitis and oesophagitis; (4) mouth breathing; and (5) the sight of other patients who are eating (Padilla *et al.*, 1979). A distinct disadvantage of the nasogastric route is its increase in upper airway resistance, thereby interfering with ventilatory exchange. This is of consequence in a patient with marginal respiratory status. Under these circumstances an alternate route, as outlined below, is best selected.

Pharyngostomy and oesophagostomy

Pharyngostomy or cervical oesophagostomy (hypopharyngotomy) is indicated when a feeding tube in the nasopharynx is intolerable or contra-indicated, e.g. borderline respiratory status, or when feedings in the hospital setting are necessary for prolonged periods. Either method is particularly useful in patients with prior: (1) subtotal gastrectomy or oesophago-gastrectomy; (2) head and neck operations; and (3) chronic obstructive pulmonary disease. The advantages of these procedures are that feeding can be provided via a stoma whose proximity to a potentially contaminated tracheotomy site does not pose a sepsis problem to the patient. Formal oesophagostomy (mucosal incision below the crico-pharyngeus) as described by Montgomery (1973) is generally performed in conjunction with head and neck procedures. For long-term home enteral feeding, a permanent sinus can be performed allowing the feeding tube to be removed between meals.

Minor problems associated with the use of a pharyngostomy or oesophagostomy include: access site skin or soft tissue irritation, and accidental extubation because of excess length of the exteriorly placed tube. Major complications may include: pulmonary aspiration due to vomiting from reflux oesophagitis, stricture of the distal oesophagus secondary to acid reflux around the tube, and arterial erosion with exsanguination, particularly in patients with heavily irradiated necks.

Gastrostomy

The advantages of a tube gastrostomy for feeding purposes, include easy access to the stomach with advantage as a reservoir and bypassing more proximal oesophageal mechanical, surgical or functional obstructions. Two basic types exist, which are placed surgically either under general anaesthesia or using local anaesthesia supplemented by intravenous sedation. In the first, a simple feeding tube is placed directly into the stomach via an abdominal wall stoma at operation under either general or local anaesthesia. It is intended for temporary use and the stoma tends to close promptly when the tube is removed (Stamm, 1894). The second type is a permanent gastrostomy, in which a formal mucocutaneous ostomy is surgically fashioned (Depage-Janeway) (Depage, 1901). This procedure is more complex but has the advantage of not requiring the presence of a mechanical tube between feedings. It is indicated for permanent gastrostomy feedings. Some methods provide a valve within the gastrostomy (Spivack, 1980) or interpose a reverse jejunal segment between the gastric ostium and the anterior abdominal wall, to maintain gastrostomy continence (Lopez, Suavez & Santiago-Delpin, 1977). Both types are useful for home enteral nutrition programmes (Campos, Butters & Meguid, 1990).

Percutaneous endoscopic gastrostomy

This method is indicated for patients requiring long term enteral feeding, who are considered poor risks for general anaesthesia and laparotomy. Under local anaesthesia, supplemented by intravenous sedation, a gastro-scope is advanced into the stomach which is distended with air, to appose the stomach to the anterior abdominal wall. A cannula is inserted via the abdominal wall into the stomach, maintaining the apposition of these two structures, and providing a portal for enteral feeding (Chung, 1985).

Contra-indications for percutaneous gastrostomy tube placement include ascites; morbid obesity; oesophageal stricture, reflux or obstruction; oesophageal or gastric varices; and previous gastric surgery. Complication rates in reported series are about 7% to 10% and included wall infections, pericatheter leakage, pneumoperitoneum, intra-abdominal extravasation, gastrocolic fistula, cutaneous stomal enlargement, and subcutaneous infections (Ponsky, 1986; Hull *et al.*, 1993).

Jejunostomy

A tube jejunostomy needs to be placed via an operation, usually under general anaesthesia and is indicated when prolonged enteral nutritional support is anticipated, generally starting in the early post-operative period. The size of the catheter is usually relatively small (No. 8 French), and its use is indicated when there is a proximal obstruction of fistula in the gastrointestinal tract, in the absence of a stomach, or when recovery of small bowel motility is anticipated long before recovery of gastric motility. Several advantages of jejunostomy over gastrostomy exist: (1) less stomal leakage and skin erosion; (2) less gastric and pancreatic secretion because the stomach and duodenum are bypassed; (3) less nausea, vomiting and bloating compared to gastric or duodenal feeding; and (4) reduced risk of pulmonary aspiration. As with nasoduodenal or nasojejunal feedings, a continuous infusion of isotonic formula is the optimal method of using this portal (Widiss & Meguid, 1981). A potential problem with intra-jejunal feeding is that there may be inadequate mixing of the nutrients with bile and pancreatic enzymes, resulting in incomplete digestion and hence malabsorption. This problem can be obviated by the use of an elemental diet.

Use of a needle catheter jejunostomy has been popularised, in which a 16 gauge polyvinyl catheter is passed into the jejunum through a 14-gauge needle (Page, Ryan & Haff, 1976). The catheter is first introduced into the bowel through the needle, along a long intramural tunnel and then it is brought through the anterior abdominal wall with the same needle. The catheter is secured to the bowel with a purse-string suture and to the abdominal wall with another suture. Even with operatively placed jejunostomy tubes, Gastrografin (meglumine diatrizoate) should be injected and X-rays taken intra-operatively to ensure the intraluminal position of the catheter prior to the start of feedings. Contra-indications to the use of a 'fine needle' catheter jejunostomy include peritonitis, ascites, regional enteritis and morbid obesity.

More recently, jejunostomy feeding tubes are being placed laparoscopically. Data on this technique and its complications are currently being collected.

Complications of enteral nutrition

Mechanical complications

Those associated with nasogastric pharyngostomy and oesophagostomy tubes fall into two broad categories: (1) low frequency–high morbidity complications, and (2) high frequency–low morbidity complications (Butters, Campos & Meguid, 1992).

Low frequency–high morbidity mechanical complications occurred in less than 5% of patients. However, because of their dramatic nature and the notoriety they attract, many of these have appeared as single case reports and overshadow the general usefulness of this route of feeding. These include injury along the nasogastric tube insertion site, arterial erosion, perforation of the gastrointestintal tract, and aspiration pneumonitis. Mucosal injury along the introduction tract occurs most frequently in the nasopharynx and the oesophagus. In the nasopharynx, profuse bleeding may occur (Siermers & Reinke, 1976) while perforation along the introduction tract leads to the nasogastric tube reaching unforeseen and unexpected sites (Wolff & Kessler, 1973), incuding pleural intubation through either the mediastinum (Kassner *et al.*, 1977) or the tracheobronchial tree (Eldar & Meguid, 1984). Intubation may be especially hazardous when the patient is unco-operative or unconscious (Siermers

& Reinke, 1976) or has lost the cough reflex (Olivaries, Segovia & Revuelta 1974); when the tube is iced to make it semirigid for ease of insertion; or with the use of a rigid stillet. Any difficult or unsuccessful nasogastric intubation (or bloody aspirate from the tube), followed by chest or upper abdominal pain, should heighten the awareness of a possible complication (Eldar & Meguid, 1984).

High frequency–low morbidity mechanical complications occur in more than 50% of patients (Payne-James *et al.*, 1990; Butters, Campos & Meguid, 1992) and consists mostly of dislodgement of feeding tubes of the type with both weighted and unweighted tips, as well as the red rubber tubes. This complication can range from a minor annoyance to a major problem associated with impaired nutrient intake secondary to missed feedings, extra time and problems/risks to reinsert a tube after surgery and increased cost of supplies if a new tube is required. Replacement of a feeding tube is potentially a high morbidity complication, e.g. accidental removal of a gastrostomy or jejunostomy tube within 24 hours of operative placement or of a nasogastric tube placed across a fresh oesophageal anastomosis.

A common mechanical problem related to gastrostomy use occurs when a Foley catheter is used for a gastrostomy tube. Progressive deflation of the balloon leads to dislodgment of the feeding catheter. Other complications include, discharge of gastric juice from the gastrostomy's stoma site which irritates the surrounding skin, and anastomotic leaks that may cause local infection, abscess formation or peritonitis. Reported complication rates range from 6.5% to 15.7% with mortality rates of 6.1% to 37%, reflecting the underlying condition of patients considered for this procedure (Meguid & Williams, 1979; Shellito & Malt, 1985).

Among the list of complications reported for jejunostomy use are free peritoneal leak, small bowel fistulisation, small bowel obstruction, pneumatosis intestinalis and jejunal varices (Edington, Zajko & Reilly, 1983).

Metabolic complications

The type and their frequency include: fluid overload 31%, electrolyte imbalance 30%, hyperglycaemia 30% and uraemia and dehydration 15% (Vanlandingham *et al.*, 1981). Symptoms of abdominal bloating, cramps and diarrhoea are related to high rates of feeding and to the high caloric density of the formula (*i.e.* high fat content), although paralytic ileus and side effects of parasympathomimetic drugs must be excluded. These symptoms are less common when feedings are administered via a bolus method. Their frequency can be decreased when enteral feeds are administered on a continuous basis. Although the pathogenesis of tube-feeding diarrhoea is not entirely clear, a number of factors have been implicated, including the use of contaminated tube feedings (Schreiner *et al.*, 1979), lactose intolerance, intolerance of high osmotic loads, inappropriate release of gastrointestinal polypeptide hormones, concomitant antibiotic therapy, and the ingestion of laxatives and hypoalbuminaemia (Silk, 1989). The use of pectin or mucilaginous hydrophilic colloid bulk laxatives (Metamucil) to promote formed but soft stools (Frank & Greene, 1979) reduces the diarrhoea associated with isotonic tube feedings (Zimmaro *et al.*, 1989). For many years, it was not possible to mix fibre with enteral feedings because the two were incompatible. Recently, a number of formulae containing non-viscous, water-insoluble fibre polysaccharides have been marketed. They are designed to bring the benefits of fibre to the hospitalised and chronically tube-fed patient, while optimising normal bowel function.

However, caution must be exercised in selecting patients to receive fibre-containing products. In certain patients, dietary fibre may be contraindicated (Emerson, 1987). Risk factors include quantity of fibre ingested, previous gastric surgery, organic stricture, concomitant illness or medications affecting bowel function and diabetic gastroparesis (Canivet *et al.*, 1980; Emerson, 1987). In these patients, the added bulk may not be tolerated and can contribute to fibre bezoars that might need to be surgically removed (McIvor *et al.*, 1990).

Infectious complications

One of the most commonly reported side effects of enteral tube feeding is diarrhoea, at times thought to be related to bacterial contamination of the enteral nutrient solution (Flynn, Norton & Fisher, 1987). Bacterial contamination of the enteral nutrient solution has been reported to occur in 30–90% when using open enteral feeding systems. Other factors which contribute to potential contamination include the use of enteral powders requiring mixing (Freedland *et al.*, 1989) and the use of either sterile or tap water to dilute the formula (Perez & Brandt, 1989). As a consequence of this high rate of contamination which generally leads to diarrhoea and its associated increased morbidity related to fluid and electrolyte losses, modifications to the basic delivery system have been made. The use of a closed delivery system is recommended to minimise potential contamination of enteral nutrient solutions. Other modifications include the introduction of a pre-packed sterile enteral formula and the use of a sterile administration set.

Standardized enteral order forms

There are many instances in daily medical practice, when the provision of enteral nutrition is suboptimal because the patient's caloric goals are not reached. The reasons for this are primarily attributable to the user's lack of awareness and/or familiarity of: (1) the patient's appropriate nutrient needs, (2) the most suitable type or composition of enteral formulae, and (3) their correct use in relation to a particular clinical setting (Abernathy *et al.*, 1989). By using the standardised enteral nutrition order forms, a decrease in the number of days needed to meet a patient's caloric goal occurs, thereby achieving the desired nutrient goals and therapeutic benefits sooner (Chapman, Cartas & Meguid, 1992). In addition, they serve as an educational tool for the house staff and consulting staff, and their use ensures a consistent level of care, as determined by nursing, nutritional and metabolic standards.

For consistent and effective delivery of enteral nutrients, enteral nutrition order forms for the continuous (Fig. 12.3) and the bolus (Fig. 12.4) delivery of enteral products are used. These order forms list the enteral formulary stocked by the hospital (which is reviewed yearly for necessary changes), and advancement schedule of formulae based on osmolality, whether the feeding would be given continuously or intermittently, and standing orders to nursing and dietary staff and for obtaining blood work to monitor tolerance. Such standardised forms ensure quality control in the care and delivery of this form of therapy.

Types of enteral diets

Fig. 12.5 summarises a representative cross section of enteral products commercially available. In general, enteral nutrition formulae can be broadly classified into disease specific diets, elemental diets, meal replacements, supplements and modular components. The disease specific diets address the metabolic needs for the stressed patients (e.g. Sustacal HC, Ensure Plus, Isocal HCN, TwoCal HN), hepatic failure (e.g. Hepatic-Aid, Travasorb Hepatic), diabetes (e.g. Glucerna, Osmolite), the immune compromised patient (e.g. Impact, Immun-Aid, Alitraq), the acute and chronic renal patient (e.g. Amin-Aid, Nepro, Suplena, Travasorb Renal), and for chronic obstructive pulmonary disease (e.g. Pulmocare, NutriVent). Elemental diets (e.g.Vivonex TEN/Alitraq), are non-residue balanced diets with protein components reduced to their basic elements. Meal replacement diets (e.g. Ensure, Osmolite, Isocal, Enrich, Jevity) consist of

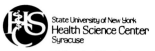

State University of New York
Health Science Center
Syracuse

University Hospital
CONTINUOUS ENTERAL NUTRITION
ORDER FORM

CHECK THE DESIRED ROUTE OF ADMINISTRATION AND FORMULA. FOLLOW THE SCHEDULE AS OUTLINED BELOW.

☐ JEJUNOSTOMY   ☐ NASODUODENAL   ☐ NASOGASTRIC   ☐ GASTROSTOMY

ISOTONIC - SCHEDULE A		HYPERTONIC - SCHEDULE B	
PRODUCT	**CALORIES/ml**	**PRODUCT**	**CALORIES/ml**
☐ Glucerna	1.0	☐ ALITRAQ*	1.0
☐ Impact	1.0	☐ Ensure Plus	1.5
☐ Lipisorb*	1.0	☐ Isocal HCN	2.0
☐ Osmolite	1.06	☐ Nepro	2.0
☐ Osmolite HN	1.06	☐ Pulmocare	1.5
☐ Ultracal	1.06	☐ Sustacal HC	1.5
		☐ Travasorb Hepatic*, ♦	1.1
		☐ Vivonex TEN*	1.0

1. Begin full strength at 25 ml/h.	1. Begin 1/2 strength at 25 ml/h x 6h.
2. Advance 10 ml/h q 6h as tolerated to goal of _____ ml/h.	2. Increase as tolerated to 3/4 strength at 25 ml/h x 6h.
	3. Increase as tolerated to full strength at 25 ml/h x 6h.
	4. Advance 10 ml/h q 6h as tolerated to goal of _____ ml/h.

ENTERAL NUTRITION ORDERS

1. **Pre-NG Feeding:** If small bore feeding tube is used, obtain chest x-ray to verify feeding tube in stomach.
2. **Nursing:**   ● Keep patient's head elevated at 30° at all times.
       ● Give formula at room temperature, hang-time 8h.
       ● Check residual per nursing protocol.
       ● q shift: check position of NG-tube, I/O, urine S/A or fingerstick glucose. (Call if fingerstick > 200).
       ● q day: weight, cumulative I/O.
3. **Dietary:** Daily calorie count per dietitian.
4. **Lab Values:** Day 1: Nutrition Panel I, II, and III
       Day 2, 3: Nutrition Panel I
    Thereafter: q Tuesday: Nutrition Panel I, II, and III
       q Friday: Nutrition Panel I
       Notify MD if glucose ≥ 200 mg/dl.
5. Problems of persistent nausea, diarrhea, and vomiting: contact members of Nutrition Support Team.

NUTRITION PANELS
I - Na, K, HCO$_3$, Cl, Glucose
II - ALP, CRE, BUN, PO$_4$, Alb, Ca, Mg
III - Chol, Trig

MODULAR COMPONENTS (WHEN SPECIAL REQUIREMENTS ARE NEEDED)

Establish tolerance to designated enteral formula at goal rate before adding modular component. Select the desired modular component and follow the schedule below.

SCHEDULE C (MODULAR ADDITION)

PRODUCT	**CALORIES**	
☐ Polycose (CHO)*	23/Tbsp	1. Add _____ per 1000 ml enteral formula. If a second component: add _____ to above.
☐ Promod (PRO)*	17/Tbsp	2. Mix thoroughly.
☐ Microlipid (FAT)*	4.5/ml	3. Run mixture at _____ ml/hr.
☐ MCT Oil (FAT)*	7.6/ml	4. Follow enteral nutrition orders above.
		5. Note osmotic effect that Polycose and Promod have on enteral prescription.
		6. Establish tolerance to one modular component before addition of a second.

*Mixed and delivered by dietary   ♦Requires approval of Nutrition Support Team

Noted by_____   Signature_____M.D.

Date_____ Time_____   Date_____ Time_____

CLINICAL DATA SERVICES (7/92)   G3.00

Fig. 12.3. Continuous enteral nutrition order form.

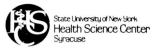

State University of New York
Health Science Center
Syracuse

University Hospital
BOLUS ENTERAL NUTRITION
ORAL SUPPLEMENTATION ORDER FORM

CHECK THE DESIRED ROUTE OF ADMINISTRATION AND FORMULA. FOLLOW THE SCHEDULE AS OUTLINED BELOW.
☐ **NASOGASTRIC** ☐ **GASTROSTOMY**

ISOTONIC ENTERAL PRODUCTS SCHEDULE A		HYPERTONIC ENTERAL PRODUCTS SCHEDULE B	
PRODUCT	**CALORIES/ml**	**PRODUCT**	**CALORIES/ml**
☐ Glucerna	1.0	☐ ALITRAQ*	1.0
☐ Impact	1.0	☐ Ensure Plus	1.5
☐ Lipisorb*	1.0	☐ Isocal HCN	2.0
☐ Osmolite	1.06	☐ Nepro	2.0
☐ Osmolite HN	1.06	☐ Pulmocare	1.5
☐ Ultracal	1.06	☐ Sustacal HC	1.5
		☐ Travasorb Hepatic*, ♦	1.1
		☐ Vivonex TEN*	1.0

STAGE	AMOUNT/FEED	STRENGTH	TIME	STAGE	AMOUNT/FEED	STRENGTH	TIME
I				I	120 ml	1/2	06-10-14-18-22
II				II	120 ml	3/4	06-10-14-18-22
III	120 ml	Full	06-10-14-18-22	III	120 ml	Full	06-10-14-18-22
IV	240 ml	Full	06-10-14-18-22	IV	240 ml	Full	06-10-14-18-22
V	360 ml	Full	06-10-14-18-22	V	360 ml	Full	06-10-14-18-22
VI	400 ml	Full	06-10-14-18-22	VI	400 ml	Full	06-10-14-18-22
VII	480 ml	Full	06-10-14-18-22	VII	480 ml	Full	06-10-14-18-22

ENTERAL NUTRITION ORDERS

1. Advance one stage q 24h as tolerated until a final stage of (check one): ☐ Stage VII or ☐ Stage _____ (Specify)
2. Maximum volume/feeding is 480 ml. If in 24h more formula is needed, additional bolus feedings can be provided. Indicate specific times when to administer the additional feedings. _____
3. Flush tube **before** and **after** each feeding with 50 ml water.
4. Check position of NG feeding tube (if appropriate) per nursing protocol.
5. **Nursing:** ● During feeding and for 60 min. after, patient to sit upright at ≥ 45°, 90° preferred.
   ● Give formula at room temperature.
   ● Check residual. If > 100 ml, refeed 100 ml, discard rest and notify MD.
   ● Daily weight, I/O.
6. **Dietary:** Daily calorie count per dietitian.
7. **Lab Values:** Nutrition Panel-I q Tuesday and Friday
8. Call Nutrition Support Team for problems of persistent nausea, diarrhea and vomiting.

NUTRITION PANEL-I
Na, K, HCO₃, Cl, Glucose

ORAL SUPPLEMENTS - SCHEDULE C

SELECT PRODUCT TYPE/FLAVOR   **SELECT AN ADMINISTRATION SCHEDULE**

PRODUCT: FLAVORS AVAILABLE	CALORIES
☐ Ensure Plus: Vanilla, Chocolate, Strawberry, Eggnog	1.5 ml
☐ Ensure Pudding: Vanilla*	250/can
☐ Fortified Clear Liquid Drink: Punch*	136/8 oz serving
☐ Fortified Shake: Vanilla, Chocolate, Strawberry*	290/8 oz serving
☐ Pulmocare: Vanilla	1.5/ml
☐ Sustacal HC: Chocolate	1.5/ml
☐ Vivonex TEN: Variety of Flavor Packets*	10-15.5/Packet

PROVIDE PRODUCT:		
With Meals:	☐ TID	☐ BID
Between Meals:	☐ TID	☐ BID
Evening Snack:	☐	

*Mixed and delivered by dietary   ♦Requires approval of Nutrition Support Team

Noted by _____   **Signature** _____ **M.D.**

Date _____ **Time** _____   **Date** _____ **Time** _____

CLINICAL DATA SERVICES (7/92)   G3.00

Fig. 12.4. Bolus enteral nutrition oral supplementation order form.

ENTERAL NUTRITION FORMULAS
(Analysis/1000 ml)

Formula	Form	Kcal/ml	gm/L PRO	gm/L CHO	gm/L FAT	Non-Pro Kcal:gmN	mg/mEq/L Na	mg/mEq/L K	mg/L Ca	mg/L Mg	mg/L Phos	mOsm/Kg H2O	ml for RDA	Fiber gm/L	Indications for Use
ALITRAQ	Powder	1.0	52.6	165	15.5	94:1	1000/44	1200/31	734	267	734	575	1500	---	Glutamine enriched for stressed patient with impaired GI function
Ensure Plus	Liquid	1.5	55	200	53	146:1	1141/50	2113/54	706	283	706	690	1420	---	High nitrogen formula for increased calories in limited fluid volume
Glucerna	Liquid	1.0	42	94	56	125:1	928/40	1561/40	704	282	704	375	1422	13.7	Formula for patient with diabetes or glucose intolerance
Impact	Liquid	1.0	56	132	28	71:1	1100/48	1300/33	800	270	800	375	1500	---	Formula for immunocompromised patient
Isocal HCN	Liquid	2.0	75	200	102	145:1	800/35	1690/43	1010	400	1010	640	1000	---	Very high calorie and nitrogen formula in limited fluid volume
Lipisorb	Powder	1.0	35	116.7	47.9	160:1	733/32	1248/32	699	300	699	320	2000	---	A readily absorbed fat blend with MCT to improve fat absorption (86% of fat as MCT)
Nepro	Liquid	2.0	69.9	215.2	95.6	157:1	829/36.1	1057/27	1373	211	686	635	947	---	Moderate protein, calorically-dense product for patient requiring fluid and electrolyte restrictions
Osmolite	Liquid	1.06	37	145	39	153:1	640/28	1020/26	530	212	530	300	1887	---	Isotonic formula, 50% of fat from MCT
Osmolite HN	Liquid	1.06	44	141	37	125:1	930/40	1570/40	758	304	758	300	1321	---	Isotonic formula with increased protein
Pulmocare	Liquid	1.5	63	106	92	125:1	1310/57	1902/49	1057	423	1057	490	947	---	High fat formula for pulmonary disease (CO$_2$ retainers)
Sustacal HC	Liquid	1.5	61	190	58	134:1	850/37	1480/38	850	340	850	650	1200	---	High nitrogen formula for increased calories in limited fluid volume
Travasorb Hepatic	Powder	1.1	29	213	15	211:1	233/10	873/22	1000	400	1000	600	2040	---	High BCAA, low aromatic AA formula for patient with hepatic failure (encephalopathy)
Ultracal	Liquid	1.06	44	123	45	128:1	930/39.7	1610/41.7	850	340	850	310	1250	14.4	Isotonic formula with fiber (oat and soy)
Vivonex TEN	Powder	1.0	38	206	3	149:1	460/20	782/20	500	200	500	630	2000	---	Elemental formula (predigested)

ORAL SUPPLEMENTS

Formula	Form	Kcal	gm PRO	gm CHO	gm FAT	mg/mEq Na	mg/mEq K	mg Ca	mg Mg	mg Phos	mOsm/Kg H2O	ml for RDA	Fiber gm/L	Indications for Use
Fortified Clear Liquid Drink	Powdered Drink Mix 8 oz	136	8	30	< 1g	120/5.1	170/4.4	300	80	200	450	---	---	High calorie, high protein liquid supplement
Fortified Pudding (Ensure Pudding)	Pudding 5 oz can	250	6.8	34	9.7	240/10.2	330/8.5	200	68	200	---	---	---	High calorie, high protein liquid supplement appropriate for supraglottic diet
Fortified Shake	Powdered Shake Mix 8 oz	290	17	37	8	240/7.5	810/20.8	550	100	450	730-820	960	---	High calorie, high protein liquid supplement

MODULAR COMPONENTS

Formula	Form	Kcal	gm PRO	gm CHO	gm FAT	mg/mEq Na	mg/mEq K	mg Ca	mg Mg	mg Phos	mOsm/Kg H2O	ml for RDA	Fiber gm/L	Indications for Use
Polycose	Powder	23/tbsp	0	6/tbsp	0	110/4.8/100 gms	10/< 1/100 gms	30/100 gms	---	5/100 gms	40/tbsp	---	---	Carbohydrate source, glucose polymers
Promod	Powder	17/tbsp	3/tbsp	< 0.5/tbsp	< 0.5/tbsp	227/10/100 gms	985/25/100 gms	880/100 gms	---	660/100 gms	18/tbsp	---	---	Protein source (whey)
Microlipid	Liquid	4.5/ml	0	0	500/L	---	---	---	---	---	60	---	---	Long chain fat source that stays in suspension
MCT Oil	Liquid	7.6/ml	0	0	384/L	---	---	---	---	---	---	---	---	Medium chain triglycerides source

Fig. 12.5. A listing of various enteral nutrition formulas.

Table 12.6. *Data on 93 patients with carcinoma of bladder receiving peripheral vein parenteral nutrition*

Solution infused	Osmolality (m.osmol/l)	Total kcal per day	% Ideal body weight		Frequency of IV site change in 9 days	Complication frequency	
			Initial	Final		Infiltration	Phlebitis
3%AA/H$_2$O[a] (n = 33)	475	340	108 ± 3	102 ± 3	6.0	57%	40%
3%AA/5%DW (n = 30)	740	860	107 ± 3	102 ± 3	5.6	56%	44%
5%DW (n = 30)	370	510	108 ± 3	103 ± 3	5.5	59%	40%

[a] Solutions contained average 40 meq KCl & NaCl; MVI, and 1 g Keflin qid.
Adapted from Massar *et al.*, 1983. Data expressed as M ± SE.

balanced proportions of protein, carbohydrate and fat with vitamins and electrolytes. Supplements contain protein, carbohydrate and fat with particular emphasis on either protein or carbohydrates (e.g. Sustacal, Ensure Plus, Carnation Instant Breakfast). Modular components contain only one component (e.g. microlipid, MCT oil, polycose, promod), allowing these to be added to standard formulae to fortify a diet calorically or nitrogenously to meet the patient's particular metabolic needs.

Venous access for parenteral nutrition

Peripheral vein cannulation

The peripheral route is usually selected over the central venous route allegedly because it is easier to establish, avoids the potential hazards of central venous catheter placement, and is associated with a lower frequency of patient problems. These assumption are tenuous, as exemplified by the data shown in Table 12.6 which underlie the limitations of peripheral nutritional support (Massar *et al.*, 1983). The limited number of calories delivered is insufficient to meet the caloric requirements of the mildly catabolic post-operative state. In this study, all patients were initially well nourished but lost an average of 6% body weight while receiving peripheral parenteral nutrition for a mean of nine days. The incidence of subcutaneous perivascular infiltration and mild to severe phlebitis were unacceptably high at 56–60% and 40%, respectively.

Infusion thrombophlebitis can be produced by a number of factors: (1) site (Fonkalsrud *et al.*, 1968), (2) duration of infusion (Medical Research

Council Report, 1957), (3) types of drugs infused (Thomas, Evers & Raez, 1970), (4) cannula and needle types (Dinely, 1976), and (5) osmolality of intravenous fluids infused, and infection (Swinscow, 1976). The low frequency of thrombophlebitis with butterfly stainless steel cannulas was shown to be due to their short duration of use. The incidence of phlebitis increases markedly with solutions of osmolality greater than 600 m osmol/l, irrespective of the duration of infusion. The addition of heparin does not prevent or decrease the incidence of phlebitis (Gazitua *et al.*, 1979). The addition of low dose hydrocortisone and heparin reduced the frequency of thrombophlebitis during peripheral TPN by 9% (Roohgpisuthipong, Puchaiwatananon & Songchitsomboon, 1993).

Whether parenteral nutrition via a peripheral vein is beneficial or indicated in mildly stressed but nourished patients, for periods of up to 16 days as in the study by Masser *et al.*, (1983), is of questionable therapeutic and cost benefit. There are inherent limitations to the use of peripheral alimentation by the amount of nutrients which can be delivered and by the incidence of morbidity as exemplified from the summarised data in Table 12.6.

Central venous cannulation

A description of the techniques for placing central venous catheters can be found in a surgical atlas. Two sites are most commonly used: (1) infraclavicular subclavian vein route, and (2) supraclavicular internal jugular vein route. Both routes are popular and permit the delivery of hypertonic nutrient solutions in a dependable manner. The indication for the use of either route is to provide nutrients for a period greater than five days, during which adequate nutrient intake to meet the patient's full nutrient requirements cannot be assured. The benefits of TPN via these routes are legion (Meguid, Campos & Hammond, 1990*a,b*; Meguid & Muscaritoli, 1993) and greatly outweigh the complications which are all too frequently stressed.

Right atrial catheters

Superior vena cava A more versatile device for long-term venous access for patients requiring home nutrition or chemotherapy, is the centrally placed silastic Broviac catheter and the longer Hickman catheter. These can be single, double, or even triple lumen. Catheters are placed centrally into the proximal superior vena cava just above the right atrium by cut-down or by percutaneous means under local or general anaesthesia. These silastic catheters can be used for multiple purposes including the

Table 12.7. *Catheter maintenance protocol*

Cutdown site	Dry sterile dressing until wound heals. Then no dressing.
Catheter exit site	Daily skin cleansing with alcohol and 3% H_2O_2. Apply povidone-iodine (Betadine) on dry sterile dressing.
Catheter	Heparin flush following blood sampling. Daily change. No millipore filter.

Reproduced with permission from Meguid *et al.* (1985). *Cancer* **55**, 279.

infusion of TPN, blood products and medications, and are also used to sample the patient's blood. Numerous studies have shown that infectious complications are infrequent even in the immunocompromised cancer patient and that multiple uses of the catheter because of its reliable venous access route, greatly outweigh its potential complications (Meguid, Akahoshi & Hill, 1986). Catheters were meticulously cared for on a daily basis using an aseptic/antiseptic technique outlined in a catheter maintenance protocol, as in Table 12.7.

Inferior vena cava Vascular access can often become problematic when continued nutritional support and other types of intravenous therapy are required during extended periods of hospitalisation. Insertion of a central silastic catheter with access sites on the upper torso may be contra-indicated in some clinical conditions: (1) thrombosis of the subclavian vein; (2) burns or trauma of the upper torso; (3) the need for upper torso radiation therapy; (4) median sternotomy with wound infection; or (5) fresh tracheostomy. In such patients, insertion of a silastic Hickman catheter for long-term use, by way of a vein in the lower extremity is a rational alternative, as illustrated in Fig. 12.6 (Curtas, Bonaventura & Meguid, 1989).

Concern has been expressed about exposing patients with thrombosis of the superior vena cava to the potential risk of inferior vena cava thrombosis from a long term inferior vena cava catheter. The incidence of thrombosis from such central catheters, however, has been shown to be reduced by the addition of 1 unit of heparin per ml to all solutions infused through the catheter (Fabri *et al.*, 1982). The early stage of pericatheter thrombosis, as manifested by increased resistance to infusion and the inability to draw blood, does not now mandate immediate removal of the catheter especially in patients for whom the solutions infused represent essential therapy. Rather, the presence of pericatheter

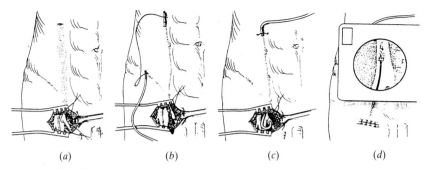

(a)   (b)   (c)   (d)

Fig. 12.6. Technique of cannulation of the inferior vena cava is shown. (a) A tributary of the greater saphenous vein is isolated; (b) a subcutaneous tunnel is made; (c) the catheter is inserted through the venotomy; and (d) the catheter is passed into the inferior vena cava under fluoroscopic visualisation. (Reproduced with permission, from Curtas *et al.* (1989). *SGO*, **168**, 121.)

thrombus formation mandates early initiation of vigorous treatment with thrombolytic agents through the catheter (Smith *et al.*, 1985). The catheter should not be removed until thrombolytic therapy has proved unsuccessful, indicating that the thrombosis is adherent to the vein and unlikely to migrate.

Port An extension of the concept of immediate, continuous and *ad libitum* access to the venous system is a subcutaneous implantable injection port. This is an alternative means of safe and reliable central venous access with improved patient convenience and cosmetic acceptability. Ports are placed in the upper torso, utilising the same upper venous system as with subclavian or right atrial catheters. Single and double ports are available and are placed under either local or general anaesthesia at operation. Antibiotics, blood components and intravenous solutions can be administered though these ports. The system remains functioning for a long time. Occlusion of the small bore catheter is common (90%), but this does not occur with the large bore catheter.

Peripherally inserted central (PIC) catheters The PIC catheter is a soft, super thin catheter 40–60 cm long [(1.5 to 5.0 French (23–16 gauge)], made of silicone elastomer (silastic and polyurethane) and is available in a single or multiple lumen. It is inserted via the antecubital fossa into either the basilic vein, which is relatively large and has a good blood flow or into the cephalic vein which is smaller and has a more sluggish blood flow and floated proximally into the superior vena cava. It is used for most infusion therapies, being comfortable for patients and does not restrict arm movements or normal activity and can remain in place for up to three months, sparing the patient multiple vein punctures. It can be used with an infusion pump.

The indications for the use of a PIC catheter include: (1) limited vascular access; (2) for irritating/vesicant drug therapy and hyperosmolar nutrient solution requiring central venous dilution; (3) for short-term nutritional support and chemotherapy. It is an ideal catheter in patients with hyperemesis gravidarum, anorexia, and ARC or AIDS. Its benefits include: (1) fewer insertion related complications such as pneumothorax, haemo-thorax, and cardiac arrhythmias because it is inserted via the antecubital fossa; (2) decreased cost: 80% less than other long-term access devices; and (3) lower complication rates of catheter-related sepsis, peripheral phlebitis, and deep vein thrombosis.

In a recent study by Rountree (1991), 410 PIC catheters were placed during 11 months in patients with medical–surgical and critical care problems. PIC catheters were used for 1 to 91 days (mean of 12 days/catheter). The indications for their use were: (1) difficult venous access – 73%; (2) antibiotic therapy – 77%; (3) TPN – 5%; (4) chemo-therapy – 1%; (5) intravenous fluids – 42%; and (6) other intravenous drugs – 41%. PIC catheters were removed because: (1) therapy was completed in 69%; (2) it was dislodged by patient in 7%; (3) clotted in 15%; (4) catheter-related complications in 5%; and (5) catheter tip migrations in 1%. The complications encountered were: (1) phlebitis – 1%; (2) swollen arm – 1%; (3) pain in arm – 1%; and (4) catheter-related sepsis – 1%. Similar experiences were reported by Elliott, D'Abrera & Dutton (1988) and Hilton *et al.* (1988).

Complications of central venous access

The complications related to the insertion and use of the central venous catheter fall broadly into three categories: mechanical, septic and metabolic (see Table 12.8).

Mechanical complications The rate of mechanical complications is inversely proportional to the skill and experience of the catheter inserter. The average frequencies of complications in 2050 patients were: mechanical 6.7%, septic 4.7% and metabolic 25.7% (Padberg *et al.*, 1981; Weinsier, Bacon & Butterworth, 1982; Jones *et al.*, 1984; Wolfe *et al.*, 1986). Other factors contributing to complications include the site of the catheter

Table 12.8. *Complications associated with the use of TPN*

Type of complication	Nature	Frequency
Mechanical	o Catheter tip malposition	6%
	o Arterial laceration	1.4%
	o Pneumo-hydro-haemo-thorax	1.1%
	o Subclavian or SVC thrombosis	0.3%
	o Thrombophlebitis	0.1%
	o Catheter embolism	0.1%
Septic	o Catheter-related sepsis	7.4%
Metabolic:		
Acute	o Hyperglycaemia/hypoglycaemia	Avoidable
	o Blood electrolyte abnormalities	
	o Fluid overload	
	o Hyperlipidaemia	
Chronic	o Metabolic bone disease	Rare
	o Alterations in bile composition	
	o Deterioration of liver function	

Modified from Meguid & Muscaritoli (1993).

insertion and the type of material of which the catheter is made. In a world review of 39 180 central venous catheters (Burri & Ahnefeld, 1977), the most frequent mechanical complication experienced with successful insertion of a subclavian central venous catheter, was malposition (6%), followed by arterial injury (1.4%), pneumo-hydro-hemo-thorax (1.1%), vessel thrombosis (0.3%), thrombophlebitis (0.1%) and catheter embolism (0.1%). The death rate related to all these complications was 1.2%. The safest method of obtaining central venous access is via the internal jugular vein, although this is not the most widely used route.

Catheter material thrombogenicity influences the outcome (Linder *et al.*, 1984). The frequencies of thrombophlebitis and radiological vessel thrombosis using a polyurethane catheter were 6% and 94%, respectively, compared to 36% and 66% using a silicone elastomer catheter. The duration of catheter placement also influenced the frequency of these two complications, being greater the longer the duration of the catheter was *in situ*.

To minimise the frequency of subclavian vein thrombosis, heparin is added to TPN solutions. Based on a number of studies (Bailey, 1979; Fabri *et al.*, 1982; Imperial *et al.*, 1983), a patient population at high risk of thrombus formation exists, who have a deficiency of Antithrombin III factor. These include patients with inflammatory bowel disease, cancer, pancreatitis and sepsis (Imperial *et al.*, 1983). In these patients the vessel thrombosis rate was 52% and the addition of 6000 units of heparin to TPN, infused continuously decreased the thrombosis frequency. In patients with normal Antithrombin III factor, the frequency of thrombosis was only 14% and the addition of 1 unit of heparin per ml of TPN appeared sufficient to prevent thrombosis.

Catheter sepsis According to the Center for Disease Control in Atlanta, Georgia, the frequency of catheter sepsis in the US is 7.4%. The most effective method of diagnosis is via the use of the quantitative blood culture method, for determining *in situ* sepsis. In all cases, when the catheter is incriminated by culture data, removal of the central venous catheter led to patient improvement. In no instance, when the central venous catheter was deemed 'innocent', did its removal lead to clinical improvement (Mosca *et al.*, 1987). Following removal for catheter-related sepsis, data now suggest that it is safe to re-insert a new sterile catheter in 12 hours (Paston *et al.*, 1993). In certain clinical situations (e.g. critically ill patients for whom removal of the central venous catheter may not be a viable option), treating an established catheter-related sepsis episode with antibiotics can eradicate the catheter colonisation, thereby prolonging the life and usefulness of the catheter (Douard *et al.*, 1991).

Metabolic complications Since TPN can be regarded as a sophisticated form of fluid and electrolyte therapy, many of the reported metabolic complications have resulted from errors of omission. Thus, the complications due to an excess or a deficit of electrolytes, vitamins or trace elements are potentially avoidable, and therefore will not be emphasised. The introduction of a safe and reliable fat source has obviated the metabolic complications derived from a glucose-based TPN (Meguid *et al.*, 1984*a*); hyperglycaemia, hypoglycaemia, hyperosmolar syndromes, hypertriglyceridaemia, abnormal lipid profiles, hyperinsulinaemia, elevated epinephrine, elevation of liver function tests, hypercarbia (Askanazi *et al.*, 1979), essential fatty acid deficiencies and venous thrombosis.

Safety: the nutritional support team

In the final report and statement of the Georgetown University Technology Assessment and Practice Guidelines Forum on the Evaluation of Total Parenteral Nutrition published in 1990, it was concluded: 'based on available data, it is recommended that the most safe and cost-effective care and delivery of nutritional support to patients in the hospital or home setting, either as TPN or using the enteral route, should be provided and supervised by knowledgeable health care professionals. These are the essential goals of safety (the least mechanical, metabolic, and septic complications), improved quality of care and of cost-effective nutritional support, as best attained by utilisation of a multi-disciplinary team approach of interested and appropriately trained professionals' (Evaluating TPN: Core Statement, 1990).

Nutrition support teams have had the greatest impact in reducing all types of complications, as related to the delivery of nutrients to hospitalised patients. Prior to the advent of the nutrition support team, the average mechanical, septic and metabolic complications in one study were 33%, 21% and 36%, respectively. After the team, these fell dramatically to 3.2%, 6.5% and 3%, respectively. These representative data elegantly demonstrate the effectiveness and cost benefits of a nutrition support team (Nehme, 1980).

Standardised TPN order form

Physicians, from consultant staff to house staff, differ greatly in their levels of nutrition education and in their familiarity with ordering parenteral solutions. As the use of TPN continues to spread in clinical practice, there is a need to establish prescription standards. To aid in the delivery of a consistent level of nutritional support care, a parenteral nutrition order form is used (Fig. 12.7). This form is designed for ease of physician use, providing more precise guidelines for the prescription of TPN, including standard orders for the starting and the stopping of TPN and for the comprehensive nursing and dietary care of the patient.

The form is based on the single delivery system of the total nutrient admixture concept (Campos, Paluzzi & Meguid, 1990) and offers the following features: (1) a standard formula concentration (15 g of glucose, 5 g of amino acids, and 20 g of lipids per 100 ml) or a space for individualised solutions; (2) the average daily recommendations for electrolytes (Na, K, phosphate, Mg, Ca), vitamins, and trace elements (Zn, Cu, Mn, Cr, Se, Mo) in paediatric and adult dosages; (3) the addition of heparin to prevent catheter thrombosis (Imperial *et al.*, 1983); (4) the addition of weekly vitamin K; (5) the option to add insulin; (6) nursing and dietary orders to start and stop TPN; and (7) laboratory tests for electrolytes, glucose, liver function, cholesterol, and triglycerides to monitor the patient's immediate and long-term tolerance of TPN.

The standardised order form provides the additional benefit of acting

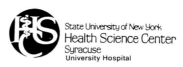

State University of New York
Health Science Center
Syracuse
University Hospital

**PARENTERAL NUTRITION
ORDER FORM**

TPN: a 3 in 1 admixture bag for a 24 hour period

ORDERS: CHECK ONE

Orders must be sent to pharmacy by 1400 hours

Weight _____ Kg

☐ INDIVIDUALIZED

☐ STANDARDIZED

		Amino Acids	50 g/l	1000 ml
_____ gm/day				
_____ gm/day or	Carbohydrate (dextrose)	177 g/l	approx.
_____ kcal/day		601 kcal/l	1
_____ gm/day or	Fat (lipid emulsion 20%)	40 g/l	kcal/ml
_____ kcal/day	500 ml supplies (100g) 1000 Kcal	400 kcal/l	

_____ kcal/KG _____ gm/Prot./KG **BAG NUMBER** _____ **INFUSION RATE** _____ml/hr for 24 HR

ADDITIVES

Amount Per 24 Hours	DAILY		ROUTINE		SPECIAL (Circle)	
	Sodium Chloride	mEq	Heparin	U/ml	Ascorbic Acid	500mg
Na 100mEq	Sodium Acetate*	mEq	Vitamin K₁	mg	Folic Acid	1mg
	Potassium Chloride	mEq	Regular Human Insulin	units	Selenium	120mcg
K 60-120mEq	Potassium Acetate*	mEq	Albumin (for serum<3gm/dl)	gm	Thiamine	100mg
PO₄ 10-22mmol	Phosphate (as potassium salt) 1mmol phosphorus = 1.5mEq K)	mmol	Ranitidine	mg	Zinc	10mg
Mg 8-20mEq	Magnesium Sulfate	mEq				
Ca 10-15mEq	Calcium Gluconate	mEq				

| | | | **LAB VALUES** | Date _____ | |

Vitamin (MVI-12) 10ml	MVI-12	10ml
Trace Elements(Conc.) 1ml	Trace Elements (Zn.Cu.Mn.Cr.Se)	1ml
Molybdenum 25 mcg = 1ml	Molybdenum Elemental	25 mcg

Na	Cl	BUN		Ca
			Gluc	PO₄
				Mg
				Alb
				Trig

*Substitute acetate salts in hyperchloremic acidosis

TPN STANDING ORDERS:

Lab Values: DAY 1:Nutrition Panel I, II & III
DAY 2,3: Nutrition Panel I
Thereafter, q TUESDAY: Nutrition Panel I, II & III
Lab values: q FRIDAY: Nutrition Panel I & II

Nursing:
• Daily weights, cumulative I/O
q SHIFT: I/O, fingerstick glucose, Notify MD if > 200 mg/dl
• Change catheter dressing q M _____ W _____ F _____ and prn ___
• Infuse daily TPN from 1900 to 1900 Hrs
DIETARY:
• Daily calorie counts during transitional feeding (tube feeding/po) or as per nutrition support team

NUTRITION PANELS: PANEL I: Na, K, HCO₃, Cl, Glucose
PANEL II: ALP, Cre, BUN, PO₄, Alb, Ca, Mg
PANEL III: Chol, Trig

4230 Rev 8-92

METHOD OF DISCONTINUING: CHECK ONE

☐ ROUTINE: When 60% of caloric requirements is provided by po diet or tube feeding, decrease TPN to 1/2 of current rate for one hour. Then discontinue TPN.

☐ PRE-OP AND ACUTE DISCONTINUATION: Infuse D10W at TPN rate through central catheter. If central catheter is removed, infuse D10W peripherally at TPN rate.

☐ FOR persistent fever of unkown etiology: a. draw isolator blood cultures from all ports of central catheter and also via peripheral route.
b. discontinue TPN as above and remove central catheter if clinically indicated.

SIGNATURE	MD	DATE	TIME
NOTE BY		DATE	TIME

CLINICAL DATA SERVICES G3.00

Fig. 12.7. Parenteral nutrition order form.

as an educational tool (Mitchell *et al.*, 1990), because the form provides not only prescription guidelines for the appropriate use of TPN, but reflects a philosophy of the use of TPN. This approach is particularly useful for inexperienced house staff in providing nutritional support practice guidelines, without compromising the quality of patient care (Fogel *et al.*, 1987).

The standardised form with appropriate guidelines facilitated the ordering of TPN and assisted house staff in writing appropriate orders, with a reduction in prescription errors. The form translates into a decrease in non-patient-related nursing and pharmacy time and an overall reduction in the total cost of patient nutritional care, because of less waste. In addition, the form is labour saving and decreases the need for refrigerator storage space.

All-in-one delivery system

The introduction of 3-litre bags made of ethyl vinyl acetate, has made the admixture of a fat emulsion to dextrose and amino acid possible. These mixtures can be prepared up to 30 days prior to use. Daily requirements of vitamins, trace elements and electrolytes can be added just before infusion is started. Using this method, between 30% and 50% of nonprotein calories are supplied as lipid.

The advantages of this approach are numerous: (1) a cost saving during preparation, handling, and delivery; (2) more uniform administrations of a balanced solution containing the three macronutrients plus micronutrients over a 24-hour period, thus circumventing the metabolic disadvantages of a single energy-substrate system; (3) less manipulation and consequently less risk of contamination; (4) obviation of care for peripheral catheters used solely for the administration of lipids in order to avoid inserting a central venous catheter; (5) decreased lipid toxicity because of the greater dilution of the lipid emulsion and the longer duration of its infusion; (6) ease of delivery and storage for patients on home nutritional support programmes; (7) the option of delivering nutritional support peripherally; and (8) reduced long-term hepatic accumulation of triglycerides, in part attributed to glucose-based TPN (Campos, Paluzzi & Meguid, 1990).

Types of parenteral formulations

In general, the majority of patients are well served using a standard TPN formula. The selection of nutrient solutions for different catabolic states, largely centres on the admixture of the major substrates: carbohydrate, fat and protein. Total parenteral nutrition implies a decision to administer all the calories and nitrogen which a patient can effectively utilise. Examples of clinical conditions requiring modification of solutions, are shown below given a hypothetical patient. As outlined in the previous section, once energy needs have been determined, TPN orders can be written, as illustrated in the case example shown below.

Case Study

A 48-year-old well-nourished male with cancer of the colon is post-colectomy. Based on the experience summarised in Table 12.1, it is anticipated that gastro-intestinal function will not be normal for about 8 days if no complications occur, or 12 days if a complication does occur. His weight is 77.2 kg, and his height is 150 cm.

Energy needs based on Harris–Benedict equation:
   BEE $\times$ 1.1 (activity factor) $\times$ 1.2 (injury factor = major surgery)
      $= 1688 \times 1.1 \times 1.2 = 2201$ kcal/day.

Formulation to be used: Stock Solution $= 50$ g/100 ml glucose, 20 g/100 ml fat, 11 g/100 ml amino acid

Relative nutrient composition	kcal	g	ml	% solution
50% glucose	1102	324	648	15
30% fat	660	66	330	330 ml of 20% fat
20% amino acid	439	107	973	5
	2201		1951	
			150 (electrolytes)	
			2101	

However, there exist a number of clinical conditions in which the standard formulation cannot be used, leading to modification of the TPN prescription. Some examples are given:

1. Chronic obstructive pulmonary disease and cystic fibrosis: decreased glucose and increased fat, but amino acids unchanged

Relative nutrient composition	kcal	g	ml	% solution
20% glucose	440	129	258	6.3
60% fat	1320	132	660	660 ml of 20% fat
20% amino acid	440	107	972	5.2
	2200		1890	
			150 (electrolytes)	
			2040	

2. Diabetes: increased fat and decreased glucose, but amino acids unchanged

Relative nutrient composition	kcal	g	ml	% solution
30% glucose	660	194	388	9.4
50% fat	1100	110	550	550 ml of 20% fat
20% amino acid	440	107	972	5.2
	2200		1910	
			150	(electrolytes)
			2060	

Concentrated stock solution = 70 g/100 ml glucose, 20 g/100 ml fat, 15 g/100 ml amino acid.

3. Congestive cardiac falure: decreased volume, increased concentration of nutrients

Relative nutrient Composition	kcal	g	ml	% solution
50% glucose	1000	294	420	19.1
34% fat	680	68	340	340 ml of 20% fat
16% amino acid	320	94	626	6.1
	2000		1386	
			150	(electrolytes)
			1536	

4. Acute renal disease: concentrated solution, increased glucose and fat, but decreased amino acid concentration and decreased volume

Relative nutrient composition	kcal	g	ml	% solution
50% glucose	800	235	336	20.3
35% fat	560	56	280	280 ml of 20% fat
15% amino acid	240	59	393	5.1
	1600		1009	
			150	(electrolytes)
			1159	

5. Hepatic disease: glucose and fat content remain unchanged, but decreased aromatic amino acid and increased branched chain amino acids are needed.

- Use Hepatamine with same nutrient concentrations as above.
- Volume will be increased as amino acid concentration in Hepatamine is only 8 g/100 ml.

Monitoring the patient on total parenteral nutrition

Table 12.9 summarises the indexes monitored to ensure safe use of TPN. Recently, serum CPK has been used to monitor the response to TPN in catabolic surgical patients (Antonas, Curtas & Meguid, 1987). Stringent

Table 12.9. *Monitoring the patient on total parenteral nutrition*

Clinical data checked daily:
Patient's sense of well-being: symptoms suggesting fluid overload, high or low blood glucose, electrolyte imbalance, etc.
Patient's strength as judged by graded activity: getting out of bed, walking, stair climbing.
Vital signs: temperature, blood pressure, pulse rate and respiratory rate.
Fluid balance: weight. Fluid input (intravenous ± enteral) versus fluid output (urine, stool, gastric suction, etc.).
Delivery equipment for TPN: composition of nutrient solution, tubing, pump, filter catheter, dressing (skin checked for local infection at time of dressing change)

Laboratory data:
Urine quantitative glucose 4 × day

Blood glucose	Daily until glucose infusion load and patient
$Na^+, K^+, Cl^-. HCO_3^-$	stable, then 2 × week
Blood urea nitrogen	

Serum albumin, transferrin (or TIBC)	
Liver function studies	
Serum creatinine	Baseline, then 2 × week
Ca^{2+}, PO_4, Mg^{2+}	
Hb/Ht, WBC	

NH_3 and prothrombin time – baseline, then weekly
Micronutrient tests as indicated (see text)

Reproduced with permission from Howard & Meguid (1981). *Cin. Lab. Med.*, **1**, 611.

monitoring is required because mechanical, metabolic and infectious complications may develop rapidly and can be life threatening.

Advantages of feeding a patient peri-operatively

A solid database exists concerning therapeutic triumphs of enteral and parenteral nutritional support. This includes: increased survival with renal failure (Abel *et al.*, 1973); decreased mortality with severe pancreatitis (Feller *et al.*, 1974); improved tolerance and response to chemotherapy (Copeland *et al.*, 1975); increased survival of the infants unable to feed orally (Heird, MacMillan & Winters, 1976); increased survival, accelerated healing and shorter hospitalisation with extensive burns (Bartlett *et al.*, 1977); and more favourable clinical outcome of severely burned and traumatised patients (Alexander *et al.*, 1980). Other benefits include: a reduction in perineal wound healing time after prostatectomy with a reduction in hospital stay (Collins, Oxby & Hill, 1978); successful nourishment of patients with short bowel syndrome at home (Dudrick *et al.*, 1979); improvement of alcoholic hepatitis (Nasrallah & Galambos, 1980); decreased morbidity and mortality in patients with gastrointestinal cancer (Muller *et al.*, 1982); decreased complications of inflammatory bowel disease (Rombeau *et al.*, 1982); improved objective muscle function following operation (Delone *et al.*, 1987); earlier recovery and hospital discharge following head injury (Rapp *et al.*, 1983); earlier ambulation and hospital discharge after femoral fracture (Bastow, Rawlings & Allison, 1983); increased rate of spontaneous closure of gastrointestinal fistula with decreased mortality (O'Morain, Segal & Levi, 1984); low incidence of ventricular arrhythmias, and low vasopressor dependence and no transmural myocardial infarction post coronary artery bypass graft operation (Lolley *et al.*, 1985); earlier discharge after radical cystectomy for cancer (Askanazi *et al.*, 1986); as well as improvement in mood states (McNair, Lorr & Droppleman, 1971), subjective symptoms of depression, anxiety and hostility (Derogatis, 1978), as well as fatigue (Christenson, Bendix & Kehlet, 1982).

In reviewing these data in detail, it will become clear to the reader that the initially malnourished patient is less able to successfully withstand the adverse effects of vigorous therapy and/or severe illness, than is the well-nourished patient. Hence correction of malnutrition either before initiating therapy or concomitant with the treatment, in order to reduce the chances of complication to the level occurring in well-nourished hospitalised patients undergoing similar procedures is desirable. It is also reasonably clear that substantial nutritional support has little or no direct effect on the pathogenesis of many diseases in which the discontinuance of oral intake may well have a beneficial effect on the basic disease process. However, the provision of enteral or parenteral nutrition gives the patient an optimal opportunity to marshal host defences in support of healing on convalescence. In organ system failures, e.g. acute renal failure, liver failure and pulmonary failure, appropriate nutritional support may assist the patient in coping with the abnormal intermediary metabolism resulting from such failure, until satisfactory organ system function returns. The current guidelines for the appropriate use of enteral and parenteral nutritional support to the hospitalised patients are summarised in Table 12.10.

If one were to accept that peri-operative nutrition would be solely of benefit for reducing post-operative complications in the malnourished patients, one would falsely conclude that well-nourished patients are rarely, if ever, candidates for peri-operative nutritional support. In certain clinical situations, the indication for peri-operative nutritional support may be based on the primary diagnosis, regardless of the patient's nutritional status at the time of hospitalisation. General examples include: the certain expectation of a prolonged period before adequate resumption of normal oral intake following operation (embodying the concept of IONIP; Meguid *et al.*, 1986; Meguid *et al.*, 1988*b*), because of a considerable delay which may occur in the resumption of normal gastrointestinal tract function, or situations in which the patient develops an acute clinical condition with concomitant non-function of the gastrointestinal tract. Such patients are often potential candidates for one or more operations because of the unpredictable clinical course of their primary diagnosis.

Severe pancreatitis resulting from acute biliary disease illustrates this situation well. It usually occurs in a previously healthy and well-nourished patient. The disorder frequently warrants long periods of bowel rest and one or more operations. The early institution of TPN in these patients, may prevent the well-documented severe nutritional depletion that often occurs during severe protracted pancreatitis (Blackburn *et al.*, 1976). Even though TPN may have no particular effect on the acute disease process in the pancreas, it is important in maintaining the nutritional status of patients with protracted gastrointestinal tract dysfunction secondary to pancreatitis and its associated morbidity. TPN should be started once the diagnosis is established and the reported evidence indicates that prompt and vigorous initiation of TPN may be crucial to the survival of these severely ill patients, particularly if one or more operative interventions are likely to be needed.

Sometimes, a previously well-nourished patient may develop a gastrointestinal fistula after an abdominal operation for trauma, cancer or a benign condition. These patients are at high risk of developing early malnutrition. Furthermore, between 20% and 70% of gastrointestinal fistula patients require an operation to assist fistula closure (McIntyre *et al.*, 1984). Because the eventual need for operation is often unpredictable, nutritional support is indicated in anticipation of prolonged functional starvation due to a long period without a normally functioning gastrointestinal tract, as outlined in Fig. 12.8. In addition, there is also evidence that nutritional support may promote spontaneous closure of enterocutaneous fistulas in 20% to 80% of the patients, thus avoiding an

Table 12.10. *Guidelines for the use of peri-operative feeding*

Condition	Recommended TPN use
Peri-operative *Pre-operatively:*	o 2 to 3 days of TPN before operation does not improve surgical outcome. o Improvement observed with 5 to 7 days of TPN. o Significant reduction in major post-operative complications and mortality is achieved with 7 to 10 days of TPN before operation.
Post-operatively:	o TPN given when anticipated period of post-operative functional starvation exceeds 5 days.
Critical care	o Of benefit in well-nourished critically ill patients with survivable injury unable to eat or attain adequate enteral intake within 5 to 7 days. o In previously malnourished patients in whom the initiation of TPN would be of benefit prior to the hypermetabolic phase. o Of little benefit in critically ill whose hypermetabolic phase is less than 4 to 5 days or when adequate enteral nutrition anticipated during such time. o Of no benefit in patients with nonsurvivable injury where its use might prolong dehumanised state.
Closed head injury	o In the first 10 to 12 days, TPN should be given irrespective of nutritional state. Enteral nutrition is not well tolerated during this time. Nutritional support is given to maintain nutritional status. Early TPN versus enteral nutrition leads to few complications and is associated with improved survival in hospital and at 1 year.
Cancer	o Is not routinely indicated in well-nourished or mildly malnourished patients undergoing operation, chemotherapy or radiation therapy. o Useful for severely malnourished patients or patients whose severe gastrointestinal or other toxicities preclude adequate enteral intake for 7 days or longer. o Should be given prior to or in conjunction with the institution of cancer therapy. o Seldom indicated in patients with advanced cancer who have significant deterioration of performance status or in patients unresponsive to anti-neoplastic therapy. o Not indicated in terminal disease or when no further anti-neoplastic therapy is available. o Beneficial in malnourished patients with cancer who can be expected to have a normal or near-normal period of greater than six months.

Table 12.10 – *Cont.*

Condition	Recommended TPN use
Cardiac surgery	o For overnight use before coronary artery bypass graft surgery to increase myocardial glycogen content and decrease post-operative morbidity and mortality.
Obstetrics	o Of benefit in hyperemesis gravidarium. o In exacerbation of pre-existing conditions, e.g. IBD, pancreatis; traumatic maternal death with viable foetus.
Femoral fracture	o Overnight nasogastric feeding in the malnourished patient leads to shorter rehabilitation time and shorter hospital stay. Mortality rate is reduced.
Inflammatory bowel disease	o Of benefit in Crohn's patients with gut failure and in paediatric populations with growth failure. o Can induce remissions in 60% to 70% of patients with acute flare-ups of Crohn's disease. o Does not influence outcome in severe flare-ups of chronic ulcerative colitis. o Indicated as adjuvant therapy in patients with chronic ulcerative colitis and malnutrition who cannot otherwise meet their nutritional needs. o Enteral feeding, using defined formula diet, is of benefit and is preferred to TPN in active Crohn's disease.
Gastrointestinal fistulas	o Stop oral intake and start TPN to prevent malnutrition, while correcting volume, electrolyte and acid–base deficits with intravenous fluid and electrolytes; obtain fistula imaging to ascertain the number of fistulas, the site of origin and their route. o Control and reduce fistula output with TPN and Somatostatin, while preventing or treating local skin complications and systemic metabolic and septic complications.
Pancreatitis	o Not required if anticipated period of its administration is < 5 days. o If outcome not predictable and may be protracted, start TPN on admission. o Effective as nutritional support in necrotising pancreatitis. TPN not curative but of benefit if complications are present or arise. o Data exist indicating safety of use of fat emulsions with TPN in patients with acute pancreatitis in whom increased cholesterol and triglyceride levels exist.
Acute renal failure	o To assist patients in coping with the abnormal intermediate metabolism of acute renal failure until satisfactory renal function returns. o Use of EAA-enriched formulas not unequivocally accepted.

continued

Table 12.10 – *Cont.*

Condition	Recommended TPN use
Advanced chronic liver failure	o In nutritionally depleted patients unable to tolerate nutrition. o To prevent secondary effects of starvation on general metabolism and the liver. o If patient cannot tolerate 60–80 g of amino acids as regular TPN due to grade 3 and 4 hepatic encephalopathy, use BCAA-enriched TPN solution to achieve the 60–80 g amino acid intake and avoid the complications of hepatic encephalopathy.
Paediatrics	o In the absence of, or in insufficient enteral nutrition, to prevent severe negative influence on growth and organ development. o Use if after 3 days adjunctive enteral feedings are not tolerated and cannot meet minimal caloric requirements.
Short bowel syndrome	o Essential for survival of critical and stormy post-operative period in order to achieve long-term stability. Ensures survival. o Temporary or for life, depending upon adaptation of remaining functional gut.

operation altogether (Meguid & Campos, 1993). The indications for the use of TPN should be according to those outlined in Table 12.10.

A third specific example for peri-operative nutritional support based on diagnosis alone is inflammatory bowel disease (see Table 12.10), particularly Crohn's disease. Some acute complications of inflammatory bowel disease are conditions in which operative intervention may be needed. A prospective randomised study showed that 35% to 47% of the patients required surgical procedures (Dickinson *et al.*, 1980). The benefits from TPN include bowel rest, maintenance of nutritional status or even replenishment of nutritionally depleted patients. In a retrospective study including 30 patients with Crohn's disease, those who received pre-operative TPN for $\geqslant 5$ days had significantly fewer post-operative complications than those who did not: all complications that occurred were in patients who had severe protein depletion (Rombeau *et al.*, 1982). In another study, 44 patients with severe active Crohn's disease and abdominal masses, fistula, and/or obstruction, received pre-operative TPN for a mean period of 33 days (Gouma *et al.*, 1988). Significant improvements were observed in body weight, plasma albumin, and total

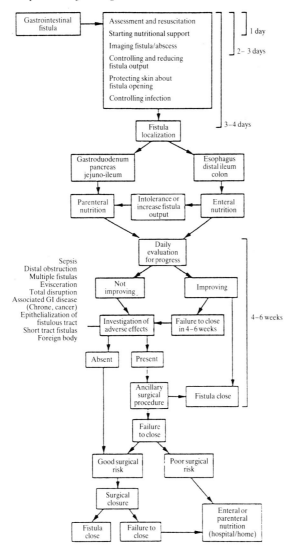

Fig. 12.8. Schema of the clinical and nutritional management of gastro-intestinal fistulas. (Reproduced with permission, from Meguid *et al.* (1990). *Am. J. Surg.*, 159, 427.

protein and remissions in the active inflammatory process. No deaths occurred and the major complication rate was only 6%. Although the beneficial effects of pre-operative TPN reported in these retrospective studies have not been confirmed in prospective randomised studies, they

Table 12.11. *Post-operative complications (%) in relation to myocardial glycogen content in 312 elective coronary artery surgery patients*

Index	Oral intake (PO)	PO + 10% DEX	PO + 20% DEX	PO + 10% FAT	PO + 10% FAT + 20% DEX
Glycogen (mg)	880	1180	1270	1509	1486
Atrial arrythmias					
None	77.8	79.2	78.5	78.6	82.8
Mild	11.1	13.4	15.4	14.3	10.0
Severe	11.1	7.4	6.1	8.1	7.2
Ventricular arrythmias					
None	55.5	58.2	55.5	56.2	84.0
Mild	20.4	19.4	9.2	14.0	7.2
Severe	5.6	7.5	12.3	7.0	4.4
Malignant	18.5	14.9	23.0	22.8	4.4
Vasopressor dependency					
None	40.6	67.2	69.2	82.5	68.2
Mild	35.2	14.9	27.7	12.7	27.5
Severe	24.2	17.9	3.1	5.2	4.3
Transmural myocardial infarction	4	3	0	0	0

DEX = dextrose.
Modified from Lolley *et al.* (1985).

strongly suggest that peri-operative nutritional support may be an important adjunct to the surgical treatment of inflammatory bowel disease.

Glycogen is an indicator of myocardial nutrition status. Efforts to increase cardiac glycogen concentration by intravenous glucose and fat loading in the immediate pre-operative period, favourably affect cardiac glycogen levels (Iyengar *et al.*, 1976). Providing TPN overnight before coronary artery bypass graft operation, increases myocardial glycogen concentrations, affording protective myocardial function and enhancing survival, as summarized in Table 12.11. Increased myocardial glycogen leads to fewer intra- and post-operative severe atrial arrhythmias, severe and malignant ventricular arrhythmias, less vasopressor dependency, fewer transmural myocardial infarctions, and greater post-operative survival (Lolley *et al.*, 1978).

Thus, three examples of gastrointestinal disease and a fourth of non-gastrointestinal disease are given in which the advantages of peri-operative TPN are evident. There are other early advantages of nutritional support which are summarized in Fig. 12.9.

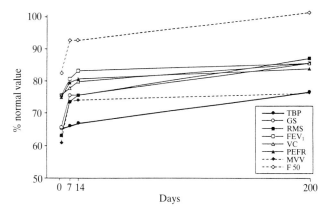

Fig. 12.9. The average changes in physiological function and total body protein that occurred during a study. TBP, total body protein; GS, maximal voluntary group strength; RMS, respiratory muscle strength; FEV, forces expiratory volume in 1 second; VC, vital capacity; PEFR, peak expiratory flow rate; MVV, maximal voluntary ventilation, F50, force at 50 Hz or maximal involuntary force. (Reproduced with permission, from Christie & Hill (1990). *Gastroenterology*, **99**, 730.)

Disadvantages of feeding a patient peri-operatively

These fall into two major groups; safety and cost of peri-operative nutritional support. Peri-operative nutritional support is indicated on an elective basis for patients who will be submitted to a well-planned operation and therefore the risks of mechanical, septic or metabolic complications associated with TPN in such patients, are probably low. The argument for the use of peri-operative nutritional support on an elective basis, is reinforced by studies reported in which few complications directly related to the nutritional support occurred. In the meta-analysis reported by Detsky *et al.* (1987), the risk of developing an iatrogenic complication secondary to TPN intervention was 6.7%. Although most of these are minor complications, they are, nevertheless, potentially harmful. In comparison, the risk of complications as a result of not providing peri-operative nutritional support, is significantly greater.

The second potential disadvantage of the use of peri-operative nutritional support is the cost. This requires consideration of the cost-effectiveness of this treatment. Before invoking the fear of cost as a reason for not giving nutritional support, the reader should be reminded of the estimated annual cost of not providing nutritional support, to either a malnourished patient, or one whose treatment might interfere with adequate nutrient intake exacerbating nutritional status with the sequelae of malnutrition. It is estimated that the cost of prolonged hospitalisation due to malnutrition and its sequelae, is $18 billion per year in the US (Meguid, 1993). The direct costs of TPN include those of catheter insertion, Roentgenograms, intravenous solutions, heparin, laboratory tests and hospital stay. The additional costs exclusively related to TPN in hospitalised patients, were reported to range from $75 to $503 per day (Anderson & Steinberg, 1986). The cost-effectiveness of preoperative TPN has been estimated to reduce (Twomey & Patching, 1985) or to increase (Detsky & Jeejeebhoy, 1984) the total hospitalisation cost per patient. The cost-effectiveness ratio improves when the attributed benefit of TPN in risk reduction of a certain disease state improves. According to Detsky & Jeejeebhoy (1984), the costs of TPN are substantially higher, if a low estimate for risk reduction (i.e. 20%) is used. Therefore, these calculations stress the need for careful patient selection in order to improve the cost-effectiveness of peri-operative nutritional support. Finally, cost reflects purchase agreements with manufacturers, volume of purchases, as well as the degree of product price mark-up. Hence, comparing costs is a tricky task, in which one should avoid comparing apples with oranges.

Acknowledgement

We thank Ms. Darlene Thompson for editorial assistance.

References

Abel, R. M., Beck, C. H., Jr., Abbott, W. M. et al. (1973). Improved survival from acute renal failure after treatment with intravenous essential L-amino acids and glucose. *New England Journal of Medicine*, **288**, 695–9.

Abernathy, G. B., Heizer, W. D., Holcombe, B. J. et al. (1989). Efficacy of tube feeding in supplying energy requirements of hospitalized patients. *Journal of Parenteral and Enteral Nutrition*, **13**, 387–91.

Abraham, E., Bland, R. D., Coho, J. C. et al. (1984). Sequential cardiorespiratory patterns associated with outcome in septic shock. *Chest*, **85**, 75–80.

Alexander, J. W., MacMillan, B. G., Stinett, J. O. et al. (1980). Beneficial effects of aggressive protein feeding in severely burned children. *Annals of Surgery*, **192**, 505–17.

AMA Department of Food and Nutrition. (1975). Guidelines for Multivitamin Preparations for Parenteral Use. A Statement by an expert panel. Chicago, Illinois; December.

AMA Department of Food and Nutrition. (1979). Guidelines for Essential Trace Element Preparations for Parenteral Use. A statement by an expert panel. *Journal of the American Medical Association*, **241**, 2051–4.

Anderson, G. F. & Steinberg, E. P. (1986). DRGs and specialized nutrition support: prospective payment and nutritional support: the need for reform. *Journal of Parenteral and Enteral Nutrition*, **10**, 3–8.

Antonas, K. N., Curtas, M. S., & Meguid, M. M. (1987). Use of serum CPK-MM to monitor response to nutritional intervention in catabolic surgical patients. *Journal of Surgical Research*, **42**, 219–26.

Askanazi, J., Rosenbaum, S. H., Hyman, A. I. *et al.* (1979). Effects of total parenteral nutrition on gas exchange and breathing patterns. *Critical Care Medicine*, **7**, 125 (abstract).

Askanazi, J., Rosenbaum, S. H., Hyman, A. I. *et al.* (1980a). Respiratory changes induced by the large glucose loads of total parenteral nutrition. *Journal of the American Medical Association*, **243**, 1444–7.

Askanazi, J., Carpentier, Y. A., Elwyn, D. H. *et al.* (1980b). Influence of total parenteral nutrition on fuel utilization in injury and sepsis. *Annals of Surgery*, **191**, 40–6.

Askanazi, J., Hensle, T. W., Starker, P. M. *et al.* (1986). Effect of immediate postoperative nutritional support on length of hospitalization. *Annals of Surgery*, **203**, 236–39.

Bailey, M. J. (1979). Reduction of catheter-associated sepsis in parenteral nutrition using low-dose intravenous heparin. *British Medical Journal*, **1**, 1671–3.

Bartlett, R. H., Allyn, P. A., Medley, T. & Wetmore, N. (1977). Nutritional therapy based on positive caloric balance in burn patients. *Archives of Surgery*, **112**, 974–80.

Bastow, M. W., Rawlings, J. & Allison, S. P. (1983). Benefits of supplementary tube feeding after fractured neck of femur: a randomized controlled trial. *British Medical Journal*, **287**, 1589–92.

Blackburn, G. L., Williams, L. F., Bistrian, B. R. *et al.* (1976). New approaches to the management of severe acute pancreatitis. *American Journal of Surgery*, **131**, 114–24.

Border, J. R., Hassett, J., LaDuca, J. *et al.* (1987). The gut origin septic states in blunt multiple trauma (ISS = 40) in the ICU. *Annals of Surgery*, **206**, 427–45.

Brozek, J. (1990). Effects of generalized malnutrition on personality. *Nutrition*, **6**, 389–95.

Burke, J. F., Wolfe, R. R., Mullany, C. J. *et al.* (1979). Glucose requirements following burn injury. *Annals of Surgery*, **190**, 274–83.

Burri, C. & Ahnefeld, F. W. (1977). *The Caval Catheter*. New York: Springer-Verlag.

Butters, M., Campos, A. C. & Meguid, M. M. (1992). High frequency-low morbidity mechanical complications of tube feeding: a prospective study. *Clinical Nutrition*, **11**, 87–92.

Campos, A. C. L., Butters, M. & Meguid, M. M. (1990). Home enteral nutrition via gastrostomy in advanced head and neck cancer patients. *Head and Neck*, **12**, 137–42.

Campos, A. C. L. & Meguid, M. M. (1992). A critical appraisal of the usefulness of perioperative nutritional support. *American Journal of Clinical Nutrition*, **55**, 117–30.

Campos, A. C. L., Paluzzi, M. & Meguid, M. M. (1990). The clinical use of total nutritional admixtures. *Nutrition*, **6**, 347–56.

Canivet, B., Creisson, G., Freychet, P. & Dageville, X. (1980). Fibre, diabetes and risk of bezoar. *Lancet*, **ii**, 862.

Chandra, R. K. (1989). Immune responses in undernutrition and overnutrition: basic considerations and applied significance. *Nutrition*, **5**, 297–302.

Chapman, G., Curtas, S. & Meguid, M. M. (1992). Standardized enteral orders attain caloric goals sooner: a prospective study. *Journal of Parenteral and Enteral Nutrition*, **16**, 149–51.

Christenson, T., Bendix, T. & Kehlet, H. (1982). Fatigue and cardiorespiratory function following abdominal surgery. *British Journal of Surgery*, **69**, 417–19.

Chung, R. S. (1985). Surgical treatment of morbid obesity. *Nutrition International*, **1**, 3–10.

Collins, J. P., Oxby, C. B. & Hill, G. L. (1978). Intravenous amino acids and intravenous hyperalimintation as protein-sparing therapy after major surgery. *Lancet*, **i**, 789–91.

Committee on Dietary Allowances, Food and Nutrition Board, National Research Council. (1980). *Recommended Dietary Allowances*, ed. 9, National Academy of Sciences, Washington, DC.

Copeland, E. M., MacFadyen, B. V., Jr., Lanzotti, V. J. et al. (1975). Intravenous hyperalimentation as an adjunct to cancer chemotherapy. *American Journal of Surgery*, **129**, 167–73.

Curtas, S., Bonaventura, M. & Meguid, M. M. (1989). Cannulation of the inferior vena cava for long term central venous access: techniques and results. *Surgery, Gynecology & Obstetrics*, **168**, 121–4.

Daws, T. A., Consolazio, C. F., Hilty, S. L. et al. (1972). Evaluation of cardiopulmonary function of work performance in man during caloric restriction. *Journal of Applied Physiology*, **33**, 211–17.

Delone, J. B., Curtas, S., Jeejeebhoy, K. N. & Meguid, M. M. (1987). Effect of operation and nutrient intake on muscle function and enzymes. *Surgical Forum*, **37**, 36–9.

Depage, A. (1901). Nouveau proiède pour la gastrostmie. *Journal de Chirurgie et Annales de la Société* Belge de Chirurgie, **1**, 715–18,

Derogatis, L. R. (1978). *SCL-90. Administration, Scoring and Procedures Manual.* Johns Hopkins University, Baltimore.

Detsky, A. S., Baker, J. P., O'Rurke, K. & Goel, V. (1987). Perioperative parenteral nutrition: a meta-analysis. *Annals of Internal Medicine*, **107**, 195–203.

Detsky, A. S. & Jeejeebhoy, K. N. (1984). Cost-effectiveness of preoperative parenteral nutrition in patients undergoing major gastrointestinal surgery. *Journal of Parenteral and Enteral Nutrition*, **8**, 632–7.

Dickinson, R. J., Ashton, M. B., Axon, A. T. R. et al. (1980). Controlled trial of intravenous hyperalimentation and total bowel rest as an adjunct to the routine therapy of acute colitis. *Gastroenterology*, **79**, 1199–204.

Dinely, R. J. (1976). Venous reactions related to indwelling plastic cannulae: a prospective clinical trial. *Current Medical Research and Opinion*, **3**, 607–17.

Douard, M. D., Arlet, G., Leverger, G. et al. (1991). Quantitative blood cultures for diagnosis and management of catheter-related sepsis in pediatric hematology and oncology patients. *Intensive Care Medicine*, 17, 30–5.

Dudrick, S. J., Copeland, E. M., Daly, J. M. et al. (1979). A clinical review of nutritional support of the patient. *Journal of Parenteral and Enteral Nutrition*, **3**, 444–51.

Edington, H., Zajko, A. & Reilly, J. J. (1983). Jejunal variceal hemorrhage: An unusual complication of needle catheter jejunostomy. *Journal of Parenteral and Enteral Nutrition*, **7**, 489–91.

Eldar, S. & Meguid, M. M. (1984). Pneumothorax following attempted nasogastric intubation for nutritional support. *Journal of Parenteral and Enteral Nutrition*, **8**, 450–2.

Elliott, T. S., D'Abrera, V. C. & Dutton, S. (1988). The effect of antibiotics on bacterial colonisation of vascular cannulae in a novel *in-vitro* model. *Journal of Medical Microbiology*, **26**, 229–35.

Emerson, A. P. (1987). Foods high in fiber and phytobezoar formation. *Journal of the American Dietetic Association*, **12**, 1675–7.

Evaluating Total Parenteral Nutrition: Core Statement of the Technology Assessment and Practice Guidelines Forum. (1990). Georgetown University, January 10–11, 1990. *Nutrition*, **6**, 475–91.

Fabri, P. J., Mirtallo, J. M., Ruberg, R. L. *et al.* (1982). Incidence and prevention of thrombosis of the subclavian vein during total parenteral nutrition. *Surgery, Gynecology & Obstetrics*, **155**, 238–40.

Feller, J. H., Brown, R. A., Toussaint, G. P. & Thompson, A. G. (1974). Changing methods in the treatment of severe pancreatitis. *American Journal of Surgery*, **127**, 196–201.

Flynn, K. T., Norton, L. C. & Fisher, R. L. (1987). Enteral tube feeding: indications, practices and outcomes. *Image Journal of Nursing Scholarship*, **19**, 16–19.

Fogel, R. S., O'Brien, J. M., Kay, B. G. *et al.* (1987). Try this simple TPN order form. *Nursing*, **17**, 58–9.

Fonkalsrud, F. W., Pederson, B. M., Murphy, J. & Beckerman, J. H. (1968). Reduction of infusion thrombophlebitis with buffered glucose solutions. *Surgery*, **63**, 280–4.

Frank, A. F. & Greene, C. G. (1979). Successful use of a bulk laxative to control the diarrhea of tube feedings. *Scandinavian Journal of Plastic and Reconstructive Surgery*, **13**, 193–4.

Freedland, C. P., Roller, R. D., Wolfe, B. M. & Flynn, N. M. (1989). Microbial contamination of continuous drip feedings. *Journal of Parenteral and Enteral Nutrition*, **13**, 18–22.

Gazitua, R., Wilson, K. Bistrian, B. R. *et al.* (1979). Factors determining peripheral vein tolerance to amino acid infusions. *Archives of Surgery*, **114**, 897–901.

Giovannini, I., Goldrini, G., Castagneto, M. *et al.* (1983). Respiratory quotient and patterns of substrate utilization in human sepsis and trauma. *Journal of Parenteral and Enteral Nutrition*, **7**, 226–30.

Gouma, D. J., von Meyenfeldt, M. F., Rouflart, M. & Soeters, P. B. (1988). Preoperative total parenteral nutrition (TPN) in severe Crohn's disease. *Surgery*, **103**, 648–52.

Hanson, R. L. (1979). Predictive criteria for length of nasogastric tube insertion for tube feeding. *Journal of Parenteral and Enteral Nutrition*, **3**, 160–3.

Hartline, J. V. & Zachman, R. D. (1976). Vitamin A delivery in total parenteral nutrition solutions. *Pediatrics*, **58**, 448–51.

Heird, W. C., MacMillan, R. W. & Winters, R. W. (1976). Total parenteral nutrition in the pediatric patient. In *Total Parenteral Nutrition*, ed. J. E. Fischer, pp. 253–84, Little, Brown and Company, Boston.

Hilton, E., Haslet, T. M., Borenstein, M. T. *et al.* (1988). Central catheter infection: single- versus triple-lumen catheters. Influence of guide wires on infection rates when used for replacement of catheters. *American Journal of Medicine*, **84**, 667–72.

Howard, L., Chu, R., Feman, S. *et al.* (1980). Vitamin A deficiency from long-term parenteral nutrition. *Annals of Internal Medicine,* **93**, 576–7.

Hull, M. A., Rawlings, J., Murray, F. E. *et al.* (1993). Audit of outcome of long-term enteral nutrition by percutaneous endoscopic gastrostomy. *Lancet,* **341**, 869–72.

Imperial, J., Bistrian, B., Bothe, A. *et al.* (1983). Limitation of central vein thrombosis in total parenteral nutrition by continuous infusion of low-dose heparin. *Journal of the American College of Nutrition,* **2**, 63–73.

Iyengar, S. R. K., Charrette, E. J. P., Iyengar, G. K. S. & Wasan, S. (1976). Myocardial glucogen in prevention of perioperative injury of the heart: a preliminary report. *Canadian Journal of Surgery,* **19**, 246–51.

Jeejeebhoy, K. N. (1986). Muscle function and nutrition. *Gut,* **27**, 25–39.

Jeejeebhoy, K. N., Anderson, G. H., Nakhooda, A. F. *et al.* (1976). Metabolic studies in total parenteral nutrition with lipid in man. *Journal of Clinical Investigation,* **57**, 125–36.

Jones, K. W., Seltzer, M. H., Slocum, B. A. *et al.* (1984). Parenteral nutrition complications in a voluntary hospital. *Journal of Parenteral and Enteral Nutrition,* **8**, 385–90.

Kassner, E. G., Baunstank, A., Balsam, D. *et al.* (1977). Passage of feeding catheters into the pleural space: a radiographic sign of trauma to the pharynx and esophagus in the newborn. *American Journal of Roentgenology,* **128**, 19–22.

Larsson, J., Akerlind, I., Permert, J. *et al.* (1993). The relation between nutritional status and quality of life in surgical patients. *European Journal of Surgery,* in press.

Liggett, S. B., St. John, R. E. & Legrak, S. S. (1987). Determination of resting energy expenditure utilizing the thermodilution pulmonary artery catheter. *Chest,* **91**, 562–6.

Linder, L. E., Curelaru, I., Gustavsson, B. *et al.* (1984). Material thrombogenicity in central venous catheterization: a comparison between soft, antebrachial catheters of silicone elastomer and polyurethane. *Journal of Parenteral and Enteral Nutrition,* **8**, 399–406.

Lolley, D. M., Ray, J. F., Myers, W. O. *et al.* (1978). Reduction of intra-operative myocardial infarction by means of exogenous anaerobic substrate enhancement. *Annals of Thoracic Surgery,* **26**, 515–24.

Lolley, D. M., Myers, W. O., Jefferson, F. R. *et al.* (1985). Clinical experience with preoperative myocardial nutrition management. *Journal of Cardiovascular Surgery,* **26**, 236–43.

Long, J. M., Wilmore, D. W., Mason, A. D. *et al.* (1977). Effects of carbohydrate and fat intake on nitrogen excretion during total intravenous feeding. *Annals of Surgery,* **185**, 417–22.

Lopez, R., Suavez, A. & Santiago-Delpin, E. A. (1977). A reversed jejunal segment interposition as feeding gastrostomy. *Archives of Surgery,* **112**, 343–4.

Macfie, J., Smith, R. C. & Hill, G. L. (1981). Glucose or fat as a nonprotein energy source? A controlled clinical trial in gastroenterological patients requiring intravenous nutrition. *Gastroenterology,* **80**, 103–7.

Massar, E. L., Daly, J. M., Copeland, E. M. *et al.* (1983). Peripheral vein complications in patients receiving amino acid/dextrose solutions. *Journal of Parenteral and Enteral Nutrition,* **7**, 159–62.

McIntyre, P. B., Rithie, J. K., Hawley, P. R. *et al.* (1984). Management of enterocutaneous fistulas: a review of 132 cases. *British Journal of Surgery,* **71**, 293–6.

McIvor, A. C., Meguid, M. M., Curtas, S. *et al.* (1990). Intestinal obstruction from cecal bezoar; a complication of fiber-containing tube feedings. *Nutrition*, **6**, 115–17.

McNair, D. M., Lorr, M. & Droppleman, L. F. (1971). *Profile of Mood States. Manual 1971.* Education and Industrial Testing Services, San Diego.

Medical Research Council Report. (1957). Thrombophlebitis following intravenous infusions: a trial of plastic and rubber-giving sets. *Lancet*, **i**, 595–7.

Meguid, M. M. (1993). Open letter to Hillary Rodham Clinton. *Nutrition*, **9**, ix–xi.

Meguid, M. M., Akahoshi, M. P. & Hill, L. R. (1986). Evaluation of the practice of using a hyperalimentation catheter for multiple purposes. *Nutrition International*, **2**, 45–52.

Meguid, M. M., Akahoshi, M., Jeffers, S. *et al.* (1984*a*). Amelioration of metabolic complications of conventional TPN: a prospective randomized study. *Archives of Surgery*, **119**, 1294–8.

Meguid, M. M., Campos, A. C. & Hammond, W. G. (1990*a*). Nutrition support in surgical practice: current knowledge and research needs, Part I. *American Journal of Surgery*, **159**, 345–58.

Meguid, M. M., Campos, A. C. & Hammond, W. G. (1990*b*). Nutrition support in surgical practice: current knowledge and research needs, Part II. *American Journal of Surgery*, **159**, 427–43.

Meguid, M. M. & Campos, A. C. L. (1993). Gastrointestinal fistulas: clinical and nutritional management. In *Parenteral Nutrition*, ed. J. Rombeau & M. Caldwell, 2nd edn. W. B. Saunders Co., Philadelphia.

Meguid, M. M., Landel, A. M., Terz, J. J. & Akrabawi, S. S. (1984*b*). Effect of elemental diet on albumin and urea synthesis: comparison with partially hydrolyzed protein diet. *Journal of Surgical Research*, **37**, 16–24.

Meguid, M. M., Campos, A. C. L., Meguid, V. *et al.* (1988*b*). IONIP: A criterion of surgical outcome and patient selection for perioperative nutritional support. *British Journal of Clinical Practice*, **42**, 8–14.

Meguid, M. M., Debonis, D., Meguid, V. *et al.* (1988*a*). Complications of abdominal operations for malignant disease. *American Journal of Surgery*, **156**, 341–5.

Meguid, M. M., Mughal, M. M., Debonis, D. *et al.* (1986). Influence of nutrional status on the resumption of adequate food intake in patients recovering from colorectal cancer operations. *Surgical Clinics of North America*, **66**, 1167–76.

Meguid, M. M. & Muscaritoli, M. (1993). Current uses of total parenteral nutrition in clinical practice. *American Family Physician*, **47**, 383–94.

Meguid, M. M. & Williams, L. F. (1979). The use of gastrostomy to correct malnutrition. *Surgery, Gynecology & Obstetrics*, **149**, 27–32.

Mitchell, K. A., Jones, E. A., Curtas, S. & Meguid, M. M. (1990). A standardized TPN order form reduces staff time and potential for error. *Nutrition*, **6**, 457–60.

Montgomery, W. W. (1973). *Surgery of the Upper Respiratory System*, Vol. 2. Lea & Febiger, Philadelphia.

Mosca, R., Curtas, S., Forbes, B. & Meguid, M. M. (1987). The benefits of isolator cultures in the management of suspected catheter sepsis. *Surgery*, **102**, 716–21.

Muller, J. M., Dienst, C., Brenner, U. & Pichlmaier, H. (1982). Preoperative parenteral feeding in patients with gastrointestinal carcinoma. *Lancet*, **i**, 68–72.

Nasrallah, S. M. & Galambos, J. T. (1980). Amino acid therapy of alcoholic hepatitis. *Lancet*, **ii**, 1276–7.

Nehme, A. B. (1980). Nutritional support of the hospitalized patient: The team concept. *Journal of the American Medical Association*, **243**, 1906–8.

Nutrition Advisory Group, American Medical Association Department of Foods and Nutrition, 1975. (1979). Multivitamin preparations for parenteral use: A statement by the Nutrition Advisory Group. *Journal of Parenteral and Enteral Nutrition*, **3**, 258–62.

Olivaries, L., Segovia, A. & Revuelta, R. (1974). Tube feeding and lethal aspiration in neurological patients: a review of 720 autopsy cases. *Stroke*, **5**, 654–6.

O'Morain, C., Segal, A. W. & Levi, A. J. (1984). Elemental diet as primary treatment of acute Crohn's disease: a controlled trial. *British Medical Journal*, **288**, 1859–62.

Padberg, F. T., Jr., Ruggiero, J., Blackburn, G. L. & Bistrian, B. R. (1981). Central venous catheterization for parenteral nutrition. *Annals of Surgery*, **193**, 264–70.

Padilla, G. V., Grant, M., Wong, H. *et al.* (1979). Subjective distresses of nasogastric tube feeding. *Journal of Parenteral and Enteral Nutrition*, **3**, 53–7.

Page, C. P., Ryan, J. A. & Haff, R. L. (1976). Enteral catheter administration of an elemental diet. *Surgery, Gynecology & Obstetrics*, **142**, 184–8.

Paston, M. J., Meguid, R. A., Muscaritoli, M. *et al.* (1993). Dynamics of central venous catheter-related sepsis in the rat. *Journal of Clinical Microbiology*, **31**, 1652–5.

Payne-James, J. J., Rees, R. G. P., Doherty, J. & Silk, D. B. A. (1990). 7 g weighted versus unweighted polyurethane nasoenteral tubes – spontaneous transpyloric passage and clinical performance: a controlled randomised trial. *Clinical Nutrition*, **9**, 102–12.

Perez, S. K. & Brandt, K. (1989). Enteral feeding contamination: comparison of diluents and feeding bag usage. *Journal of Parenteral and Enteral Nutrition*, **13**, 306–8.

Peters, C. & Fischer, J. E. (1980). Studies on calorie nitrogen ratio for total parenteral nutrition. *Surgery, Gynecology & Obstetrics*, **151**, 1–9.

Ponsky, J. L. (1986). Evolving trends in enteral alimentation. *Surgery Annual*, **18**, 327–38.

Rapp, R. P., Young, B., Twyman, D. *et al.* (1983). The favorable effect of early parenteral feeding on survival of head-injured patients. *Journal of Neurosurgery*, **58**, 906–12.

Rombeau, J. L., Barot, L. R., Williamson, C. W. & Mullen, J. L. (1982). Preoperative total parenteral nutrition and surgical outcome in patients with inflammatory bowel disease. *American Journal of Surgery*, **143**, 139–43.

Roongpisuthipong, C., Puchaiwatananon, O. & Songchitsomboon, S. (1993). The influence of hydrocortisone and heparin on intravenous infusion. *Nutrition*, **9**, November/December, in press.

Rountree, D. (1991). The PIC catheter: a different approach. *American Journal of Nursing*, **91**, 22–8.

Rudman, D., Millikan, W. J., Richardson, T. J. *et al.* (1975). Elemental balances during intravenous hyperalimentation of underweight adult subjects. *Journal of Clinical Investigations*, **55**, 94–104.

Rutten, P., Blackburn, G. L., Flatt, J. P. *et al.* (1975). Determination of optimal hyperalimentation infusion rate. *Journal of Surgical Research*, **18**, 477–83.

Saffle, J. R., Medina, E., Raymond, J. *et al.* (1985). Use of indirect calorimetry in the nutritional management of burned patients. *Journal of Trauma*, **25**, 32–9.

Schreiner, R., Eitzen, H., Gfell, M. *et al.* (1979). Environmental contamination of continuous drip feedings. *Pediatrics*, **63**, 232–7.

Shellito, P. C. & Malt, R. A. (1985). Tube gastrostomy: techniques and complications. *Annals of Surgery*, **201**, 180–5.

Shoemaker, W. C. Appel, P., Gzer, L. S. C. *et al.* (1980). Pathogenesis of respiratory failure (ARDS) after hemorrhage and trauma: I. Cardiorespiratory patterns preceding the development of ARDS. *Critical Care Medicine*, **8**, 504–12.

Siermers, P. T. & Reinke, R. T. (1976). Perforation of the nasopharynx by nasogastric intubation: a rare cause of left pleural effusion and pneumomediastinum. *American Journal of Roentgenology*, 127, 341–3.

Silk, D. B. A. (1989). Fibre and enteral nutrition. *Gut*, **30**, 246–64.

Sim, A. J. W., Wolfe, B. M., Young, V. R. *et al.* (1979). Glucose promotes whole body protein synthesis from infused amino acids in fasting man. *Lancet*, **13**, 68–72.

Smith, N. L., Ravo, B., Soroff, H. S. & Khan, S. A. (1985). Successful fibrinolytic therapy for superior vena cava thrombosis secondary to long term total parenteral nutrition. *Journal of Parenteral and Enteral Nutrition*, **9**, 55–7.

Spivack, J. L. (1980). Gastrostomy. In *Developments in Digestive Diseases*, ed. J. E. Berk, Lea & Febiger, Philadelphia.

Stamm, M. (1894). Gastrostomy: a new method. *Medical News*, **54**, 324–6.

Studley, H. O. (1936). Percentage of weight loss: a basic indicator of surgical risk in patients with chronic peptic ulcer. *Journal of the American Medical Association*, **106**, 458–60.

Swinscow, T. D. V. (1976). Contaminated infusion fluids. *British Medical Journal*, **2**, 547–8.

Thomas, E. T., Evers, W. & Raez, G. B. (1970). Post-infusion phlebitis. *Anesthesia and Analgesia*, 49, 150–9.

Thompson, J. S., Vaughan, W. P., Forst, C. F. *et al.* (1987). The effect of the route of nutrient delivery on gut structure and diamine oxidase levels. *Journal of Parenteral and Enteral Nutrition*, **11**, 28–32.

Twomey, P. L. & Patching, S. C. (1985). Cost-effectiveness of nutritional support. *Journal of Parenteral and Enteral Nutrition*, 9, 3–10.

Van Lanschot, J. J. B., Feenstra, B. W. A., Vermeij, O. G. *et al.* (1986). Calculation versus measurement of total energy expenditure. *Critical Care Medicine*, **24**, 981–5.

Vanlandingham, S., Simpson, S., Daniel, P. & Newmark, S. R. (1981). Metabolic abnormalities in patients supported with enteral tube feeding. *Journal of Parenteral and Enteral Nutrition*, **5**, 322–4.

Weinsier, R. L., Bacon, J. & Butterworth, C. E., Jr. (1982). Central venous alimentation: a prospective study of the frequency of metabolic abnormalities among medical and surgical patients. *Journal of Parenteral and Enteral Nutrition*, **6**, 421–5.

Widiss, T. L. & Meguid, M. M. (1981). The enteral alternative: update. *Contemporary Surgery*, **19**, 75–95.

Wolfe, B. M., Ryder, M. A., Nishikawa, R. A. *et al.* (1986). Complications of parenteral nutrition. *American Journal of Surgery*, **152**, 93–9.

Wolff, A. P. & Kessler, S. (1973). Iatrogenic injury to the hypopharynx and cervical esophagus: An autopsy study. *Annals of Otolaryngology*, **82**, 778–83.

Zimmaro, D. M., Rolandelli, R. H., Koruda, M. J. *et al.* (1989). Isotonic tube feeding formula induces liquid stool in normal subjects: reversal by pectin. *Journal of Parenteral and Enteral Nutrition*, **13**, 117–23.

13

How I feed the starving patient

S. P. ALLISON

Introduction

Before describing how I feed the starving patient, it is important to define starvation in a clinical sense. Colloquially, we say that we feel starving when we have had a busy day and have missed lunch. On the other hand, our health is not impaired by such an experience. If we are of normal weight or slightly overweight and undergo uncomplicated abdominal surgery, involving a week of relative starvation and weight loss of 2 or 3 kg, this is unlikely to impair our recovery and trials have shown what we know intuitively, that nutritional support has no value in such patients. The reason why so many controlled trials of nutritional support were negative in the 1970s and 1980s may have been due to inclusion of patients who did not need the treatment and the failure to focus upon groups of patients with clinically significant malnutrition (Allison, 1992). What, then, is clinically significant? Let us first consider four trials of nutritional support to see whether they give us a clue to this question.

The first of these was carried out by Bastow in my unit in 1980 and 1981 (Bastow, Rawlings & Allison, 1983). It involved the administration of an overnight nasogastric feed of 1000 calories to old ladies who had sustained fractured femur. The patients were divided anthropometrically on admission into normal, thin and very thin, by relating their arm circumference and triceps skinfold thickness to a reference population of the same age and sex. Normal, was defined as within 1 standard deviation of the reference mean, thin, as 1–2 standard deviations below and very thin, more than 2 standard deviations, below the mean. Those in the thin and very thin groups, were randomised to receive overnight nasogastric feeding, as well as a ward diet. The controls received the ward diet only. The time to full mobility was measured by the physiotherapist, as the ability to get out of bed unaided and walk across the ward. The normally nourished took 10 days, the thin took 12 days which was reduced to 10 by feeding, but the very thin took 24 days, which was reduced to 16 days by feeding. This illustrates the fact that malnutrition has to be quite severe in order to impair recovery and that the effect of nutritional support is only demonstrable in those who are severely malnourished.

The recently published Veterans' Affairs Total Parenteral Nutrition Study Group (1991) trial of peri-operative parenteral nutriton and the Maastricht trial (Von Meyenfeldt *et al.* (1992)) of enteral and parenteral nutrition produced similar results. In those with a recent weight loss of less than 10%, parenteral nutrition was associated with either no improvement or a worse outcome, compared with controls. In those who had lost more than 10% of their body weight, both infectious and non-infectious complications of surgery were reduced by the treatment. From these trials, therefore, we might conclude that patients who start with a normal weight, can tolerate up to 10% weight loss without impairment of outcome or benefit from nutritional support. Clinically, important malnutrition requiring treatment may therefore be defined in these terms.

The problems of the long-stay elderly are illustrated by the study of Larsson *et al.* (1990) of 501 elderly patients in hospital for up to 28 weeks. They divided their patients on admission into those who were well nourished and those who were under nourished, and randomised each category of patient into a group who received supplements in addition to the ward diet, and those who received the ward diet alone. Among those who were initially malnourished, there was a greater discharge rate and lower mortality among the supplemented group. On the other hand, among those who were initially well nourished, there was a gradual decline in nutritional state unless supplements were given, reflecting the difficulty of adequately nourishing long-stay elderly patients, and highlighting length of stay as an important predisposing factor in malnutrition.

Our definition of important malnutrition may also be refined by considering studies which relate changes in body weight and composition to function and to survival. The famous study of Keys *et al.* (1950), in young, healthy, male volunteers, showed that partial starvation was associated with 23% weight loss over 24 weeks and serious reductions in mental and physical function. Even after 20 weeks of refeeding, fat-free mass had not returned to normal and muscle function, mood and stamina were still impaired. If this is true in healthy volunteers, it is likely to be even more of a problem in our patients who suffer not only starvation but the effects of disease. The price therefore of nutritional neglect may be increased morbidity and greatly prolonged convalescence. The 30 IRA

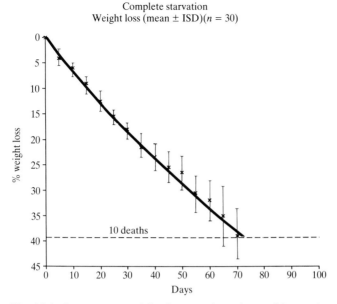

Fig. 13.1. Percentage weight loss against time with total starvation during hunger strike. (From Allison, 1992.)

hunger strikers provide an example of total starvation for 60 days (Allison, 1992; Love, A. G., personal communication). During that time they lost on average 38% of their body weight and 30% of them died (see Fig. 13.1). This illustrates the absolute limits of survival from starvation alone. When this is combined with disease, weight loss may be even more poorly tolerated.

Survival is not the only consideration, however. Between 10 and 15% weight loss, progressive deterioration in function can be measured (Russell *et al.*, 1984; Pichard & Jeejeebhoy, 1988; Church, Choong & Hill, 1984; Hill, 1992; Arora & Rochester, 1982; Kelsen, Ference & Kapoor, 1985; Lewis *et al.*, 1986; Lewis & Sieck, 1990; Doekel, Zwillich & Scroggin, 1976; Kelly *et al.*, 1984; Bassili & Deitel, 1981; Jeejeebhoy, 1988; Murciano *et al.*, 1990; Shizgal, 1981; Chandra, 1988; Windsor & Hill, 1988; Levine *et al.*, 1974). Muscle strength diminishes and fatiguability increases. The fast-twitch muscle fibres are preferentially lost, with consequent impairment in respiratory muscle strength and respiratory function. Wound healing, immune responses and resistance to infection are also reduced. Autonomic changes occur with impairment in thermoregulation. Gut mucosal atrophy and increased permeability may result from total absence of oral intake for long periods. Some of these changes may be more directly related to the body protein mass than to changes in total body weight, or adipose tissue. Hill (1992) related weight to body protein and showed that a reduction in body protein of up to 20% can be tolerated with only a small decline in function, but thereafter muscle and respiratory functions decline rapidly. The relationship between structure and function may not therefore be linear but a curve with an inflexion and steep decline at 20% total body protein loss (approximately equal to 15% weight loss).

The studies carried out by the Jewish Physicians in the Warsaw Ghetto (Winick, 1979) not only constitute a fitting memorial to their courage but also an invaluable documentation of the physiological consequences of severe famine disease. Most of their subjects had lost 35% of their body weight and were within three weeks of death. They showed extreme apathy and weakness. Cardiac function and autonomic responses were impaired. Gastrointestinal dysfunction, achlorhydria and diarrhoea were observed. Famine oedema developed with the incapacity to excrete an excess salt and water load, which is characteristic of the response not only to acute illness and injury, but also to starvation. Some authors have drawn an analogy between the changes seen in malnourished patients and those seen in starved children with marasmus and kwashiorkor, according to whether oedema, hypoalbuminaemia and protein deficiency predominate. Such analogies may be helpful in an illustrative sense but are imprecise comparisons when the details of the conditions are examined closely.

The accumulated therapeutic and physiological evidence, therefore, suggests that starvation or malnutrition become clinically important during illness, at a weight loss between 10 and 15%, assuming the patient starts at a normal weight. Obese patients who, by controlled dieting, reduce their weight in preparation for surgery, are excluded. More severe degrees of weight loss, i.e. >35%, may be fatal.

Measurement

Weight and anthropometrics

The value of weighing patients as a clinical tool can scarcely be over-estimated. The knowledge of the patient's normal weight provides an invaluable baseline against which to measure changes. Serial measurements allow calculation of the percentage weight loss, as well as the rate of weight loss in response to starvation or gain in response to re-feeding. Weight allows calculation not only of drug dosage, but also of metabolic expenditure and hence likely nutritional requirements. Its interpretation in terms of real tissue weight gain or loss may be distorted by acute changes in fluid balance, but this, of itself, may be of clinical value, since day-to-day changes in weight may be interpreted in terms of water balance, thereby assisting fluid management. Weight may also be related to normal tables for the patient's height, age and sex. The weight in kilograms divided by the square of the height in metres provides the body mass index, with a normal range of 18–25. Particularly in elderly or injured patients, the measurement of height is problematical. A useful surrogate is the demispan, measured from the suprasternal notch to the web between the third and fourth fingers of the hand with the arm stretched laterally. Tables relating weight to demispan have been devised (Lehmann *et al.*, 1991). Measurements of weight may be enhanced by anthropometric assessment (Durnin & Womersley, 1974; Collins, McCarthy & Hill, 1979; Bastow, 1982); mean arm circumference is measured using a tape-measure at the mid point between the acromion and olecranon. The triceps skinfold thickness, measured by Harpenden callipers, assesses the thickness of the fat layer. By subtraction of the latter from the former value, the relative proportions of fat and lean body mass may be estimated using the formula of Durnin and Womersley (1974). Mean arm circumference is a fairly robust parameter, but there is considerable inter-observer variation in the triceps skinfold thickness, which is more prone to error. An alternative method of measuring body composition is by the bioimpedance technique which is cheap and easily carried out by the bedside. Unfortunately, it also has some inherent errors and is less reliable in very sick patients (Elia, 1992). More sophisticated methods of measuring body composition, such as neutron activation, the dexa radiological method and densitometry, are much more accurate but are research tools rather than day-to-day bedside clinical methods.

Voluntary oral intake

Second only to weight and anthropometric measurements as practical predictors of malnutrition, is the measurement of voluntary oral intake by a good dietitian. When done over several days, it is possible to calculate whether the intake is appropriate to the patient's estimated metabolic requirements and furthermore, whether that intake is increasing or decreasing. Its predictive value is illustrated in Fig. 13.2, in which voluntary oral intake and a decision-making box are superimposed on the values of weight loss in Fig. 13.1. Most patients undergoing surgery may starve for a few days and have an associated fall in weight. Within

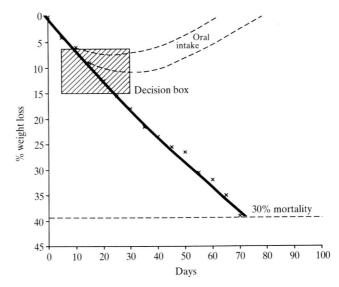

Fig. 13.2. Percentage weight loss against time during total starvation. The theoretical recovery rate is shown if oral intake is resumed between 5 and 10% weight loss. A decision box is shown to emphasise the importance of providing nutritional supplements before 15% weight loss (see text). (From Allison, 1992.)

a week, however, their voluntary oral intake usually starts to increase and their body composition returns to normal over a period of time, as shown by the dotted lines. Should oral intake not be possible for prolonged periods, or be inadequate for one reason or another, then the patient will progress down the weight loss curve and a clinical decision will have to be made whether he or she is going to require nutritional support. The decision box allows a short period of assessment, but emphasises the necessity for introducing nutritional support before the patient reaches 15% weight loss and emerges from the box in a downward direction. It is at this point that serious functional abnormalities start to appear and morbidity increases. The weight loss curve in this Figure of course shows total starvation. Many of our patients undergo partial starvation, in which case the rate of weight loss is correspondingly more gradual. On the other hand, if they are suffering from the catabolic response to injury or sepsis, weight loss will be accelerated. In general, however, three weeks with minimal or no food intake results in a serious reduction in body composition and function which is of clinical significance and should be prevented. In Benedict's (1915) classical study, for example, 15% weight loss occurred with three weeks' total starvation. Meguid *et al.* (1988) has used this principle to decide whether to give their post-operative patients nutritional support. He has defined the inadequate oral nutrient intake period (IONIP) as the time to recover an oral intake which is 60% of estimated requirements. If this exceeds 10 days, then the patient is given nutritional support. The emphasis should be upon anticipating clinically important malnutrition and preventing it occurring.

Plasma proteins

Although the biochemical measurement of levels of vitamins, minerals and trace elements, may be invaluable in demonstrating specific deficiencies associated with disease and assessing whether long-term nutritional support is adequate, it is rarely necessary to have such measurements in order to make the initial clinical decision to give nutritional support. The plasma proteins albumin, thyroid-binding prealbumin and transferrin have also been described as nutritional indicators. Unfortunately, their concentrations in plasma are more profoundly affected by disease than by malnutrition. In anorexia nervosa and other examples of pure starvation, it is extremely rare to find any change in plasma protein concentrations. Fleck (1988) has pointed out, for example, that the daily exchange of albumin between the intravascular and extravascular space is ten times the albumin synthesis rate. Disease therefore, tends to have a greater effect on albumin distribution, although the recovery from hypoalbuminaemia or a low level of thyroid-binding prealbumin may be impaired by malnutrition. Measurements of plasma proteins may therefore be useful in monitoring the response to nutritional support, but of little value in making the initial decision. Similar criticisms may be aimed at tests of immunological function, whether they be the lymphocyte count or skin responses to injected antigens. When all these are combined in so-called nutritional indices, the opportunities for confusion are multiplied. The combination of a low albumin, a low lymphocyte count, impaired skin responses and a function of weight, can make an excellent risk index and predict the outcome of surgery. The element of risk which is purely nutritional and reversible by nutritional treatment may be negligible. All these parameters, therefore, as well as those of muscle strength and respiratory function may be useful in monitoring recovery, but when it comes to nutritional support, most clinicians are thrown back to the basic concepts of changes in weight, body composition, voluntary oral intake and a knowledge of the natural history of disease. This concept is summarised in Table 13.1.

Table 13.1. *Making the clinical decision to give nutritional support using simple assessment methods*

Question	Measurement
1. Where does the patient start?	Weight. Reference weight Previous weight Height, demispan Anthropometrics Oral intake
2. Is the patient deteriorating?	Serial weight and oral intake
3. How fast is the patient deteriorating?	Serial weights Oral intake Knowledge of the natural history of disease

How to treat

Having decided who to treat and defined the starving patient, for present purposes, as one in whom the clinical benefit of nutritional treatment can be demonstrated, I will now move to the question of how to treat. In broad terms, the answer to this is simple. If the gut works, use it.

Oral intake

Food intake among children and the elderly particularly, may be impaired by poor appetite and failure to provide preferred food in the most appropriate manner. It is of no use, for example, placing the meal tray on the right side of a patient with a right hemiplegia, or wrapping up the food in a manner which an arthritic patient cannot undo. It is important to pay attention to the patient's food preferences, and to provide food in a palatable and attractive manner. It is also important to remember that, as people get older, they often eat smaller meals, supplemented by nibbling between meals. The bringing in of fruit, sweets, biscuits, etc., by the relatives should not be discouraged. Most children enjoy ice-cream, which can be made very high in both energy and protein. I once looked after a publican with a 40% burn, and we met his fluid and food requirements partly by having a barrel of beer, delivered from the brewery, which he kept by his bedside and to which he helped himself liberally! Since nurses abandoned the task of serving meals and delegated them to orderlies, patient nutrition has received diminished attention from nurses, who are in the best position to improve matters. We have adopted a link nurse system, whereby a nurse with a nutritional interest is identified on each ward in the hospital. Under the auspices of the nutrition team, these nurses meet with their colleagues at regular intervals to discuss nutritional problems. Improved nursing training and improved links between nurses and dietitians are needed.

Tube feeding

Among those who are unable or unwilling to swallow, but in whom the gastrointestinal tract is functioning, tube feeding should be tried. For periods of less than two or three weeks, nasogastric tube feeding may be the treatment of choice, but for longer periods of time it may be appropriate to use a percutaneous endoscopic gastrostomy (PEG) or needle catheter jejunostomy. A recent controlled trial (Park *et al.*, 1992) or nasogastric versus PEG feeding in patients with neurological dysphagia, showed a high failure rate for nasogastric feeding and a greater effectiveness of the gastrostomy approach.

Particularly in patients with intense anorexia associated with disease, nasogastric feeding may not only support the patient nutritionally until the anorexia recovers, but of itself appears to stimulate the appetite. It was found that, in a group of such patients, fed 2000 calories during 12 hours overnight by continuous pump, voluntary oral intake by day improved rapidly, to the point where nasogastric feeding could be withdrawn after 1–4 weeks (Bastow, Rawlings & Allison, 1985).

We have recently reviewed four years' experience of using percutaneous endoscopic gastrostomy, in the management of patients with mainly neurological disorders of swallowing (Hull *et al.*, 1993). The robust nature of gastrostomies and their usefulness in long-term home enteral feeding are confirmed, providing that such patients are supported by an expert nutrition team, to whom they can refer in the event of complications. Half our patients had no complications at all, and the remainder had minor complications, e.g. line blockage or hub fracture, which could be resolved at home. Patients with motor neurone disease, for example, are followed by a dietitian from the time of diagnosis, in order to identify patients who develop dysphagia of sufficient degree to cause weight loss. We have found, by measuring voluntary oral intake, that those whose intake exceeds $1.5 \times$ their estimated BMR, maintain their weight. Those who take less than this have a gradual decline in weight. Before they have lost 10%, these patients are offered a PEG, not only to provide fluid and food, but also necessary drugs. This form of palliative support seems to be of value in about one-fifth of patients with motor neurone disease, in whom it prevents the weakness of starvation being added to the weakness of their neurological deficit. A PEG or jejunostomy may also be of value in malignant disease where there is obstruction of the upper gastrointestinal tract. This method of feeding allows the patient to be discharged home for palliative care.

Parenteral nutrition

This is the treatment of gastrointestinal failure and needs an expert nutrition team to oversee it, otherwise its complication rate is high. Technical details can be obtained from appropriate texts (Allison, 1992).

Summary and conclusions

Starvation may be defined for clinical purposes as prolonged lack of food sufficient to cause 10–15% weight loss or 20% whole body protein loss, at which point the changes in body composition are associated with significant deterioration in important functions such as muscle strength, respiration, immune responses and healing. These impair recovery from acute illness and when taken to extremes may be fatal. A knowledge of the nutritional history of disease and measurement of weight and oral intake, may be sufficient to enable the clinician to decide when nutritional support should begin. Treat by the simplest and most effective route possible. Use tempting and well-presented food first. Secondly, consider oral supplements of a proprietary defined formula feed. If swallowing is impaired or anorexia extreme, use enteral tube feeding. Parenteral nutrition is the management of gastrointestinal failure. Detection of developing malnutrition at an early stage by well-trained staff, allows prevention of severe malnutrition. Prevention is better than cure.

References

Allison, S. P. (1992). The uses and limitations of nutritional support. *Clinical Nutrition*, **11**, 319–30.

Arora, N. S. & Rochester, D. F. (1982). Effect of body weight and muscularity on human diaphragm muscle mass, thickness and area. *Journal of Applied Physiology*, **52**, 64–70.

Bassili, H. R. & Deitel, M. (1981). Effect of nutritional support on weaning patients off mechanical ventilation. *Journal of Parenteral and Enteral Nutrition*, **5**, 161–3.

Bastow, M. D. (1982). Anthropometrics revisited. *Proceedings of the Nutrition Society*, **41**, 381.

Bastow, M. D., Rawlings, J. & Allison, S. P. (1983). Benefits of supplementary tube feeding after fractured neck of femur: a randomised controlled trial. *British Medical Journal*, **287**, 1589–92.

Bastow, M. D., Rawlings, J. & Allison, S. P. (1985). Overnight nasogastric tube feeding. *Clinical Nutrition*, **4**, 7–11.

Benedict, E. G. (1915). *A Study of Prolonged Fasting*. Carnegie Inst. 1915. Washington Publ. No. 203.

Chandra, R. K. (1988). Immunity and infection. In *Nutrition and Metabolism in Patient Care*, ed. J. M. Kinney, K. N. Jeejeebhoy, G. L. Hill & O. E. Owen, pp. 598–604. W. B. Saunders Co., Philadelphia.

Church, J. M., Choong, S. Y. & Hill, G. L. (1984). Abnormalities of muscle metabolism and histology in malnourished patients awaiting surgery: effect of a course of intravenous nutrition. *British Journal of Surgery*, **71**, 563–9.

Collins, J. P., McCarthy, I. D. & Hill, G. L. (1979). Assessment of protein nutrition in surgical patients – the value of anthropometrics. *American Journal of Clinical Nutrition*, **32**, 1527–30.

Doekel, R. C. Jr., Zwillich, C. W. & Scroggin, C. H. (1976). Clinical semi-starvation: Depression of hypoxic ventilatory response. *New England Journal of Medicine*, **295**, 358–61.

Durnin, J. V. G. A. & Womersley, J. (1974). Body fat assessed from body density and its estimation from skinfold thickness: measurements on 481 men and women aged from 16–72 years. *British Journal of Nutrition*, **32**, 77–97.

Elia, M. (1992). Body composition analysis: an evaluation of 2 component models, multicomponent models and bedside techniques. *Clinical Nutrition*, **11**, 114–27.

Fleck, A. (1988). Plasma proteins as nutritional indicators in the perioperative period. *British Journal of Clinical Practice*, **42**, Suppl. **63**, 20–4.

Hill, G. L. (1992). *Disorders of Nutrition and Metabolism in Clinical Surgery*. Churchill Livingstone, Edinburgh.

Hull, M. A., Rawlings, J., Murray, F. E. *et al.* (1993). Au audit of outcome of long-term enteral nutrition using percutaneous endoscopic gastrostomy. *Lancet*, **341**, 869–72.

Jeejeebhoy, K. N. (1988). Bulk or bounce – the object of nutritional support. *Journal of Parenteral and Enteral Nutrition*, **12**, 539–49.

Kelly, S. M., Rosa, A., Field, S. *et al.* (1984). Inspiratory muscle strength and body composition in patients receiving total parenteral nutrition therapy. *American Review of Respiratory Disease*, **130**, 33–7.

Kelsen, S. G., Ference, M. & Kapoor, S. (1985). Effects of prolonged undernutrition on structure and function of the diaphragm. *Journal of Applied Physiology*, **58**, 1354–9.

Keys, A., Brozek, J., Henschel, A., Michelson, O. & Taylor, H. L. (1950). In *The Human Biology of Human Starvation*, Vol. 1, pp. 703–48, Vol. 2, pp. 819–18. University of Minnesota Press, Minneapolis, MN.

Larsson, J., Unosson, M., Ek, A.-C., Nilsson, L., Thorslund, S. & Bjurulf, P. (1990). Effect of dietary supplement on nutritional status and clinical outcome in 501 geriatric patients – a randomised study. *Clinical Nutrition*, **9**, 179–84.

Lehmann, A. B., Bassey, E. J., Morgan, K. & Dalloso, H. M. (1991). Normal values for weight, skeletal size and body mass indices in 890 men and women aged over 65 years. *Clinical Nutrition*, **10**, 18–22.

Levine, G. M., Deren, J. J., Steiger, E. & Zinno, R. (1974). Role of oral intake in maintenance of gut mass and disaccharidase activity. *Gastroenterology*, **67**, 975–82.

Lewis, M. I., Sieck, G. C., Fournier, M. & Belman, M. J. (1986). Effect of nutritional deprivation on diaphragm contractility and muscle fibre size. *Journal of Applied Physiology*, **60**, 596–603.

Lewis, M. I. & Sieck, G. C. (1990). Effect of acute nutritional deprivation on diaphragm structure and function. *Journal of Applied Physiology*, **68**, 1938–44.

Meguid, M. M., Campos, A. C. L., Meguid, V., Debonis, D. & Terz, J. J. (1988). IONIP, a criterion of surgical outcome and patient selection for perioperative nutritional support. *British Journal of Clinical Practice*, Suppl. **63**, 8–14.

Murciano, D., Armengauk, M. H., Rigand, D. *et al.* (1990). Effect of renutrition on respiratory and diaphragmatic function in patients with severe mental anorexia. *Annual Review of Respiratory Diseases*, **141**, A 547.

Park, R. H. R., Allison, M. C., Lang, J. *et al.* (1992). Randomised comparison of percutaneous endoscopic gastrostomy and naso-gastric tube feeding in patients with persisting neurological dysphagia. *British Medical Journal*, **304**, 1406–9.

Pichard, C. & Jeejeebhoy, K. N. (1988). Muscle dysfunction in malnourished patients. *Quarterly Journal of Medicine*, **260**, 1021–45.

Russell, D. M., Walker, P. M., Leiter, L. A. *et al.* (1984). Metabolic and structural changes in muscle during hypocaloric dieting. *American Journal of Clinical Nutrition*, **39**, 503–13.

Shizgal, H. M. (1981). Nutrition and immune function. *Surgery Annals*, **12**, 15–29.

Veterans Affairs Total Parenteral Nutrition Study Group (1991). Perioperative total parenteral nutrition in surgical patients. *New England Journal of Medicine*, **325**, 525–32.

Von Meyenfeldt, M. F., Meijerink, W. J. H. J., Rouflart, M. M. J., Buil-Maassen, M. T. H. J. & Soeters, P. B. (1992). Perioperative nutritional support: a randomised clinical trial. *Clinical Nutrition*, **11**, 180–6.

Windsor, J. A. & Hill, G. L. (1988). Risk factors for postoperative pneumonia: the importance of protein depletion. *Annals in Surgery*, **208**, 209–14.

Winick, M. (ed.) (1979). *Hunger Disease: Studies by the Jewish Physicians in the Warsaw Ghetto.* Wiley, New York.

14

Intensive care management

I. T. CAMPBELL AND R. A. LITTLE

Following an episode of trauma or sepsis a number of complex physiological and endocrinological events occur. Classically, these have been classified into 'ebb' and 'flow' phases (Barton, 1987). The ebb phase is a period of reduced metabolic activity immediately following the injury; spontaneous activity is reduced and body temperature may be diminished. It merges into the 'flow' phase – a period of regeneration and repair, of increased metabolic rate and elevation in body temperature; appetite is depressed and energy and protein requirements are met in part from endogenous stores. Energy is provided principally by the oxidation of fat (Little, Stoner & Frayn, 1981) and the ongoing need for glucose by certain tissues, such as wound tissue and the central nervous system, is met by glucose supplied by hepatic gluconeogenesis. The gluconeogenic substrates come principally from amino acids supplied by breakdown of lean tissue.

If the injury is of limited extent no complications ensue and the patient recovers; he or she enters the anabolic phase. Food intake increases, lean tissue is laid down and normal function resumes, but usually with a reduced body mass (Frayn, 1986). If the traumatic or septic insult is overwhelming, or physiological reserves are reduced, perhaps by a preceding period of illness or undernutrition, or blood loss is overwhelming and not treated, organ systems fail and death ensues from a process that has been termed necrobiosis (Stoner, 1986). In clinical practice, if deemed appropriate, it is now possible to support or replace organ function – the lungs by mechanical ventilation, renal function by haemodiafiltration and the myocardium by inotropic drugs. Many patients are kept alive by artificial means, often for prolonged periods until treatment results in recovery, or until he or she dies. Metabolic processes occurring in multiple systems organ failure, are similar to those seen with a discrete episode of trauma and sepsis, but do not follow a well-defined pattern.

The ebb phase

The ebb phase involves metabolic, thermoregulatory and hormonal changes, with an alteration in the central control of a number of physiological mechanisms (Barton, 1987). There is evidence from animal work for abnormalities of thermoregulation in the ebb phase, with an impairment of the ability to respond to and withstand a cold stress (Tabor & Rosenthal, 1947). This is exacerbated by hypovolaemia and nociceptive stimuli from injured tissue and appears to be under central control. In man, there is also some evidence for an abnormality in thermoregulation, in that body temperature is diminished after severe injury (Little & Stoner, 1981) and injured individuals prefer a higher ambient temperature for thermal comfort than do controls (Little *et al.*, 1986).

Metabolic rate is reduced in animals, but the evidence for such a reduction following injury in man is not very convincing. Some very low values have been recorded, although relatively few measurements have been made. Little (1985), reviewed the available data and found a wider spread of values than for a normal control population. Calculating oxygen consumption from cardiac output measurements, Edwards and colleagues showed that the majority of patients after severe multiple injury had higher levels of oxygen consumption than normal (Edwards *et al.*, 1988).

The hypothalamic–pituitary–adrenal axis is activated following trauma, with rises in circulating cortisol and in vasopressin, the latter from the neurohypophysis. The relationship between severity of injury and cortisol, however, is complex (Frayne *et al.*, 1985); moderate injuries cause greater rises in circulating cortisol levels than minor ones, but with severe injury cortisol levels are often lower than expected, possibly due to hypoperfusion of the adrenal cortex.

There is an increase in sympathetic activity and a rise in circulating adrenaline from the adrenal medulla and noradrenaline from sympathetic nerve endings. Adrenaline often inhibits insulin release and low blood insulin levels are a common finding in acute injury, despite quite marked hyperglycaemia (Frayn *et al.*, 1987).

Sympathetic activity and adrenaline release result in glucose mobilisation from glycogen stores in the liver and skeletal muscle. Adrenaline stimulates lactate release from muscle, which is recycled via the liver to form glucose.

A number of 'acute phase' plasma proteins, such as C reactive protein and fibrinogen, rise after injury and this is associated with a fall in albumin. These changes are thought to be due to increases in release of the cytokine interleukin-6 (IL-6) from activated macrophages, with the increase occurring about 6 hours after the injury (Gauldie *et al.*, 1987).

The flow phase

During the 'flow' phase, energy expenditure is said to be elevated to a degree that is proportional to the extent of the injury; 0–5% after elective surgery, 20–30% following major trauma or sepsis and 100% after major burn injury (Wilmore, 1977; Matsuda *et al.*, 1977).

Increases in energy expenditure are inevitably associated with elevations in cardiac output and ventilation. Failure to achieve these increases necessitates the use of artificial (positive pressure) ventilation, or myocardial support with inotropic drugs. However, measurement of metabolic rate in some patients, particularly those ill for prolonged periods, often does not show the expected hypermetabolism, as the picture may be confused by periods of bed rest, failure to provide adequate nutritional support and a reduced lean body mass.

The cause of the hypermetabolism is also not entirely clear. An upward setting of (central) metabolic control has been suggested, stimulated by cytokines from the injured tissue and mediated by sympathoadrenal mechanisms. Other possibilities include increased substrate recycling, such as the glycolysis–gluconeogenesis cycle and the triglyceride fatty acid cycle (Wolfe *et al.*, 1987). The precise contribution of such processes, however, is difficult to assess.

The wound itself (fracture, burn, abscess, etc), may have quite a major effect on energy expenditure (Wilmore, 1986). This depends on fibroblasts, polymorphonuclear leukocytes, endothelial/epithelial cells, etc, all of which are metabolically very active. Blood supply is independent of normal control and burn wounds particularly have been shown to be consumers of large amounts of glucose. This is metabolised to lactate, then passed to the liver, where it is converted to glucose via the Cori cycle – a process which consumes energy (Wilmore *et al.*, 1980).

Changes occur in whole body and muscle protein kinetics with sepsis and trauma. Measurements of protein turnover after elective surgery and moderate injury, have generally shown a depression of protein synthesis and no change in rate of breakdown (Clague *et al.*, 1983). However, after severe trauma or sepsis and in multiple organ failure, both synthesis and breakdown of whole body protein are elevated (Arnold *et al.*, 1993).

Skeletal muscle is the principal protein 'reservoir' and provides gluco-neogenic precursors for tissues that have an obligatory need for glucose, such as the central nervous system. It is, in addition, a source of amino acids for synthesis of protein involved in immune defence and wound healing. Contributions of other tissues to nitrogen excretion such as the gut, lungs, skin, etc may also be substantial.

In severe injury and sepsis, skeletal muscle is broken down and quite characteristic changes occur in intracellular muscle amino acid con-centrations, with increases in branch chain amino acids and a decrease in glutamine (Vinnars *et al.*, 1975; Milewski *et al.*, 1982). Plasma levels of a number of amino acids fall, particuarly alanine and the hepatic extraction of alanine increases with the elevation in gluconeogenesis (Barton, Frayn & Little, 1990). This increase in gluconeogenesis occurs despite elevations in blood levels of glucose and insulin. The glutamine released from muscle is an important fuel for the lymphocyte and macro-phages activated by injury. It also features in the maintenance of the integrity of the gut mucosa which may be impaired after injury (O'Dwyer *et al.*, 1989).

The insulin resistance has been shown using glucose/insulin clamp techniques, with decreases in both the maximum response achieved with insulin infusion and also in insulin sensitivity. This suggests changes in both insulin receptor binding and in cellular metabolism (Henderson *et al.*, 1991; Black *et al.*, 1982; White *et al.*, 1987). Classically it has always been thought that the stress hormones – glucagon, cortisol and adrenaline were responsible for the insulin resistance and the negative nitrogen balance. Indeed features of the flow phase have been reproduced in normal volunteers, by infusion of all three hormones simultaneously (Bessey *et al.*, 1984), but the degree of 'catabolism' (i.e. negative nitrogen balance) produced was less than that seen in clinical practice. Also at the time the greatest degree of catabolism is seen after a discrete injury, concentrations of these hormones have returned almost to normal values. Frayn observed that at the time of the greatest degree of negative nitrogen balance, i.e. 10 days after injury, insulin is at its highest (Frayn, 1986).

Attention has now turned to the cytokines, specifically IL-1, IL-6 and tumour necrosis factor, as mediators of the acute and flow phase responses (Van der Poll *et al.*, 1991; Roh *et al.*, 1987). They have been shown to reproduce many of the changes seen – stimulation of the pituitary–adrenal axis, alterations in stress hormone concentrations, central resetting of metabolic activity and changes in glucose metabolism.

Energy intake, energy expenditure and energy balance

In life, energy requirements are met by oxidation of foodstuffs – carbohydrate, fat and protein. If energy intake exceeds expenditure, either because intake is increased or expenditure diminished, or both, the individual gains body mass, normally in the form of adipose tissue. If expenditure exceeds intake, either because intake is diminished or expenditure elevated, this is normally manifest as a decrease in body mass. Although fat, in the form of adipose tissue, is the principal storage tissue of the body, there is, in the starving or semi-starving individual, an ongoing need for glucose and this is derived by gluconeogenesis, principally from amino acids.

In simple starvation, a number of complex biochemical adjustments occur, which minimise the extent of the breakdown of lean tissue and as far as possible conserve lean tissue mass. Urinary nitrogen excretion decreases. Protein oxidation, running at 75 g/24 h in the first week of starvation, diminishes to 20 g/day by week three and glucose consumption by the brain decreases from 140 g/day to 40 g/day. The metabolic responses to trauma and sepsis modify the adaptation to simple starvation but the two are often inextricably related, as appetite is normally diminished following trauma and energy and protein intake are inadequate for requirements.

Energy expenditure

Energy expenditure is normally estimated by measuring the oxygen consumed and making assumptions about the energy expenditure, that the consumption of 1 litre of oxygen denotes. This is usually in the range of 4.6–5 kcal, dependent on the nutrients being oxidised. There are now a number of commercially available indirect calorimeters, which enable energy expenditure to be measured as a routine clinical procedure (Regan, Snowdon & Campbell, 1990; Takala *et al.*, 1989). Combined with measurement of urinary nitrogen excretion, indirect calorimetry can be used to quantify nutrient oxidation in terms of weight of carbohydrate fat and protein oxidised. There are, however, a number of practical problems with the technique. These include the ease with which naive subjects, such as patients, tolerate the apparatus, factors other than nutrient oxidation that affect respiratory exchange ratios, the problem with $\dot{V}O_2$ measurements in the presence of a high inspired oxygen concentration (F_IO_2) and the validity of taking a brief measurement of

$\dot{V}O_2$, as an indication of true 24-hour energy expenditure. Included in all of this is the question of whether measurements of 24 h energy expenditure are actually an indication of what the patient ought to be fed.

Indirect calorimetry apparatus can be connected to patients to collect expired air in a number of ways. A mouthpiece and nose clip is one of the simplest techniques, but patients unused to the apparatus often do not tolerate this very well, particularly, those who are seriously ill. Loose fitting masks and hoods are a better option and in ventilated patients the calorimeter can be connected to the ventilator circuitry.

Inspired and expired volumes are normally different, because less CO_2 is expired than oxygen consumed. They can both be measured, but this is a cumbersome procedure and it is more usual to measure one and calculate the other from the measured volume and the ratio of the inspired and expired nitrogen concentrations – the so called Haldane transformation. Thus, if expired volume (V_E) is measured

$$V_I = V_E \times N_E/N_I$$

where V_I is inspired volume and N_I and N_E are inspired and expired nitrogen concentrations respectively.

This technique works very well for measuring $\dot{V}O_2$ in subjects breathing room air, but it is self evident that as the F_IO_2 increases, the amount of nitrogen in the system diminishes, such that at an F_IO_2 of 1 (i.e. with a patient breathing 100% oxygen), it will break down completely. This has been discussed at some length by Ultman and Bursztein (1981), but in practice most indirect calorimetry systems run into problems with accuracy at around an F_IO_2 of 0.7. One system has the facility to assume a respiratory exchange ratio/respiratory quotient, thus making assumptions about the inspired and expired volumes and, within the limitations of this assumption, is accurate at least up to an F_IO_2 of 0.8 (Regan *et al.*, 1990). Above this level it is more accurate to measure inspired and expired volumes separately (Ultman & Bursztein, 1981; Svensson, Sonander & Stenqvist, 1990).

Factors that affect the respiratory quotient or respiratory exchange ratio (RER) include hyper- and hypo-ventilation. In the critically ill, however, disturbances of acid base balance may be more of a problem than normal, acidosis raising CO_2 production and thus raising the RER and alkalosis depressing it.

Another question is that of how closely measurements of oxygen consumption made over brief periods, reflect true 24 h energy expenditure. In ventilated patients, expenditure can, potentially, be measured continuously; all of the patients' expired air passes out via the ventilator circuitry, so it can be analysed continuously. To do so, however, requires that the calorimeter be dedicated exclusively to one particular ventilator and thus, effectively to one particular patient. Such systems do exist (Regan *et al.*, 1990) but others can be moved from ventilator to ventilator (Takala *et al.*, 1989), measurements made for an hour or so and the results extrapolated to 24 hours. The indications are that such estimates will generally be within 10–20% of the true energy expenditure (Green *et al.*, 1990*a*).

Body mass and composition

There are a variety of methods of assessing body composition. All of them have quite severe limitations in critical illness, usually in relation to abnormal fluid retention, but also in terms of the practicality of, for example, moving a patient attached to a ventilator and a haemodialysis machine into a total body counter (Beddoe, Streat & Hill, 1984).

In normal circumstances, body weight is the usual technique for assessing increases and decreases in body mass. In the normal adult this varies by up to 0.5 kg/day, although daily variations of up to 1 kg are normal due to variations in body water (Adam, Best & Edholm, 1961). In serious illness, large quantitites of fluid may be given during resuscitation and are retained in the interstitial tissue and manifest as oedema. Respiratory problems arise when the fluid retention affects the lungs and impairs gas exchange. Surprisingly little information is available as to how much fluid critically ill patients do actually retain. The few figures that are available, suggest that it may be up to 20 litres, with quantities in excess of 10 litres being quite common (Hall, Pollard & Campbell, 1992; Streat, Beddoe & Hill, 1987). By comparison, fluid retention after major elective surgery is usually in the region of 1–2 litres (Hill, 1992).

The two commonest techniques for measuring body composition are the derivation of percentage body fat from skinfold measurements and the measurement of body water with assumptions made about the body water/lean body mass relationship. The limitations of assessing body composition from skinfold thickness in the presence of gross oedema are obvious. Fluid is 'squeezed' out of the subcutaneous skinfolds to varying degrees during measurement and the indeterminate quantity of retained fluid is within both adipose tissue and visceral tissue, to degrees which again are indeterminable. Estimating lean body mass from measurements of total body water are open to the same criticism.

A more recent technique of assessing body composition is total body impedance. This relies on measuring the electrical resistance, or more correctly impedance, that the body presents to an alternating electrical current. The current is generated by a very low voltage and is undetectable by the subject. On the assumption that conduction of the current occurs only via body water, lean body mass can be derived using the same assumptions as outlined above. In the presence of oedema this, too is obviously limited, as a method of measuring lean body mass.

Other indices of lean tissue mass such as naturally occurring ^{40}K total body potassium or total body nitrogen measured using neutron activation analysis (Beddoe et al., 1984), are probably the most satisfactory ways of measuring body composition in the presence of large amounts of oedema fluid. They require, however, that the patient be placed in a whole body counter and this presents obvious practical difficulties. Neutron activation analysis also involves the administration of significant amounts of radiation, so the measurement cannot be repeated frequently, although one such specialised facility has been built for the use of intensive care patients (Beddoe et al., 1984).

Energy and nitrogen intake

Energy intake is normally quite a difficult parameter to measure because of the variability in the nutrient content of food and the social problems associated with trying to make accurate measurements of intake. In critical illness, nutritional support is normally given enterally or parenterally and is homogeneous and the measurement of protein and energy intake is relatively easy. Problems in the provision of adequate nutritional support arise from two sources. One is the difficulty of enteral feeding when the gastrointestinal tract does not function adequately. The other is the problem of feeding adequate quantities of energy and amino acids intravenously when the patient already has problems with fluid balance and an overloaded circulation and the potential for further problems with oedema and pulmonary gas exchange. Many patients are on intensive care because of abdominal sepsis and in these circumstances the gastrointestinal tract often ceases to function. Also, many are given dopamine as a means of renal and cardiovascular support and this too has an adverse effect on gastric emptying (Valenzuela, 1976; Hartley et al., 1992).

Multiple organ systems failure

When the physiological reserves are unable to cope with the pathological insult, or the pathological insult is overwhelming, the various organ systems fail and require artificial support. The commonest are ventilatory and cardiovascular failure requiring artificial ventilation and inotropic support of the myocardium. Multiple organ systems failure, unlike elective surgery, does not follow a predestined course of 'ebb and flow'. The appearance generally is that of a patient stuck in the flow phase, but some are hypometabolic and the course of the illness is generally unpredictable. Patients suffering multiple organ failure all appear remarkably similar, no matter what the precipitating condition (Beale & Bihari, 1993). They often have the appearance of being septic with myocardial depression and a low peripheral resistance but with no identifiable infection. It has been suggested that translocation of bacteria and endotoxins from the gut may be the cause of this 'septic' state (Deitch & Bridges, 1987) and strategies have been devised for sterilizing the gut (McClelland *et al.*, 1990) but the outcome so far has generally been disappointing (Vandenbroucke-Grauls & Vandenbroucke, 1991).

Patients undergoing intermittent positive pressure ventilation have the advantage that energy expenditure can be measured continuously. In order to determine 24 hour energy expenditure it is not therefore necessary to extrapolate from brief periods of measurement. It is also difficult to predict energy expenditure on clinical grounds, whereas in patients suffering uncomplicated burns, multiple trauma, acute sepsis, etc, energy expenditure is, to an extent, predictable from the severity of illness. There are a variety of sickness scores available to quantify severity of illness in multiple organ failure, but their reliability is still uncertain and the values they produce bear no relationship to energy expenditure (Murray *et al.*, 1990).

Probably the major factor affecting energy expenditure in ventilated patients is the degree of sedation, muscle relaxation and spontaneous muscle activity, commensurate with their ability to tolerate the ventilator. Weissman and colleagues investigated this in detail and showed that energy expenditure was affected by turning the patient, by the presence of visitors, positioning for X-rays etc. and increased by up to 30–40% of resting expenditure (Weissman *et al.*, 1986*a, b*). They also pointed out, however, that such episodes were relatively short-lived and actually contributed little to the overall 24-hour expenditure. The same group also demonstrated that 'resting expenditure' measured for a limited period and extrapolated to 24 hours was often greater than 24-hour expenditure as actually measured. This occurred because of the unpredictable effects and timing of sedation and muscle relaxation.

Despite these problems, a number of measurements have been made of energy expenditure in patients ventilated for varying periods and suffering from a variety of illnesses (Weissman *et al.*, 1986*a*, *b*; Weissman, Kemper and Hyman, 1989; Dickerson *et al.*, 1991; Lanschott *et al.*, 1966). Most have shown an average figure for energy expenditure of around 120–130% of basal predicted from age, height and weight, but with a very wide spread of values, sometimes down to 50% of predicted basal to around 200%. None of these workers, however, has quantified the role that muscle tone and activity have contributed to the total figure.

Only two studies have attempted to measure changes in body composition in patients suffering multiple organ failure (Streat *et al.*, 1987; Green *et al.*, 1990*b*). One used neutron activation analysis to estimate changes in body mass and composition (Streat *et al.*, 1987). They failed to measure energy expenditure, but showed that patients lost 12.5% of their total body protein stores, despite an energy intake of about 42 kcal/kg lean body mass (2350 kcal for a 70 kg adult, 20% body fat) and a nitrogen intake of around 20 g/24 h. Body fat increased, so one must assume that energy intake was adequate for requirements. Total body water decreased by 10–14 litres in those patients who recovered. The other study measured intake and expenditure and related the findings to changes in arm circumference. This of course was partly confounded by the abnormal fluid retention. They did, however, demonstrate that energy balance (i.e. the apparent adequacy of feeding), bore no relationship to the rate of loss of arm circumference (Green *et al.*, 1990*b*) and this decreased steadily no matter how apparently adequate the intake. The arm circumference figures were confirmed by changes in measurements of muscle fibre area taken at biopsy.

Studies with isotope tracers have demonstrated that providing energy substrate for patients who are highly catabolic (i.e. with high rates of gluconeogenesis), decreases the rate at which gluconeogenesis proceeds by about 50%, but does not suppress it completely (Shaw, Klein & Wolfe, 1985). Whether this conclusion is borne out in practice in terms of feeding the patient, is as yet unproven, largely because of the difficulties involved in making reliable body composition measurements.

It is probable that feeding patients with multiple organ failure makes little or no difference to rates of loss of lean tissue, although intuitively it is difficult to believe that feeding has no beneficial effect on the patients' physiological and immunological mechanisms. It is probable that eventually specific protein and energy substrates such as glutamine (Wilmore, 1991), will provide a means of maintaining lean tissue mass in these patients and/or various methods of pharmacological manipulation will also be required. Obvious candidates that have already undergone some experimental evaluation include growth hormone (Ward, Halliday & Sim, 1987), somatostatin, histamine antagonists (Shaw & Wolfe, 1988) and in animals, beta 2 stimulants (Emery *et al.* 1984).

References

Adam, J. M., Best, T. W. & Edholm, O. G. (1961). Weight changes in young men. *Journal of Physiology*, **156**, 38P.

Arnold, J., Campbell, I. T., Samuels, T. A. *et al.* (1993). Increased whole body protein breakdown predominates over increased body protein synthesis in multiple organ failure. *Clinical Science*, **84**, 655–61.

Barton, R. N. (1987). The neuroendocrinology of physical injury. Ballière's *Clinical Endocrinology Metabolism*, **1**, 355–74.

Barton, R. N., Frayn, K. N. & Little, R. A. (1990). Trauma, burns and surgery. In *The Metabolic and Molecular Basis of Acquired Disease* Vol I, ed. R. D. Cohen, N. Lewis, K. G. M. M. Alberti & A. M. Denman, pp. 684–717. Ballière Tindall, London.

Beale, R. & Bihari, D. J. (1993). Editorial; Multiple organ failure: the pilgrim's progress. *Critical Care Medicine*, **21**, S1–S3.

Beddoe, A. H., Streat, S. J. & Hill, G. L. (1984). Evaluation of an in vivo prompt gamma neutron activation analysis facility for body composition studies in critically ill intensive care patients: results on 41 normals. *Metabolism*, **33**, 270–80.

Bessey, P. Q., Watters, J. M., Aoki, T. T. & Wilmore, D. W. (1984). Combined hormonal infusion simulates the metabolic response to injury. *Annals of Surgery*, **200**, 264–80.

Black, P. R., Brooks, D. C., Bessey, P. A. *et al.* (1982). Mechanisms of insulin resistance following injury. *Annals of Surgery*, **196**, 420–35.

Clague, M. B., Keir, M. J., Wright, P. D. & Johnston, I. D. A. (1983). The effects of nutrition and trauma on whole-body protein metabolism in man. *Clinical Sciences*, **65**, 165–75.

Deitch, E. A. & Bridges, R. M. (1987). Effect of stress and trauma on bacterial translocation from the gut. *Journal of Surgical Research*, **42**, 536–42.

Dickerson, R. N., Vehe, K. L., Mullen, J. L. & Feurer, I. D. (1991). Resting energy expenditure in patients with pancreatitis. *Critical Care Medicine*, **19**, 484–8.

Edwards, J. D., Redmond, A. D., Nightingale, P. & Wilkins, G. (1988). Oxygen consumption following trauma – a reappraisal in severely injured patients requiring mechanical ventilation. *British Journal of Surgery*, **75**, 690–2.

Emery, P. W., Rothwell, N. J., Stock, M. J. & Winter, P. D. (1984). Chronic effects of beta 2 adrenergic agonists on body composition and protein synthesis in the rat. *Bioscience Reports*, **4**, 83–91.

Frayne, K. N. (1986). Hormonal control of metabolism in trauma and sepsis. *Clinical Endocrinology*, **24**, 577–99.

Frayn. K. N., Little, R. A., Maycock, P. F. & Stoner, H. B. (1985), The relationships of plasma catecholamines to acute metabolic and hormonal responses to injury in man. *Circulatory Shock*, **16**, 229–35.

Frayn, K. N., Maycock, P., Little, R. A. *et al.* (1987). Factors affecting the plasma insulin concentration shortly after accidental injury in man. *Archives in Emergency Medicine*, **4**, 91–9.

Gauldie, J., Richards, C., Harnish, *et al.* (1987). Interferon beta2/B-cell stimulatory factor type 2 shares identity with monocyte-derived hepatocyte-stimulating factor and regulates the major acute plasma protein response in liver cells. *Proceedings of the National Academy of Sciences, USA*, **84**, 7251–5.

Green, C. J., Phillips, B., McClelland, P. & Campbell, I. T. (1990*a*). For how long and how often should oxygen consumption be measured in the ventilated patient to assess 24 h energy expenditure. *Proceedings of the Nutrition Society*, **49**, 185A.

Green, C. J., Helliwell, T. R., McClelland, P. *et al.* (1990*b*). Arm circumference and energy balance in acute illness. *Proceedings of the Nutrition Society*, **49**, 17A.

Hall, I., Pollard, B. J. & Campbell, I. T. (1992). Daily body weight changes in critical illness. *Proceedings of the Nutrition Society*, **51**, 126A.

Hartley, M. N., Sarginson, R. F., Green, C. J. *et al.* (1992). Gastric pressure response to low dose dopamine infusion in normal man. *Clinical Nutrition*, **11**, 23–9.

Henderson, A. A., Frayn, K. N., Galasko, C. S. B. & Little, R. A. (1991). Dose response relationships for the effects of insulin on glucose and fat metabolism in injured patients and control subjects. *Clinical Science*, **80**, 25–32.

Hill, G. L. (1992). *Disorders of Nutrition and Metabolism in Clinical Surgery. Understanding and Management*, pp. 19–32. Churchill Livingstone, Edinburgh.

Lanschott, J. B. V., Feenstra, B. W. A., Vermeij, C. G. *et al.* (1966). Calculation versus measurement of total energy expenditure. *Critical Care Medicine*, **14**, 981–5.

Little, R. A. (1985). Heat production and injury. *British Medical Bulletin*, **41**, 226–31.

Little, R. A. & Stoner, H. B. (1981). Body temperature after accidental injury. *British Journal of Surgery*, **68**, 221–4.

Little, R. A., Stoner, H. B. & Frayn, K. N. (1981). Substrate oxidation shortly after accidental injury in man. *Clinical Science*, **61**, 789–91.

Little, R. A., Stoner, H. B., Randall, P. & Carlson, G. (1986). An effect of injury on thermoregulation in man. *Quarterly Journal of Experimental Physiology*, **71**, 295–306.

McClelland, P., Murray, A. E., Williams, P. S. *et al.* (1990). Reducing sepsis in severe combined acute renal and respiratory failure by selective decontamination of the digestive tract. *Critical Care Medicine*, **18**, 935–9.

Matsuda, T., Clarke, N., Hariyani, G. D., Bryant, R. S., Hanumadass, M. L., Kagan, R. J. (1977). The effect of burn wound size on resting energy expenditure. *Journal of Trauma*, **27**, 115–18.

Milewski, P. J., Threlfall, C. J., Heath, D. F., Holbrook, I. B., Wilford, K. & Irving, M. H. (1982). Intracellular free amino acids in undernourished patients with or without sepsis. *Clinical Science*, **62**, 83–91.

Murray, A. E., Bell, M., Green, C. J., McClelland, P., Mostafa, S. M., Campbell,

I. T. (1990). C-reactive protein, sickness scores and energy expenditure in critical illness. *Proceedings of the Nutritional Society*, **49**, 184A.

O'Dwyer, S. T., Smith, R. J., Hwang, T. L. & Wilmore, D. W. (1989). Maintenance of small bowel mucosa with glutamine enriched parenteral nutrition. *Journal of Parenteral and Enteral Nutrition*, **13**, 579–85.

Regan, C. J., Snowdon, S. L. & Campbell, I. T. (1990). Laboratory evaluation and use of the Engstrom Metabolic Computer in the clinical setting. *Critical Care Medicine*, **18**, 871–7.

Roh, M. S., Drazenovich, K. A., Barbose, J. J., Dinarello, C. A. & Cobb, C. F. (1987). Direct stimulation of the adrenal cortex by interleukin-1. *Surgery*, **102**, 140–6.

Shaw, J. H. F., Klein, S. & Wolfe, R. R. (1985). Assessment of alanine, urea and glucose inter-relationships in normal subjects and severely septic patients. *Surgery*, **97**, 557–62.

Shaw, J. H. F. & Wolfe, R. R. (1988). Metabolic intervention in surgical patients. *Annals of Surgery*, **207**, 274–82.

Stoner, H. B. (1986). Metabolism after trauma and in sepsis. *Circulatory Shock*, **19**, 75–87.

Streat, S. J., Beddoe, A. H. & Hill, G. L. (1987). Aggressive nutritional support does not prevent protein loss despite fat gain in septic intensive care patients. *Journal of Trauma*, **27**, 262–6.

Svensson, K. L., Sonander, H. G. & Stenqvist, O. (1990). Validation of a system for measurement of metabolic gas exchange during anaesthesia with controlled ventilation in an oxygen consuming lung model. *British Journal of Anaesthesia*, **64**, 311–19.

Tabor, H. & Rosenthal, S. M. (1947). Body temperature and oxygen consumption in traumatic shock and haemorrhage in mice. *American Journal of Physiology*, **149**, 499–64.

Takala, J., Keinanen, O., Vaisanen, P. & Kari, A. (1989). Measurement of gas exchange in intensive care: laboratory and clinical validation of a new device. *Critical Care Medicine*, **17**, 1041–7.

Ultman, J. S. & Bursztein, S. (1981). Analysis of error in the determination of respiratory gas exchange at varying FIO_2. *Journal of Applied Physiology (Respiratory, Environmental, Exercise Physiology)*, **30**, 210–16.

Van der Poll, T., Romijn, J. A., Endert, R., Borm, J. J., Buller, H. R. & Sauerwein, H. P. (1991). Tumour necrosis factor mimics the metabolic response to acute infection in healthy humans. *American Journal of Physiology*, **261**, E457–65.

Vandenbroucke-Grauls, C. M. J. E. & Vandenbroucke, J. P. (1991). Effective selective decontamination of the digestive tract on respiratory tract infections and mortality in the intensive care unit. *Lancet*, **338**, 859–62.

Valenzuela, J. (1976). Dopamine as a possible neurotransmitter in gastric relaxation. *Gastroenterology*, **71**, 1019–22.

Vinnars, E., Bergstrom, J. & Furst, P. (1975). Influence of the postoperative state on the intracellular free amino acids in human muscle tissue. *Annals of Surgery*, **182**, 665–71.

Ward, H. C., Halliday, D. & Sim, A. J. W. (1987). Protein and energy metabolism with biosynthetic human growth hormone after gastrointestinal surgery. *Annals of Surgery*, **206**, 56–61.

Weissman, C., Kemper, M. & Hyman, A. I. (1989). Variation in the resting metabolic rate of mechanically ventilated critically ill patients. *Anesthesia and Analgesia*, **68**, 457–61.

Weissman, C., Kemper, M., Elwyn, D. H. *et al.* (1986*a*). The energy expenditure of the mechanically ventilated critically ill patient. An analysis. *Chest*, **89**, 254–9.

Weissman, C., Kemper, M., Askanazi, *et al.* (1986*b*). Resting metabolic rate of the critically ill patient: measured versus predicted. *Anesthesiology*, **64**, 673–9.

White, R. H., Frayn, K. N., Galasko, C. S. B. *et al.* (1987). Hormonal and metabolic responses to glucose infusion in sepsis studied by the hyperglycaemic glucose clamp technique. *Journal of Parenteral and Enteral Nutrition*, **11**, 345–53.

Wilmore, D. W. (1977). *The Management of the Critically Ill*, Plenum Press, New York.

Wilmore, D. W. (1986). The wound as an organ. In *The Scientific Basis for the Care of the Critically Ill*, eds R. A. Little & K. N. Frayn, pp. 45–59. Manchester University Press, Manchester.

Wilmore, D. W. (1991). Catabolic illness strategies for enhancing recovery. *New England Journal of Medicine*, **365**, 695–702.

Wilmore, D. W., Goodwin, C. W., Aulick, L. H. *et al.* (1980). Effect of injury and infection on visceral metabolism and circulation. *Annals of Surgery*, **192**, 491–502.

Wolfe, R. R., Herndon, D. N., Jahoor, F. *et al.* (1987). Effect of severe burn injury on substrate cycling by glucose and fatty acids. *New England Journal of Medicine*, **317**, 403–8.

15

The role of the liver in nutrition

M. S. LOSOWSKY AND P. N. BRAMLEY

Introduction

The liver is uniquely situated between two blood supplies, the hepatic artery from the systemic circulation and the portal venous system which carries blood and absorbed nutrients from the intestines.

The liver acts as the major processor of the fat, protein and carbohydrate together with the micronutrients such as vitamins and minerals, present in the diet.

The hepatocytes are a major storage site for nutrients and synthesise carrier proteins to deliver the processed nutrients to other tissues.

The liver is metabolically extremely active, accounting for over 20% of the body's resting energy expenditure. It is the major site for the intermediate metabolism of macronutrients absorbed from the bowel as well as detoxifying waste products and metabolising hormones produced within the body.

The liver has a large functional reserve and a prodigious regenerative capacity so that acute damage must be very severe to impair its ability to perform crucial homeostatic functions.

In chronic liver disease, changes occur in the ability of the hepatocytes to carry out their normal metabolic functions. The blood system and biliary drainage from the liver may be affected. Different patterns of damage are seen. If the main effect is loss of hepatocytes by inflammation and/or necrosis, then the damage is termed hepatocellular. If the damage predominantly affects the biliary drainage from the liver, the damage is termed cholestatic. This distinction has important implications for the pattern of disturbances of the body in absorption and metabolism of nutrients.

In this chapter, the relationship between nutrition and liver disease will be discussed, in terms of how the liver can be affected by dietary factors and how liver disease can cause malnutrition.

Dietary causes of liver disease

A significant proportion of liver disease may be caused by nutritional factors. By far the commonest cause of diet-induced liver disease is excessive ingestion of alcohol.

Alcohol

The prevalence of alcoholic liver disease correlates closely with ethanol consumption. In France, the country with the world's highest *per capita* intake of alcohol, strict wine rationing during World War II was reflected in a rapid reduction in cirrhosis-related mortality, in the period 1940 to 1946, with the death rate dropping from 17.2 to 6.9 per 100 000 population. The increase in alcohol consumption which followed the end of the war, was matched by a corresponding increase in cirrhosis mortality to 32.5 deaths per 100 000 total population in 1956 (Lelbach, 1985).

Although the average alcohol intake in alcoholics with cirrhosis is 180 g/day, intakes as low as 40 g/day for men and 20 g/day for women, are associated with an increased risk of cirrhosis (Pequignot & Tuyns, 1980). Cirrhosis may be seen after only five or six years, or may not become evident for many years.

However, as only a small proportion of heavy drinkers go on to develop cirrhosis, other factors such as nutrition, hormonal balance, environmental factors and genetic predisposition may have a role to play in the pathogenesis.

Ethanol causes predictable changes in liver histology, the earliest change being fatty liver, with the intracellular deposition of fat, abnormal liver function tests and hepatomegaly. This is a relatively benign condition and totally reversible. With continued alcohol ingestion, gradually increasing deposition of collagen around the sinusoids and the hepatic venules eventually leads to fibrosis and subsequent cirrhosis.

In some people, acute inflammation of the hepatic parenchyma (alcoholic hepatitis) occurs, associated with a high mortality and this often follows an increase in ethanol ingestion. Alcoholic hepatitis is a definite precursor of cirrhosis. Hepatocellular carcinoma is a well documented sequel to alcoholic cirrhosis.

If the patient remains abstinent, it is possible to see reversal of the histological changes of fatty liver and alcoholic hepatitis and there is an improvement in the prognosis in established cirrhosis.

Malnutrition

For many years it was postulated that malnutrition was a direct cause of cirrhosis in man (Himsworth, 1947) by analogy with the fact that animal models of nutritional deficiency lead to cirrhosis. It is now clear that the protein deficiency state of kwashiorkor accounts for histological changes of fatty liver and eventually a degree of fibrosis, but not cirrhosis (Cook & Hutt, 1967). In those countries where kwashiorkor is common, there is also an increase in viral hepatitis, such as hepatitis B, to account for an apparent relationship with chronic liver disease.

In marasmus, in which both protein and calorie intake are low, non-specific histological changes may occur in the liver, but fibrosis and cirrhosis do not occur. In developed countries, a state of protein-energy malnutrition, such as occurs in various diseases, does not lead to chronic liver disease. There is, however, little doubt that, if there is pre-existing liver disease, malnutrition can adversely affect the potential of the liver to regenerate and may lead to a worsening of the prognosis.

Obesity

Patients with morbid obesity often have fatty liver and, in particularly severe and chronic cases, a degree of inflammation and mild peri-central and peri-cellular fibrosis. These findings are often associated with mildly abnormal liver function tests (Galambos, 1976). Liver biopsy is often required to exclude other pathology. If weight loss is achieved through dieting, liver function tests can return to normal.

Starting about 30 years ago, jejuno-ileal bypass had a brief vogue in resistant obesity, to promote weight loss. This operation is almost invariably associated with fatty liver and also carries the risk of serious hepatic and metabolic complications, with increased fatty infiltration, inflammation and fibrosis in 50% of patients. One study reported 3 out of 88 patients also developed liver cirrhosis (Marubbio *et al.*, 1976). Bacterial production of a hepatotoxic substance in the colon or in the bypassed loop has been postulated to account for these findings, but there is also the possibility of subtle nutritional deficiencies.

Total parenteral nutrition (TPN)

Abnormal liver function tests frequently occur within a few weeks of starting TPN. In some cases, there is a fatty liver, perhaps related to carbohydrate excess, but in others, particularly young children, the serum bilirubin and alkaline phosphatase become elevated in a predominantly cholestatic picture. Ursodeoxycholic acid may be of help in the latter (Lindor & Burnes, 1991). In some cases metronidazole appears to be of benefit, perhaps overcoming bacterial contamination of bowel or bile.

Even as short a course as a few weeks of TPN has been found to cause biliary sludging detectable on ultrasound examination, these changes being reversible on stopping the TPN (Messing *et al.*, 1982). Continuation of TPN may lead to gallstones. Provision of enteral stimulation by some oral intake, injections of cholecystokinin to increase gall-bladder contraction, or the use of intravenous amino acids (Zoli *et al.*, 1993), have been proposed in this situation.

Of more significance, is development of inflammatory change, fibrosis, cirrhosis and liver failure in children and adults who require long-term TPN for the short-bowel syndrome. This occurs in only a small percentage of cases. The cause is not clear. There have now been cases of multi-visceral transplantation as a treatment for this condition, though the mortality is still high (Starzl *et al.*, 1989).

Other dietary factors

Certain constituents of food may cause acute or chronic liver injury. This may be due to the hepatotoxin naturally present in a particular foodstuff, or to contamination of the food by toxin or infective agent.

Plants and fungi

Mycotoxins: The mushroom *Amanita phalloides* (death cap) is found throughout Europe. It contains two toxins, amanitotoxin and phalloidin which, even in small doses, can cause severe fatty change and hepatic necrosis leading to fulminant hepatorenal failure.

Aflatoxins are derived from aspergillus following contamination of stored foods and grains and have been demonstrated in food consumed in Africa and Asia. An association between chronic aflatoxin consumption and the development of hepatic tumours has been described in Uganda and Kenya. In animal models, there is a strong relationship between aflatoxin exposure and hepatocellular carcinoma.

Plant alkaloids: In the Caribbean and South America there is a tradition of using 'Bush Tea' and infusion of plants for medicinal purposes. Plants of the genera Crotolaria and Senecio cause centrilobular fibrosis leading to cirrhosis. The incidence of hepatocellular carcinoma in these areas is not high.

Contaminants

Infective agents: Hepatitis A (infective hepatitis) is transmitted by ingestion of contaminated water and foods, particularly seafood. Hepatitis E (endemic non-A, non-B hepatitis) is responsible for outbreaks of oral–faecal transmitted hepatitis in Asia and is thought to be spread by contaminated foodstuffs.

There are various parasitic infestations which occur mainly in under-developed countries, where one stage of the life cycle of the parasite can be transmitted to humans, either in undercooked fish or meat, or in vegetables washed in contaminated water. An example of this is the liver fluke (*Fasciola hepatica*) which can be transmitted by eating contaminated watercress, its usual definitive hosts being sheep and cattle.

Metal: Excessive ingestion of iron, through the use of iron cooking utensils and fermenting beverages in iron pots, is recognised to cause excessive iron deposition within the liver parenchyma. This is best docu-mented as the Bantu hepatic siderosis.

Vitamins

Dietary vitamin A, while essential in moderation, has been implicated in hepatic damage, cirrhosis and portal hypertension, if ingested in excessive amounts for long periods.

Nutritional consequences of liver disease (Table 15.1)

Malnutrition is commonly found in advanced liver cirrhosis, with nausea and anorexia occurring in 55% and 87% of patients respectively (Achord, 1987). However, the majority of work has been carried out in alcoholic liver disease and it is possible that disease-specific changes occur.

Protein

Many of the complications of liver disease are associated with the development of a state of negative nitrogen balance. Clinical studies of metabolism in liver disease have concentrated on patients in a stable compensated state. However, as liver disease advances, most patients spend longer periods of time in a decompensated condition, with hospitalisation,

Table 15.1. *Causes of malnutrition in chronic liver disease*

---

1. *Decreased dietary intake*
   Anorexia, nausea and vomiting due to disease or treatment.
   Iatrogenic dietary restriction during investigations.
   Chronic restrictions on dietary fat, protein or fluid.
   Empty calories of an exclusive diet of ethanol.

2. *Gastrointestinal malabsorption*
   Cholestasis leading to luminal bile salt deficiency.
   Pancreatic insufficiency secondary to alcohol abuse.
   Enteropathy secondary to alcohol abuse.
   Chronic purgation and neomycin treatment.

3. *Negative energy balance*
   Secondary to increased energy consumption, due to liver disease or complications such as sepsis, ascites or bleeding.

4. *Negative protein balance*
   Secondary to increased protein breakdown during periods of decompensation such as listed in 3 above.

5. *Disturbance of normal metabolic homeostasis*
   Altered metabolism of fat, protein and carbohydrate in the fasting and post-prandial state, secondary to hepatocyte damage and hormonal derangement.

---

variceal bleeding, anorexia, sepsis, ascites and encephalopathy all leading to a decrease in protein intake and impaired protein balance.

Studies in protein breakdown give conflicting results, depending to some extent on the methodology used to determine the protein degradation rate. Techniques that use the urinary excretion of the end products of nitrogen metabolism consistently show increased protein breakdown. However, using a representative amino-acid such as leucine to determine the rate of amino-acid oxidation by steady-state tracer techniques, protein degradation rates are normal. Both of these techniques do need standardising against the mass of metabolically active tissue, which is decreased in cirrhosis. When defined per unit of metabolically active tissue, protein degradation is increased regardless of which technique is used (McCullough & Tavill, 1991). This is one reason why chronic liver disease is associated with an increased dietary protein requirement.

On the other side of the protein balance equation, is the synthesis rate of protein: plasma proteins, particularly albumin and clotting factors, are low due to diminished synthesis. Muscle wasting in liver disease may result from decreased protein synthesis (Morrison *et al.*, 1990).

Acute liver diseases such as alcoholic hepatitis and fulminant liver failure, in which tissue injury leads to release of cytokines including tumour necrosis factor and the interleukins, may produce reduced protein synthesis as well as enhanced breakdown (McClain & Cohen, 1989).

Carbohydrate

In patients with cirrhosis, there is altered carbohydrate metabolism, due to the reduced glycogen storage capacity within the liver. The source of fuel is altered and there is rapid development of a catabolic state following an overnight fast, with preferential use of calories from fat instead of from carbohydrate oxidation (Green, Bramley & Losowsky, 1991). This represents the state normally seen in healthy subjects who have have been fasting for a period of 2–3 days (Owen *et al.*, 1983). This is thought to be due to the decreased availability of glucose from liver glycogen, leading to increased gluconeogenesis (and contributing to enhanced wasting of metabolically active tissue) and increased lipolysis and fatty acid oxidation to provide the necessary energy for the fasting patient.

Most patients with chronic liver disease have glucose intolerance. The circulating level of insulin is raised, with increased insulin resistance in the peripheral tissues secondary to decreased binding to insulin receptors and defective post-receptor mechanisms (Petrides & DeFronzo, 1989), together with the antagonistic action of hyperglucagonaemia (Smith-Laing *et al.*, 1980).

Fat

In cholestatic liver disease, delivery of bile salts to the lumen of the small intestine is reduced and hence micelle formation is defective and absorption of fat and fat soluble vitamins diminished. In parenchymal liver disease, defective synthesis of bile salts leads to a similar but milder defect, dependent on the severity of the hepatocellular dysfunction (Walker, Kelleher & Losowsky, 1969).

Plasma lipid concentrations are high in patients with cholestasis, particularly in primary biliary cirrhosis. This probably depends on several mechanisms including diminished biliary lipid excretion, regurgitation of biliary lipid into the blood and diminished hepatic synthesis of the enzyme lecithin – cholesterol acyl transferase (LCAT), which esterifies cholesterol and hence makes it less soluble. Deposition of lipid in the eyelids (xanthelasma) is common: deposition of lipid elsewhere in the skin and in peripheral nerves is much less common (Walker, Kelleher & Losowsky, 1969).

Energy

The use of indirect calorimetry in patients with chronic liver disease has produced conflicting results, probably due to inadequacies in design of the studies. As described above, there is, however, a measure of agreement that the respiratory quotient at rest is lower than normal, indicating preferential use of fat.

Whether or not a patient with chronic liver disease is reported as having increased energy expenditure (EE), appears to depend on how the EE is expressed. When related to lean body mass there is increased EE compared to controls (Schneeweiss *et al.*, 1991; Bramley, Green & Losowsky, 1992); perhaps increased gluconeogenesis contributes to this (Owen *et al.*, 1981). However, the measurement of body composition and hence lean body mass in patients with cirrhosis is fraught with technical difficulties. There are also problems in obtaining well-matched control subjects.

Vitamins

In patients with liver disease, in addition to inadequate intake of the main dietary energy sources, specific deficiencies of micronutrients can occur (Morgan *et al.*, 1976). This may arise from changes directly caused by liver impairment, as well as from inadequate supply due to poor diet or defective absorption.

A study of nutritional parameters in the first one hundred patients undergoing liver transplantation at the Mayo clinic documented the range of vitamin deficiencies found, and of interest was that patients with recent onset of liver disease due to acute hepatitis, as well as patients with non-cholestatic chronic liver disease, had reductions in both water-soluble and fat-soluble vitamins (Dicecco *et al.*, 1989).

Water-soluble vitamins

Deficiencies may occur secondary to reduced dietary intake, increased demand (thiamine), reduced hepatic storage (thiamine, B12, folate, ribo-flavin), reduction in pathways for metabolising vitamins into more active forms (thiamine, B6, B12), reduced production of plasma carrier proteins (folate, B12), or impaired absorption (thiamine – particularly in alcoholics). Drugs, e.g. cholestyramine, taken by the patient to treat complications of liver disease, may interfere with vitamin absorption (ascorbic acid, folate).

Clinical and sub-clinical deficiencies of most water soluble vitamins are documented as much more common in alcoholic than in non-alcoholic liver disease.

Fat-soluble vitamins

Absorption depends on the presence of bile salts within the small intestinal lumen to combine with free fatty acids and monoglycerides to form hydrophilic micelles in which vitamins and cholesterol are dissolved. These are then taken across the mucosal cells. Monoglycerides and fatty acids can be absorbed without the micellar phase. When the delivery of bile salts to the intestinal lumen is reduced, either by cholestasis or liver cell damage, absorption of fatty acids can occur to some extent, but fat-soluble vitamins cannot be absorbed, leading to deficiency states.

Vitamin A: This is taken up from the intestinal lumen as retinol, which is then esterified and transported within chylomicrons, via the lymphatics, finally being stored in the liver. It is released to the tissues bound to retinol-binding protein which is itself bound to pre-albumin.

Vitamin A deficiency can occur in long-standing cholestasis. Reduction in hepatocyte mass can interfere with vitamin A metabolism, as retinol-binding protein production or pre-albumin production is depressed.

Vitamin A deficiency causes impaired glycosylation of proteins, reduction in spermatogenesis, skin rashes, decreased dark adaptation and night blindness. Replacement by regular intramuscular injection is required in chronic cholestasis.

Vitamin D: This deficiency depends on climatic as well as dietary factors. Cholecalciferol (D3) is converted from 7-dehydrocholesterol, by ultraviolet radiation within the skin. If there is sufficient sunlight all the requirements for vitamin D can be met. However, in northern climes, and in people not exposed to sun, dietary sources of D3 are required.

The cholecalciferol (D3) is hydroxylated into more active forms in two stages, to 25 hydroxycholecalciferol in the liver (perhaps surprisingly, this stage is not affected by chronic liver disease) and then to 1–25 dihydroxycholecalciferol in the renal parenchyma. The active 25 OH vitamin D and 1–25 OH_2 vitamin D alter the absorption, release and retention of calcium from the bowel, bone and kidney and, together with parathyroid hormone and calcitonin, regulate calcium and phosphorus homeostasis. Deficiency of vitamin D causes osteomalacia in adults and rickets in children, in which bone matrix (osteoid) remains unmineralised. If micelle formation is reduced, as in cholestatic liver disease, vitamin D supplementation is required. Regular intramuscular injections correct the osteomalacia of cholestatic liver disease, but have no beneficial effect on the usual bone problem of chronic liver disease, which appears to be a low-turnover osteoporosis. The aetiology of this condition is not certain.

Vitamin E: This deficiency is now recognised as being clinically relevant. Vitamin E is an important anti-oxidant, which prevents cellular damage by free radicals, thus having a protective effect in sepsis and other forms of cellular damage.

Long-standing deficiency, as occurs in chronic cholestasis, causes increased red cell fragility and haemolytic anaemia, nerve conduction defects and cerebellar signs, particularly in children.

Vitamin K: This is the first of the fat soluble vitamins to become depleted, due to the small reserves present in the body. It plays a key role in the synthesis of clotting factors II, VII, IX and X.

Deficiency in cholestatic liver disease is common, with prolongation of the prothrombin time, which is readily reversed with intramuscular vitamin K. If, however, there is severe hepatic damage, synthesis of the precursor factors may also be reduced.

Minerals

The liver plays an important role in the metabolism of minerals, as it is the first organ to be perfused by newly absorbed minerals and is responsible for the synthesis of specific carrier proteins or plasma proteins, which bind the minerals for transport around the body. Changes in the synthesis of these carrier proteins can alter the potential toxicity of the mineral. The liver can act as the major storage organ for minerals absorbed in excess. Liver disease can cause total body excess or deficiency of minerals and genetically determined abnormal metabolism of certain minerals can lead to chronic liver disease.

Zinc

Zinc is essential for normal protein metabolism, forms a component of over 200 enzymes and is involved in normal immune function and wound healing (McClain, Kasarkis & Allen, 1985). Zinc deficiency causes a wide variety of dysfunctions including impaired wound healing, the skin lesions and diarrhoea of acrodermatitis enteropathica, hypogonadism, retinal abnormalities and impaired taste leading to anorexia.

Low serum zinc levels have been found in the various types of liver disease (Walker *et al.*, 1973). This may be due to reduced zinc intake, or secondary to reduced protein intake as in alcoholic liver disease. There is also evidence for depressed absorption by the increased production of metallothionein, a zinc-binding protein which blocks uptake by the enterocytes (Cousins & Leinart, 1988).

Selenium

This element appears to function as an anti-oxidant and as part of enzyme systems. There are three forms of selenium found in plasma, glutathione peroxidase and selenoprotein P (both compounds acting as free-radical scavengers) and selenomethionine, which is derived from the diet and has no known physiological function. The measurement of total plasma selenium can therefore be misleading, as the majority is in the form of selenomethionine and a low plasma level probably reflects the preceding diet, rather than a true deficiency state (McClain *et al.*, 1991).

There have been reports noting a reduction in plasma selenium in liver disease, particularly alcoholic liver disease (Thuluvath & Triger, 1987).

Copper

The liver plays a central role in copper metabolism. Fifteen percent of total body copper is stored within the liver, caeruloplasmin produced by the liver is responsible for binding copper in the plasma and excess copper is excreted via the biliary system.

Hepatic toxicity secondary to copper excess is of clinical importance. Wilson's disease, which is an autosomal recessive inherited disorder with a prevalence of approximately 1 in 30 000, causes tissue damage directly as a result of excess tissue copper. The primary defect is located within the liver, as liver transplantation reverses all the abnormalities of copper metabolism. Hepatic copper overload also occurs in the cholestatic liver diseases, such as primary biliary cirrhosis and chronic extrahepatic biliary obstruction.

Iron

The liver plays a central role in the homeostasis of this mineral, producing the iron transport protein transferrin and acting as the major storage organ; the iron being within hepatocytes mainly as ferritin and haemosiderin (Bacon & Tavill, 1984).

Chronic hepatic iron overload results in hepatic fibrosis, cirrhosis and hepatocellular carcinoma. An example of this is haemochromatosis, which is an autosomal dominant inherited disorder, leading to the accumulation of iron throughout the body. As a relationship exists between the amount of excess hepatic iron and the degree of tissue damage, chelation therapy and venesection have proved useful in reducing total body iron and limiting the amount of tissue damage.

Nutritional assessment in liver disease

Nutritional assessment is based on an overview of history (including dietary history), physical signs, pertinent laboratory values and anthropometric measurements. However, liver disease itself and its consequences can directly affect such methods of evaluating nutritional status.

The accumulation of body fluid makes reliance on body weight or body mass indices unreliable, often masking the loss of lean body mass that is characteristic of severe liver disease.

Reductions in plasma albumin and other proteins in liver cirrhosis are a reflection of the decrease in the hepatic synthetic capacity, but may also reflect protein depletion secondary to malnutrition. It is not possible to quantify the contribution of each process.

The immunocompetence of a patient is often taken as an index of nutritional status, lymphocyte counts and skin anergy tests usually being used. The presence of liver disease depresses many of the functional tests of immunocompetence.

Assessment of fat and lean tissue is most useful, if performed serially during the patient's illness. Fat stores can be evaluated using fat fold thicknesses, provided it is appreciated that subclinical oedema may lead to an overestimation. Muscle mass can be estimated using mid-arm muscle circumference.

Advances have been made in the assessment of changes in body composition that occur in chronic liver disease, using techniques such as *in vivo* neutron activation analysis, dual energy X-ray absorptiometry and isotopic labelling of body fluid compartments. These remain research tools.

The presence of ascites has recently been shown to be associated with increased energy expenditure in liver cirrhosis, with the possibility that patients who have significant ascites for prolonged periods of time may develop protein-calorie malnutrition, due to negative energy balance (Dolz *et al.*, 1991).

Principles of nutritional therapy in liver disease

Chronic liver disease

Using standard equations based on body size (Harris–Benedict equation), it is possible to predict resting energy consumption (Harris & Benedict, 1991). Normally, supplying approximately 175% of this value should prevent negative energy balance. However, patients with chronic liver disease can rapidly become catabolic during periods of stress, such as sepsis or bleeding and require increased energy intake at a time when they are least able to tolerate increased enteral nutrition. The importance of preventing negative energy balance is to preserve the lean body mass, because amino acids will be mobilised from muscle for gluconeogenesis, and protein synthesis will decrease during periods of reduced energy intake. It is necessary to supply the energy in a form that is efficiently handled by the body, as a balanced supply of nitrogen and calories to optimise protein synthesis and reduce gluconeogenesis. It may, however, be difficult to supply sufficient protein if the patient develops hepatic encephalopathy and requires a low protein diet to reverse the deterioration in mental function. It is also important not to increase energy intake to such an extent, or in such a form, that fat deposition occurs within hepatocytes, putting further strain on the damaged liver.

Patients with chronic liver disease have a defect in synthesis of hepatic glycogen. For this and other reasons they have impaired glucose tolerance and appropriate dietary manipulation is indicated.

Of total energy requirements, 40–50% should be provided by carbohydrate either enterally (preferably as high fibre foods) or parenterally (Munoz, 1991). It may be necessary to use insulin to maintain normoglycaemia.

Some patients may be intolerant of fat, particularly those with cholestatic liver disease with associated steatorrhoea. However, most patients can tolerate an unrestricted fat diet. Attention must be paid to the possibility of deficiencies of fat-soluble vitamins. In cholestatic liver disease parenteral administration is necessary. If parenteral feeding is required, then non-protein calories are most appropriately supplied by dextrose and lipid infusions, with insulin as required. Using intravenous lipid has the advantage that this is metabolised extrahepatically and provides high energy content in low volume.

Most well compensated patients in an early stage of their disease, without any recent complications, are in reasonable nitrogen balance, and have normal protein requirements. These patients do not require protein restriction. Patients who are malnourished and affected by complications are almost certainly in negative nitrogen balance. Those with hepatic encephalopathy may be unable to tolerate a normal protein intake. The policy in these patients is to start at a low protein intake, 20–40 g protein per day, and increase every other day in 10–20 g increments, until the development or worsening of encephalopathy. Using such regimes, with the protein supplied as part of enteral feeding (Smith *et al.*, 1982), or as parenteral nutrition, it is usually possible to increase protein intake to over 100 g per day, even in patients awaiting liver transplantation (Munoz, 1991).

Branched chain amino-acids (BCAA) have been extensively studied as treatment for hepatic encephalopathy. There are theoretical reasons why they may be advantageous in the nutritional support of patients with chronic liver disease who are unable to tolerate standard protein. BCAA inhibit muscle protein breakdown and increase the synthesis of hepatic and muscle proteins and as a protein precursor act as an energy source for muscle. However, the studies which have reported the use of BCAA as a nutritional therapy are divided on the efficacy compared to standard protein diets (Weber *et al.*, 1990). As they are expensive (10–14 times the equivalent standard protein) and the case for these supplements is not proven, more detailed clinical trials over longer periods need to be undertaken.

Other forms of protein in the diet have been investigated. Vegetable protein diets have been used in resistant encephalopathy, but the evidence for improved mental status is not conclusive. The unpalatability of a vegetable protein-based diet of over 50 g protein per day, the gastro-intestinal intolerance and increased stool output, render these diets impracticable (Weber *et al.*, 1985). Casein based diets are useful in providing high caloric content (1500 to 2000 kcal/litre) and high nitrogen (60 to 70 g protein/litre) content in low volumes and are particularly useful for patients requiring fluid restriction. They have the advantage of easy absorption from enteral tube feeding.

Ascites and oedema are common manifestations of fluid retention in patients with chronic liver disease. At the time of active accumulation of fluid such patients excrete very little of the dietary salt intake and retain water accordingly. Severe salt restriction stops further fluid accretion. In the minority of patients who develop marked hyponatraemia, fluid restriction is also required. Diuretics are necessary, in addition, to clear excess fluid.

Fulminant hepatic failure (FHF)

These patients demonstrate rapid onset of muscle loss and protein-energy malnutrition. The metabolic consequences of FHF are not well character-ised. Profound hypoglycaemia may occur, requiring large amounts of concentrated dextrose solutions to maintain normoglycaemia. This may be related to the inability of the liver to maintain any significant glycogen reserves and reduction in gluconeogenesis, due to loss of active liver cell mass.

Lipid and dextrose infusions form the mainstay of calorie support (Forbes *et al.*, 1987), supplying approximately 35 to 50 kcal/kg body weight per day; with amino-acid solutions providing the equivalent nitrogen content of 40 to 60 g/protein per day. There have been few controlled trials in this condition, but the rationale of providing sufficient calories and protein to prevent lean tissue loss is the same as for patients with chronic liver disease.

Conclusion

It has become increasingly recognised that the nutritional status of a patient with liver disease has important implications for prognosis and treatment.

With the increasing indications for liver transplantation in liver disease of whatever aetiology, acute as well as chronic, the challenge to maintain the patient in the best possible nutritional state has never been greater.

References

Achord, J. L, (1987). Malnutrition and the role of nutritional support in alcoholic liver disease. *American Journal of Gastroenterology*, **82**, 1–7.

Bacon, B. R. & Tavill, A. S. (1984). Role of the liver in normal iron metabolism. *Seminars in Liver Disease*, **4**, 181–92.

Bramley, P. N., Green, J. H. & Losowsky, M. S. (1992). The incidence of hypermetabolism in liver cirrhosis of different aetiologies. *Hepatology*, **16** (2), 518 [Abst].

Cook, G. C. & Hutt, M. S. R. (1967). The liver after Kwashiorkor. *British Medical Journal*, **3**, 454–7.

Cousins, R. J. & Leinart, A. S. (1988). Tissue-specific regulation of zinc metabolism and metallothionein genes by interleukin 1. *FASEB Journal*, **2**, 2884–90.

Dicecco, S. R., Weiners, E. J., Weisner, R. H. et al. (1989). Assessment of nutritional status in patients with end-stage liver disease undergoing liver transplantation. *Proceedings of the Mayo Clinic*, **65**, 95–102.

Dolz, C., Raurich, J. M., Ibanez et al. (1991). Ascites increases the resting energy expenditure in liver cirrhosis. *Gastroenterology*, **100**, 738–44

Forbes, A., Wicks, C., Marshall, W. et al. (1987). Nutritional support in fulminant hepatic failure: The safety of lipid solutions. *Gut*, **28**, A1347–8.

Galambos, J. T. (1976). Jejuneal bypass and nutritional liver injury. *Archives of Pathology and Laboratory Medicine*, **100**, 229–31.

Green, J. H., Bramley, P. N. & Losowsky, M. S. (1919). Are patients with primary biliary cirrhosis hypermetabolic? A comparison between patients before and after liver transplantation and controls. *Hepatology*, **14**, 464–72.

Harris, J. A. & Benedict, F. G. (1991). A biometric study of basal metabolism in man. Washington DC: Carnegie Institute Publications, **279**, 1–266.

Himsworth, H. P. (1947). *Lectures on the Liver and its Diseases*. Blackwell, Oxford.

Lelbach, W. K. (1985). Continental Europe. In *Alcoholic Liver Disease*, 1st edn, ed. P. Hall. pp. 130–42. Edward Arnold Ltd, London.

Lindor, K. D. & Burnes, J. (1991). Ursodeoxycholic acid for the treatment of home parenteral nutrition-associated cholestasis. *Gastroenterology*, **101**, 250–3.

McClain, C. J., Kasarkis, E. J. & Allen, I. J. (1985). Functional consequences of zinc deficiency. *Progress in Food Nutrition Science*, **19**, 185–226.

McClain, C. J. & Cohen, D. A. (1989). Increased TNF production by monocytes in alcoholic hepatitis. *Hepatology*, **9**, 349–51.

McClain, C. J., Marsano, L., Burk, R. & Bacon, B. (1991). Trace metals in liver disease. *Seminars in Liver Disease*, **11**, 321–39.

McCullough, A. J. & Tavill, A. S. (1991). Disordered energy and protein metabolism in liver disease. *Seminars in Liver Disease*, **11**, 265–77.

Marubbio, A. T., Buchwald, H., Schwartz, M. Z. & Varco, R. (1976). Hepatic lesions of central pericellular fibrosis in morbid obesity and following jejunoileal bypass. *American Journal of Clinical Pathology*, **66**, 684–91.

Messing, B., Bories, C., Kunstlinger, F. & Bernier, J. J. (1982). Does parenteral nutrition induce a lithogenic gallbladder bile? *Journal of Parenteral & Enteral Nutrition*, **5**, 560.

Morgan, A. G., Kelleher, J., Walker, B. E. et al. (1976). Nutrition in cryptogenic cirrhosis and chronic aggressive hepatitis. *Gut*, **17**, 113–18.

Morrison, W. L., Bouchier, I. A. D., Gibson, J. N. A. & Rennie, M. J. (1990). Skeletal muscle and whole body protein turnover in cirrhosis. *Clinical Science*, **78**, 613–19.

Munoz, S. J. (1991). Nutritional therapies in liver disease. *Seminars in Liver Disease*, **11**, 278–91.

Owen, O. E., Reichle, F. A., Mozzoli, M. A. et al. (1981). Hepatic, gut and renal substrate flux rates in patients with hepatic cirrhosis. *Journal of Clinical Investigation*, **68**, 240–52.

Owen, O. E., Trapp, V. E., Reichard, G. A. et al. (1983). Nature and quantity of fuels consumed in patients with alcoholic cirrhosis. *Journal of Clinical Investigation*, **72**, 1821–32.

Pequignot, G. & Tuyns, A. J. (1980). Compared toxicity of ethanol on various organs. In *Alcohol and the Gastro-intestinal Tract*, ed. C. Stock & H. Sarles, Paris: INSERM, **85**, 17–32.

Petrides, A. S. & DeFronzo, R. A. (1989). Glucose and insulin metabolism in cirrhosis. *Journal of Hepatology*, **8**, 107–14.

Schneeweiss, B., Graninger, W., Ferenci, P. *et al.* (1991). Energy metabolism in patients with acute and chronic liver disease. *Hepatology*, **11**, 387–93.

Smith, J., Horowitz, J., Henderson, J. M. *et al.* (1982). Enteral hyperalimentation in undernourished patients with cirrhosis and ascites. *American Journal of Clinical Nutrition*, **35**, 56–72.

Smith-Laing, G., Orskov, H., Gore, M. B. R. *et al.* (1980). Hyperglycemia in cirrhosis. *Diabetologia*, **19**, 103–8.

Starzl, E. T., Rowe, M. I., Todo, S. *et al.* (1989). Transplantation of multiple organ viscera. *Journal of the American Medical Association*, **261**, 1449–57.

Thuluvath, P. J. & Triger, D. R. (1987). Selenium in primary biliary cirrhosis. *Lancet*, **ii**, 219.

Walker, B. E., Kelleher, J. & Losowsky, M. S. (1969). The steatorrhoea of chronic liver disease without jaundice. *Scandinavian Journal of Gastroenterology*, **4**, 341–4.

Walker, B. E., Dawson, J. B., Kelleher, J. *et al.* (1973). Plasma and urinary zinc in patients with malabsorption syndromes or hepatic cirrhosis. *Gut*, **14**, 943–8.

Weber, F. L., Minco, D., Fresard, K. M. *et al.* (1985). Effects of vegetable diets on nitrogen metabolism in cirrhotic subjects. *Gastroenterology*, **85**, 538–44.

Weber, F. L., Bagby, B. S., Licate, L. *et al.* (1990). Effects of branched chain Amino-acids on nitrogen metabolism in patients with cirrhosis. *Hepatology*, **11**, 942–50.

Zoli, G., Ballinger, Anne, Healy, Jeremiah *et al.* (1993). Promotion of gallbladder emptying by intravenous amino acids. *Lancet*, **341**, 1240–1.

16

Nutritional deficiencies in inflammatory bowel disease

P. DUANE AND R. V. HEATLEY

Ulcerative colitis (UC) and Crohn's disease (CD) are the disorders collectively referred to as inflammatory bowel disease (IBD). The inflammation in ulcerative colitis is superficial, being confined to the mucosal surface except in the most severe cases and affects the large bowel alone. Unlike ulcerative colitis, the inflammation in Crohn's disease is not necessarily continuous and areas of ulceration may be interspersed by relatively normal mucosa. Crohn's disease can affect any part of the intestine from the mouth to the anus, although the most common site to be involved is the terminal ileum. The inflammatory process extends deep to the mucosal surface and can affect all layers of the gut wall. The ulceration heals by fibrosis which may lead to stricture formation. When deep, the ulceration can cause fissures and eventually fistulae between affected areas of bowel and adjacent organs, or skin.

While the presentation and pathological processes of these two diseases are different, the effects on the nutritional status of the patient are often quite similar yet frequently distinct. During prolonged or severe exacerbations of their disease patients can become obviously wasted. Chronic undernourishment is, however, more commonly seen in Crohn's disease (CD) (Harries et al., 1982a; Harries & Heatley, 1986). Weight loss and emaciation were major clinical features in the original description of Crohn's disease (Crohn, Ginzburg and Oppenheimer, 1932). In chronic CD, weight loss has been reported in several series to affect up to 70–80% of patients. (Crohn & Yarnis, 1958; Mekhjian et al., 1979). Even patients with CD who are not acutely ill, may have a considerable degree of undernutrition. About 20% of 106 unselected, consecutive outpatients with CD were below 90% of their ideal weight (Harries et al., 1982a). Lanfranchi et al. (1982) found that 40% of 44 outpatients with CD were below ideal weight.

350

Table 16.1. *Prevalence of nutritional insufficiency in Crohn's disease*[a]

	Prevalence (%)
Weight loss	65–75
Hypoalbuminaemia	25–80
Intestinal protein loss	65–80
Negative nitrogen balance	55–75
Anaemia	
Iron deficiency	35–50
Folate deficiency	50–65
B12 deficiency	35–45
Calcium deficiency	10–20
Magnesium deficiency	14–35
Potassium deficiency	5–20
Zinc deficiency	40–55
Vitamin C deficiency	10–30
Vitamin D deficiency	60–80
Vitamin K deficiency	10–25

[a] Reference Russell, 1991.

The range of nutritional disturbances found in patients with IBD is wide. Undernourished patients are at risk of multiple deficiencies (Table 16.1) which can have significant effects on the patients in response to their illness or any therapeutic intervention. In common with other chronic illnesses, undernourished patients with inflammatory bowel disease are probably more prone to complications such as poor wound healing, depressed cellular and humoral immunity and increased susceptibility to infections. Furthermore, many of these complications will remit with nutritional therapy alone. Unfortunately, however, the importance of nutritional factors in individual patients with inflammatory bowel disease, except in extreme cases, is frequently ignored by physicians and surgeons alike. Difficulties in recognising the extent of the nutritional deficiencies and equivocal evidence that giving nutritional treatment actually affects the long-term outcome of the disease, undoubtedly are some of the reasons which may account for these omissions.

Pathogenesis of malnutrition

The multiple aetiological factors involved in the development of malnutrition are outlined in Table 16.2. Frequently more than one factor is

Table 16.2. *Aetiological factors involved in the development of malnutrition*

Inadequate food intake	Anorexia (disease/drugs)
	Fear of eating from abdominal pain
	Restrictive diet
Increased requirements	Fever
	Sepsis
	Fistulae
	Surgery
	Increased intestinal cell turnover
	Rapid gastrointestinal transit
Increased intestinal losses	Blood loss
	Protein losing enteropathy
	Bile salt losing enteropathy
	Electrolytes, minerals, trace elements
Malabsorption	Extensive disease
	Extensive resection (short bowel syndrome)
	Disturbed enterohepatic circulation (ileal resection)
	Bacterial overgrowth (fistulae, strictures)
	Small intestine bypass (fistulae)
	Drugs
	Corticosteroids (calcium)
	Sulphasalazine (folate)
	Cholestyramine (fat and fat soluble vitamins)

responsible at any one time. The most important causes of malnutrition are probably reduced food intake, active inflammation and enteric loss of nutrients. Such factors take on more importance at times when the disease is active.

Protein-calorie malnutrition

Longstanding inadequate calorie intake leading to growth retardation, is particularly important in children and adolescents with IBD (Seidman *et al.*, 1991; Seidman, 1989). Growth abnormalities often dominate the clinical picture with up to a third of paediatric patients having depressed linear growth prior to the onset of gastrointestinal symptoms (O'Donoghue & Dawson, 1977; Homer, Grand & Colodny, 1977). Abnormalities in growth pattern are generally accompanied by delays in sexual maturation. Increased energy expenditure associated with active inflammation has been thought to be one cause of weight loss in patients with CD. Although, predictably, patients with the lowest weights when expressed as percentages of ideal body weight, had the greatest resting energy expenditure per kilogram of body weight, most CD patients without fever or sepsis do not have increased resting energy expenditure (Chan *et al.*, 1986). It is likely, therefore, that decreased growth is an adaptive response to longstanding caloric restriction (Motil *et al.*, 1982). This insufficient intake is often attributed to anorexia caused by the presence of a chronic illness or fear of precipitating abdominal pain. Certainly, the growth retardation can be reversed with total parenteral nutrition (Strobel, Byrne & Ament, 1979) or by therapy with oral supplementation using either an elemental (Seidman *et al.*, 1987) or polymeric diet (Kirschner *et al.*, 1981; Harries *et al.*, 1983; Kirschner, Voinchet & Rosenberg, 1978). Surgery to resect localised disease in CD often allows a symptom-free period when nutrient intake may be markedly increased and can result in improved growth (McLain *et al.*, 1990; Davies *et al.*, 1990).

It has recently been suggested that the chronic elevation of cytokines, such as tumour necrosis factor (TNF)-α, as occurs in active inflammatory bowel disease, may be factors contributing to the anorexia and growth failure (MacDonald *et al.*, 1990). Cytokines are known to have a direct effect on the appetite centres in the central nervous system (Plata-Salaman, Oomura & Kai, 1988). They may also effect peripheral signals to the feeding centres, since TNF-α leads to a transient inhibition of gastric emptying (Patton *et al.*, 1987). The results of studies looking at TNF-α in IBD at present are contradictory. One showed elevated serum levels of TNF-α in active disease (Murch *et al.*, 1991) while another did not (Hyams *et al.*, 1991). The conflicting findings in these studies may have been due to different techniques in preparing the serum and in the method of analysis. It is, however, becoming increasingly clear that cytokines released during inflammation have major metabolic effects (Evans, Argiles & Williamson, 1989; Wan, Haw & Blackburn, 1989), and thus can directly influence nutritional status (Ramadori *et al.*, 1988; Audus *et al.*, 1988; Duane *et al.*, 1991).

Major loss of body protein mass in IBD is less common than weight loss, which is more attributable to loss of body water and fat (Powell-Tuck, 1986). Hypoalbuminaemia, on the other hand, is a very common finding in patients with IBD. Such low serum albumin concentrations are, however not necessarily related to protein undernutrition. Gastrointestinal protein loss is probably the most important cause of hypoproteinaemia (Beeken, Bursch & Sylwester, 1972), although increased catabolism, due to disease activity and reduced hepatic albumin synthesis, may contribute (Powell-Tuck, 1986).

Changes in whole-body protein turnover in inflammatory bowel disease, which can result in a negative nitrogen balance, occur because of a generalised effect on several tissues within the body. Increase in whole-body protein synthesis and breakdown correlate with disease activity (Powell-Tuck *et al.*, 1984) which will have major adverse effects on protein metabolism (Silk & Payne-James, 1989). It is important to realise that large losses of nitrogen will occur in patients with IBD treated with corticosteroids in the absence of adequate protein intake (O'Keefe *et al.*, 1989).

Fat and carbohydrate absorption

Malabsorption of fat is a common finding in patients with Crohn's disease, occurring in up to a third of patients (Heatley, 1986). The degree of steatorrhoea is determined by the extent of small bowel involvement in Crohn's disease and the extent of any surgical small bowel resection (Lenz, 1975). The loss of bile acids because of extensive involvement or resection of the terminal ileum in severe Crohn's disease will add to malabsorption of fats and fat soluble vitamins. Furthermore, malabsorption of bile acids is a significant physiological factor in the pathogenesis of diarrhoea in CD (Krag & Krag, 1976).

Dietary carbohydrate malabsorption is seldom severe enough to produce undernourishment. Malabsorbed carbohydrate passes into the colon where it undergoes bacterial fermentation to short-chain fatty acids and gas. There, short-chain fatty acids, particularly butyrate, are preferentially used by colonic enterocytes as a fuel source (Rombeau & Kripke, 1990).

Anaemia

Anaemia is a common finding in patients with IBD and can affect over three quarters of patients with Crohn's disease. Frequently the anaemia is multifactorial due to deficiencies of haematinics, or simply due to chronic inflammation (Harries & Heatley, 1983; Heatley, 1986). Iron and folate deficiency anaemia occurs in both CD and UC, whereas B_{12} deficiency occurs only in CD (Table 16.3).

Electrolyte deficiencies

Hypokalaemia can occur in association with profuse diarrhoea. Hyponatraemia and hypochloraemia are uncommon but can become major problems in patients with short bowel syndrome, extensive small bowel involvement, or high small bowel fistulae in CD. Anorexia in patients

Table 16.3. *Anaemia in inflammatory bowel disease*

Type	Causes	UC	CD
Iron deficiency	Inadequate intake	$\pm$	$+$
	Bacterial overgrowth	$-$	$+$
	Small bowel resection	$-$	$+$
	Blood loss	$+$	$+$
Folic acid	Inadequate intake	$\pm$	$+$
	Increased utilisation	$+$	$+$
	Sulphasalazine	$+$	$+$
B_{12}	Bacterial overgrowth	$-$	$+$
	Ileal resection	$-$	$+$
	Extensive ileal disease	$-$	$+$
Anaemia of chronic disease	Chronic inflammation	$+$	$+$

with active IBD may interfere with the normal thirst response to electrolyte deficiency and so cause dehydration. Low serum calcium levels are usually associated with hypoalbuminaemia, thus true hypocalcaemia is uncommon. Calcium balance in CD does not appear to be associated with intestinal fat excretion, D-xylose malabsorption, bacterial colonisation of the jejunum, or glucocorticosteroid therapy (Krawitt, Beeken & Janney, 1976). Hypomagnesaemia in ill patients on the other hand is very common, occurring in over 80% of patients as judged by serum and urine levels (Main *et al.*, 1981).

Minerals and trace elements

Zinc deficiency has been implicated in the anorexia, poor wound healing and impaired growth which occurs in patients with Crohn's disease (Aggett & Harries, 1979). Although low plasma zinc levels may be found in up to 40% of patients (Harries & Heatley, 1983), the low levels may simply reflect the reduced serum albumin, as serum zinc correlates well with serum albumin concentrations (Sturniolo *et al.*, 1980). The true extent of zinc deficiency remains unclear because of a lack of any reliable way of assessing zinc status. Impaired ^{65}Zn Cl_{12} absorption in patients with IBD is evident only in undernourished persons with moderate or severe disease activity, biochemical evidence of zinc deficiency has been reported to be uncommon, and clinical features of zinc depletion are not usually encountered (Valberg *et al.*, 1986).

Deficiencies of other trace elements such as copper (Fujita *et al.*, 1989) and selenium (Reeves *et al.*, 1989) have been described in patients with CD, but these are very rare and virtually confined to patients receiving inadequate total parenteral nutrition.

Vitamin deficiencies

Overt osteomalacia due to vitamin D deficiency is rare in IBD, being reported in 5% of patients with Crohn's disease (Cooke, 1972). While it is likely that 25-hydroxy D_3 is lost through an interrupted enterohepatic circulation in CD, levels of the active metabolite, 1.25 dihydroxy D_3 are kept within normal range by the action of parathormone due to secondary hyperparathyroidism (Harries *et al.*, 1982*b*).

It has been emphasised, however, that attempts should be made to improve the vitamin D nutrition of patients with CD who are significantly undernourished (mid-arm circumference below 90% of the ideal standard), as it is these patients who are most likely to have secondary hyperparathyroidism and thus be at risk of vitamin D deficiency (Harries *et al.*, 1985). Furthermore, even in the face of normal vitamin D metabolism, patients with small bowel resection show markedly reduced trabecular bone mass and therefore have increased risk of spontaneous fractures (Hessov *et al.*, 1984).

Deficiencies of water soluble B vitamins producing syndromes resembling beriberi and pellagra have been described in patients with Crohn's disease (Harries & Heatley, 1983). Vitamin C supplements have been shown to improve T-cell hypofunction in patients with CD (Animashaun *et al.*, 1990). Whether this influence was nutritional could not be ascertained as lymphocyte ascorbic acid measurements were not available and none of the patients was vitamin C 'deficient' when plasma levels were compared to normal values. It has been suggested that patients with CD have an accelerated demand for vitamin C and, indeed, scurvy with low leucocyte ascorbate levels has been reported (Linaker, 1979). Low serum or leucocyte ascorbate levels are relatively common in patients with active or inactive CD and these abnormalities are due in part to the reduced intake of dietary ascorbate (Imes *et al.*, 1986). Patients with fistulae appear to be unable to concentrate as much ascorbate in their diseased intestine as patients without fistulae (Pettit & Irving, 1987). It has been suggested that ascorbate deficiency could be a factor in the pathogenesis of fistula formation because of the importance of ascorbate in collagen synthesis. However, recent evidence suggests that ascorbic acid absorption is normal in patients with both fistulating and non-fistulating Crohn's disease, thus routine supplements of vitamin C are not necessary unless oral intake is low (Pettit *et al.*, 1989).

Vitamin A deficiency is also associated with disease activity in CD. It does not appear to be related to vitamin B_{12} absorption, to the localization of disease or to previous ileal resection (Schoelmerich *et al.*, 1985). Nutritional amblyopia has been reported in a patient with Crohn's disease (Iansek and Edge, 1985), and it has been suggested that patients with extensive small bowel CD who are less than 80% of ideal weight should have plasma retinol measured. Those who have plasma retinol concentrations less than 0.8 µmol/l (less than 22.9 micrograms %) run a high risk of night blindness and it has been recommended they should be given vitamin supplements (Main *et al.*, 1983).

Effects of drugs

Certain drugs used in the treatment of IBD can also have undesirable side effects which will add to the malabsorption of nutrients. Sulphasalazine reduces folate absorption (Franklin & Rosenberg, 1973). Broad spectrum antibiotics, used to treat secondary infections in patients with IBD, can cause diarrhoea and may add to the patient's anorexia. Upper abdominal discomfort, a well recognised side effect of sulphasalazine and cortico-steroids, may adversely affect the patient's ability to eat sufficient nourishment in the face of increased demands. Olsalazine, the azo-linked dimer of 5-aminosalicylic acid is of proven value in the management of patients with UC, but can cause diarrhoea in a significant number of patients (Wadworth and Fitton, 1991). This diarrhoea is distinguishable from that usually associated with inflammatory bowel disease by the high water content and absence of blood, and may cause problems in patients with inadequate fluid intake. Corticosteroids, which are known to suppress absorption of calcium, may have important effects on bone formation. Corticosteroids also increase the rate of protein metabolism. This, how-ever, occurs at the expense of body protein stores, with substantial losses of nitrogen (O'Keefe *et al.*, 1989). Those patients with significant under-nourishment (Harries *et al.*, 1985), or small bowel resection (Hessov *et al.*, 1984), appear to be particularly at risk. Cholestyramine, a bile salt chelating agent, used to treat bile salt-related diarrhoea in patients with ileal resection or extensive ileal involvement due to CD, may put such patients at a greater risk of developing significant steatorrhoea and fat soluble vitamin malabsorption. Osteomalacia and, on rare occasions, a haemorrhagic diathesis, are both reported with cholestyramine impairment of vitamin D and vitamin K absorption, respectively (Knodel and Talbert, 1987; Hathcock, 1985).

Treatment of nutritional deficiencies

It is clear that it is important to recognise nutritional disturbances in patients with IBD, in order that nutritional support can be instituted early in the course of their illness (Heatley, 1988). Patients with CD, particularly, should be monitored for signs of undernutrition. High risk patients are those who relapse frequently and require repeated courses of cortico-steroids, who have had small bowel surgical resections, or who have complications such as strictures, fistulae or abscesses. Prophylactic parenteral B_{12} is required in patients with extensive ileal disease or those who have had resection of the terminal ileum for CD. In most cases undernutrition can be avoided, or corrected, if adequate intake of nutrients is maintained. Diet counselling (Imes, Pinchbeck & Thompson, 1988) or supplementing a normal diet with high calorie and high protein liquid feeds (Harries *et al.*, 1983), will help those at risk of undernutrition. The severely undernourished patient with IBD may require more intensive nutritional therapy with total parenteral nutrition (TPN) or total enteral nutrition (TEN) with liquid diets.

Nutritional support is frequently supplied temporarily as an adjunct to conventional medical or surgical therapy. However, as treatment failures may be due to nutritional deficiencies, limiting the body's immune responses and reparative processes, considerable interest has now developed in the application of nutritional support as primary treatment to facilitate disease remission. It is extremely difficult to make an objective analysis of the numerous trials and papers on the value or otherwise of nutritional therapy in IBD, as these are often non-randomised, retro-spective reviews of prospective studies on small numbers of patients. Total nutritional therapy, which is invariably expensive, complex and labour-intensive as compared to drug therapy, is frequently restricted to patients who are resistant to other forms of medical therapy, particularly steroids. Patients with IBD, especially CD, are a very heterogeneous group which limits the evaluation of therapy (Kirsner, 1990). Concerns have also been expressed as to the appropriate control group in trials of nutritional therapy (Matuchansky, 1986; Powell-Tuck *et al.*, 1986; Lennard-Jones, 1992). In spite of these reservations, important facts on the value of nutritional therapy in IBD are emerging.

For patients with acute ulcerative colitis, nutritional support is limited

Table 16.4. *Total parenteral nutrition versus enteral diets in Crohn's disease*[a]

Series (n)	Patients	Remission <3 months	Remission 12 months
TPN $(n = 24)$[a]	637	68%	48%
TEN $(n = 17)$[a]	448	67%	49%

[a] Reference Greenberg, 1992.

Table 16.5. *Enteral diets versus prednisolone in Crohn's disease*[a]

		Elemental or polymeric diet	
	Prednisolone 0.5–0.75 mg/kg/day	Total number	After withdrawal for non-palatability
Patients	146	163	129
Remission	119 (81%)	93 (57%)	93 (72%)

[a] Reference Greenberg, 1992.

to a supportive role. When drug treatment fails in severe ulcerative colitis, remission rates are not influenced by concurrent administration of TPN or TEN (Greenberg, 1992). In contrast, there is evidence to support the role of TPN or TEN as adjunctive or primary therapy in Crohn's disease. Medical therapy, although effective in the majority of patients in achieving remission in active CD, is unsatisfactory in the long term. Relapse after therapy with corticosteroids occurs in 62%–80% of patients within one year (Summers *et al.*, 1979; Malchow *et al.*, 1984). In those who relapse, repeated treatment with high doses of corticosteroids increases the risk of serious side effects (O'Keefe *et al.*, 1989). Furthermore, medical therapy does not improve nutritional status. Alternative therapy, in particular nutritional therapy, has therefore been advocated for the acute phase of CD (Tables 16.4 and 16.5).

Available information now seems to suggest that most of the benefits of TPN in CD are related to the improvement in nutritional status rather than a primary therapy. Its use should therefore be restricted to the treatment of specific complications of CD, such as intestinal obstruction related to stricture formation, or short bowel syndrome following repeated resection (Perry, Hanft and Chzanowski, 1990; Silk, 1992).

Increased use of enteral formulae can be expected in the future management of IBD. Enteral nutrition costs less than parenteral nutrition, maintains gut integrity and stimulates immunocompetence (Lowen, Greene and McClave, 1992). Components of the diet which may have particular relevance to mucosal immunity and the pathogenesis of IBD include polyunsaturated fatty acids, nucleotides and amino acids such as glutamine and arginine (Seidman *et al.*, 1991). Preliminary studies on the use of dietary supplements of marine-oil-derived omega-3 fatty acids, have also indicated a beneficial effect in IBD patients (Lorenz *et al.*, 1989; O'Morain *et al.*, 1989).

It is becoming accepted that active CD patients remit, in the short-term, with TEN whether this is in the form of an elemental diet (O'Morain, Segal & Levi, 1984), or polymeric diet (Rigaud *et al.*, 1991). However, much controversy still surrounds such nutritional therapy, as there are doubts about the efficacy of TEN compared to conventional drug therapy and little is known about the long-term effects of TEN (Clark, 1986; Rhodes & Rose, 1986; Whittaker, 1987; Singleton, 1991). The European Co-operative Crohn's Disease (ECCD) study group have found that a regimen of drug treatment with corticosteroids or a combination of corticosteroids and sulphasalazine, is better than a polymeric diet at inducing remission in patients with active CD (Lochs *et al.*, 1991).

Some doubt exists over the efficacy of a polymeric diet compared to an elemental one, as a recent study found that a polymeric diet did not offer an effective therapeutic alternative to an elemental diet (Giaffer, North & Holdsworth, 1990). Although the findings of this study have been questioned (Klein, 1990), available evidence favours elemental diets as long as they are tolerated by the patient. Elemental diets have been shown to help refractory CD patients or those dependent on corti-costeroids (O'Brien *et al.*, 1991). Furthermore, elemental feeding reverses growth arrest while decreasing corticosteroid requirements and CD activity index in paediatric CD patients prior to puberty (Sanderson *et al.*, 1987a; Belli *et al.*, 1988), improves altered intestinal permeability (Sanderson *et al.*, 1987b; Teahon *et al.*, 1991), and reduces gastrointestinal protein and lymphocyte loss from diseased intestine (Logan *et al.*, 1981). The beneficial effects are likely to be restricted to the short term, with high relapse rates by one year, this being particularly so in patients with distal Crohn's proctocolitis and fistulae (Teahon *et al.*, 1990).

Despite its efficacy and lack of serious side effects, elemental diet is not widely used for treatment of active CD. So far, the only consistently mentioned adverse effect limiting treatment with elemental diets has been their poor palatability. This can be improved by serving the drinks ice cold with a straw. There are also many flavours available which can be added according to the patient's taste (Teahon & Levi, 1989). In the very ill patients, who cannot tolerate the volumes required and in those who are unwilling to drink it, fine bore nasogastric tube feeding may be required. Furthermore, it has been shown that it is safe to administer undiluted, hypertonic, elemental diets by constant nasogastric infusion, thus leading to increased nutrient intake and improved nitrogen balance (Rees *et al.*, 1986). Scepticism based on a lack of understanding as to how elemental diets exert a therapeutic effect (Rhodes & Rose, 1986) is, no doubt, another reason why such diets have not been universally accepted.

An elemental diet is made up of oligosaccharides, amino acids and short-chain fatty acids and no normal food is usually given concurrently. The beneficial effects may therefore be related to removal of antigenic load from food proteins, but also probably from modifications of intestinal flora (Boumous & Devroede, 1974). Bowel rest does not appear to be a significant factor (Greenberg *et al.*, 1988). Restoration of the integrity of inflamed intestinal mucosa has been suggested as a possible mechanism by which elemental diet achieves remission in active CD (Teahon *et al.*, 1991; Lowen, Greene & McClave, 1992). This may be due to the provision of glutamine, an amino acid which is a crucial fuel substrate in time of stress for enterocytes and lymphocytes (Dudrick & Souba, 1991). Glutamine is a very important energy substrate for the small bowel. It can be utilised from the arterial or luminal side of the intestinal epithelium and therefore has important implications in small bowel metabolism (Heatley & Johnson, 1988). Current TPN solutions are glutamine free, which may explain in part the development of villous atrophy in patients receiving long-term TPN (O'Dwyer *et al.*, 1989). Short-chain fatty acids, another component of elemental diets, are an important fuel source for colonic enterocytes (Rombeau & Kripke, 1990), and may therefore promote healing of the large bowel (Culpepper-Morgan & Floch, 1991).

Dietary restrictions

Because of the relapsing nature of their disease, patients with IBD frequently inquire whether certain food should be avoided, or, because of misguided advice, adopt unusual dietary habits. Studies have shown that patients with UC and CD consume a lower residue diet than controls

(Gilat *et al.*, 1987). Women in particular, have poorer diets than men and consume less meat than the general population (Gee *et al.*, 1985). Patients with CD tend to eat more refined sugar and less raw fruit and vegetables than controls (Thornton, Emmett & Heaton, 1979). A large multi-centre prospective study found, however, no clear difference in the clinical course of CD among patients randomly allocated to a diet unrestricted in sugar and low in fibre or a diet with little or no sugar and increased fibre (Richie *et al.*, 1987).

Low-residue diets have been recommended for patients with obstructive symptoms due to stricturing CD, without much scientific evidence to back up such dietary restriction (Levenstein *et al.*, 1985). Low fat diets, in contrast, may be effective therapy for regulation of steatorrhoea following small bowel excisional surgery for CD (Andersson *et al.*, 1982). If such dietary restrictions are used, it is important to replace the calories from other sources such as medium chain triglycerides, or protein, or carbo-hydrate supplementation, to ensure the diet remains nutritionally adequate (Russell, 1991).

Lactose intolerance has been implicated in the diarrhoea associated with IBD and thus restriction in lactose intake has been advised in patients with IBD. However, in CD, lactose deficiency has been found to be rare and thus lactose restriction should not be routinely recommended for patients with CD (Park, Duncan & Russell, 1990). Exclusion and elimination diets have been suggested as a valuable way in which to prolong the remission period in patients with CD treated initially with TPN and TEN (Alun Jones *et al.*, 1985; Alun Jones, 1987; Giaffer, Cann & Holdsworth, 1991). Occasional successes, when single food substances such as wheat or dairy produce provoke symptoms, have been reported (Workman *et al.*, 1984). However, there is a real danger that a very restricted diet and occasionally iatrogenic malnutrition will ensue when multiple food intolerances are identified (Teahon & Levi, 1989). It is, therefore, considered essential to distinguish between specific food intolerance and psychological food aversion with double-blind challenge testing (Giaffer, Cann & Holdsworth, 1991).

Conclusion

The nutritional complications of IBD, in particular CD can be protean. Although still not fully documented, these must have a significant impact on the general health and well-being of patients suffering from these disorders. Much more remains to be discovered about the nutritional impact of these diseases and for a full realisation of the consequences of malnutrition upon IBD patients. Nevertheless, we already have considerable insight into a range of nutritional problems that can occur in both active and long-standing disease and yet, in many sufferers, these complications are not recognised or acted upon. The need is pressing for all those concerned with the treatment of patients with IBD, to be familiar with the nutritional aspects of their management.

There is now steadily accumulating evidence to implicate nutritional factors in the pathogenesis of CD and to demonstrate that nutritional therapy has a role in clinical management. Unfortunately, this appears not to have captured the imagination of many clinicians involved in patient care. No doubt, this is because of our general lack of understanding of how nutritional influences could bear on the mucosal inflammation occurring in these disorders. Further insight will come only from future research which, hopefully, will help to increase our knowledge of the pathogenic mechanisms involved in these enigmatic conditions. There is, however, no evidence to date to incriminate dietary constituents in the development of IBD. Patients should, therefore, be encouraged to eat essentially normal diets apart from modifications which may be recommended on entirely nutritional or therapeutic lines.

References

Aggett, P. J. & Harries, J. T. (1979). Current status of zinc in health and disease states. *Archives of Disease in Childhood*, **54**, 909–17.

Alun-Jones, V. (1987). Comparison of total parenteral nutrition and elemental diet in the induction of remission of Crohn's disease. Long-term maintenance of remission by personalized food exclusion diets. *Digestive Diseases and Sciences*, **32**, 100s–7s.

Alun-Jones, V., Dickinson, R. J., Workman, E., Wilson, A. J., Freeman, A. H. & Hunter, J. O. (1985). Crohn's disease: maintenance of remission by diet. *Lancet*, **ii**, 177–80.

Andersson, H., Bosaeus, I., Hellberg, R. & Hulten, L. (1982). Effect of a low-fat diet and anti-diarrhoeal agents on bowel habit after excisional surgery for classical Crohn's disease. *Acta Chirurgica Scandinavica*, **148**, 285–90.

Animashaun, A., Kelleher, J., Heatley, R. V., Trejdosiewicz, L. K. & Losowsky, M. S. (1990). The effect of zinc and vitamin C supplementation on the immune status of patients with Crohn's disease. *Clinical Nutrition*, **9**, 137–46.

Audus, T., Geiger, T., Hirano, T., Kishimoto, T. & Heinrich, P. C. (1988). Action of recombinant human interleukin 6, interleukin 1 beta and tumour necrosis factor alpha on the mRNA induction of acute-phase proteins. *European Journal of Immunology*, **18**, 739–46.

Beeken, W. L., Busch, H. J. & Sylwester, D. L. (1972). Intestinal protein loss in Crohn's disease. *Gastroenterology*, **62**, 207–15.

Belli, D. C., Seideman, E., Bouthillier, L. *et al.* (1988). Chronic intermittent elemental diet improves growth failure in children with Crohn's disease. *Gastroenterology*, **94**, 603–10.

Boumous, G. & Devroede, G. J. (1974). Effects of an elemental diet on human fecal flora. *Gastroenterology*, **14**, 790–3.

Chan, A. T., Fleming, C. R., O'Fallon, W. M. & Huizenga, K. A. (1986). Estimated versus measured basal energy requirements in patients with Crohn's disease. *Gastroenterology*, **91**, 75–8.

Clark, M. L. (1986). Role of nutrition in inflammatory bowel disease: an overview. *Gut*, **27** (suppl. 1), 72–5.

Cooke, W. T. (1972). Survey of results of treatment of Crohn's disease. *Clinics in Gastroenterology*, **1**, 521–31.

Crohn, B. B. & Yarnis, H. (1958). *Regional Ileitis*, 2nd edn. Grune & Stratton, London.

Crohn, B. B., Ginzburg, L. & Oppenheimer, G. D. (1932). Regional ileitis, a pathologic and clinical entity. *Journal of the American Medical Association*, **99**, 1323–8.

Culpepper-Morgan, J. A. & Floch, M. H. (1991). Bowel rest or bowel starvation: defining the role of nutritional support in the treatment of inflammatory bowel diseases. *The American Journal of Gastroenterology*, **86**, 269–71.

Davies, G., Evans, C. M., Shand, W. S. & Walker-Smith, J. A. (1990). Surgery for Crohn's disease in childhood: influence of site on disease and operative procedure on outcome. *British Journal of Surgery*, **77**, 891–4.

Duane, P. D., Teahon, K., Crabtree, J. E., Levi, A. J., Heatley, R. V. & Bjarnason, I. (1991). The relationship between nutritional status and serum soluble interleukin-2 receptor concentrations in patients with Crohn's disease treated with elemental diet. *Clinical Nutrition*, **10**, 222–7.

Dudrick, P. S. & Souba, W. W. (1991). The role of glutamine in nutrition. *Current Opinion in Gastroenterology*, **7**, 299–305.

Evans, R. D., Argiles, J. M. & Williamson, D. H. (1989). Metabolic effects of tumour necrosis factor-α (cachectin) and interleukin-1. *Clinical Science*, **77**, 357–64.

Franklin, J. L. & Rosenberg, H. H. (1973). Impaired folic acid absorption in inflammatory bowel disease: effects of salicylazosulfapyridine (Azulfidine). *Gastroenterology*, **64**, 517–25.

Fujita, M., Itakura, T., Takagi, Y. & Okada, A. (1989). Copper deficiency in total parenteral nutrition; clinical analysis of three cases. *Journal of Parenteral and Enteral Nutrition*, **13**, 421–5.

Gee, M. I., Grace, M. G., Wensel, R. H., Sherbaniuk, R. W. & Thompson, A. B. (1985). Nutritional status of gastroenterology outpatients: comparison of inflammatory bowel disease with functional disorders. *Journal of the American Dietetic Association*, **85**, 1591–9.

Giaffer, M. H., Cann, P. & Holdsworth, C. D. (1991). Long-term effects of elemental and exclusion diets for Crohn's disease. *Alimentary Pharmacology and Therapeutics*, **5**, 115–25.

Giaffer, M. H., North, G. & Holdsworth, C. D. (1990). Controlled trial of polymeric versus elemental diet in treatment of active Crohn's disease. *Lancet*, **335**, 816–19.

Gilat, T., Hacohen, D., Lilos, P. & Langman, M. J. (1987). Childhood factors in ulcerative colitis and Crohn's disease. An international co-operative study. *Scandinavian Journal of Gastroenterology*, **22**, 1009–24.

Greenberg, G. R., Fleming, C. R., Jeejeebhoy, K. N., Rosenberg, I. H., Sales, D.

& Tremaine, W. J. (1988). Controlled trial of bowel rest and nutritional support in the management of Crohn's disease. *Gut*, **29**, 1309–15.

Greenberg, G. R. (1992). Nutritional support in inflammatory bowel disease: current status and future directions. *Scandinavian Journal of Gastroenterology*, **27** (suppl. 192), 117–22.

Harries, A. D., Jones, L. A., Heatley, R. V. & Rhodes, J. (1982*a*). Malnutrition in inflammatory bowel disease; an anthropometric study. *Human Nutrition; Clinical Nutrition*, **36 C**, 307–13.

Harries, A. D., Brown, R., Heatley, R. N., Woolhead, S. & Rhodes, J. (1982*b*). vitamin D deficiency in Crohn's disease; an association with undernutrition. *Scandinavian Journal of Gastroenterology*, **17** (suppl. 78), 151A.

Harries, A. D., Jones, L. A., Danis, V. *et al.* (1983). Controlled trial of supplemented oral nutrition in Crohn's disease. *Lancet*, **i**, 887–90.

Harries, A. D. & Heatley, R. V. (1983). Nutritional disturbances in Crohn's disease. *Postgraduate Medical Journal*, **59**, 690–9.

Harries, A. D., Brown, R., Heatley, R. V., Williams, L. A., Woolhead, S. & Rhodes, J. (1985). Vitamin D status in Crohn's disease; association with nutrition and disease activity. *Gut*, **26**, 1197–203.

Harris, A. D. & Heatley, R. V. (1986). Nutrition in inflammatory bowel disease. In *Clinical Nutrition in Gastroenterology*, ed. R. V. Heatley, M. S. Losowsky & J. Kelleher, pp. 146–61. Churchill Livingstone, Edinburgh.

Hathcock, J. N. (1985). Metabolic mechanisms of drug–nutrient interactions. *Federation Proceedings*, **44**, 124–9.

Heatley, R. V. (1986). Assessing nutritional state in inflammatory bowel disease. *Gut*, **27**, **S1**, 61–6.

Heatley, R. V. (1988). Inflammatory bowel disease. In *Current Therapy in Nutrition*, ed. K. N. Jeejeebhoy, pp. 155–65. B. C. Dekker Inc., Toronto, Philadelphia.

Heatley, R. V. & Johnson, A. W. (1988). Changing requirements? The small bowel as a metabolic organ. *British Journal of Clinical Practice*, **42** (Suppl. 63), 89–92.

Hessov, I., Mosekilde, L., Melsen, F. *et al.* (1984). Osteopenia with normal vitamin D metabolites after small bowel resection for Crohn's disease. *Scandinavian Journal of Gastroenterology*, **19**, 691–6.

Homer, D. R., Grand, R. J. & Colodny, A. H. (1977). Growth, course and prognosis after surgery for Crohn's disease in children and adolescents. *Paediatrics*, **59**, 717–25.

Hyams, J. S., Tream, N. R., Eddy, E., Wyzga, N. & Moore, R. E. (1991). Tumour necrosis factor-α is not elevated in children with inflammatory bowel disease. *Journal of Paediatric Gastroenterology & Nutrition*, **12**, 233–6.

Iansek, R. & Edge, C. J. (1985). Nutritional amblyopia in a patient with Crohn's disease. *Journal of Neurology, Neurosurgery and Psychiatry*, **48**, 1307–8.

Imes, S., Dinwoodie, A., Walker, K., Pinchbeck, B. & Thompson, A. B. (1986). Vitamin C status in 137 outpatients with Crohn's disease. Effect of diet counselling. *Journal of Clinical Gastroenterology*, **8**, 443–6.

Imes, S., Pinchbeck, B. R. & Thompson, A. B. (1988). Diet counselling modifies nutrient intake of patients with Crohn's disease. *Journal of the American Dietetic Association*, **87**, 457–62.

Kirschner, B. S., Voinchet, O. & Rosenberg, I. H. (1978). Growth retardation in inflammatory bowel disease. *Gastroenterology*, **75**, 504–11.

Kirschner, B. S., Klich, J. R., Kalman, S. S., De Favaro, M. V. & Rosenberg,

I. H. (1981). Reversal of growth retardation in Crohn's disease with therapy emphasizing oral nutritional restitution. *Gastroenterology*, **80**, 10–15.

Kirsner, J. B. (1990). Limitations in the evaluation of therapy in inflammatory bowel disease: suggestions for future research. *Journal of Clinical Gastroenterology*, **12**, 516–24.

Klein, S. (1990). Elemental versus polymeric feeding with Crohn's disease – is there really a winner? *Gastroenterology*, **99**, 893–4.

Knodel, L. C. & Talbert, R. L. (1987). Adverse effects of hypolipidaemic drugs. *Medical Toxicology*, **2**, 10–32.

Krag, E. & Krag, B. (1976). Regional ileitis (Crohn's disease). I. Kinetics of bile acid absorption in the perfused ileum. *Scandinavian Journal of Gastroenterology*, **II**, 481–6.

Krawitt, E. L., Beeken, W. L. & Janney, C. D. (1976). Calcium absorption in Crohn's disease. *Gastroenterology*, **71**, 251–4.

Lanfranchi, G. A., Brignola, C., Campieri, M., Bazzocchi, G., Pasquali, R. & Baraldi, G. (1982). Malnutrition in patients with Crohn's disease in remission. Effects of an elemental diet. *Clinical Nutrition*, **1** (special suppl. 44), F38.

Lennard-Jones, J. E. (1992). Inflammatory bowel disease: medical therapy revisited. *Scandinavian Journal of Gastroenterology*, **27** (suppl. 192), 110–16.

Lenz, K. (1975). The effect of the site of lesion and extent of resection on duodenal bile acid concentration and Vitamin B12 absorption in Crohn's disease. *Scandinavian Journal of Gastroenterology*, **10**, 241–8.

Levenstein, S., Prantera, C., Luzi, C. & D'Ubaldi, A. (1985). Low residue or normal diet in Crohn's disease: a prospective controlled study in Italian patients. *Gut*, **26**, 989–93.

Linaker, B. D. (1979). Survey of Vitamin C in Crohn's disease. *Postgraduate Medical Journal*, **55**, 26–9.

Lochs, H., Steinhardt, H. T., Klaus-Wentz, B. *et al.* (1991). Comparison of enteral nutrition and drug treatment in active Crohn's disease. Results of the European Co-operative Crohn's disease. Study IV. *Gastroenterology*, **101**, 881–8.

Logan, R. F., Gillon, J., Ferrington, C. & Ferguson, A. (1981). Reduction of gastrointestinal protein loss by elemental diet in Crohn's disease of the small bowel. *Gut*, **22**, 383–7.

Lorenz, R., Weber, P. C., Szimnau, P., Heldwein, V., Strasser, T. & Loeschke, K. (1989). Supplementation with n-3 fatty acids from fish oil in chronic inflammatory bowel disease. A randomized, placebo-controlled, double-blind cross-over trial. *Journal of Internal Medicine* (suppl.), **225**, 225–32.

Lowen, C. C., Greene, L. M. & McClave, S. A. (1992). Nutritional support in patients with inflammatory bowel disease. *Postgraduate Medicine*, **91**, 407–74.

MacDonald, T. T., Hutchings, P., Chey, M. Y., Murch, S. & Cooke, A. (1990). Tumour nucrosis factor-alpha and interferon-gamma production measured at the single cell level in normal and inflamed human intestine. *Clinical & Experimental Immunology*, **81**, 301–5.

Main, A. N. H., Morgan, R. J., Russell, R. I. *et al.* (1981). Mg deficiency in chronic inflammatory bowel disease and requirements during intravenous nutrition. *Journal of Parenteral and Enteral Nutrition*, **5**, 15–19.

Main, A. N., Mills, P. R., Russell, R. I. *et al.* (1983). Vitamin A deficiency in Crohn's disease. *Gut*, **24**, 1169–75.

Malchow, K., Ewe, K., Brandes, J. W. *et al.* (1984). European co-operative

Crohn's disease study (ECCDS): results of drug treatment. *Gastroenterology*, **86**, 249–66.

Matuchansky, C. (1986). Parenteral nutrition in inflammatory bowel disease. *Gut*, **27** (suppl. I), 81–4.

McLain, B. I., Davidson, P. M., Stokes, K. B. & Beasley, S. W. (1990). Growth after gut resection for Crohn's disease. *Archives of Disease in Childhood*, **65**, 760–62.

Mekhjian, H. S., Switz, D. M., Melnyk, C. S., Rankin, G. D. & Brooks, R. K. (1979). Clinical features and natural history of Crohn's disease. *Gastroenterology*, **77**, 898–906.

Motil, K. J., Grand, R. J., Maletskos, C. J. & Young, V. R. (1982). The effect of disease, drug and diet on whole body protein metabolism in adolescents with Crohn's disease and growth failure. *Journal of Paediatrics*, **101**, 345–51.

Murch, S. H., Lamkin, V. A., Savage, M. O., Walker Smith, J. A. & MacDonald, T. T. (1991). Serum concentrations of tumour necrosis factor alpha in childhood chronic inflammatory bowel disease. *Gut*, **32**, 913–17.

O'Brien, C. J., Giaffer, M. H., Cann, P. A. & Holdsworth, C. D. (1991). Elemental diet in steroid-dependent and steroid refractory Crohn's disease. *American Journal of Gastroenterology*, **86**, 1614–18.

O'Donoghue, D. P. & Dawson, A. M. (1977). Crohn's disease in childhood. *Archives of Disease in Childhood*, **52**, 627–32.

O'Dwyer, S. T., Smith, R. J., Hwang, T. L. & Wilmore, D. W. (1989). Maintenance of small bowel mucosa with glutamine enriched parenteral nutrition. *Journal of Parenteral and Enteral Nutrition*, **13**, 579–85.

O'Keefe, S. J., Ogden, J., Rund, J. & Potter, P. (1989). Steroids and bowel rest versus elemental diet in the treatment of patients with Crohn's disease. The effect on protein metabolism and immune function. *Journal of Parenteral and Enteral Nutrition*, **13**, 455–60.

O'Morain, C., Segal, A. W. & Levi, A. J. (1984). Elemental diet as primary treatment of acute Crohn's disease: a controlled trial. *British Medical Journal*, **288**, 1859–62.

O'Morain, C., Tobin, A., Suzuki, Y. & O'Riordan, T. (1989). Risk factors in inflammatory bowel disease. *Scandinavian Journal of Gastroenterology* (supplement) **170**, 58–60.

Park, R. H. R., Duncan, A. & Russell, R. I. (1990). Hypolactasia in Crohn's disease. A myth. *American Journal of Gastroenterology*, **85**, 708–10.

Patton, J. S., Peters, P. M., McCabe, J. *et al.* (1987). Development of partial tolerance to the gastrointestinal effects of recombinant tumour necrosis factor-α in rodents. *Journal of Clinical Investigation*, **80**, 1587–96.

Perry, S., Hanft, R. & Chzanowski, R. (1990). Role of parenteral nutrition in inflammatory bowel disease, acute renal failure and hepatic encephalopathy. *International Journal of Technology Assessment in Health Care*, **6**, 655–62.

Pettit, S. H. & Irving, M. H. (1987). Does local intestinal ascorbate deficiency predispose to fistula formation in Crohn's disease. *Diseases of the Colon and Rectum*, **30**, 552–7.

Pettit, S. H., Shaffer, J. L., Johns, C. W., Bennett, R. J. & Irving, M. H. (1989). Ascorbic acid absorption in Crohn's disease. Studies using L-[carboxyl-14C] ascorbic acid. *Digestive Diseases and Sciences*, **34**, 559–66.

Plata-Salaman, C. R., Oomura, Y. & Kai, Y. (1988). Tumour necrosis factor and interleukin 1B; suppression of food intake by direct action in the central nervous system. *Brain Research*, **448**, 106–14.

Powell-Tuck, J. (1986). Protein metabolism in inflammatory bowel disease, *Gut*, **27** (suppl. 1), 67–71.

Powell-Tuck, J., Garlick, P. J., Lennard-Jones, J. & Waterlow, J. C. (1984). Rates of whole body protein syntheses and breakdown increase with severity of inflammatory bowel disease. *Gut*, **25**, 460–4.

Powell-Tuck, J., MacRae, K. D., Healy, M. J. R., Lennard-Jones, J. E. & Parkin, R. A. (1986). A defence of the small clinical trial: evaluation of three gastrointestinal studies. *British Medical Journal*, **292**, 599–602.

Ramadori, G., Van Damme, J., Rieder, H. & Buschenfield, K. H. M. (1988). Interleukin-6, the third mediator of acute-phase reaction modulates hepatic protein synthesis in human and mouse. Comparison with interleukin 1 beta and tumour necrosis factor-a. *European Journal of Immunology*, **18**, 1259–64.

Rees, R. G., Keohane, P. P., Grimble, G. K., Frost, P. G., Attrill, H. & Silk, D. B. (1986). Elemental diet administered nasogastrically without starter regimens to patients with inflammatory bowel disease. *Journal of Parenteral and Enteral Nutrition*, **10**, 258–62.

Reeves, W. C., Marcuard, S. P., Willis, S. E. and Movahed, A. (1989). Reversible cardiomyopathy due to selenium deficiency. *Journal of Parenteral and Enteral Nutrition*, **13**, 663–5.

Rhodes, J. & Rose, J. (1986). Does food affect acute inflammatory bowel disease? The role of parenteral nutrition, elemental and exclusion diets. *Gut*, **27**, 471–4.

Richie, J. K., Wadsworth, J., Lennard-Jones, J. E. & Rogers, E. (1987). Controlled multicentre therapeutic trial of an unrefined carbohydrate, fibre rich diet in Crohn's disease. *British Medical Journal*, **295**, 517–20.

Rigaud, D., Cosnes, J., Le Quintrec, Y., Rene, E., Gendre, J. P. & Mignon, M. (1991). Controlled trial comparing two types of enteral nutrition in treatment of active Crohn's disease: elemental *v* polymeric diet. *Gut*, **32**, 1492–7.

Rombeau, J. L. & Kripke, S. A. (1990). Metabolic and intestinal effects of short-chain fatty acids. *Journal of Parenteral and Enteral Nutrition*, **5**, S181–5.

Russell, R. I. (1991). Review article; dietary and nutritional management of Crohn's disease. *Alimentary Pharmacology and Therapeutics*, **5**, 211–22.

Sanderson, I. R., Udeen, S., Davies, P. S., Savage, M. O. & Walker-Smith, J. A. (1987*a*). Remission induced by an elemental diet in small bowel Crohn's disease. *Archives of Diseases in Childhood*, **62**, 123–7.

Sanderson, I. R., Boulton, P., Menzies, I. & Walker-Smith, J. A. (1987*b*). Improvement of abnormal lactulose/rhamnose permeability in active Crohn's disease of the small bowel by an elemental diet. *Gut*, **28**, 1073–6.

Schoelmerich, J., Bechner, M. S., Hoppe-Seyler, P. *et al.* (1985). Zinc and Vitamin A deficiency in patients with Crohn's disease is correlated with activity but not with localization of extent of the disease. *Hepato-Gastroenterology*, **32**, 34–8.

Seidman, E. G. (1989). Nutritional management of inflammatory bowel disease. *Gastroenterology Clinics of North America*, **18**, 129–55.

Seidman, E. G., Roy, C. C., Weber, A. M. & Morin, C. L. (1987). Nutritional therapy of Crohn's disease in childhood. *Digestive Diseases and Sciences*, **32** (suppl. 12), 82–8.

Seidman, E., Leleiko, N., Ament, M. *et al.* (1991). Nutritional issues in paediatric inflammatory bowel disease. *Journal of Paediatric Gastroenterology & Nutrition*, **12**, 424–38.

Silk, D. B. (1992). Medical management of severe inflammatory disease of the rectum: nutritional aspects. *Baillière's Clinical Gastroenterology*, **6**, 27–41.

Silk, D. B. A. & Payne-James, J. (1989). Inflammatory bowel disease: nutritional implications and treatment. *Proceedings of the Nutritional Society*, **48**, 355–61.

Singleton, J. W. (1991). Enteral feeding versus drug therapy in Crohn's disease: a continuing story. *Gastroenterology*, **101**, 1127–8.

Strobel, C. T., Byrne, W. J. & Ament, M. E. (1979). Home parenteral nutrition in children with Crohn's disease: an effective management alternative. *Gastroenterology*, **77**, 272–9.

Sturniolo, G. C., Molokhia, M. M., Shields, R. & Turnberg, L. A. (1980). Zinc absorption in Crohn's disease. *Gut*, **21**, 387–91.

Summers, R. W., Switz, D. M., Sessions, J. T. Jr. *et al.* (1979). National co-operative Crohn's disease study: result of drug treatment. *Gastroenterology*, **77**, 847–69.

Teahon, K. & Levi, A. J. (1989). Dietary management. In *Current Management of Inflammatory Bowel Disease*, ed. T. N. Bayless, pp. 223–30. Decker, Toronto.

Teahon, K., Bjarnason, I., Pearson, M. & Levi, A. J. (1990). Ten years' experience with an elemental diet in the management of Crohn's disease. *Gut*, **31**, 1133–7.

Teahon, K., Smethurst, P., Pearson, M., Levi, A. J. & Bjarnason, I. (1991). The effect of elemental diet on intestinal permeability and inflammation in Crohn's disease. *Gastroenterology*, **101**, 84–9.

Thornton, J. R., Emmett, P. M. & Heaton, K. W. (1979). Diet and Crohn's disease: Characteristics of the pre-illness diet. *British Medical Journal*, **2**, 762–4.

Valberg, L. S., Flanagan, P. R., Kertez, A. & Bondy, D. C. (1986). Zinc absorption in inflammatory bowel disease. *Digestive Diseases and Sciences*, **31**, 724–31.

Wadworth, A. N. & Fitton, A. (1991). Olsalazine, a review of its pharmacodynamic and pharmacokinetic properties, and therapeutic potential in inflammatory bowel disease. *Drugs*, **41**, 647–64.

Wan, J. M. F., Haw, M. P. & Blackburn, G. L. (1989). Nutrition, immune function and inflammation, an overview. *Proceedings of the Nutritional Society*, **48**, 315–35.

Whittaker, J. S. (1987). Nutritional therapy of hospitalized patients with inflammatory bowel disease. *Digestive Diseases and Sciences*, **32** (suppl. 12), 89S–94S.

Workman, E. M., Alun Jones, V., Wilson, A. J. & Hunter, J. O. (1984). Diet in the management of Crohn's disease. *Human Nutrition – Applied Nutrition*, **38**, 469–73.

17

Short bowel syndrome

J. E. LENNARD-JONES

Introduction

Consensus about the consequences and clinical management of patients with a short length of small intestine anastomosed to colon was achieved with the classic studies of Booth and his colleagues (Booth 1961; Booth, MacIntyre & Mollin, 1964). Since then, a different type of short bowel syndrome has become more common, namely resection of much of the small intestine and the whole of the colon leaving residual jejunum ending at a stoma. Furthermore, techniques have been developed for improving absorption and for by-passing the intestine with nutrients given intravenously by patients at home. This chapter will concentrate on the pathophysiology and management of a high jejunostomy and these new developments.

Physiological consequences of a jejunostomy

Water and electrolyte losses

The jejunum differs from the ileum and colon in its handling of water and sodium. It is characterised by greater permeability, rapid fluxes of water and sodium from lumen to plasma and vice versa, and dependence on concentration gradients. Sodium absorption can take place against only a small concentration gradient, it is greatly influenced by water movement and increased by the concurrent absorption of glucose, galactose and some amino acids.

Effects of sodium depletion

Loss of sodium leads progressively to reduction in the extra-cellular fluid volume with loss of body weight, decreased tissue turgor, postural hypotension, pre-renal failure and vascular collapse. The speed at which these changes can occur, and their potential danger, means that sodium balance must take priority when caring for a patient with a stoma.

Magnitude of sodium losses

Jejunostomy effluent has a surprisingly constant sodium concentration of 90 mmol/l (Ladefoged & Ølgaard, 1979) and daily sodium loss therefore bears a linear relation to stomal output. Many patients lose 2 l of fluid daily from the stoma and a few lose 3–5 litres. There is an obligatory loss of fluid even when the patient is fasting, and losses increase with food and drink. Sodium losses of 100–200 mmol daily can be replaced by mouth, but larger losses usually require intravenous replacement.

Effect of water or dilute sodium solutions on stomal loss

Experimental studies in animals and man show that when water or dilute sodium solutions enter the jejunum, sodium is secreted into the lumen. The lumenal concentration below which sodium is secreted varies in different studies between 60 and 100 mmol/l (Lifshitz & Wapnir, 1985; Saunders & Sillery, 1985). In health, the sodium secreted in the jejunum is re-absorbed lower in the gut, but when there is a jejunostomy the sodium is lost from the body (Griffin *et al.*, 1982; Newton *et al.*, 1985). Thus, a patient with a high jejunostomy must restrict water and dilute sodium solutions by mouth because they literally wash sodium out of the body as illustrated in Fig. 17.1.

Effect of dilution of food by exocrine digestive secretions

Studies using non-absorbable markers in healthy subjects have shown that nutrients are diluted two- or three-fold by digestive juices as they pass through the duodenum (Borgström *et al.*, 1957; Fordtran & Locklear, 1966). On entering the jejunum, absorption of water and sodium begins but dilution of the original meal is still detectable 100 cm or more distal to the duodeno–jejunal flexure. Thus, if a patient has a stoma situated in the proximal 100 cm of jejunum, the volume which emerges after a meal is likely to be greater than the volume taken by mouth. Balance studies show that this is the case (Fig. 17.2) and patients with a high jejunostomy can be divided into two groups (Nightingale *et al.*, 1990). One group is in constant negative balance and cannot convert to positive balance by increasing oral intake. These patients usually have less than 100 cm of residual jejunum and they all need intravenous supplements. The second group is in positive balance and they can increase absorption by ingesting more (Fig. 17.3).

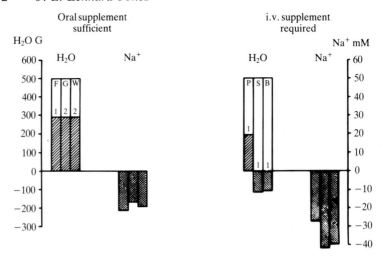

Fig. 17.1. Six fasting patients with a high jejunostomy, three maintained on an oral regime and three who needed intravenous supplements, took 500 ml of water to drink (with a PEG marker) and the effluent from the stoma was collected over 6 hours with over 80% marker recovery. The hatched colums show absorption or secretion of water and sodium. The patients absorbed about 60% of the water but each *lost* sodium (from data of Newton *et al.*, 1985, with permission).

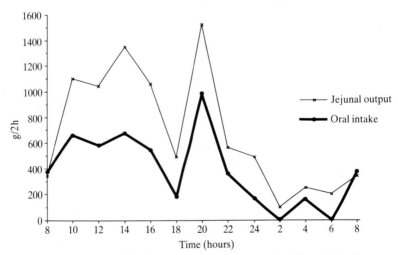

Fig. 17.2. The jejunal output was compared with oral intake at two hourly intervals throughout the 24 hours in a patient with a jejunostomy situated 30 cm distal to the duodeno–jejunal flexure. In every period jejunal output exceeded oral intake, differences were greatest during waking hours when food was taken but also persisted during the night (from Nightingale *et al.*, 1990, with permission).

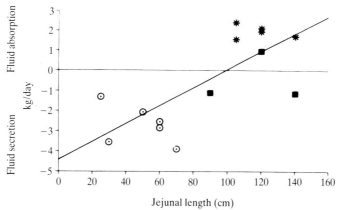

Fig. 17.3. The figure shows the net intestinal balance (wet weight) when patients with a jejunostomy took a freely chosen diet over 24 hours (mean of two periods). Eight of the patients were in negative balance and all these patients required parenteral supplements. Seven patients were in positive balance and all but one of these patients were maintained without intravenous supplements on an oral regime. ⊙ = required parenteral nutrition, ■ = required parenteral electrolytes but not nutrition, * = maintained on an oral regime (from Nightingale *et al.*, 1990, with permission).

Effect of drugs on decreasing jejunostomy output

Since part of the jejunostomy effluent comprises digestive secretions, drugs which decrease their output should decrease its volume. Octreotide, a somatostatin analogue, given by injection does reduce the losses of fluid and sodium, but not sufficiently to allow positive balance (Shaffer *et al.*, 1988; Rodrigues *et al.*, 1989a; Nightingale *et al.*, 1989; Ladefoged *et al.*, 1989). A few patients use this preparation before meals to reduce the social disability of a large stomal output after food and to decrease the volume of saline needed for intravenous replacement. Gastric anti-secretory drugs have an equivalent effect suggesting that most of the action of octreotide is on gastric secretion. Proton pump inhibitors, such as omeprazole, are often effective but are not always well absorbed (Nightingale *et al.*, 1991); H2 blockers are also effective and should be tried as the first choice (Jacobsen *et al.*, 1986). Neither octreotide, nor gastric antisecretory drugs reduce stomal output when the patient is already in positive intestinal fluid and sodium balance.

Anti-diarrhoeal drugs such as diphenoxylate, loperamide and codeine phosphate decrease the output of water and sodium from an ileostomy (Newton, 1978). The mode of action of such drugs is complex and involves

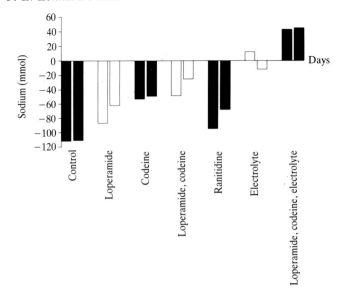

Fig. 17.4. The effect of various therapeutic measures on sodium balance in a patient with a jejunostomy who had given herself a parenteral infusion of saline daily for 14 years. On each day of the study she took a constant diet and each period lasted two days. On the control day there was negative intestinal sodium balance. Loperamide 4 mg qds and codeine phosphate 60 mg qds, separately or together caused some improvement over the control day. Ranitidine 300 mg had little effect. An oral glucose–electrolyte solution 1 litre daily restored balance. A satisfactory positive balance was achieved by using both the glucose electrolyte solution and anti-diarrhoeal drugs. On this regime she has been able to discontinue the daily parenteral infusion (from Nightingale *et al.*, 1992*a*, with permission).

both effects on motility (see below) and on exocrine secretions (Remington, Fleming & Malagelada, 1982). An effect is difficult to demonstrate in patients with a high jejunostomy (Rodrigues *et al.*, 1989*a, b*) but they can be effective (Fig. 17.4) in individual patients (Nightingale *et al.*, 1992*a*).

The optimum concentrations of glucose and sodium to promote absorption

The ratio of sodium chloride and glucose in an isotonic solution which leads to greatest absorption of sodium has been studied in animals and in man. Perfusion of a jejunal segment in rats showed maximal absorption with 120 mmol/l of sodium and 60 mmol/l of glucose (Saunders & Sillery, 1985). Data from perfusion of jejunal segments in man showed

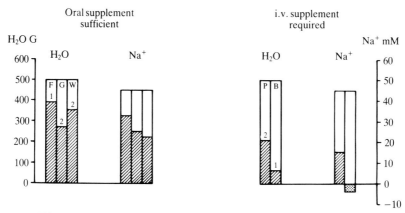

Fig. 17.5. Five of the patients shown in Fig. 17.1 took 500 ml of a solution containing sodium chloride (90 mmol/l) and glucose (100 mmol/l). On this occasion water absorption was little changed but four of the five patients *absorbed* sodium (from data of Newton *et al.*, 1985, with permission).

maximal sodium absorption in the range 105–142 mmol/l of sodium with corresponding glucose concentrations of 84–14 mmol/l of glucose (Sladen & Dawson, 1969). Another study has shown that sodium absorption was twice as great when the concentration in the perfusate was increased from 80 to 120 mmol/l and the corresponding glucose concentration reduced from 130 to 30 mmol/l. The same study showed that there is no advantage in replacing part or all of the chloride by bicarbonate (Fordtran, 1975). Results of balance studies in patients with a high jejunostomy have shown sodium loss with a drink containing sodium 60 mmol/l but absorption (Fig. 17.5) when the concentration was raised to 90 or 120 mmol/l (Newton *et al.*, 1985; Rodrigues *et al.*, 1988).

It is apparent from these data that a solution to promote greatest sodium absorption contains sodium in a concentration of over 100 mmol/l with a corresponding concentration of glucose to maintain isotonicity. Absorption occurs at lower concentrations but 90 mmol/l (Spiller, Jones & Silk, 1987) is a critical level below which absorption is either minimal or sodium loss begins.

Potassium and divalent cations

Potassium losses from a jejunostomy are about 15 mmol/l and an oral supplement is rarely needed (Ladefoged & Ølgaard, 1979). Magnesium and calcium balances are precarious (Ladefoged & Ølgaard, 1979; McIntyre,

Fitchew & Lennard-Jones, 1986; Woolf *et al.*, 1987). Some patients with a jejunostomy who can be stabilised on an oral regime need a magnesium supplement and others can manage without (Woolf *et al.*, 1987); a check should be kept on serum magnesium levels. Both magnesium and calcium absorption are promoted by vitamin D (Selby, Peacock & Bambach, 1984). Serum levels of 25-hydroxyvitamin D are often low and may be undetectable in patients with a jejunostomy (Compston & Creamer, 1977; Selby, Peacock & Bambach, 1984), possibly due not only to poor absorption but also to interruption of an entero-hepatic circulation. Patients who need intra-venous nutrients need parenteral magnesium, calcium and zinc (Ladefoged & Ølgaard, 1979). Zinc losses correlate with intestinal output from a high stoma at a concentration of about 3 mg/l (Wolman *et al.*, 1979); those stabilised on an oral regime rarely need a supplement (Woolf *et al.*, 1987).

Nutrient absorption

In normal subjects, intubation studies suggest that absorption of most carbohydrate and protein occurs within the upper 100–200 cm of jejunum (Borgström *et al.*, 1957). These observations may explain why a hydrolysed liquid feed, composed of peptides and oligosaccharides is not absorbed better than a feed containing whole protein and polysaccharides in patients with a high jejunostomy (McIntyre, Fitchew & Lennard-Jones, 1986). However, major losses of nitrogen and carbohydrate occur (Ladefoged, Nicolaidou & Jarnum, 1980; Woolf *et al.*, 1987; Ameen, Powell & Jones, 1987).

Fat malabsorption occurs in patients with a jejunostomy but absorption is a constant proportion of the intake. There is no evidence that excess fat in the jejunostomy effluent is harmful or offensive (Simko *et al.*, 1980; Woolf *et al.*, 1983, 1987; McIntyre, Fitchew & Lennard-Jones, 1986).

As an overall measure of energy absorption, measurement of oral intake and stomal losses can be made by bomb calorimetry (Woolf *et al.*, 1983, 1987). As expected, the total energy absorption is reduced and correlates with residual intestinal length (Nightingale *et al.*, 1990). In general, patients who absorb less than 30–40% of their energy intake (Fig. 17.6) require intravenous nutritional supplements to maintain health (Rodrigues *et al.*, 1989*b*; Nightingale *et al.*, 1990).

Metabolic consequences of a major resection with enterocolic anastomosis

There are specific receptor sites for vitamin B12 and bile salts in the distal ileum which are lost if this is resected.

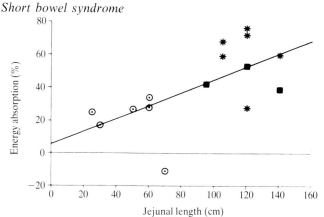

Fig. 17.6. Net intestinal energy balance (% absorbed) when 15 patients with a jejunostomy took a freely chosen diet over 24 hours (mean of two periods). Five of 7 patients with energy absorption of less than 40% required parenteral nutritional supplements. ⊙ = required parenteral nutritional supplements; ■ = required parenteral electrolytes but not nutrition;∗ = maintained on an oral regime.

If a short length of small intestine is anastomosed to the colon, unabsorbed nutrients enter the large bowel. Fatty acids and bile salts in the lumen promote colonic secretion of water and electrolytes, so aggravating diarrhoea. Fatty acids bind divalent ions, especially calcium and magnesium, so increasing losses; calcium is no longer available for combination with oxalate, a factor contributing to excess oxalate absorption. The presence of fatty acids and bile salts in the colon also promotes oxalate absorption. Many of these effects can be reduced by a low fat diet.

Liability to renal stones

In a comparative study, a quarter of patients with a residual jejunal length of less than 200 cm anastomosed to colon developed symptomatic renal stones, whereas a comparable group of patients with a jejunostomy did not experience this problem (Nightingale *et al.*, 1992*b*). Increased urinary excretion of oxalate and intestinal fluid losses leading to concentrated urine are important factors.

General metabolic consequences of major small bowel resection

Interruption of the entero-hepatic circulation

Diminished bile acid reabsorption leads to depletion of the bile salt pool and a reduced concentration of bile salts in bile. These changes reduce the capacity of bile to dissolve cholesterol (Dowling, Bell & White, 1972). A survey has shown that 40% of patients with resection of the ileum and distal jejunum had gall stones (Nightingale *et al.*, 1992*b*), though these were often symptomless.

Depletion of the bile salt pool may also reduce the concentration of bile acids in the jejunum below that needed for micelle formation, so impairing fat absorption.

D-*lactic acidosis*

A very rare complication of a short gut is a severe metabolic acidosis due to high concentrations of D-lactic acid in the blood. The usual L-isomer of lactic acid is metabolised rapidly by L-lactate dehydrogenase which is isomer specific. D-lactic acid is most probably generated by bacterial action on unabsorbed nutrients in the colon and accumulates because it is metabolised slowly (Oh *et al.*, 1979; Hudson, Pocknee & Mowat, 1990). The neurological and neuro-psychiatric features associated with D-lactic acidosis may not all be due to D-lactic acid, other unidentified compounds may also be involved.

Motility disturbances

Experimental studies show that increased transit rate through the small intestine can lead to decreased absorption. In health the presence of unabsorbed nutrients in the ileum, especially fat, delays transit through the jejunum, an effect likely to be lost if the ileum is removed. A comparative study in patients with an ileostomy has shown that small bowel transit of a meal was faster in five patients with an ileal resection of 50–70 cm than in eight patients with a resection of less than 10 cm (Neal *et al.*, 1984). A motility study in seven patients with a small bowel resection of 102–209 cm has shown that the inter-digestive motor complex was shorter than in controls due mainly to a reduced phase 2. Less segmenting activity and more frequent migrating motor complexes in which propulsion is associated with exocrine secretion, are both factors likely to increase output from a stoma or worsen diarrhoea (Remington *et al.*, 1983).

Intestinal adaptation

Experimentally, intestinal resection is followed by increased crypt cell production-rate in the remaining intestine with elongation of villi and increased numbers of cells lining them. This hyperplasia leads to an increased absorptive area, increased mucosal enzyme activity per unit length of gut, and enhanced absorption (Bristol & Williamson, 1988). These adaptive changes are greater in distal than in proximal small bowel. The response is dependent on the passage of nutrients and pancreatico–biliary secretions through the lumen.

Adaptation takes place proximal to a resection line which suggests a hormonal mechanism, the most favoured being enteroglucagon released from the distal gut. Among possible growth factors are polyamines formed by the action of ornithine decarboxylase. The possible roles of glutamine, epidermal growth factor, pituitary growth hormone, and other growth factors in treatment await definition.

In man, biopsy studies have failed to show lengthening of jejunal villi but a greater number of cells than normal has been observed lining each villus (Porus, 1965; Weinstein *et al.*, 1969; O'Keefe *et al.*, 1992). Functional adaptation over time with increased jejunal absorption of water and sodium (Weinstein *et al.*, 1969), glucose (Dowling & Booth, 1966) and calcium (Gouttebel *et al.*, 1989) has been recorded. There was little evidence of a reduced requirement for intravenous supplements in patients with less than 200 cm of jejunum, with or without a colon, during the period 6 months to 5 years after resection (Nightingale, Lennard-Jones & Walker, 1992).

Early post-operative management of the short gut

Step 1. Gaining stability and assessment of needs

The first objectives after major bowel resection are to gain control of fluid and electrolyte balance, measure basal output from the gut, assess major nutritional deficiencies, and plan future care based on the length and type of gut remaining.

Fluid and electrolyte balance

Fluid and electrolyte requirements should be supplied intravenously until balance is achieved and the basal output from the intestine has been assessed. A careful fluid balance chart is essential. The patient should be weighed and the blood pressure measured daily. Sodium loss from a stoma can be estimated for clinical purposes as 100 mmol/l; stomal losses should be largely replaced by normal saline. Measurement of the sodium concentration in random samples of urine gives a simple guide to sodium depletion; normally the concentration is greater than 5 mmol/l.

Assess major deficiencies

Nutritional assessment is needed based on previous intake, clinical observation (Baker *et al.*, 1982) and laboratory measurements.

Plan for future care

A patient with less than about 100 cm of jejunum is likely to need intravenous nutritional support for many weeks at least (Gouttebel *et al.*, 1986; Nightingale *et al.*, 1992). Conversely, a patient with distal or mid-small bowel resection and anastomosis is likely to do well with oral replacements. The presence of intra-abdominal sepsis or an entero-cutaneous fistula suggests that parenteral nutritional support will be needed initially.

Step 2. Gradual transfer to oral fluids and nutrients

Additions are made one at a time and their effect on intestinal output assessed. Intravenous water and electrolyte supplements are continued to prevent thirst and pressure to drink. Oral fluids are started in small quantities, 500 ml daily initially, and food is introduced slowly. The possible need for a glucose electrolyte solution is assessed. Loperamide 2–4 mg or larger doses, and/or codeine phosphate 30–60 mg, may be tried and given one hour before meals as a liquid, easily dispersable tablet or powder. If there is a high jejunostomy, a gastric anti-secretory drug such as oral ranitidine, 300 mg twice daily, may be tried. These drugs should not be given as a routine, but their effect should be measured in each patient so that an optimal regime can be established.

Step 3. Complete transfer to enteral feeding if possible

Hopefully, a simple regime with few or no restrictions or supplements may be sufficient. Oral fluid intake may need to be controlled (see below); electrolyte and/or nutritional supplements may be needed; drug therapy may be required. Only if all these measures fail should long-term intravenous supplements be continued.

Long-term management

The following paragraphs outline possible measures needed to maintain health and permit full rehabilitation. The simplest possible regime should be worked out for each patient.

Oral supplements

Sodium

Patients with stoma losses of less than 1200 ml daily can usually maintain sodium balance by adding extra salt to the limit of palatability at the table and when cooking. When losses are greater, gelatine capsules each containing sodium chloride 0.5 G (8.5 mmol) can be given with food but these cause nausea in some patients (Nightingale *et al.*, 1992*a*). Alternatively, a glucose electrolyte solution should be sipped in small quantities at frequent intervals throughout waking hours. Convenient solutions are

Sodium chloride	60 mmol (3.5 G)
Sodium citrate	30 mmol (2.9 G)
Glucose	110 mmol (20 G)

or

Sodium chloride	120 mmol (7.0 G)
Glucose	44 mmol (8.0 G)

both made up to 1 litre with tap water. The salt and glucose may be measured at home using appropriate scoops; sodium citrate improves palatability.

Magnesium

Patients with high stoma losses frequently become deficient in magnesium manifested by paraesthesiae, tetany, and occasionally fits. A convenient and effective oral supplement is magnesium oxide 4 mmol (160 mg) in gelatine capsules, giving 12–24 mmol daily. In addition, 1α-OH vitamin D_3, by mouth, may be needed for intractable deficiency (Selby, Peacock & Bambach, 1984).

Calories and protein

Calorie-protein malnutrition causes muscular weakness, loss of body fat with a sense of coldness, apathy, depression and irritability. Many patients simply need to take more nutrients by mouth to compensate for reduced absorption. They should be taught which foods are high in energy and advised to take them frequently, often as snacks, and in larger quantities than normal. The extra food intake can be supplemented by liquid sip feeds of a palatable polymeric diet taken between meals and at bedtime.

Slow infusion of a polymeric liquid feed through a fine-bore nasogastric tube at night, enables the short length of gut to be used for 24 hours a day, which adds at least 1000 kcal to the daily intake. Many patients are able to dispense with a tube feed once weight is regained and intestinal adaptation has occurred. The few patients who need a tube feed indefinitely are helped by an endoscopically inserted fine-bore gastrostomy tube which is socially more acceptable and is more comfortable.

Vitamins and trace elements

A supplement of water soluble vitamins or trace elements is rarely needed by patients maintained on an oral regime. It is possible that some patients who need parenteral nutrients could take oral vitamins and/or trace elements by mouth so simplifying the regime.

The need for an oral supplement of vitamin D is uncertain. Low plasma levels of 25-hydroxyvitamin D can occur (Compston & Creamer, 1977; Selby *et al.*, 1984) and osteomalacia has been shown by bone biopsy when serum levels of calcium, phosphorus and alkaline phosphatase were normal (Compston *et al.*, 1978). Although vitamin D absorption is impaired, evidence suggests that vitamin D_3 is absorbed almost as well as 25-hydroxyvitamin D_3, and there may be no advantage in using the latter (Davies, Mawer & Krawitt, 1980). It is probably wise to give an oral supplement of vitamin D, 400–900 IU daily, using the higher dose to compensate for malabsorption (Davies, Mawer & Krawitt, 1980).

Restriction of oral intake

Water

Sodium (and water) depletion lead to thirst and a patient with a high jejunostomy may drink large volumes of water, and equivalent drinks in an effort to quench it. To avoid aggravating sodium depletion, such patients should be advised to restrict consumption of water and similar drinks to 1 litre daily and substitute a glucose–electrolyte solution. Very often in this situation, it is necessary to give normal saline intravenously over a day or two until sodium deficiency is corrected.

Fat

Restriction of dietary fat benefits patients in whom a shortened small bowel is anastomosed to colon. However, fat is a high energy source and makes food palatable; a compromise is necessary between a dietary fat intake that is acceptable and reduction of diarrhoea.

Oxalate

Patients with steatorrhoea and an intact colon should be advised to limit not only fat, but also rhubarb, spinach, tomatoes, strawberries, chocolate and tea.

By-passing the gut

Vitamins and iron by injection

Vitamin B_{12} is needed as hydroxocobalamin, 1000 µg every 2 months, if more than 100 cm of distal ileum has been resected. Vitamin K as phytomenadione, 10 mg monthly, is advisable in patients receiving long-term parenteral nutrition. There is usually no need for regular injections of vitamin D. Iron injections as iron dextran, 100 mg, may be needed if deficiency develops, unresponsive to oral supplements.

Fluid and electrolytes without nutrients

Some patients are able to maintain nutrient balance by oral intake but are subject to chronic or episodic sodium depletion. Infusion at home of normal saline (150 mmol/l) daily or a few times a week can maintain sodium balance. Such infusions require an in-dwelling venous cannula but are simpler and cheaper than nutritional supplements. If magnesium deficiency is unresponsive to an oral supplement, magnesium sulphate, 12 mmol (3 G of $MgSO_{4.7}H_{20}$) can be added to each litre of normal saline.

Fluid, electrolytes and nutrients

All patients continue to eat and parenteral nutrients are used as a supplement. The usual indication for intravenous nutritional supplement is persistent malnutrition despite all efforts at oral replacement. A less common indication is great social disability due to incapacitating diarrhoea or stomal output after food. Parenteral nutrients may enable such patients to eat just enough at meals to maintain social life but little enough to avoid an embarrassing and disabling high intestinal effluent.

Every effort should be made to minimise the inconvenience of self-administered infusions at home. Thorough education of patients and those closest to them is essential. Infusions should be given overnight to allow freedom of activity by day.

Surgical treatment

A reversed small bowel segment can slow intestinal transit but there is a risk of causing functional obstruction. A technique for lengthening the gut has been used occasionally in childhood but not in adults (Pokorny & Fowler, 1991). Intestinal transplantation has been successful in a few patients and may become a routine procedure (Wood, 1992), even so it may be applicable to only a proportion of patients with the short bowel syndrome (Clark *et al.*, 1992).

Therapeutic goals

With modern management, patients with even the shortest lengths of gut should be able to live an active life appropriate to their age, physique and underlying disease. Gut losses should, if possible, be less than 2 litres daily, urine volume be greater than 1 litre daily with a sodium content > 5 mmol/l, and the body weight be within 10% of normal. The patient should not suffer from thirst or symptoms of dehydration, should enjoy normal energy and strength, and should appear normally nourished. The simplest possible regime should be worked out so that there is minimal restriction of social life.

References

Ameen, V. Z., Powell, G. K. & Jones, L. A. (1987). Quantitation of fecal carbohydrate excretion in patients with short bowel syndrome. *Gastroenterology*, **92**, 493–500.

Baker, J. P., Detsky, A. S., Wesson, D. E., Wolman, S. L., Stewart, S., Whitewell, J., Langer, B. & Jeejeebhoy, K. N. (1982). Nutritional assessment: A comparison of clinical judgement and objective measurements. *New England Journal of Medicine*, **306**, 969–72.

Booth, C. C. (1961). The metabolic effects of intestinal resection in man. *Postgraduate Medical Journal*, **37**, 725–39.

Booth, C. C., MacIntyre, I. & Mollin, D. L. (1964). Nutritional problems associated with extensive lesions of the distal small intestine in man. *Quarterly Journal of Medicine*, **33**, 401–20.

Borgström, B., Dahlqvist, A., Lundh, G. & Sjövall, J. (1957). Studies of intestinal digestion and absorption in the human. *Journal of Clinical Investigation*, **36**, 1521–36.

Bristol, J. B. & Williamson, R. C. N. (1988). Nutrition, operations, and intestinal adaptation. *Journal of Parenteral and Enteral Nutrition*, **12**, 299–309.

Clark, C. L., Ingham, Lear, P. A., Wood, S., Lennard-Jones, J. E. & Wood, R. F. M. (1992). Potential candidates for small bowel transplantation. *British Journal of Surgery*, **79**, 676–9.

Compston, J. E. & Creamer, B. (1977). Plasma levels and intestinal absorption of 25-hydroxyvitamin D in patients with small bowel resection. *Gut*, **18**, 171–5.

Compston, J. E., Ayers, A. B., Horton, L. W. L., Tighe, J. R. & Creamer, B. (1978). Osteomalacia after small-intestinal resection. *Lancet*, **i**, 9–12.

Davies, M., Mawer, E. B. & Krawitt, E. L. (1980). Comparative absorption of vitamin D_3 and 25-hydroxyvitamin D_3 in intestinal disease. *Gut*, **21**, 287–92.

Dowling, R. H. & Booth, C. C. (1966). Functional compensation after small-bowel resection in man. *Lancet*, **i**, 146–7.

Dowling, R. H., Bell, G. D. & White, J. (1972). Lithogenic bile in patients with ileal dysfunction. *Gut*, **13**, 415–20.

Fordtran, J. S. (1975). Stimulation of active and passive sodium absorption by sugars in the human jejunum. *Journal of Clinical Investigation*, **55**, 728–37.

Fordtran, J. S. & Locklear, T. W. (1966). Ionic constituents and osmolality of gastric and small intestinal fluids after eating. *American Journal of Digestive Diseases*, **11**, 503–21.

Gouttebel, M. C., Saint-Aubert, B., Astre, C. & Joyeux, H. (1986). Total parenteral nutrition needs in different types of short bowel syndrome. *Digestive Diseases and Sciences*, **31**, 718–23.

Gouttebel, M. C., Saint Aubert, B., Colette, C., Astre, C., Monnier, L. H. & Joyeux, H. (1989). Intestinal adaptation in patients with short bowel syndrome. *Digestive Diseases and Sciences*, **34**, 709–15.

Griffin, G. E., Fagan, E. F., Hodgson, H. J. & Chadwick, V. S. (1982). Enteral therapy in the management of massive gut resection complicated by chronic fluid and electrolyte depletion. *Digestive Diseases and Sciences*, **27**, 902–8.

Hudson, M., Pocknee, R. & Mowat, N. A. G. (1990). D-lactic acidosis in short-bowel syndrome; an examination of possible mechanisms. *Quarterly Journal of Medicine*, **74**, 157–63.

Jacobsen, O., Ladefoged, K., Stage, J. G. & Jarnum, S. (1986). Effects of cimetidine on jejunostomy effluents in patients with severe short-bowel syndrome. *Scandinavian Journal of Gastroenterology*, **21**, 824–8.

Ladefoged, K., Christensen, K. C., Hegnhøj, J. & Jarnum, S. (1989). Effect of a long acting somatostatin analogue SMS 201–995 on jejunostomy effluents in patients with severe short bowel syndrome. *Gut*, **30**, 943–9.

Ladefoged, K., Nicolaidou, P. & Jarnum, S. (1980). Calcium, phosphorus, magnesium, zinc, and nitrogen balance in patients with severe short bowel syndrome. *American Journal of Clinical Nutrition*, **33**, 2137–44.

Ladefoged, K. & Ølgaard, K. (1979). Fluid and electrolyte absorption and renin–angiotensin–aldosterone axis in patients with severe short-bowel syndrome. *Scandinavian Journal of Gastroenterology*, **14**, 729–35.

Lifshitz, F. & Wapnir, R. A. (1985). Oral hydration solutions: experimental optimization of water and sodium absorption. *Journal of Pediatrics*, **106**, 383–9.

McIntyre, P. B., Fitchew, M. & Lennard-Jones, J. E. (1986). Patients with a jejunostomy do not need a special diet. *Gastroenterology*, **91**, 25–33.

Neal, D. E., Williams, N. S., Barker, M. C. J. & King, R. F. G. (1984). The effect of resection of the distal ileum on gastric emptying, small bowel transit and absorption after proctocolectomy. *British Journal of Surgery*, **71**, 666–70.

Newton, C. R. (1978). Effect of codeine phosphate, Lomotil and Isogel on ileostomy function. *Gut*, **19**, 377–83.

Newton, C. R., Gonvers, J. J., McIntyre, P. B., Preston, D. M. & Lennard-Jones, J. E. (1985). Effect of different drinks on fluid and electrolyte losses from a jejunostomy. *Journal of the Royal Society of Medicine*, **78**, 27–34.

Nightingale, J. M. D., Lennard-Jones, J. E., Walker, E. R. & Farthing, M. J. G. (1990). Jejunal efflux in short bowel syndrome. *Lancet*, **336**, 765–8.

Nightingale, J. M. D., Lennard-Jones, J. E., Walker, E. R. & Farthing, M. J. G.

(1992*a*). Oral salt supplements to compensate for jejunostomy losses: comparison of sodium chloride capsules, glucose electrolyte solution, and glucose polymer electrolyte solution. *Gut*, **33**, 759–61.

Nightingale, J. M. D., Lennard-Jones, J. E., Gertner, D. J., Wood, S. R. & Bartram, C. I. (1992*b*). Colonic preservation reduces the need for parenteral therapy, increases the incidence of renal stones but does not change the high prevalence of gallstones in patients with short bowel. *Gut*, **33**, 1493–7.

Nightingale, J. M. D., Lennard-Jones, J. E. & Walker, E. R. (1992). A patient with jejunostomy liberated from home intravenous therapy after 14 years; contribution of balance studies. *Clinical Nutrition*, **11**, 101–5.

Nightingale, J. M. D., Walker, E. R., Burnham, W. R., Farthing, M. J. G. & Lennard-Jones, J. E. (1989). Octreotide (a somatostatin analogue) improves the quality of life in some patients with a short intestine. *Alimentary Pharmacology and Therapeutics*, **3**, 367–73.

Nightingale, J. M. D., Walker, E. R., Farthing, M. J. G. & Lennard-Jones, J. E. (1991). Effect of omeprazole on intestinal output in the short bowel syndrome. *Alimentary Pharmacology and Therapeutics*, **5**, 405–12.

O'Keefe, S. J. D., Shorter, R. G., Bennet, W. M. & Haymond, M. W. (1992). Villous hyperplasia is uncommon in patients with massive intestinal resection. *Gastroenterology*, **102**, A231.

Oh, M. S., Phelps, K. R., Traube, M., Barbosa-Saldivar, J. L., Boxhill, C. & Carroll, H. J. (1979). D-lactic acidosis in a man with the short-bowel syndrome. *New England Journal of Medicine*, **301**, 249–52.

Pokorny, W. J. & Fowler, C. L. (1991). Isoperistaltic intestinal lengthening for short bowel syndrome. *Surgery Gynecology and Obstetrics*, **172**, 39–43.

Porus, R. L. (1965). Epithelial hyperplasia following massive small bowel resection in man. *Gastroenterology*, **48**, 753–7.

Remington, M., Fleming, C. R. & Malagelada, J.-R. (1982). Inhibition of postprandial pancreatic and biliary secretion by loperamide in patients with short bowel syndrome. *Gut*, **23**, 98–101.

Remington, M., Malagelada, J., Zinsmeister, A. & Fleming, C. R. (1983). Abnormalities in gastrointestinal motor activity in patients with short bowels; effect of a synthetic opiate. *Gastroenterology*, **85**, 629–36.

Rodrigues, C. A., Lennard-Jones, J. E., Thompson, D. G. & Farthing, M. J. G. (1988). What is the ideal sodium concentration of oral rehydration solutions for short bowel patients? *Clinical Science*, **74** (Suppl. 18), p. 69.

Rodrigues, C. A., Lennard-Jones, J. E., Walker, E. R., Thompson, D. G. & Farthing, M. J. G. (1989*a*). The effects of octreotide, soy polysaccharide, codeine and loperamide on nutrient, fluid and electrolyte absorption in the short bowel syndrome. *Alimentary Pharmacology and Therapeutics*, **3**, 159–69.

Rodrigues, C. A., Lennard-Jones, J. E., Thompson, D. G. & Farthing, M. J. G. (1989*b*). Energy absorption as a measure of intestinal failure in the short bowel syndrome. *Gut*, **30**, 176–83.

Saunders, D. R. & Sillery, J. K. (1985). Absorption of carbohydrate–electrolyte solutions in rat duodenojejunum: Implications for the composition of oral electrolyte solutions in man. *Digestive Diseases and Sciences*, **30**, 154–60.

Selby, P. L., Peacock, M. & Bambach, C. P. (1984). Hypomagnesaemia after small bowel resection: treatment with 1α-hydroxylated vitamin D metabolites. *British Journal of Surgery*, **71**, 334–7.

Shaffer, J. L., O'Hanrahan, T., Rowntree, S., Shipley, K. & Irving, M. H. (1988). Does somatostatin analogue (SMS201–995) reduce high output stoma effluent? A controlled trial. *Gut*, **29**, A1432–3.

Simko, V., McCarroll, A. M., Goodman, S., Weesner, R. E. & Kelley, R. E (1980). High-fat diet in a short bowel syndrome. Intestinal absorption and gastroenteropancreatic hormone responses. *Digestive Diseases and Sciences*, **25**, 333–9.

Sladen, G. E. & Dawson, A. M. (1969). Inter-relationships between the absorptions of glucose, sodium and water by the normal human jejunum. *Clinical Science*, **36**, 119–32.

Spiller, R. C., Jones, B. J. M. & Silk, D. B. A. (1987). Jejunal water and electrolyte absorption from two proprietary enteral feeds in man: importance of sodium content. *Gut*, **28**, 681–7.

Weinstein, D. L., Shoemaker, C. P., Hersh, T. & Wright, H. K. (1969). Enhanced intestinal absorption after small bowel resection in man. *Archives of Surgery*, **99**, 560–2.

Wolman, S. L., Anderson, G. H., Marliss, E. B. & Jeejeebhoy, K. N. (1979). Zinc in total parenteral nutrition: Requirements and metabolic effects. *Gastroenterology*, **76**, 458–67.

Wood, R. F. M. (1992). Small bowel transplantation. *British Journal of Surgery*, **79**, 193–4.

Woolf, G. M., Miller, C., Kurian, R. & Jeejeebhoy, K. N. (1983). Diet for patients with a short-bowel: High fat or high carbohydrate? *Gastroenterology*, **84**, 823–8.

Woolf, G. M., Miller, C., Kurian, R. & Jeejeebhoy, K. N. (1987). Nutritional absorption in short bowel syndrome: Evaluation of fluid, calorie, and divalent cation requirements. *Digestive Diseases and Sciences*, **32**, 8–15.

18

Nutrition in cystic fibrosis

J. M. LITTLEWOOD and S. P. WOLFE

Nutrition and growth

In the past, cystic fibrosis (CF) children had suboptimal growth, poor weight for height and delayed puberty (Schwachman & Kulczycki, 1958; Sproul & Huang, 1965; Mearns, 1984). The eventual weight and height of CF adults has been below average (Mitchell-Heggs, Mearns & Batten, 1976) and this is still a problem for many CF adults today. In the United States the majority of CF patients are short of stature and underweight; 50% are below the tenth centile for height and 53% below the tenth centile for weight (Fitzsimmons, 1993). Fortunately with modern dietary advice, more efficient pancreatic enzyme extracts and more aggressive treatment of the chest infection, most CF individuals should now grow normally and be well nourished (Crozier, 1974).

The fine details of nutritional and respiratory management are of great importance in achieving normal growth; the advice to take 'a high energy diet, pancreatic enzymes and vitamin supplements' is open to many different interpretations. Consequently, there are marked differences in the nutritional state of CF patients, even those attending different specialised CF clinics. For example, both the nutritional state and survival of CF patients attending the Toronto CF clinic were significantly better than those treated in the Boston CF unit (Corey et al., 1988). In the United Kingdom many patients have no regular contact with a specialised CF clinic (British Paediatric Association, 1986). When such patients receive appropriate advice, there is usually a significant improvement in their nutritional state (Littlewood et al., 1984, 1988). Respiratory function and survival are better in those with sufficient pancreatic function to achieve normal fat absorption (Gaskin et al., 1982). A better nutritional state is associated with an improved prognosis (Kraemer et al., 1978).

Reasons for nutritional and growth problems

A number of factors commonly contribute to the poor nutritional state including an inadequate energy intake, the often severe and rarely completely controlled intestinal malabsorption, the increased energy demands of chest infections and a variable intrinsic increase in resting energy expenditure (REE) even in those who appear to have little or no chest involvement (Vaisman *et al.*, 1987; Buchdahl *et al.*, 1988). This suggests that the presence of the CF mutation itself results in increased energy expenditure (O'Rawe *et al.*, 1992).

Energy intake

Until the mid-1980s, before the introduction of effective pancreatic enzymes, it was customary to advise a low fat diet in order to reduce the symptoms of malabsorption, which often persisted despite the use of the older pancreatic extracts. Unfortunately, fat restriction compromised the total energy intake and many patients were consuming even less than the recommended intake for normal individuals (Chase, Long & Lavin, 1979; Hubbard, 1985). Many CF patients still eat less than the estimated average requirement for energy (EAR) for healthy individuals of the same age (Department of Health, 1991). Even with no restriction of dietary fat and the use of acid-resistant pancreatic enzymes, the self-determined energy intake of many CF individuals may still be quite inadequate to maintain normal nutrition and growth (Bell, Durie & Forstner, 1984; Daniels, Davidson & Martin, 1987; Littlewood *et al.*, 1988; Murphy *et al.*, 1991; Ellis, Bond, Wootton, 1992).

Reasons for the poor energy intake

In young children, the understandable parental insistence on an adequate energy intake may perpetuate the negative attitude to feeding common even in many unaffected children. In older patients, anorexia and aversion to eating is often associated with increasing activity of the chest infection and physical debility. There is commonly depression and an increasing realisation of the full implications of having the disease, in addition to the usual adolescent behavioural problems. Although advice to restrict dietary fat is unusual and unnecessary nowadays, some older patients have become accustomed to a low fat diet and find a normal intake unpalatable. There are still many CF individuals who do not receive the appropriate advice to achieve an adequate energy intake.

Sub-optimal control of intestinal malabsorption from incorrect administration or inadequate doses of pancreatic enzymes will result in abdominal pain and distension and even episodes of distal intestinal obstruction – symptoms which will reduce appetite.

The high energy diet recommended for CF patients is expensive and difficult for families with a low income to provide (Hanes & MacDonald, 1988).

The widespread advice in the media recommending a diet low in fat and high in fibre as 'healthy', has caused many CF patients and their parents to question the advice to take a diet high in fat and low in fibre. As malabsorption is rarely completely controlled, it is unlikely that a normal fat intake will impair health.

Finally, professional workers, inexperienced in CF nutrition, may give inappropriate advice, e.g. CF patients who develop diabetes mellitus may be advised on carbohydrate and fat restriction, thus compromising energy intake (MacDonald, 1992).

Gastrointestinal malabsorption

The malabsorption is severe in the majority of untreated patients (Schmerling, Forrer & Prader, 1970). Even in CF patients considered to be on an adequate dose of pancreatic enzymes, there is often a significant malabsorption (Littlewood *et al.*, 1988; Murphy *et al*, 1991; Littlewood, 1991).

Some pancreatic damage is present in all CF individuals by the time of birth. Most have histological abnormalities (Oppenheimer & Easterly, 1975; Sturgess, 1984) caused by a relative deficiency of fluid in the pancreatic ducts, secondary to the basic secretory defect (Kopelman *et al.*, 1985) (see Fig. 18.1(*a*) and (*b*)). Pancreatic insufficiency is present in the majority of infants (Bronstein *et al.*, 1992). The pancreatic damage is progressive (Couper *et al.*, 1992) and present in approximately 95% of patients.

Factors other than pancreatic enzyme insufficiency contribute to the intestinal malabsorption (Durie & Forstner, 1989; Zentler-Munro, 1989). Diminished pancreatic bicarbonate secretion increases duodenal acidity, causing both inactivation of pancreatic enzymes and precipitation of bile salts. The bile salt precipitation impairs lipid solubilisation (Zentler-Munro *et al.*, 1985); there is also excessive loss of bile salts in the faeces. The subsequent compensatory production of bile salts contains a relative increase of glycine conjugates which further contributes to the problem (Roy *et al.*, 1977; Carey, 1984; Setchell *et al.*, 1985). Protein absorption is

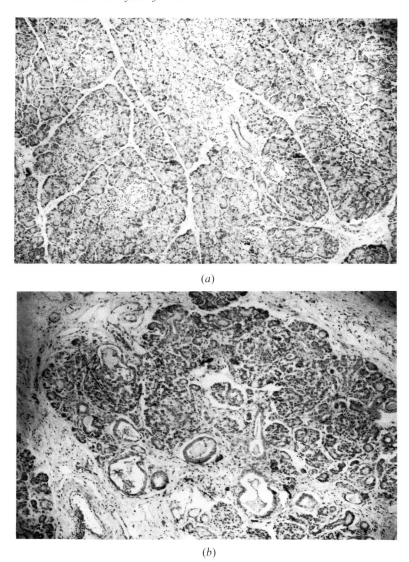

(a)

(b)

Fig. 18.1. (a) Pancreas of a newborn infant who did not have cystic fibrosis showing normal acinar pattern and islets of Langerhans. (b) Pancreas of a newborn CF infant. Already there is extensive fibrosis and distortion of the normal architecture.

usually adequately controlled with acid-resistant pancreatic enzymes (Beverley *et al.*, 1987). Carbohydrate absorption is not a problem as carbohydrate appears to be transported across the intestinal epithelium more efficiently than in normals (Baxter *et al.*, 1990). Ion transport abnormalities are present in the epithelium of the jejunum (Taylor *et al.*, 1988; Baxter *et al.*, 1989), ileum and colon (Berschneider *et al.*, 1988) and rectum (Goldstein *et al.*, 1988).

As the patient becomes older, there are other factors which may have an adverse effect on metabolism and nutrition; diabetes mellitus (DM) and liver disease are of particular importance.

Diabetes mellitus

Estimates of prevalence vary between 2.5% and 12% of CF patients. Of the 212 patients, attending the Leeds CF clinics 17 (8%) have DM – 3% of these less than 16 years old and 12.5% of the CF adults. In Copenhagen, 32% developed DM by the age of 25 years (Lanng *et al.*, 1991) which is the experience of most large CF clinics. For some years before the onset of clinical DM, the developing glucose intolerance has an adverse effect on the patient's condition (Lanng *et al.*, 1992). Treatment of the glucose intolerance before the development of clinical DM offers a potential therapeutic approach which requires further investigation (Zipf *et al.*, 1991).

Liver disease

Some 20% of CF individuals at some time have biochemical, ultrasound or clinical evidence of liver disease. Approximately 5% eventually have clinical evidence of liver involvement – rising from 0.3% in the under-five-year-olds to 9% in those over 16 years old (Scott-Jupp, Lama & Tanner, 1991).

The recent observation that administration of ursodeoxycholic acid improves both the abnormal liver function tests (Colombo *et al.*, 1990, 1992; O'Brien, Fitzgerald & Heggarty, 1992) and hepatobiliary excretion demonstrated by scintigraphy (Colombo *et al.*, 1992) represents an important advance.

Increased resting energy expenditure

Initial observations on the increased energy expenditure in undernourished CF adolescents and adults (Pencharz *et al.*, 1984) led to a study, using indirect calorimetry. This demonstrated increased resting energy expenditure (REE) in patients with mild chest disease (Vaisman *et al.*, 1987). Many subsequent studies have confirmed REE is increased (Buchdahl *et al.*, 1988; O'Rawe *et al.*, 1992). There is discussion as to the relative importance of the type of CF mutation and the severity of the chest infection (O'Rawe *et al.*, 1992; Fried *et al.*, 1991). Certainly the REE is reduced during antibiotic treatment of the chest infection.

Evaluation and monitoring of nutrition

The patient attends the CF clinic every one to three months – usually every two months if well. As the condition of the chest is so closely related to the nutritional state, they are considered together. The patient sees the dietitian at most clinic visits and always if weight progress is unsatisfactory.

The following information is obtained at every visit.

- Appetite/food intake/energy supplementation/nutritional support, e.g. enteral feeding.
- Abdominal symptoms particularly pain and distension.
- Bowel frequency and characteristics of the stools.
- Pancreatic extract – type, dose, method of taking.
- Vitamin supplement doses are checked.
- Consideration is given to patient compliance.
- Weight and length are plotted on the growth chart.
- Percentage weight and height for age are calculated.
- Percentage weight for height is calculated.
- Abdominal contour is noted (fullness suggests persisting malabsorption).
- Abdominal masses are felt (presence suggests inadequate enzymes).
- Abnormalities of liver (firmness or enlargement) and the presence of palpable spleen are noted.
- Condition of the chest carefully evaluated by history, clinical examination, spirometry, pulse oximetry and sputum culture.
- Urine is tested for glucose.

Dietary assessment

The seven-day weighed inventory is regarded as the most accurate method of assessing food intake (Bingham, 1987). Its use, however, is mainly restricted to research purposes and we regard a five-day prospective dietary record, using household measures and weights where convenient, to be the best way of obtaining nutritional intake data in clinical practice.

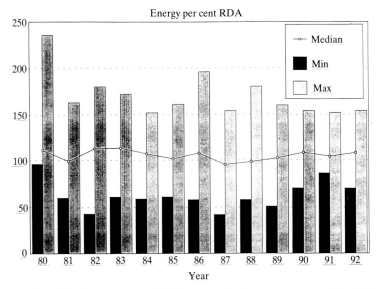

Fig. 18.2. Recommended daily amount of energy consumed by 365 new CF patients when referred for first assessment. There was no evidence of a trend in values over the years 1981 to 1992. Those assessed in 1980 were already attending the unit for full care.

The data are analysed using the McCance and Widdowson data (Paul & Southgate, 1978) and the 'Microdiet' computer programme ('Microdiet' system, University of Salford, 1988). Until recently the results were calculated as a percentage of the recommended daily amount (RDA) of energy for age (DHSS, 1979). Now the estimated average requirement (EAR) is used as the normal standard.

The energy intakes of CF patients referred to the Leeds Regional CF Unit from many different general hospitals are likely to be representative of those in the United Kingdom. There has been no significant improvement in energy intake from 1981 to 1992; there are still many patients who are taking less than 120% of that recommended for age (see Fig. 18.2).

Nutritional state

The weight and height are plotted on a growth chart at every clinic visit (Tanner & Whitehouse, 1976); they are also used to calculate the percentage of each for age and the percentage weight for height using a

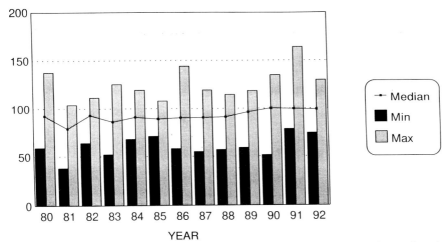

Fig. 18.3. Percentage weight for age of 397 CF patients when referred for first assessment. There was a significant improvement between 1981 and 1992 ($p < 0.001$).

Cole's rule (Cole, Donnett & Stanfield, 1981). Any slowing in the rate of growth or deterioration of the weight for height is carefully evaluated both from the gastrointestinal and respiratory aspects. The weight for height should remain above 85% and ideally be over 90%.

The mid upper arm circumference (MUAC) is a useful simple clinical measurement of nutritional status. Estimation of body fat from measurement of skinfold thickness (Frisancho, 1981) is unreliable in CF (Johnston *et al.*, 1988; Newby, Keim & Brown, 1990). These methods have been superseded by more direct methods which are not usually used for routine clinical monitoring (Johnston *et al.*, 1988; Heymsfield *et al.*, 1982; Gregory *et al.*, 1991).

There has been an improvement in the nutritional state of patients referred to the CF Unit over the past decade (see Figs. 18.3, 18.4 and 18.5). A normal fat diet, the availability of acid resistant pancreatic enzymes from the mid-1980s, and more aggressive treatment of chest infections have all contributed.

Laboratory investigations

Haematology

The haemoglobin is usually normal although the serum iron and ferritin are commonly low (Erdhardt, Miller & Littlewood, 1987). The total white

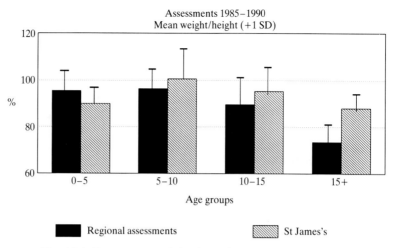

Fig. 18.4. Percentage weight for height of patients when referred for assessment..

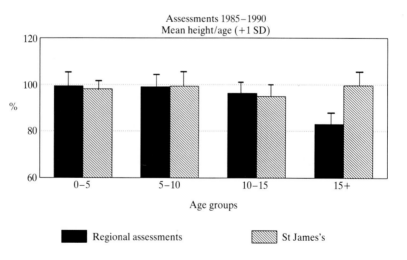

Fig. 18.5. Percentage height for age of 397 CF patients when referred for first assessment.

cell and neutrophil count and also the plasma viscosity are helpful in assessing the activity of the chest infection. It has been suggested that iron supplements may favour bacterial growth (Brown, Anwar & Lambert, 1984). Thus, we administer iron only when deficiency is associated with anaemia.

Albumin

Pre-albumin may be a more sensitive indication of nutritional status. However, serum albumin is more readily available and is usually within the normal range. Low values may occur in young infants at diagnosis (Fleischer *et al.*, 1964), in those with severe liver disease and in patients with advanced pulmonary damage.

Liver function tests

Standard liver function tests are performed annually.

Urea and electrolytes

The excessive loss of salt in the sweat may lead to chronic electrolyte depletion and pseudo Bartter's syndrome (Devlin, Beckett & David, 1989; Kennedy *et al.*, 1990). The low electrolyte content of both breast milk and infant formulae may lead to chronic sodium chloride depletion (Laughlin, Brady & Elgen, 1981). A similar syndrome occurs in some older patients if the salt intake is inadequate, especially in hot climates. Plasma electrolytes are checked if progress is not entirely satisfactory.

Vitamin A

Low plasma vitamin A levels are common in CF patients even if they are receiving supplements (Congdon *et al.*, 1981) (see Fig. 18.6). The plasma level usually correlates with that of the retinol-binding protein (Rasmussen *et al.*, 1986). Clinical evidence of vitamin A deficiency is rarely recognised. However, in one recent study of 43 older CF Patients, eight had abnormal dark adaptation (Rayner *et al.*, 1989); two of these and one additional patient had conjunctival xerosis (Vernon *et al.*, 1989). In infancy, vitamin A deficiency may present with raised intracranial pressure (Abernathy, 1976; Eid *et al.*, 1990). In our experience, correction of vitamin A deficiency is associated with an improved general condition and clinical course. Vitamin A levels are checked annually.

Vitamin D

Clinical evidence of vitamin D deficiency is rare, although rickets (Scott *et al.*, 1977) and osteomalacia have been reported (Friedman, Ingman &

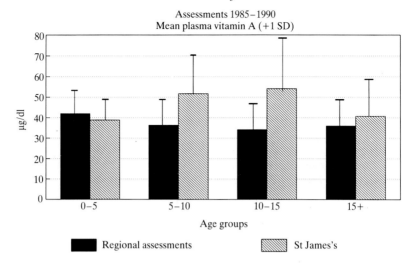

Fig. 18.6. Plasma vitamin A levels of new CF referrals and of patients attending the CF unit (St James) where plasma levels are monitored regularly. Normal range 37–110 μg/dl.

Favus, 1985). Osteoporosis and low levels of vitamin D metabolites are well documented particularly in older patients (Hanley *et al.*, 1985; Gibbens *et al.*, 1988; Stead *et al.*, 1987). Levels of vitamin D metabolites vary significantly with the exposure to sunlight (Reiter *et al.*, 1985). Reduced bone mineralisation is common and confirmed by bone photon adsorptiometry (Mischler *et al.*, 1979); however, the general osteoporosis seems to be related more to the overall nutritional state than to vitamin D levels. 25 OH cholecalciferol is measured annually.

Vitamin K

The initial presentation of CF may be with bleeding due to vitamin K deficiency (Walters & Koch, 1972). Bleeding may also occur in patients with liver disease. Plasma levels of vitamin K are usually normal and routine supplements are not given (Choonara *et al.*, 1989). However, blood coagulation studies are checked before any major surgical procedure and vitamin K given (Phytomenadione [Konakion] 5 to 10 mg by slow intravenous injection).

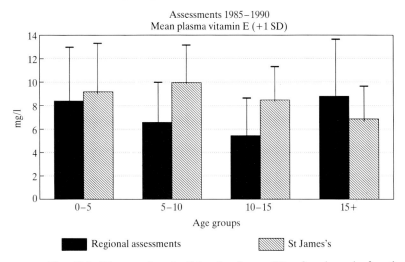

Fig. 18.7. Plasma vitamin E levels of new CF referrals and of patients attending the CF unit (St James) where levels are monitored regularly. Normal range 9–14 mg/l.

Vitamin E

Unless specifically supplemented with substantial doses of vitamin E, plasma levels will be very low (Congdon *et al.*, 1981) (see Fig. 18.7). The plasma levels fall into the first weeks in CF infants (Sokel *et al.*, 1989) and haemolytic anaemia has been reported (Farrel *et al.*, 1977). A small, but significant rise in haemoglobin has been noted after correction of vitamin E deficiency in older CF patients (Kelleher *et al.*, 1987). Neurological complications in CF adults are well documented and include loss of tendon reflexes, muscle weakness, reduced vibration and proprioceptive sensation (Sitrin *et al.*, 1987; Cynamon *et al.*, 1988). The presence of liver disease increases the likelihood of neurological complications. In severe cholestatic states in non-CF patients, vitamin E deficiency is severe, difficult to control and commonly associated with neurological complications (Elias, Muller & Scott, 1981). The role of vitamin E as an anti-oxidant in cystic fibrosis remains to be investigated but it may be of considerable importance. Vitamin E levels are checked annually.

Water soluble vitamins

These are well absorbed. In a study performed before the advent of acid-resistant pancreatic enzyme preparations, we found normal levels in contrast to frequently abnormal levels of fat soluble vitamins (Congdon *et al.*, 1981). An exception is a report of abnormal vitamin B6 status in a significant proportion of CF patients. A significant correlation between pyridoxal-5-phosphate and transaminase suggests hepatic disease may be contributing to the deficiency (Faraj *et al.*, 1986). Vitamin C has received attention in its role as an anti-oxidant which may have a favourable effect on the respiratory damage. Plasma vitamin C levels are usually normal (Congdon *et al.*, 1981). Folic acid and vitamin B12 deficiencies are not a problem except occasionally in those patients who have had extensive small intestinal resections usually for meconium ileus or other reasons. Regular measurement of the water soluble vitamins is not indicated.

Minerals and trace elements

Plasma minerals and trace element levels are usually normal (Kelleher *et al.*, 1986) although there are isolated reports of malabsorption and deficiencies of trace elements even when taking regular pancreatic enzyme supplements (Aggett *et al.*, 1979).

Symptomatic zinc deficiency has been described (Dodge & Yassa, 1978) but plasma levels are usually normal (Solomons *et al.*, 1981; Kelleher *et al.*, 1986). Both the importance of zinc as a co-factor for many enzymes and the difficulties in interpreting plasma levels as an indicator of zinc status should be borne in mind when considering the possibility of zinc deficiency.

Plasma calcium, copper and magnesium are usually normal (Kelleher *et al.*, 1986). Hypomagnesaemia has been reported as a complication of N-acetyl cysteine treatment of distal intestinal obstruction (Godson *et al.*, 1988). Selenium deficiency does not appear to be frequent or significant (Castillo *et al*, 1981). Minerals and trace elements are not checked as a routine.

Essential fatty acids

In infants, clinical evidence of essential fatty acid (EFA) deficiency has been reported. This is very rare in treated patients although abnormalities of blood lipids are common (Farrel *et al.*, 1985). Low plasma essential fatty acid levels are confined to those with pancreatic insufficiency (Forstner, Durie & Corey, 1988) and probably do not represent a primary abnormality.

Nutritional management of the CF patient

Ensuring adequate energy intake

Dietary advice to improve suboptimal energy intakes should take into consideration the reasons for poor intake already discussed in order for it to be achievable and realistic. One interview with an experienced dietitian will result in a sustained increase in energy intake over one year later (MacDonald, Kelleher & Littlewood, 1988). The recommendations given to patients who have an inadequate energy intake depend on the nutritional state and growth and include, counselling regarding psychological factors which affect the patient's appetite; simple advice to increase food intake; to lift dietary fat restrictions; to commence or increase the use of dietary supplements; to commence or increase the use of more invasive supplementary feeding techniques such as nasogastric or enterostomy feeding. Very occasionally, total parenteral nutrition may be indicated (Littlewood & MacDonald, 1987; MacDonald, Holden & Harris, 1991; Ramsey, Farrell & Pencharz, 1992).

Regular dietetic counselling

This enables advice to be given on maximising energy and protein intakes. The use of high energy and protein foods should be promoted and cooking techniques encourage the addition of extra fat, e.g. frying and basting. Full fat milk, yogurts, cheese, butter and margarine should be used. Butter or margarine should be spread thickly on bread and added to vegetables. To achieve high energy intakes, 40% of the energy should be taken as fat. Generous meat, fish and egg portions need be encouraged to improve protein intakes. Sweetened fizzy drinks and squashes, confectionery and savoury snacks are useful additional energy sources, however, the timing of these snacks should be taken into consideration so that they are not allowed to replace meals.

Nutritional supplements

If the patient has a poor intake, and is failing to gain weight despite encouraging a high energy diet, dietary supplements are an important means of improving the nutritional intake.

Carbohydrate polymer powders

Maxijul (Scientific Hospital Supplies); Polycal (Cow and Gate). These powders may be added to infant formulae and weaning foods. Because of their osmotic load we usually add up to 5 g per 100 ml of infant formula; this will provide an additional 19 calories per 100 ml. Older children may tolerate a 20% carbohydrate polymer solution in water which can be made up in advance and stored in the 'fridge for use during the day. It is most palatable if used to dilute squashes.

Carbohydrate and fat powders and liquids

Duocal (Scientific Hospital Supplies). The osmolality of this supplement is reduced by the addition of fat allowing a greater energy concentration to be achieved when added to infant formulae. Up to 8 g m per 100 ml should be used providing an additional 37 calories per 100 ml.

Fat emulsions

Calogen and Liquigen (Scientific Hospital Supplies). These emulsions can be added to infant formulae either as the sole energy supplement or in addition to a carbohydrate polymer. Calogen is a 50% solution of long-chain triglycerides (LCT) and Liquigen a 50% emulsion of medium chain triglycerides (MCT). There is little advantage in the use of Liquigen, except perhaps in infants who have undergone extensive gut resection when MCT fat may be better tolerated. An addition of 3 g/100 ml of infant formula is usually tolerated and provides an additional 13.5 calories per 100 ml. Additional pancreatic enzyme supplementation is required when fat emulsions are used.

Carbohydrate polymer liquids

Hycal (Smith Kline and Beecham) Maxijul liquid (Scientific Hospital Supplies). These concentrated carbohydrate solutions may be taken undiluted or mixed with water, squash or fizzy drinks. Because of their high osmotic load they are of little use to children under the age of three years unless taken very diluted.

Nutritionally complete protein and energy supplements

Fresubin (Fresenius), Fortisip (Cow and Gate), Ensure Plus (Abbott). These milkshake-type drinks can be taken as a supplement to the diet of any child over the age of three years. The use of high protein supplements, e.g. Fortimel (Cow and Gate) should be restricted to children over five years of age. The drinks should be given either between meals with snacks or after meals; they should not be allowed to replace meals. Many are available in a tetrabrik presentation and therefore convenient to take to school.

In order for supplement regimens to be successful, the dietitian should give clear guidelines regarding how many supplements should be taken on a daily basis and when they should be taken. Increasing supplement use during periods of acute infection when anorexia may be exacerbated is beneficial (Williams, Handy & Weller, 1989).

Enteral feeding

Enteral feeding should be considered if the weight gain is less than normal for a few months or the weight for height is less than 80 to 85%. However, the decision to start enteral feeds will be based on a detailed clinical assessment of the patient, particularly whether more aggressive treatment of the chest infection may itself significantly improve the nutritional state. Also psychosocial factors, family issues and home conditions may determine the feasibility of such nutritional support. There is significant evidence that improvement in nutritional status by enteral feeding can stabilise pulmonary function (Levy *et al.*, 1985; Shepherd, Cookley & Cooke, 1980; Shepherd *et al.*, 1986; Dalzell *et al.*, 1992).

The most commonly chosen methods of feeding are via the nasogastric or gastrostomy routes although jejunostomy feeding has been used (Thomas, Blue & Hemried, 1990; Boland *et al.*, 1986). The method to be used should be discussed between the patient and carers and a mutually acceptable route chosen.

Nasogastric feeding should involve the use of a fine bore nasogastric tube which may either be left *in situ* or repassed each time a feed is given (O'Loughlin *et al.*, 1986; Holden *et al.*, 1991). In the Leeds CF Unit nasogastric feeding has proved both acceptable to patients and effective. Gastrostomy feeding has become a more popular method of enteral feeding over the past decade. The main reasons are the introduction of more sophisticated feeding devices and the recognition that the need for this method of nutritional support may be long term (Wicks *et al.*, 1992). There are various gastrostomy devices available, e.g. Entrafeed tube (Medicina), Bower Percutaneous Endoscopic Gastrostomy (PEG) (Merck) and the button replacement gastrostomy device (Bard). Before siting a gastrostomy in a CF patient, the clinical condition must be improved as much as possible by intensive physiotherapy and a course of intravenous antibiotics. In older patients or those in whom a general anaesthetic is considered inadvisable, the PEG has the advantage of being sited under local anaesthesia.

Feeding via the nasogastric or gastrostomy route usually takes place for eight to 10 hours overnight, permitting the patient to attempt to eat as well as possible during the day. Patients with CF tolerate lower volumes of more highly concentrated feeds, e.g. Ensure Plus (Abbott) and 2 Cal HN (Abbott) better than dilute feeds fed at high rates. An alternative to these whole protein preparations are elemental feeds, e.g. Elemental 028 (Scientific Hospital Supplies). There is no conclusive evidence that elemental feeds offer any significant advantage over whole protein feeds. Improvements in body weight, body fat and total body potassium have been documented during short term feeding with elemental preparations (Pencharz *et al.*, 1984). However, others have reported that there is no difference in the rates of protein synthesis or catabolism in patients fed isocaloric amounts of elemental formula and non-elemental formula of the same protein content (Pekekanos *et al.*, 1990). Because elemental diets are expensive and are not tolerated as well as whole protein feeds we would not routinely advocate their use.

The carbohydrate content of the feed has also been subject to much debate. In patients with chronic lung disease the ventilatory response to carbon dioxide may be diminished. High carbohydrate feeds are associated with an increased ventilatory effort secondary to increased carbon dioxide production (Shepherd *et al.*, 1986; Kane & Hobbs, 1991). This increased ventilatory demand could compromise CF patients who already have muscle fatigue by leading to carbon dioxide retention and hypoxia requiring oxygen supplementation. Respiratory failure has been reported in patients who have been given very high carbohydrate feeds (Covelli *et al.*, 1981). Therefore, a low carbohydrate feed, e.g. Pulmocare (Abbott) may be preferable for patients with chronic lung disease.

Whatever the type of feed administered, careful monitoring of the patient's glycaemic control is essential. Hyperglycaemia requiring insulin therapy is common in young adults given night time enteral feeds, irrespective of their carbohydrate content (Kane & Black, 1989). This tendency is exacerbated if the patient is also receiving corticosteroids.

Pancreatic enzyme supplements are necessary with all enteral feeds including elemental preparations and those containing medium chain triglycerides (Durie *et al.*, 1980).

The dose of enzymes is usually estimated from the enzymes required with food during the day and the fat content of that food. For example, if approximately one enzyme capsule is required for each 5 g of fat and the enteral feed contains 80 g of fat, 16 capsules are given with each feed. If an elemental/MCT feed is used, it is advisable to start with half this dose and titrate up until control of symptoms is achieved. Enzymes should be taken orally and not mixed with the feed; two-thirds are taken at the beginning and one third at the end. It is better to space them out as far as possible through the feed if the patient is awake.

Parenteral nutrition

Parenteral nutrition (PN) is used for short-term support after abdominal surgery for meconium ileus in infants and other major abdominal surgery in older CF patients and also during severe gastroenteritis; more prolonged use may be required for short gut syndrome. The parenteral route has been used for short term nutritional support during acute chest exacerbations. There are relatively few reports of PN in CF patients. In an uncontrolled study, Shepherd gave 130% RDA for three weeks and demonstrated improved nutrition and respiratory function maintained at follow-up six months later (Shepherd, Cookley & Cooke, 1980).

Infant feeding

Most CF infants thrive on either breast milk or a standard infant formula (Simmonds *et al.*, 1993). A pre-digested MCT fat-containing formula, e.g. Pregestimil (Mead Johnson) may be of benefit to infants who have undergone extensive small bowel resection for meconium ileus or those who have a co-existing cows' milk intolerance (Hill *et al.*, 1989). If the infant is failing to thrive, despite adequate pancreatic enzyme administration and an adequate oral intake (up to 200 ml/kg body weight), additional energy supplements may be added to the milk. We often advocate CF infants are weaned a little earlier than is customary, at approximately two and a half months, both to satisfy the infants and achieve higher energy intakes.

Vitamin supplements

Routine supplementation of water-soluble vitamins is unnecessary. A daily supplement of the fat soluble vitamins, A, D, E is essential to achieve normal plasma levels (Congdon *et al.*, 1981). The doses are adjusted according to the plasma levels. Average daily doses required to achieve normal plasma levels are vitamin A 8000 IU (2400 µg), vitamin D 800 IU (20 mg) and vitamin E 100–200 mg/day.

Table 18.1. *Acid resistant pancreatic enzyme preparations (BP Units)*

Name	Maker	Lipase	Protease	Amylase
Creon	Duphar	8 000	210	9 000
Pancrease	Cilag	5 000	330	2 900
Nutrizyme GR	Merck	10 000	650	10 000
Creon 25 000	Duphar	25 000	467	18 000
Pancrease HL	Cilag	25 000	1250	22 500
Nutrizyme 22	Merck	22 000	1100	19 800
Nutrizyme 10	Merck	10 000	500	9 000

Administration of pancreatic enzymes

Of CF patients 95% are pancreatic insufficient and require an enzyme supplement to control their malabsorption. With adequate pancreatic enzyme replacement over 90% of the fat ingested should be absorbed. Protein and carbohydrate absorption are usually not a major problem and the lipase content of the preparation is the main consideration when assessing the adequacy of the enzyme replacement therapy. All CF patients who require enzyme supplements should now be using acid-resistant microspheres, e.g. Pancrease (Cilag), Creon (Duphar) or Nutrizym GR (Merck) (see Table 18.1). These are more effective than the older preparations although many patients require large doses to achieve a coefficient of fat absorption of over 85% (Beverley *et al.*, 1987; Stead *et al.*, 1987).

The recent introduction of preparations with a higher lipase content (Creon 25 000, Pancrease HL, Nutrizym 22) has been an advance; initially it was reported their use would permit a 50% to 60% reduction in the number of capsules required to achieve similar fat absorption (Morrison *et al.*, 1991; Bowler *et al.*, 1993*b*). However, it has become apparent that, although the number of capsules required is less, the reduction has not been as great as would have been predicted from the relative lipase activity in the standard and higher lipase preparations, e.g. a capsule reduction of only 22% on changing from Creon to Creon 25 000 and 42% on changing from Pancrease to Pancrease HL. Also, caution in the use of these new enzymes has been advised by the Committee on the Safety of Medicines, following reports of fibrous strictures of the ascending colon in 12 CF children some months after transferring to one or other of the higher lipase preparations. It is interesting that six of the patients were attending the Liverpool CF clinic (Smythe *et al.*, 1994). Most of our CF patients have been transferred to the new higher lipase preparations and we have observed no increase in the incidence of abdominal pain reported at routine clinic visits (11%). However, one 7 year-old girl who had been taking higher lipase enzymes for 18 months had variable abdominal pain. There was some narrowing and lack of distensibility of the ascending colon on barium enema.

Enzyme capsules should be administered with every meal or snack containing fat and the dose adjusted according to the amount of fat in the meal. Administration of enzymes should be started as soon as the diagnosis and pancreatic insufficiency are established even if a predigested formula is used, e.g. Pregestimil (Mead Johnson) (Ramsey, Farrell & Pencharz, 1992). The usual starting dose is one-third to half a capsule of a standard acid-resistant microsphere preparation given at the beginning of the feed and titrated upwards until clinical control of malabsorption is achieved. For infants, the enzyme capsules are opened and the microspheres taken on a spoon with a small amount of breast milk or formula milk at the beginning of the feed (Brady *et al.*, 1992). If the infant has difficulty taking the enzymes this way, they may be given with a small amount of gelatinous weaning food, e.g. fruit puree.

When weaning foods are introduced, advice on varying the dose of enzyme according to the fat content of the meal is important. At this stage, the enzyme dose should be divided – half at the beginning and half in the middle of the feed (Brady *et al.*, 1992).

Frequent dietetic advice and support at this stage is important. Mothers must be confident in their approach to the child's feeding, if enzyme taking is to be successful.

Young children less than three or four years old usually have difficulty swallowing the enzyme capsules, and it is necessary to remove the microspheres from the capsule and mix them with a small amount of liquid or food; the microspheres should not be mixed with the whole meal. The mixing to ingestion time should not be more than 30 minutes. Both chewing the microspheres and exposure to hot food or to food with a pH of less than 5.5 will reduce their eventual efficacy. Children should take the enzymes in the capsules as soon as possible; it is good that smaller capsules are now available for younger children (Nutrizym 10, Merck).

The enzyme dose is usually determined by the clinical and bio-chemical control of the malabsorption. However, the degree of pan-creatic insufficiency is very variable and a starting dose of two to three capsules of standard preparation per meal is usually advised in older

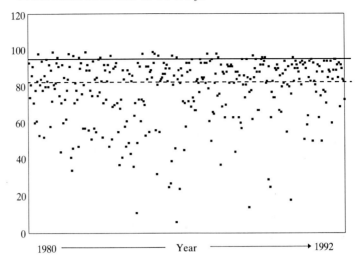

Fig. 18.8. Percentage of dietary fat absorbed by 328 new CF referrals. There was no significant change from 1980 to 1992 although there was a slight worsening of fat absorption with increasing age. ——— normal absorption >95%; ----- CF with adequate enzymes >85%.

children. In the authors' clinic, CF patients up to 16 years old take an average of 30 capsules of a standard microsphere enzyme preparation each day. This dose has been established by increasing the dose to control symptoms and signs and then checking the faecal fat output; if the coefficient of fat absorption is less than 90%, the dose of enzyme is increased (Littlewood, 1991). Regular faecal fat microscopy (Walters *et al.*, 1990), faecal fat estimations (Gilbert *et al.*, 1988) and faecal chymotrypsin estimations (Kasper *et al.*, 1982) should be used to monitor the adequacy of the enzyme dose. Most CF patients attending general clinics receive a dose of enzymes to control their symptoms without additional biochemical monitoring; often there is a significant and improvable steatorrhoea (Littlewood, 1991) (see Fig. 18.8).

Additional strategies to improve absorption

Even with the higher lipase preparations a minority, perhaps 5–10%, do not achieve an adequate fat absorption of more than 85%. For such patients, there are additional treatment strategies which may be helpful. First it is important to ensure there is no other gastrointestinal condition present (Littlewood, 1992); this is particularly important when there has been previous surgery for meconium ileus. Increasing the dose of enzymes does not appear to be effective in the majority of these patients, if the dose is already high, e.g. 10 to 15 standard capsules per meal.

Problems with compliance and the technique of taking enzymes must always be considered as explanations for poor control. Poor fat absorption and a low faecal chymotrypsin, despite allegedly taking large doses of pancreatic enzymes is suggestive of poor compliance; a low plasma vitamin E despite reasonable supplements (100 to 200 mg/day) also suggests poor compliance. Taking all the dose at the end of the feed or mixing with all the food, rather than with a small quantity which is immediately swallowed, will seriously reduce the efficiency of the enzyme.

Of the enzyme activity, 90% of the older non-acid resistant preparations was destroyed in the stomach (DiMagno, Malagelada & Go, 1977); fat absorption was improved when the gastric acid was reduced (Chalmers *et al.*, 1985). In a minority of patients, who fail to achieve adequate absorption with high doses of acid resistant pancreatic enzymes, a reduction of gastric acid will improve absorption (Gow *et al.*, 1981). Sodium bicarbonate (Braggion *et al.*, 1987) and misoprostol (Robinson, Sly & Smith, 1988) have proved effective in improving absorption in some patients.

The initial suggestion that the addition of taurine to the enzyme treatment may improve absorption (Darling *et al.*, 1985) has not been confirmed by one subsequent study (De Curtis *et al.*, 1992).

Conclusions

The nutritional consequences of untreated cystic fibrosis are severe. However, with present day treatments, many introduced over the past decade, gastrointestinal symptoms and signs should be controlled in over 90% of CF patients and their nutritional state and growth should be normal. Of particular importance has been the realisation that many have a poor dietary energy intake and that enteral feeding can restore and maintain a good nutritional state even in patients with advanced chest disease. Intestinal absorption can be well controlled in the majority and fat soluble vitamin deficiency avoided by appropriate supplementation and regular monitoring of plasma levels. As the CF population becomes older, the potential for chronic nutritional deficiencies increases, diabetes mellitus and chronic liver disease become major problems and more invasive measures may be needed to combat the nutritional consequences of the chronic chest infection. The increased resting energy expenditure, its relationship to the CF mutation present and to the chest infection are areas of intense interest. Now that it is possible to control the quantitative aspects of nutrition in most patients, it is important that these techniques are made available to all CF patients. It is now important to determine the most suitable qualitative 'fuel mix' for the CF individual at each stage of the disease.

References

Abernathy, R. S. (1976). Bulging fontanelle as presenting sign in cystic fibrosis. *American Journal of Diseases in Children*, **130**, 1360–2.

Aggett, P. J., Thorn, J. M., Delves, H. T., Harries, J. T. & Clayton, B. E. (1979). Trace element malabsorption in exocrine pancreatic insufficiency. *Monographs in Paediatrics*, **10**, 8–11.

Baxter, P. S., Wilson, A. J., Read, N. W., Hardcastle, J., Hardscastle, P. T. & Taylor, C. J. (1989). Abnormal jejunal potential difference in cystic fibrosis. *Lancet*, **i**, 464–6.

Baxter, P., Goldhill, J., Hardcastle, J., Hardcastle, P. T. & Taylor, C. J. (1990). Enhanced intestinal glucose and alanine transport in cystic fibrosis. *Gut*, **31**, 817–20.

Bell, L., Durie, P. R. & Forstner, G. G. (1984). What do children with cystic fibrosis eat? *Journal of Pediatric Gastroenterology and Nutrition*, **3**, (Suppl. 1), 137–46.

Berschneider, H. M., Knowles, M. R., Azizkhan, R. G. *et al.* (1988). Altered intestinal chloride transport in cystic fibrosis. *FASEB Journal*, **2**, 2625–9.

Beverley, D. W., Kelleher, J., MacDonald, A., Littlewood, J. M., Robinson, T. & Walters, M. P. (1987). Comparison of four pancreatic extracts in cystic fibrosis. *Archives of Disease in Childhood*, **62**, 564–8.

Bingham, S. A. (1987). The dietary assessment of individuals, methods, accuracy, new techniques and recommendations. *Nutritional Abstracts Review* (Series A), **57**, 705–42.

Boland, M. P., Stocki, D. S., MacDonald, N. E., Saucy, P. & Patrick, J. (1986). Chronic jejunostomy feeding with non-elemental formulas in undernourished patients with cystic fibrosis. *Lancet*, **i**, 232–4.

Bowler, I. M., Green, J. H., Wolfe, S. P. & Littlewood, J. M. (1993a). Resting energy expenditure and substrate oxidation rates in cystic fibrosis. *Archives of Disease in Childhood*, **68**, 754–9.

Bowler, I. M., Wolfe, S. P., Owens, H. M., Sheldon, T. A., Littlewood, J. M. & Walters, M. P. (1993b). A double blind lipase for lipase comparison of a high lipase and standard pancreatic enzyme preparation in cystic fibrosis. *Archives of Disease in Childhood*, **68**, 227–30.

Brady, M. S., Richard, K., Yu, P. Eigen, H. (1992). Effectiveness of enteric coated pancreatic enzymes given before meals in reducing steatorrhoea in children with cystic fibrosis. *Journal of the American Dietetic Association*, **92**, 813–17.

Braggion, C., Borgo, G., Faggionato, P. & Mastella, G. (1987). Influence of antacid and formulation on effectiveness of pancreatic enzyme supplementation in cystic fibrosis. *Archives of Disease in Childhood*, **62**, 349–56.

British Paediatric Association. (1986). Report of a Working Party on Cystic Fibrosis. *Bulletin of the International Pediatric Association*, **7**, 439–44.

Bronstein, M. N., Sokel, R. J., Abman, S. H. *et al.* (1992). Pancreatic insufficiency, growth, and nutrition in infants identified by newborn screening as having cystic fibrosis. *Journal of Pediatrics*, **120**, 533–40.

Brown, M. R. W., Anwar, H. & Lambert, P. A. (1984). Evidence that mucoid pseudomonas aeruginosa in the cystic fibrosis lung grows under iron restricted conditions. *FEMS Microbiology Letters*, **21**, 113–17.

Buchdahl, R. M., Cox, M., Fully, C. *et al.* (1988). Increased resting energy expenditure in cystic fibrosis. *Journal of Applied Physiology*, **64** (5), 1810–16.

Carey, M. C. (1984). Bile acids and bile salts: ionisation and solubility properties. *Histology*, **4**, 665–715.

Castillo, R., Landon, C., Eckhardt, K., Morris, V., Levander, D. & Lewiston, N. (1981). Selenium and vitamin E status in cystic fibrosis. *Journal of Pediatrics*, **99**, 583–5.

Chalmers, D. M., Brown, R. C., Miller, M. G. *et al.* (1985). Influence of long-term cimetidine as an adjuvant to pancreatic enzyme therapy in cystic fibrosis. *Acta Paediatrica Scandinavica*, **74**, 114–17.

Chase, H. P., Long, M. A. & Lavin, M. H. (1979). Cystic fibrosis and malnutrition. *Journal of Pediatrics*, **95**, 337–47.

Choonara, I. A., Winn, M. J., Park, B. K. & Littlewood, J. M. (1989). Plasma vitamin K concentration in cystic fibrosis. *Archives of Disease in Childhood*, **64**, 732–4.

Cole, T. J., Donnett, M. L. & Stanfield, J. P (1981). Weight for height indices to assess nutritional status – a new index on a slide rule. *American Journal of Clinical Nutrition*, **34**, 1935.

Colombo, C., Setchell, K. D. R., Podda, M. *et al.* (1990). Effects of ursodeoxycholic acid therapy for liver disease associated with cystic fibrosis. *Journal of Pediatrics*, 117, 482–9.

Colombo, C., Castellani, M. T., Balisteri, W. F., Segerni, E., Assaiso, M. L. & Giunta, A. (1992). Scintigraphic documentation of an improvement in hepato-biliary excretory function after treatment with ursodeoxycholic acid in patients with cystic fibrosis and associated liver disease. *Hepatology*, **15**, 677–84.

Congdon, P. J., Bruce, G., Rothburn, M. M. *et al.* (1981). Vitamin status in treated patients with cystic fibrosis. *Archives of Disease in Childhood*, **56**, 708–14.

Corey, M., McLaughlin, F. J., Williams, M. & Levison, H. A. (1988). A comparison of survival, growth and pulmonary function in patients with cystic fibrosis in Boston and Toronto. *Journal of Clinical Epidemiology*, **41**, 588–91.

Couper, R. T., Corey, M., Moore, D. J., Fisher, L. J., Forstner, G. G. & Durie, P. R. (1992). Decline of exocrine pancreatic function in cystic fibrosis patients with pancreatic insufficiency. *Pediatric Research*, **32**, 179–82.

Covelli, H. D., Black, J. W., Oslem, M. S. & Beckman, J. F. (1981). Respiratory failure precipitated by high carbohydrate loads. *Annals of International Medicine*, **95**, 579–91.

Crozier, D. N. (1974). Cystic fibrosis: a not so fatal disease. *Pediatric Clinics of North America*, **21**, 935–48.

Cynamon, H. A., Milov, D. E., Valenstein, E. & Wagner, M. (1988). Effect of vitamin E deficiency on neurological function in patients with cystic fibrosis. *Journal of Pediatrics*, **113**, 637–40.

Dalzell, A. M., Shepherd, R. W., Dean, B., Cleghorn, G. J., Holt, T. L. & Francis, P. J. (1992). Nutritional rehabilitation in cystic fibrosis: a 5 year follow-up study. *Journal of Pediatric Gastroenterology and Nutrition*, **15**, 141–5.

Daniels, L., Davidson, G. P. & Martin, A. J. (1987). Comparison of macronutrient intake of healthy control and children with cystic fibrosis on low fat and non-restricted fat diets. *Journal of Pediatric Gastroenterology and Nutrition*, **7**, 381–6.

Darling, P., Lepage, G., Leroy, C., Masson, P. & Roy, C. C. (1985). Effect of taurine supplements on fat malabsorption in cystic fibrosis. *Pediatric Research*, **19**, 578–82.

De Curtis, M., Santamaria, F., Ercolini, R., Vittoria, L., De Ritis, G., Garafalo, V. & Ciccimarra, F. (1992). Effect of taurine supplementation on fat and energy absorption in cystic fibrosis. *Ardhives of Disease in Childhood*, **67**, 1082–5.

Devlin, J., Beckett, N. S. & David, T. J. (1989). Elevated sweat potassium, hyperaldosteronism and pseudo-Bartter's syndrome: a spectrum of disorders associated with cystic fibrosis. *Journal of the Royal Society of Medicine*, **82** (Suppl. 16), 38–43.

Department of Health (1991). Dietary reference values for food and energy and nutrients for the United Kingdom. *Report of the Panel on Dietary Reference Values of the Committee on Medical Aspects of Food Policy. Report 41 on Health and Social Subjects*. HMSO, London.

DiMagno, E. P., Malagelada, J.-R. & Go, V. L. W. (1977). Fate of orally ingested enzymes in pancreatic insufficiency: comparison of two dosage schedules. *New England Journal of Medicine*, 1318–22.

Dodge, J. A. & Yassa, J. G. (1978). Zinc deficiency syndrome in a British youth with cystic fibrosis. *British Medical Journal*, **i**, 411.

Durie, P. R., Newth, C. J., Forstner, G. G. & Gall, D. G. (1980). Malabsorption of medium-chain triglycerides in infants with cystic fibrosis. Correction of pancreatic enzyme supplements. *Journal of Pediatrics*, **96**, 862–4.

Durie, P. R. & Forstner, G. G. (1989). Pathophysiology of the exocrine pancreas in cystic fibrosis. *Journal of the Royal Society of Medicine*, **82** (Suppl. 16), S2–S10.

Eid, N. S., Milov, D. E., Valenstein, E. & Wagner, M. (1990). Vitamin A in cystic fibrosis: case report and review of the literature. *Journal of Pediatric Gastroenterology and Nutrition*, **10**, 265–9.

Elias, E., Muller, D. P. R. & Scott, J. (1981). Association of spinocerebellar disorders with cystic fibrosis or chronic childhood cholestasis and low serum vitamin E. *Lancet*, **ii**, 1319–21.

Ellis, J. A., Bond, S. A. & Wootton, S. A. (1992). Energy and protein intakes of patients with cystic fibrosis. *Journal of Human Nutrition and Diet*, **5**, 333–42.

Erhardt, P., Miller, M. G. & Littlewood, J. M. (1987). Iron deficiency in cystic fibrosis. *Archives of Disease in Childhood*, **62**, 185–7.

Faraj, B. A., Caplan, D. B., Camp, V. M., Pilzer, E. & Kutner, M. (1986). Low levels of pyridoxal 5′ phospate in patients with cystic fibrosis. *Pediatrics*, **78**, 278–82.

Farrel, P. M., Bieri, J. G., Fratantoni, J. F., Wood, R. E., di Sant'Agnese, P. A. (1977). The occurrence and effects of human vitamin E deficiency. *Journal of Clinical Investigation*, **60**, 233–41.

Farrel, P. M., Mischler, E. H., Engle, M. J., Brown, D. J. & Lau, S. (1985). Fatty acid abnormalities in cystic fibrosis. *Pediatric Research*, **19**, 104–9.

Fitzsimmons, S. C. (1993). Epidemiological observations on the role of nutritional status in cystic fibrosis patients: evidence from the US cystic fibrosis patient registry. Workshop on Nutrition in Cystic Fibrosis. Bethesda.

Fleischer, D. S., Di George, A. M., Barness, L. A. & Cornfield, D. (1964). Hypoproteinemia and edema in infants with cystic fibrosis of the pancreas. *Journal of Pediatrics*, **64**, 341–8.

Forstner, G. G., Durie, P. R. & Corey, M. (1988). Cystic fibrosis, progress in gastroenterology and nutrition. 10th International Cystic Fibrosis Congress 1988. Sydney. Australia. *Excerpta Medica*, Asia Pacific Congress, Series 74, pp. 154–60.

Fried, M. D., Durie, P. R., Tsui, L. C., Corey, M., Levison, H. & Pencharz, P. B. (1991). The cystic fibrosis gene and resting energy expenditure. *Journal of Pediatrics*, **119**, 913–16.

Friedman, H. Z., Ingman, C. B. & Favus, M. J. (1985). Vitamin D metabolism and osteomalacia in cystic fibrosis. *Gastroenterology*, **88**, 808–13.

Frisancho, A. R. (1981). New norms of upper limb fat and muscle areas for assessment of nutritional status. *American Journal of Clinical Nutrition*, **34**, 2540–5.

Gaskin, K., Gurwitz, D., Durie, P. R., Corey, M., Levison, H. & Forstner, G. G. (1982). Improved respiratory prognosis in patients with cystic fibrosis with normal fat absorption. *Journal of Pediatrics*, **100**, 857–62.

Gibbens, D. T., Gilsanz, V., Boechat, M. I., Dufer, D., Carlson, M. E. & Wang, C. I. (1988). Osteoporosis in cystic fibrosis. *Journal of Pediatrics*, **113**, 295–300.

Gilbert, J., Kelleher, J., Walters, M. P. & Littlewood, J. M. (1988). Markers for faecal fat estimation in monitoring steatorrhoea in cystic fibrosis. *Gut*, **29**, 1286–8.

Godson, C., Ryan, M. P., Brady, H. R., Bourk, S. & Fitzgerald, M. X. (1988). Acute hypomagnesemia complicating the treatment of meconium ileus equivalent in cystic fibrosis. *Scandinavian Journal of Gastroenterology*, **23** (Suppl. 143), 148–50.

Goldstein, J. L., Nash, N. T., Al-Bazzaz, F., Layden, T. J. & Rao, M. C. (1988). Rectum has abnormal ion transport but normal cAMP-binding proteins in cystic fibrosis. *American Journal of Physiology*, **254**, C719–24.

Gow, R., Bradbear, R., Francis, P. & Shepherd, R. (1981). Comparative study of varying regimens to improve steatorrhoea and creatorrhoea in cystic fibrosis: effectiveness of an enteric coated preparation with and without antacids and cimetidine. *Lancet*, **ii**, 1071–4.

Gregory, J. W., Greene, S. A., Scrimgecur, C. M. & Renie, M. J. (1991). Body water measured in growth disorders: a comparison of biochemical impedance and skinfold thickness techniques with isotope dilution. *Archives of Disease in Childhood*, **66**, 220–2.

Hanes, F. A. & MacDonald, A. (1988). 'Can I afford the diet?' British Dietetic Association Position Paper. *Journal of Human Nutrition and Dietetics*, **1**, 389–96.

Hanley, J. G., McKenna, M. J., Quigley, C., Freaney, R., Muldowney, F. P. & Fitzgerald, M. X. (1985). Hypovitaminosis D and response to supplementation in older patients with cystic fibrosis. *Quarterly Journal of Medicine* (new series), **56**, 377–85.

Heymsfield, S. B., McManus. C., Smith, J., Stevens, V. & Nixon, D. W. (1982).

Anthropometric measurement of muscle mass: revised equations for calculating bone-free arm muscle mass. *American Journal of Clinical Nutrition*, **36**, 680–90.

Hill, S. M., Phillips, A. D., Mearns, M. & Walker-Smith, J. A. (1989). Cow's milk sensitive enteropathy in cystic fibrosis. *Archives of Disease in Childhood*, **64**, 1251–5.

Holden, C. E., Puntis, J. W. L., Charlton, C. P. J. & Booth, I. W. (1991). Home enteral nutrition through nasogastric tubes: acceptability and safety. *Archives of Disease in Childhood*, **66**, 148–51.

Hubbard, V. S. (1985). Nutritional considerations in cystic fibrosis. *Seminars of Respiratory Medicine*, **6**, 308–13.

Johnston, J. L., Leong, M. S., Checkland, E. G., Zuberbuhler, P. C., Conger, P. R. & Quinney, H. A. (1988). Body fat assessed from body density and estimated from skinfold thickness in normal children and children with cystic fibrosis. *American Journal of Clinical Nutrition*, **48**, 1362–6.

Kane, R. E. & Black, P. (1989). Glucose intolerance with low-, medium- and high carbohydrate formulas during nighttime enteral feedings in cystic fibrosis patients. *Journal of Pediatric Gastroenterology and Nutrition*, **8**, 321–6.

Kane, R. E. & Hobbs, P. (1991). Energy and respiratory metabolism in cystic fibrosis: the influence of carbohydrate content of nutritional supplements *Journal of Pediatric Gastroenterology and Nutrition*, **12**, 217–23.

Kasper, P., Moeller, G., Wahlefeld, A. W. & Staehler, F. A. (1982). A new photometric method for the determination of chymotrypsin in the stool. Frezenius, Zeitschrift Analytische Chemie, **311**, 391–2.

Kelleher, J., Goode, H. F., Field, H. P., Walker, B. E., Miller, M. G. & Littlewood, J. M. (1986). Essential element nutritional status in cystic fibrosis. *Human Nutrition and Applied Nutrition*, **40A**, 79–84.

Kelleher, J., Miller, M. G., Littlewood, J. M., McDonald, A. M. & Losowsky, M. S. (1987). The clinical effect of vitamin E depletion in cystic fibrosis. *International Journal of Vitamin Nutrition Research*, **57**, 253–9.

Kennedy, J. D., Dinwiddie, R., Daman-Willems, C., Dillon, M. J. & Matthew, D. J. (1990). Pseudo-Bartters, syndrome in cystic fibrosis. *Archives of Disease in Childhood*, **65**, 786–7.

Kraemer, R., Rudeberg, A., Hadorn, B. & Rossi, E. (1978). Relative under weight in cystic fibrosis and its prognostic value. *Acta Paediatrica Scandinavica*, **67**, 33–7.

Kopelman, H. R., Durie, P. R., Gaskin, K. J., Weisman, Z., Forstner, G. G. (1985). Pancreatic fluid and protein hyperconcentration in cystic fibrosis. *New England Journal of Medicine*, **312**, 329–34.

Lanng, S., Thorsteisson, B., Nerup, J. & Koch, C. (1991). Glucose tolerance in cystic fibrosis. *Archives of Disease in Childhood*, **66**, 612–16.

Lanng, S., Thorsteisson, B., Nerup, J. & Koch, C. (1992). Influence of the development of diabetes mellitus on the clinical status in patients with cystic fibrosis. *European Journal of Pediatrics*, **151**, 684–7.

Laughlin, J. L., Brady, M. S. & Elgen, H. (1981). Changing feeding trends as a cause of electrolyte depletion in infants with cystic fibrosis. *Pediatrics*, **68**, 203–7.

Levy, L. D., Durie, P. R., Pencharz, P. B. & Corey, M. L. (1985). Effects of long term nutritional rehabilitation on body composition and clinical status in malnourished children and adolescents with cystic fibrosis. *Journal of Pediatrics*, **107**, 225–30.

Littlewood, J. M., Kelleher, J., Losowsky, M. S. *et al.* (1984). Comprehensive clinical and laboratory assessment in cystic fibrosis. In *Cystic Fibrosis: Horizons*, ed. D. Lawson, p. 266. John Wiley, Chichester.

Littlewood, J. M. & MacDonald, A. (1987). Rationale of modern dietary recommendations in cystic fibrosis. *Journal of the Royal Society of Medicine*, **80** (Suppl. 15), 16–24.

Littlewood, J. M., Kelleher, J., Rawson, I. *et al.* (1988). Comprehensive assessment at a CF centre identifies suboptimal treatment and improves management, symptoms and condition. 10th International Cystic Fibrosis Congress, Sydney, p. 89. *Excerpta Medica Asia Pacific Congress* Series 74.

Littlewood, J. M. (1991). Pancreatic enzymes in cystic fibrosis. In *Pancreatic Enzymes in Health and Disease*, ed. P. G. Lankisch, Springer-Verlag, Berlin, Heidelberg.

Littlewood, J. M. (1992). Gastrointestinal complications in cystic fibrosis. *Journal of the Royal Society of Medicine*, **85** (Suppl. 18), 13–19.

MacDonald, A., Kelleher, J. & Littlewood, J. M. (1988). A normal fat diet for cystic fibrosis: is a dietitian still needed? *Scandinavian Journal of Gastroenterology* **23** (Suppl. 143), 155–9.

MacDonald, A., Holden, C. & Harris, G. (1991). Nutritional strategies in cystic fibrosis: current issues. *Journal of the Royal Society of Medicine*, **84** (Suppl. 18), 28–35.

MacDonald, A. (1992). Diet in diabetes mellitus. 11th International Cystic Fibrosis Conference. Dublin.

Mearns, M. B. (1984). Growth and development. In *Cystic Fibrosis*, ed. M. E. Hodson *et al.* Baillière Tindall, London.

Mischler, E. H., Chesney, P. J., Chesney, R. W. & Mazess, R. B. (1979). Demineralisation in cystic fibrosis. *American Journal of Diseases in Children*, **133**, 632–5.

Mitchell-Heggs, P., Mearns, M. B. & Batten, J. C. (1976). Cystic fibrosis in adolescents and adults. *Quarterly Journal of Medicine*, **45**, 479–504.

Morrison, G., Morrison, J., Redmond, A., Byers, C., McCracken, K. & Dodge, J. A. (1991). Pancreatic enzyme supplementation in cystic fibrosis. *Lancet*, **338**, 1596–7.

Murphy, J. L., Wooton, S. A., Bond, S. A. & Jackson, A. A. (1991). Energy content of stools in normal healthy controls and patients with cystic fibrosis. *Archives of Disease in Childhood*, **66**, 495–500.

Newby, M. J., Keim, N. L. & Brown, D. L. (1990). Body composition of adult cystic fibrosis patients and control subjects as determined by densitometry, bioelectrical impedance, total-body electrical conductivity, skinfold measurements, and deuterium oxide dilution. *American Journal of Clinical Nutrition*, **52**, 209–13.

Oppenheimer, E. & Easterly, J. (1975). Pathology of cystic fibrosis; review of the literature and comparison of 146 autopsied cases. In *Perspectives in Pediatric Pathology*, ed. H. S. Rosenberg & R. P. Bolande, vol. 2, pp. 241–78, Chicago Year Book.

O'Brien, S., Fitzgerald, M. X. & Heggarty, J. E. (1992). A controlled trial of ursodeoxycholic acid treatment in cystic fibrosis related liver disease. *European Journal of Gastroenterology and Hepatology*, **4**, 857–63.

O'Loughlin, E. O., Forbes, D., Parsons, H., Scott, B., Cooper, D. & Gall, G. (1986). Nutritional rehabilitation of malnourished patients with cystic fibrosis. *American Journal of Clinical Nutrition*, **5**, 732–7.

O'Rawe, A., MacIntosh, I., Dodge, J. A. *et al.* (1992). Increased energy expenditure in cystic fibrosis in associated with specific mutations. *Clinical Science*, **82**, 71–6.

Paul, A. A. & Southgate, D. A. T. (1978). In *The Composition of Foods*, ed. McCance & E. Widdowson, 4th edn, HMSO, London.

Pekekanos, J. T., Holt, T. L., Ward, L. C., Cleghorn, G. J. & Shepherd, R. W. (1990). Protein turnover in malnourished patients with cystic fibrosis: effects of elemental and non-elemental nutritional supplements. *Journal of Pediatric Gastroenterolgy and Nutrition*, **10**, 339–43.

Pencharz, P., Hill, R., Archibald, E., Levy, L. & Newth, C. (1984). Energy needs and nutritional of rehabilitation undernourished adolescents and adults with cystic fibrosis. *Journal of Pediatric Gastroenterology and Nutrition.* (Suppl. 1), S147–53.

Ramsey, B. W., Farrell, P. M. & Pencharz, P. (1992). Nutritional assessment and management in cystic fibrosis: a consensus report. *American Journal of Clinical Nutrition*, **55**, 108–16.

Rasmussen, M., Michalsen, H., Lie, S. O., Nilsson, A., Petersen, L. B. & Norum, K. R. (1986). Intestinal retinol esterification and serum retinol in children with cystic fibrosis. *Journal of Pediatric Gastroenterology and Nutrition*, **5**, 397–403.

Rayner, R. J., Tyrell, J. C., Hiller, E. J. *et al.* (1989). Night blindness and conjuctival xerosis due to vitamin A deficiency in cystic fibrosis *Archives of Disease in Childhood*, **64**, 1151–6.

Recommended Amounts of Food, Energy and Nutrients for Groups of People in the United Kingdom. (1979). *Report by Committee on Medical Aspects of Food Policy*. HMSO, DHSS.

Reiter, E. O., Brugman, S. M., Pike, J. W. *et al.* (1985). Vitamin D metabolites in adolescents and young adults with cystic fibrosis: effects of sun and season. *Journal of Pediatrics*, **106**, 21–5.

Robinson, P. J., Sly, P. D. & Smith, A. L. (1988). Effect of misoprostol on fat absorption in cystic fibrosis. *Archives of Disease in Childhood*, **63**, 1081–2.

Roy, C. C., Weber, A. M., Morin, C. L. *et al.*, (1977). Abnormal biliary composition in cystic fibrosis. Effect of pancreatic enzymes. *New England Journal of Medicine*, **292**, 1301–5.

Schmerling, D. H., Forrer, J. C. W. & Prader, A. (1970). Faecal fat and nitrogen in healthy children and in children with malabsorption and maldigestion. *Pediatrics*, **46**, 690–5.

Schwachman, H. & Kulczyki, L. L. (1958). Long term study of one hundred and five patients with cystic fibrosis. *American Journal of Diseases in Children*, **96**, 6–15.

Scott, J., Elias, E., Moult, P. J. A., Barnes, S. & Wills, M. R. (1977). Rickets in adult cystic fibrosis with myopathy, pancreatic insufficiency and proximal renal tubular dysfunction. *American Journal of Medicine*, **63**, 488–92.

Scott-Jupp, R., Lama, M. & Tanner, M. S. (1991). Prevalence of liver disease in cystic fibrosis. *Archives of Disease in Childhood*, **66**, 698–701.

Setchell, K. D. R., Smethurst, P., Giunta, A. M. & Colombo, C. (1985). Serum bile acid composition in patients with cystic fibrosis. *Clinica Chimica Acta*, **151**, 101–10.

Shepherd, R. W., Cookley, W. G. E. & Cooke, W. D. D. (1980). Improved growth and clinical, nutritional and respiratory changes in response to nutritional therapy in cystic fibrosis. *Journal of Pediatrics*, **97**, 351–7.

Shepherd, R. W., Holt, T. L., Thomas, D. J., Isles, A., Francis, P. J. & Ward, L. C. (1986). Nutritional rehabilitation in cystic fibrosis patients, controlled studies of effects on nutritional growth retardation, total body protein turnover, and course of pulmonary disease. *Journal of Pediatrics*, **109**, 788–94.

Simmonds, E. J., Wall, C. R., Wolfe, S. P. & Littlewood, J. M. (1994). A review of infant feeding practices at a regional cystic fibrosis unit. *Journal of Human Nutrition and Dietetics,* (in press).

Sitrin, M. D., Leiberman, F., Jensen, W. E., Noronha, A., Milburn, C. & Addington, W. (1987). Vitamin E deficiency and neurological disease in adults with cystic fibrosis. *Annals of Internal Medicine,* **107**, 51–4.

Smythe, R. L., van Velzen, D., Smyth, A. R. *et al.* (1994). Structures of ascending colon in cystic fibrosis and high-strength pancreatic enzymes. *Lancet,* **343**, 85–6.

Sokel, R. J., Reardon, M. C., Accurso, F. J. *et al.* (1989). Fat soluble vitamin status during the first year of life in infants with cystic fibrosis identified by screening of newborns. *Clinical Nutrition,* **50**, 1064–71.

Solomons, N.W. Reiger, C. H. L., Jacob, R. A., Rothberg, R. & Sandstead, H. H. (1981). Zinc nutrient and taste activity in patients with cystic fibrosis. *Nutrition Research,* **1**, 13–24.

Sproul, A. & Huang, N. N. (1965). Growth patterns in children with cystic fibrosis. *Journal of Pediatrics,* **65**, 644–76.

Stead, R. J., Skypala, I., Hodson, M. E. *et al.* (1987). Enteric coated microspheres of pancreatin in the treatment of cystic fibrosis: comparison with a standard enteric coated preparation. *Thorax,* **42**, 433–7.

Stead, R. J., Houlder, S., Angew, J. *et al.* (1987). Vitamin D and parathyroid hormone and bone mineralisation in adults with cystic fibrosis. *Thorax,* **43**, 190–4.

Sturgess, J. M. (1984). Structural and development abnormalities of the exocrine pancreas cystic fibrosis. *Journal of Pediatric Gastroenterology and Nutrition,* **3** (Suppl. 1), 555–66.

Tanner, J. M. & Whitehouse, R. H. (1976). Clinical longitudinal standards for height, weight, height velocity, weight velocity and stages of puberty. *Archives of Disease in Childhood,* **51**, 170–9.

Taylor, C. J., Baxter, P. S., Hardcastle, J. & Hardcastle, P. T. (1988). Failure to induce secretion in jejunal biopsies from children with cystic fibrosis. *Gut,* **29**, 957–62.

Thomas, B., Blue, B. & Hemried, L. (1990). Enteral feeding practices among cystic fibrosis centres. *Pediatric Pulmonology* (Suppl. 5), 267.

Vaisman, N., Pencharz, P. B., Corey, M., Canny, G. J. & Hahn, E. (1987). Energy expenditure in patients with cystic fibrosis. *Journal of Pediatrics,* **11**, 496–500.

Vernon, S. A., Neugehauer, M. A. Z., Brimlow, G., Tyrell, J. C. & Hiller, E. J. (1989). Conjuctival xerosis in cystic fibrosis. *Journal of the Royal Society of Medicine,* **42**, 46–7.

Walters, T. R. & Koch, H. F. (1972). Haemorrhagic diathesis and cystic fibrosis in infancy. *American Journal of Diseases in Children,* **124**, 641–7.

Walters, M. P., Kelleher, J., Gilbert, J. & Littlewood, J. M. (1990). Clinical monitoring of steatorrhoea in cystic fibrosis. *Archives of Disease in Childhood,* **63**, 99–102.

Wicks, C., Gimson, A., Vlavianos, P. *et al.* (1992). Assessment of the percutaneous endoscopic gastrostomy feeding tube as of an integrated approach to enteral feeding. *Gut,* **33**, 613–16.

Williams, J., Handy, D. J. & Weller, P. H. (1989). Improving oral intakes in older children with cystic fibrosis. *Journal of Human Nutrition,* **2**, 279–85.

Zentler-Munro, P. L., Fitzpatrick, J. W. F., Batten, J. C. & Northfield, T. C. (1985). Effects of intraduodenal acidity on aqueous phase bile acid and lipid concentrations in pancreatic steatorrhoea due to cystic fibrosis. *Gut*, **25**, 500–7.

Zentler-Munro, P. L. (1989). Pancreatic exocrine insufficiency and cystic fibrosis. *Current Opinion in Gastroenterology*, **5**, 706–10.

Zipf, W. B., Kien, C. L., Horswill, C. A., McCoy, K. S., O'Dorisio, T. & Dineyerd, B. L. (1991). Effects of tolbutamide on growth and body composition on non diabetic children with cystic fibrosis. *Pediatric Research*, **30**, 309–14.

Suggested approach to nutritional management

For the poor energy intake

- Dietetic assessment to quantify the problem and determine the important causative factors.
- Increase energy intake to $> 120\%$ recommended for age
  avoid fat restriction ($> 40\%$ energy as fat)
  give more normal food
  add dietary energy supplements
  nasogastric feeds
    enterostomy feeds
    parenteral nutrition

For the intestinal malabsorption

- Measure the severity of the malabsorption
  faecal fat estimation
  faecal fat microscopy
- Improve pancreatic enzyme treatment
  use microsphere acid resistant preparation
  higher lipase preparation if necessary
  increase dose on results of faecal fat
  when symptoms controlled, check faecal fat or microscopy and chymotrypsin
- Exclude other gastrointestinal disorders
- Acid reduction by hydrogen ion blockers
- Review patient's compliance with enzymes

To avoid deficiencies of fat soluble vitamins

- Give daily supplements in doses appropriate for CF
  Vitamin A 8000 units
  Vitamin D 800 units
  Vitamin E 50–200 mg
- Check plasma levels
- Increase doses if levels are below normal
- Give vitamin K before major surgery and with liver disease.

To minimise the increased energy expenditure

- Vigorous treatment of the respiratory infection
- Search for and control of diabetes mellitus
    routine urine glucose test
    over 10 years annual glucose tolerance test
- Consider other causes of excessive energy utilisation, e.g. salbutamol for bronchospasm

Comprehensive CF assessment

History/examination	Haemoglobin WBC platelets
Weight, height, wt/ht	Film plasma viscosity
MUAC and Skin folds	C reactive protein
Immunisation state	Plasma electrolytes
Respiratory function	Liver function tests
Bronchodilator response	Fasting glucose
Physiotherapist's assessment	Glucose tolerance > 10 years
Dietitian's assessment	HbA1 fructosamine
X-ray chest and abdomen	plasma vitamin A, D, E
Ultrasound liver, gallbladder	Prothrombin time
Sputum culture	Aspergillus pptns and RAST
Sweat test (once only)	Aspergillus skin test
DNA status (once only)	Total IgE
	Immunoglobulins IgG, IgA, Igm
	Pseudomonas IgG antibodies
	Faecal fat collection
	Faecal chymotrypsin

These investigations are performed as a 'First assessment' and also annually for a 'Birthday assessment'.

19

Diet, lipids and lipoproteins

J. P. MILLER AND A. NAYLOR

The principal interest in the influence of dietary factors on serum lipids and lipoproteins is the association, now widely accepted as causal (Steinberg, 1989), between quantitative and qualitative abnormalities of lipoprotein metabolism and atheromatous vascular disease. Detailed discussion of this relationship is beyond the scope of this review but *inter alia* it is based upon:

1. the extensive epidemiological evidence which links serum and hence low density lipoprotein (LDL) cholesterol concentrations, to risk of developing clinical coronary heart disease (CHD)
2. the greatly increased risk of developing CHD in certain single gene abnormalities of lipoprotein metabolism, most notably familial hyper-cholesterolaemia (FH) (Goldstein & Brown, 1989) and evidence that survival can be prolonged in homozygous FH by plasmapheresis (Thompson, Miller & Breslow, 1985)
3. the observation that lipids deposited in atheromatous plaques are derived from circulating lipoproteins (Nicoll, Duffield & Lewis, 1981)
4. a reduction in fatal and non-fatal CHD events in trials of cholesterol lowering achieved with diet and drugs (Holme, 1993) and partial ileal bypass (Buchwald *et al.*, 1990)
5. angiographic evidence of delayed progression or actual regression in coronary and femoral atherosclerosis after cholesterol lowering with drugs (Brown *et al.*, 1993), surgery (Buchwald *et al.*, 1990) or dietary intervention (Ornish *et al.*, 1990; Watts *et al.*, 1992)
6. a wealth of experimental data in animals linking development of atheroma and its regression to changes in serum lipoproteins.

420

The importance of diet in CHD prevention

Dietary change to modify serum lipids and thereby reduce atherosclerosis and thrombosis is, together with other lifestyle measures such as aerobic exercise and abstention from smoking, the basis of the 'population strategy' for the prevention of CHD. The ability of dietary modification to alter significantly the serum cholesterol in large numbers of free-living individuals, as opposed to smaller numbers in closely monitored trials, has recently been questioned. Ramsay, Yeo & Jackson (1991), concluded that the National Cholesterol Education Program step 1 diet (<30% calories from fat, ratio of polyunsaturated to saturated fatty acids (P/S ratio) 1.0, dietary cholesterol <300 mg/day), will lower serum cholesterol by only 2% on average. This may be an unduly pessimistic view (Miller, 1992) and in the Oslo study (Hjermann *et al.*, 1981), which used essentially a step 1 diet, serum cholesterol was reduced by 13%.

Nevertheless, it has to be conceded that, in the medium term, the reduction in serum cholesterol likely to be achieved in the general population with dietary advice, will be modest. The absolute reduction in CHD events could still be substantial. A 1% reduction in serum cholesterol, because of the statistical phenomenon of regression dilution bias, is likely to lead to a 3% reduction in CHD events (Standing Medical Advisory Committee to the Secretary of State for Health, 1990), rather than the 2% usually quoted. Where triglycerides (TG) are also reduced and high density lipoprotein cholesterol (HDL-C) increased, the reduction may be greater (Frick, *et al.*, 1987). The reduction in risk for the individual from such an approach will be small, though large numbers of CHD deaths could be prevented. A 'high risk strategy' is still required for individuals with existing vascular disease, multiple risk factors and monogenic lipoprotein disorders. They will often achieve better responses to diet under close supervision, though many will also require lipid-lowering drugs.

Body weight and serum lipids

In epidemiological studies, greater nutrient intake can be associated with lower body weight, a more desirable lipid profile and less CHD (Gordon *et al.*, 1981). Since it seems improbable that eating more will reduce both weight and CHD, the explanation for this apparent paradox is probably that those who weighed less, had higher energy expenditure. Various indices of overweight correlate positively with serum TG and negatively with HDL-C (Glueck *et al.*, 1980) and weight loss usually, but not always leads to improvements in these variables. Effects on serum and low density lipoprotein cholesterol (LDL-C) are less predictable in the individual. This may partly result from the observation that not only LDL production but also its fractional catabolic rate, can be increased in obesity and both of these may be reversed by weight loss (McNamara, 1987).

Wolf and Grundy (1983) found that, while weight reduction (8 to 56 kg) led to persistent reductions in serum triglycerides and increases in HDL-C, the tendency of total cholesterol and LDL-C to fall during weight loss was reversed during stabilisation at the lower weight. Wood *et al.* (1988) also found that weight loss, produced by calorie restriction in essentially normolipidaemic men, had no significant effect on serum cholesterol and LDL-C, though there were small reductions in TG and increases in HDL-C (about 0.2 and 0.14 mmol/l respectively). The failure of calorie restriction without change in dietary composition, in these (but not all) studies, to produce a sustained reduction in LDL-C, does not exclude the possibility that such diets may reduce LDL-C in subjects with primary hypercholesterolaemia. LDL in obese subjects tend to be relatively poor in cholesterol (Kesaniemi & Grundy, 1983; Ginsberg, Le & Gibson, 1985) and small dense (i.e. lipid depleted) LDL are believed to be particularly atherogenic (Austin *et al.*, 1988). It is conceivable, therefore, that weight loss might reduce the atherogenicity of LDL, without any measurable change in LDL-C, if this were the result of a smaller number of more lipid-rich particles.

These and other studies emphasise that overweight is frequently not associated with marked hyperlipidaemia and that the average improvement in serum lipids seen with weight reduction in such subjects may be modest. Where obesity is associated with substantial hyperlipidaemia other genetic factors may be operative. Responses vary considerably, however, and some hyperlipidaemic obese individuals can achieve very gratifying improvements by weight reduction. It does not necessarily follow that a given degree of weight reduction achieved by different dietary means or by increasing energy expenditure, will be accompanied by the same alteration in serum lipids. Wood *et al.* (1988), however, could not demonstrate significant differences between the lipid changes in men who lost weight by dieting (without altering dietary composition) and by increased exercise.

Epidemiological studies attribute significant changes in lipid and lipoprotein variables to change in weight. In a longitudinal study of the Framingham cohort, change in weight was accompanied by changes in several atherogenic traits (cholesterol, systolic blood pressure, blood sugar and serum uric acid). A 10% reduction in relative body weight in men, was associated with a 0.3 mmol/l reduction in serum cholesterol and about half that in women (Ashley & Kannel, 1974). When the effects on other risk factors were also taken into account, it was calculated that weight loss of this order was associated with about a 20% reduction in risk of developing CHD.

Denke, Sempos & Grundy (1990), calculated that weight gain contributes about 1 mmol/l in men and about 0.6 mmol/l in women, to the increase seen in serum cholesterol between the ages of 20 and 44 years. The effect was less marked at older ages and indeed serum cholesterol levels in men, but not in women, tend to plateau at about 50 years of age. Over the age range 20–74 years, an increase of about 0.9 mmol/l in TG and a decrease of about 0.25 mmol/l in HDL-C, was attributed to gain in weight. A gain of 20 lb (9 kg) was calculated to increase non-HDL cholesterol (very low density lipoproteins (VLDL) + LDL), by about 0.2 mmol/l and reduce HDL-C by about 0.07 mmol/l (Grundy, 1992).

Until recently, the literature has focussed entirely on degree of overweight and neglected its distribution. Central (upper body, truncal, android) adiposity is particularly associated with hypertriglyceridaemia, low HDL-C, hypertension, glucose intolerance and risk of CHD (Kaplan, 1989; Despres, 1991). When assessing patients for cardiovascular risk, simple calculation of body mass index is less than optimal and we should probably be paying more attention to fat distribution, as assessed by waist–hip ratio and subscapular sink fold thickness. Indeed the relationship between serum lipoprotein abnormalities and obesity seems largely to depend on the amount of intra-abdominal fat (Despres *et al.*, 1990).

Dietary cholesterol

There has been considerable controversy about the importance of dietary cholesterol in determining serum cholesterol. Much of this controversy may be related to the very varied experimental approaches to the problem including:

- free-living subjects or metabolic ward studies
- physiological or pharmacological (i.e. > 1000 mg/day) quantities of dietary cholesterol
- duration of the study
- composition of background diet (quantity and type of dietary triglyceride; formula or solid foods)
- responsiveness of the experimental subjects.

It is not always appreciated that dietary cholesterol is not the major determinant of serum cholesterol and that dietary saturated fatty acid (SFA) content is quantitatively more important (McNamara *et al.*, 1987). What then is the quantitative relationship between dietary and serum cholesterol? The classical equations of Keys and Hegsted, estimated that for a 100 mg increase in dietary cholesterol (half the yolk of a hen's egg), serum cholesterol would rise by about 0.2 mmol/l. Hegsted (1986) recently revised this to about 0.1 mmol/l. McNamara (1990*a*, *b*) reviewing 68 studies published over the last 30 years, estimates the increase to be smaller still at an average of 0.06 mmol/l.

Reduction in fractional absorption of cholesterol, normally about 55%, helps to mitigate the effects of an increase in dietary cholesterol. Reduction in endogenous synthesis, though subject to individual variability, is believed to be an important compensatory mechanism for the increased cholesterol that is absorbed (McNamara, 1987, 1990*a*). When the increase in absorbed cholesterol exceeds endogenous synthesis, clearly even complete suppression of synthesis cannot compensate and serum cholesterol may rise. Other compensatory mechanisms exist, however, such as increased conversion of cholesterol to bile acids as exemplified by a man who ate 25 eggs per day (about 5 grams of cholesterol, rather than the 300 mg usually recommended) and still had a serum cholesterol of 5.2 mmol/l and no clinically important atheroclerosis at the age of 88 years (Kern, 1991). He absorbed only 18% of the dietary cholesterol, compared to about 50% in a group of controls and further compensated for the cholesterol that he did absorb, by doubling the rate of conversion of cholesterol to bile acids. Reduction in endogenous synthesis seemed to be relatively unimportant in this man.

Thus, there are powerful regulatory mechanisms which can minimise the change in LDL cholesterol in response to changes in dietary cholesterol, so why should we worry about cholesterol intake? First, foods that are rich in cholesterol tend also to be rich in SFA, though hens' eggs, which contain some 190 mg cholesterol each but only about 1.6 g SFA, are an exception. Moreover, the efficiency of the compensatory mechanisms for absorbed cholesterol are variable and subjects have been classified as responders and non-responders or compensators and non-compensators. There is some uncertainty as to how much of this variability is experimental and how much represents reproducible biological variability (Oh & Miller, 1985; Katan *et al.*, 1986; Kestin *et al.*, 1989). One might argue that it would be enough simply to observe which individuals get a good response to dietary cholesterol restriction, but the biological and analytical variability in serum cholesterol determinations make this impracticable in a clinical setting and it is clearly irrelevant to a population strategy for reducing serum cholesterol by dietary means.

Dietary cholesterol does not contribute directly to LDL, since it is transported in the chylomicrons from the intestine into the circulation where much of the triglyceride is removed under the influence of lipoprotein lipase. The chylomicron remnants thus formed, depleted in triglyceride and relatively enriched in cholesterol, are then removed by the liver, probably by the so-called remnant or apolipoprotein E (apoE) receptor. Cholesterol delivered to the liver in chylomicron remnants can, however, in non-compensators who allow hepatocyte cholesterol to rise in response to dietary cholesterol, secondarily influence LDL cholesterol concentrations by down-regulating the activity of hepatic LDL receptors.

There is, in addition, a more subtle way in which dietary cholesterol may be atherogenic, without greatly influencing serum and LDL cholesterol. Chylomicron remnants are believed by many to be atherogenic and while not normally present in large amounts, enriching them with dietary cholesterol may increase their atherogenicity (Zilversmit, 1979). It has been suggested that dietary cholesterol may increase the risk of CHD independently of its effects on serum cholesterol (Stamler & Shekelle, 1988). It is possible that variation in a quantitatively minor but atherogenic subfraction of serum cholesterol such as the chylomicron remnant might explain this.

Some of the discrepancy in the literature over the sensitivity of serum cholesterol to changes in dietary cholesterol may relate to the duration of the studies, with greater responses in short-term (Mistry *et al.*, 1981; Packard *et al.*, 1983) than in longer-term experiments (McNamara *et al.*, 1987). Moreover dietary cholesterol and concomitant saturated fat intake might interact in their effects on serum and LDL cholesterol (Schonfeld *et al.*, 1982), though most authors have not found this (Oh & Monaco, 1985; McNamara *et al.*, 1987; Kestin *et al.*, 1989).

It seems sensible, therefore, to try to reduce dietary cholesterol somewhat and to some extent this will be a by-product of reducing saturated fat in the diet. It is doubtful if fanatical avoidance of eggs is warranted and, in longer term experiments, modest changes in egg consumption do not produce measurable changes in total cholesterol or LDL-C in subjects on a low fat diet (Porter *et al.*, 1977; Flynn *et al.*, 1979; Edington *et al.*, 1987), though the possibility of an increase in atherogenicity of chylomicron remnants, without a readily detectable change in fasting lipid levels, remains.

Dietary fatty acids

A typical Western diet may contain some 100 g of triglyceride daily, about 200 times the intake of cholesterol in terms of mass. It is not surprising therefore that fasting before estimation of serum lipids has little effect on cholesterol but may reduce triglycerides. Dietary fatty acid type and quantity are the major dietary determinants of serum and LDL cholesterol levels, though concentrations of lipoprotein(a), a species of LDL widely believed to have both atherogenic and thrombogenic properties (MBewu & Durrington, 1990), are little influenced by changes in the intake of cholesterol or of different fatty acids (Brown *et al.*, 1991).

The traditional view that SFA raise cholesterol, monounsaturates (MUFA) are 'lipid neutral' and polyunsaturates (PUFA) lower cholesterol is an oversimplification. Individual fatty acids within these classes can have different effects so that the widely used P/S ratio is at best a crude index of dietary fat composition with regard to effects on circulating lipids. Lauric, myristic and palmitic acids (C12:0, C14:0, C16:0) are indeed cholesterol-raising, but those of shorter chain length probably are not. Stearic acid (C18:0) also is not and this was suggested by the pioneering studies of Ahrens, Keys and Hegsted some 30 years ago, though largely ignored until recently. Stearate seems to be as effective as oleic acid at reducing serum and LDL-C concentrations when substituted for palmitic acid (Bonanome & Grundy, 1988). Serum triglyceride and HDL-C concentrations are unchanged. The mechanism is uncertain, but may be related to the relatively rapid conversion of stearic to oleic acid *in vivo*. The findings have implications for the development of manufactured fats, such as margarines and shortenings. Denke and Grundy (1991), for example, demonstrated that beef and cocoa butter fat, both rich in stearate, lower LDL-C when substituted for butter fat in the diet, though not as much as does oleic acid. As they suggest it would be preferable to label foods with the content of cholesterol-raising saturates (C12:0–C16:0), rather than total saturates.

Keys and Hegsted concluded that serum cholesterol was reduced more if SFA were replaced in the diet with n-6 PUFA rather than MUFA. Modern work suggests that MUFA (e.g. oleic acid, C18:1) and n-6 PUFA may be equipotent at reducing serum and LDL cholesterol (Mensink & Katan, 1989; Grundy & Denke, 1990), probably as a result of upregulation of hepatic LDL-receptors (Shepherd *et al.*, 1980; Spady & Dietschy, 1988).

Replacing SFA with PUFA is usually said to lead to a reduction in HDL-C (Grundy & Denke, 1990), but others (Oh & Monaco, 1985;

Mensink & Katan, 1989) found no change and suggested that studies which had observed this had used unusually large quantities of PUFA and in some cases had partially replaced SFA with carbohydrate. Even when substituting PUFA for SFA has had no measurable effect on total HDL-C, it has been reported to reduce those HDL subfractions (HDL2, LpA-I) which are believed to be better predictors of CHD risk (Fumeron *et al.*, 1991). The clinical significance of this is unclear.

Interest in n-3 PUFA, particularly eicosapentaenoic (20:5) and docosa-hexaenoic (22:6) derived predominantly from fish oils, began 20 years ago when Bang and Dyerberg drew attention to the apparently low incidence of CHD in Greenland Eskimos (Leaf & Weber, 1988). Recent histo-pathological evidence from Alaskan Eskimos and other native Alaskans suggests that they do indeed have a reduced tendency to develop athero-sclerosis (Newman *et al.*, 1993). Fish eaters in Western societies may also gain protection from myocardial infarction and reinfarction (Burr, 1992). When fish oils are given pharmacologically as a supplement to the normal diet they reduce serum TG but usually have little effect on total cholesterol or LDL-C (Miller *et al.*, 1988). When n-3 PUFA, or for that matter n-6 PUFA, MUFA or carbohydrate, isocalorically replace SFA in the diet, a major part of the effect will result from the withdrawal of SFA. It is clearly impossible to keep energy intake constant and change only one source of dietary energy. Where changes in LDL-C have been reported with fish oil, these have usually been associated with reduction in SFA intake (Harris, 1990). It is likely that long chain n-3 fatty acids exert their beneficial effects partly, or even principally, by virtue of their anti-thrombotic action.

Trans fatty acids (or at least elaidic acid and its isomers, trans 18:1), have unfavourable effects on serum lipoproteins, raising LDL-C and lowering HDL-C (Mensink & Katan, 1990). Milk fat contains 4–8% trans fatty acids, but larger amounts are found in vegetable and marine oils that have been hardened by hydrogenation and it is estimated that the daily intake of trans fatty acids is 6–8 g in the USA and 17 g in the Netherlands. Replacement of all *trans*-fatty acids in the US diet with *cis*-oleic acid, might reduce LDL-C by 0.1 mmol/l and increase HDL-C by 0.05 mmol/l (Mensink & Katan, 1990).

There is general agreement that replacing dietary SFA with carbo-hydrate, reduces HDL-C as well as LDL-C concentrations (Mensink & Katan, 1987; Grundy & Denke, 1990). 40–50% of the total cholesterol reduction may be in HDL (Mensink & Katan, 1987) and the ratio total:HDL-C may actually increase. The impact of this on the development of atherosclerosis is unknown. Total fat intake rather than type of fat, seems to be an important determinant of HDL-C concentrations, though trans fatty acids are an exception (Mensink & Katan, 1990). When total fat intake is profoundly reduced, the lower concentrations of HDL-C and apoA-I probably result from reduced secretion. This contrasts with the variability in HDL-C and apoA-I concentrations in subjects on a fixed diet, which seems to depend upon the fractional catabolic rate of apoA-I (and hepatic lipase activity), rather than secretion (Brinton, Eisenberg & Breslow, 1990). Since the mechanisms are different, it may not follow that reducing in HDL-C as a result of dietary modification has the same significance with respect to CHD risk, as a low HDL-C on a subject's habitual diet. If correct, this means that measurement of HDL-C for assessment of CHD risk should ideally be undertaken before the diet is changed. Some reassurance may be gained from the observation that less developed countries which consume low saturated fat diets and have low incidences of CHD, also tend to have low HDL-C levels (Knuiman, Hermus & Hautvast, 1980). The whole question is, however, controversial (Sacks & Willett, 1991).

Genetic factors in responsiveness to dietary cholesterol and fat

Not surprisingly it appears that genetic factors play a role in the individual variability in response of serum lipids to dietary change and ultimately this may involve most of the key proteins in lipoprotein metabolism – enzymes, receptors and apolipoproteins. Much of the existing work has been directed at the effects of polymorphisms in apoE and apoB (Abbey, 1992).

Katan & Beynen (1987) could not identify obvious metabolic character-istics which would allow one to identify hyper-responders (non-compensators) to dietary cholesterol in a clinical setting. Some of the variability may depend on apoE phenotype. Subjects with apoE4 tend to have higher serum and LDL-C concentrations than those with apoE2; those with the commonest isoform (apoE3) are intermediate (Davignon, Gregg & Sing, 1988). This trend is most apparent in subjects taking high cholesterol, high saturated fat diets. Subjects with the E4 allele have been said to be hyperresponsive to changes in dietary fat and cholesterol (Tikkanen *et al.*, 1990*a*; Miettinen *et al.*, 1992), though further analysis of patients from the North Karelia studies could not confirm a graded response to diet across the spectrum of apoE phenotypes (Xu *et al.*, 1990). Others too have failed to demonstrate this (Savolainen *et al.*, 1991).

Absorption of dietary cholesterol is greater in those with apoE4 than in those with apoE3 and apoE2 (Kesaniemi, Enholm & Miettinen, 1987), tending to increase hepatic cholesterol and depress endogenous synthesis and LDL receptor activity, thus leading to an increase in circulating LDL (Miettinen *et al.*, 1992). The difference between subjects with apoE4 and apoE2 is likely to be exaggerated because apoE2 binds less well to hepatic lipoprotein receptors (a key factor in the genesis of type III hyperlipo-proteinaemia), so that the cholesterol that is absorbed may be delivered less readily to the liver to exert the regulatory effects just described. Feeding 'pharmacological' (Mistry *et al.*, 1981; Packard *et al.*, 1983) or physiological (Miettinen *et al.*, 1992) amounts of cholesterol in man, appears not only to impair receptor-mediated LDL catabolism, but also to increase LDL production.

A variety of restriction fragment length polymorphisms related to the apoB gene and the apoAI–CIII–AIV gene cluster, which appear to be heterogeneous with respect to response to dietary change, have also been identified, though some results are in conflict (Tikkanen *et al.*, 1990*b*; Xu *et al.*, 1990; Abbey, 1992; Talmud *et al.*, 1992).

There is the prospect of identifying subjects who will respond especially well to particular dietary manoeuvres or who will tolerate, for example, higher cholesterol or saturated fat intakes. If combined with genetic approaches to detect those patients who are most likely to suffer vascular events, this could ultimately greatly refine our approach to the dietary management of patients with polygenic lipoprotein disorders and multiple risk factors.

Antioxidants

Reviews of the role of oxygen-free radicals in disease can be found in Dormandy (1989) and Lunec & Blake (1990). For more than a decade, interest has centred on the possibility that oxidative damage to the lipid and protein of LDL might increase its atherogenicity independently of its concentration (Steinberg *et al.*, 1989; Witztum, 1993). Briefly, peroxidation of PUFA in LDL-lipids within the subintimal space, leads secondarily to changes in apoB100. These allow the particles to be taken up in large quantities by the scavenger receptor on macrophages, generating foam cells. *In vitro* this process can be prevented by the addition of antioxidants such as vitamin E. There is evidence that the extent of angiographically assessed CHD correlates with the susceptibility of LDL to undergo oxidation *in vitro* (Regnstrom *et al.*, 1992). These observations lead to the possibility of a new approach to the prevention of atherosclerosis by means of diet or drugs. Probucol, for example, which has moderate LDL-reducing properties, resembles butylated hydroxytoluene in structure and is also a powerful antioxidant (Kita, 1991). Two recent large questionnaire-based studies suggest that men and women who take substantial vitamin E supplements are protected against major CHD events (Rimm *et al.*, 1993; Stampfer *et al.*, 1993), but the results of randomised controlled trials should be awaited before specific recommendations are made about widespread supplementation with vitamin E (Steinberg, 1993).

In simple terms, LDL oxidation may be reduced, by increasing its antioxidant content or by altering its lipid content, to render it less susceptible to oxidation (Berry, 1992). Paradoxically the desire to reduce SFA in the diet in order to reduce LDL concentration, may make LDL more susceptible to oxidation, because of the increased reactivity in this respect of both n-3 and n-6 PUFA. It is likely to be important therefore, to ensure that dietary PUFA are adequately protected by antioxidants (Kok *et al.*, 1991) and the extent to which this is achieved with common foodstuffs is uncertain. There may therefore, be an argument for limiting the extent to which SFA in the diet are replaced by PUFA and using more MUFA, which are less susceptible to oxidation (Reaven *et al.*, 1991).

Present knowledge does not however, warrant undue restriction of PUFA, which include essential fatty acids and which can have favourable effects on platelet function. Moreover, there is evidence linking CHD to inadequate intakes of n-6 PUFA (Miettinen *et al.*, 1982; Oliver *et al.*, 1989). Thus, there appear to be opposing effects of PUFA with regard to atherosclerosis and it seems reasonable to settle for modest increases only in the diet until the issue is clarified. The current UK recommendations are for total PUFA (n-3 plus n-6) not to exceed 10% of dietary energy (Committee on Medical Aspects of Food Policy, 1991).

Alcohol

The interrelationships between alcohol, CHD and changes in serum lipoproteins are controversial and complex. It is established that moderate alcohol intake is associated with a reduction in all-cause mortality, predominantly due to an inverse relationship with CHD mortality, generating a J-shaped curve. This apparent protective effect of alcohol is found in international ecological comparisons, case-control and prospective studies (Moore & Pearson, 1986; Marmot & Brunner, 1991). Whether this association is causal remains a matter of controversy. It has been argued that the excess CHD mortality in abstainers is borne by those with CHD who have given up alcohol ('sick quitters') (Shaper, Wannamethee & Walker, 1988), but where this has been examined it seems that those who have never drunk also carry an increased risk of CHD compared with moderate drinkers (Jackson, Scragg & Beaglehole, 1991; Marmot & Brunner, 1991). Other confounding variables do not appear to explain the findings and controlling for cigarette smoking strengthens the apparent protective effect of alcohol (Yano, Rhoads & Kagan, 1977). There is an increasing body of opinion that the effect is causal (Rimm *et al.*, 1991).

Mechanisms which might underlie any protective effect of alcohol, include a decreased thrombotic tendency (Meade *et al.*, 1979; Mikhailidis *et al.*, 1983) and a reduction in the development of atherosclerosis mediated through an increase in HDL (Castelli *et al.*, 1977; Moore & Pearson, 1986). It should be emphasised, however, that the basis for the well established negative relationship between HDL-C and CHD morbidity and mortality (Wilson, Abbott & Castelli, 1988), is far from understood and may have other explanations than simply efficient reverse cholesterol transport (Schmitz & Williamson, 1991; Miesenbock & Patsch, 1992). In addition the HDL subfractions which have usually been regarded as most closely associated with protection against CHD are HDL2 and LpA-I (HDL particles which contain apoA-I but not apoA-II). Alcohol has been found to increase HDL2 in some, but not all studies (Moore & Pearson, 1986). A cross-sectional study suggests that increasing alcohol intake raises LpA-I:A-II (HDL particles containing both apoA-I and A-II) but reduces LpA-I (Fruchart, 1992), though no data from non-drinkers were included.

It has not been firmly established that any particular form of alcoholic beverage exerts a greater protective effect than another (Rimm *et al.*, 1991) and most studies have simply considered total ethanol intake. There is current interest in the possibility that red wine may be especially potent in this regard and that its antioxidant properties may be important (Renaud & De Lorgeril, 1992; Frankel *et al.*, 1993). Indeed, in population studies incorporating a term for wine or for total alcohol consumption, improves the correlation between fat intake and CHD mortality and may help explain the 'French paradox' (Hegsted & Ausman, 1988; Renaud & De Lorgeril, 1992), in which there is less CHD mortality in France than would be predicted from fat consumption (Fig. 19.1). Intake of MUFA from olive oil has also been invoked to explain the low CHD mortality in Mediterranean countries, but this does not seem to be necessary if SFA, PUFA and alcohol consumption are considered (Hegsted & Ausman,

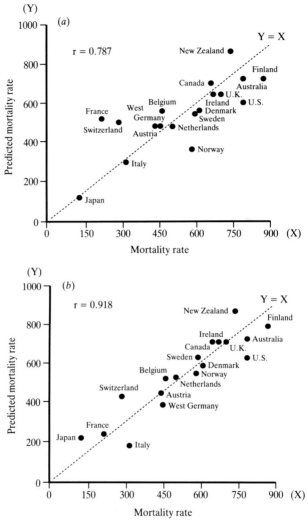

Fig. 19.1. Observed international CHD mortality rates compared with those predicted (*a*) by saturated and polyunsaturated fat intake and (*b*) by saturated and polyunsaturated fat and alcohol intake. Line of equality shown (from Hegsted & Ausman, 1988).

1988). It would, however, be unsafe to assume from this that MUFA are unimportant.

The problem posed by alcohol in the lipid clinic is rather different, in that regular substantial alcohol intake is a common cause of, or contributor to, hypertriglyceridaemia. This is mediated through an increase in hepatic fatty acid and triglyceride synthesis and secretion (Baraona & Lieber, 1979; Lieber, 1991). Clearance of triglyceride-rich lipoproteins is unaffected as judged by the intravenous fat tolerance test (Chait *et al.*, 1972) but prolonged heavy intake can lead to an increase in lipoprotein and hepatic lipase activities (Taskinen *et al.*, 1982) and to a decrease in cholesteryl ester transfer protein (Savolainen *et al.*, 1990). These changes would tend to mitigate the development of hypertriglyceridaemia but could contribute to the increase in HDL.

It has not been demonstrated that this increase in serum triglycerides increases the risk of vascular disease, but it may alert one to the possibility that an individual is taking sufficient alcohol to pose other health hazards and it would be inappropriate to prescribe lipid-lowering drugs for alcohol-mediated hypertriglyceridaemia. The most severe secondary hyper-triglyceridaemia due to alcohol is seen in those who have a moderate primary hypertriglyceridaemia and in such cases the chylomicronaemia syndrome and pancreatitis may result (Brunzell, 1989). The role of alcohol in an individual with hypertriglyceridaemia can be assessed if the subject is prepared to co-operate with a short period (one to two weeks) of abstinence, since triglycerides fall rapidly when alcohol is withdrawn (Losowsky *et al.*, 1963; Chait *et al.*, 1972).

Even if it is true that moderate alcohol intake confers some protection against CHD, this should not lead to advice to non-drinkers to take up alcohol, in view of the suggestion that increasing average consumption in a community leads to a rise in the proportion of heavy drinkers and hence of alcohol-related morbidity (Rose & Day, 1990).

Coffee

Epidemiological studies yield conflicting information about the relationship between coffee consumption and CHD risk (Tuomilheto & Pietinen, 1991). In some, but not all (LaCroix *et al.*, 1986) studies, the univariate relationship between coffee consumption disappears in multivariate analyses, which also consider cigarette smoking. The mechanisms underlying any link are uncertain, but might include effects of caffeine on blood pressure and cardiac rhythm in heavy consumers and an increase in serum and LDL-C (Tuomilheto & Pietinen, 1991). There is some epidemiological evidence that the elevation of cholesterol may not account for all the potential effects of coffee on CHD mortality (Tverdal *et al.*, 1990).

In general, consumption of 5–9 cups of coffee daily increases serum cholesterol about 5–10% (0.3–0.6 mmol/l), but this effect is more apparent in Scandinavian studies than in those from the USA and this is probably due to the method of preparation (Thelle, 1991; Tuomilheto & Pietinen, 1991). The increase in serum cholesterol seems to result mainly from boiled, rather than filtered or instant coffee (Bonaa *et al.*, 1988; Bak & Grobbee, 1989) and to be independent of other dietary factors (Lindahl *et al.*, 1991). It is probably mediated by a lipid which is retained by the filter paper (Zock *et al.*, 1990; Ahola, Jauhiainen & Aro, 1991). Caffeine does not seem to be responsible for the hyperlipidaemic effects of coffee. Instant coffee (520 mg caffeine/day) and tea (200 mg caffeine/day) had no detectable effect on serum lipids in a three-week study (Aro *et al.*, 1985). Replacement of regular filter coffee with decaffeinated coffee, has been reported to have no influence on serum lipids (van Dusseldorp, Katan & Demacker, 1990) or even to increase LDL-C (Superko *et al.*, 1991).

Dietary fibre

The cholesterol-reducing properties of dietary fibre (non-starch polysaccharides) are essentially confined to soluble fibre (fruit pectin, betaglucan in oats and guar gums), insoluble fibre (cellulose, wheat) having little or no effect (Jenkins *et al.*, 1975). There is, however, considerable controversy as to the magnitude and mechanisms underlying the effects (Connor, 1990; Topping, 1991).

Guar gum has been used pharmacologically to lower cholesterol (Todd, Benfield & Goa, 1990), but substantial doses are required for modest effects when used alone; 30 g daily reducing serum and LDL-C by about 10% (Turner *et al.*, 1990). It has also been used as an adjuvant to other lipid lowering therapies (Tuomilheto *et al.*, 1989). The predominant kinetic effect on LDL metabolism is an increase in fractional catabolic rate, compatible with a mechanisms of action similar to bile-acid sequestrating resins (Turner *et al.*, 1990). Psyllium hydrophilic mucilloid (ispaghula) when given as a dietary supplement in a dose of about 10 g daily has been reported to reduce serum cholesterol by 5–15% and LDL-C by 8–20%. Serum TG and HDL-C were unaffected (Anderson *et al.*, 1988; Bell *et al.*, 1989).

Oat bran (100 g/day), may decrease serum cholesterol by up to 19% (LDL-C by 23%) (Anderson *et al.*, 1984), but Swain *et al.* (1990) concluded that it had little direct effect and that it simply displaced saturated fat and cholesterol from the diet. This was because a 100 g supplement of a low-fibre wheat product had similar effects to oat bran. If this is correct, it is hard to understand why the literature in general, reports a cholesterol-lowering effect for soluble but not for insoluble fibre, unless it can be shown that subjects taking the former, reduce their intake of SFA to a greater extent. The study has been criticised because the oat bran group consumed more fat than the low-fibre wheat group and this might have obscured any ability of the oat bran to reduce serum lipids directly. It is far from certain that this is the explanation, however, since most of the extra fat was in the form of MUFA and PUFA, which would not have been expected to raise cholesterol. The subjects were normolipidaemic and this may have made the responses relatively small. A similar study in subjects with hyper-cholesterolaemia and more exactly balanced fat intakes would be worthwhile.

From the practical viewpoint, an increase in soluble fibre produces a modest reduction in serum and LDL-cholesterol, but not many people are going to consume 100 g oat bran (18.5 g total fibre) daily on a regular basis and in the individual who has simply switched to a plate of porridge daily (2 g total fibre), do not expect to be able to measure the difference! Soluble fibre can be an adjunct to other dietary measures but is not a panacea.

Conclusion

Knowledge of the interrelationships between diet, lipoproteins and CHD continues to grow, but much remains to be discovered. Use of the well-worn P/S ratio is simplistic and moribund as understanding of the atherogenic and thrombogenic potential of individual fatty acids improves, leading to new and more complex indices to describe dietary fat com-position (Ulbricht & Southgate, 1991). Moreover, individual fatty acids such as stearic (18:0), may have opposing effects in terms of atherogenicity and thrombogenicity (Ulbricht & Southgate, 1991).

We need a better understanding of the significance of the reductions in HDL-C which sometimes accompany reductions in LDL-C, when dietary SFA are partially replaced. Are they undesirable and is the new ratio of total:HDL-C as predictive of risk as that prior to intervention? There is still scope for better labelling of foodstuffs, for example by quoting the content of cholesterol raising fatty acids, rather than total saturates. The use of dietary supplements as 'drugs' (e.g. guar, fish oil) may have a place for high risk individuals in lipid clinics (though they have not been widely used), but for the poulation at large they are clearly inappropriate. The objective should be to incorporate their parent foodstuffs, at the expense of cholesterol-raising SFA, into the natural diet.

We need better strategies for encouraging dietary change in the population, the results of recent attempts at modifying serum lipids in large numbers of free-living populations, proving modest to say the least (Ramsay, Yeo & Jackson, 1991). National diets can change substantially, though usually slowly in the absence of economic disaster and it is likely that the dietary component of the population strategy for the prevention of CHD, will evolve gradually over a generation or more.

References

Abbey, M. (1992). The influence of apolipoprotein polymorphism on the response to dietary fat and cholesterol. *Current Opinion in Lipidology*, **3**,12–16.

Ahola, I., Jauhiainen, M. & Aro, A. (1991). The hypercholesterolaemic factor in boiled coffee is retained by a paper filter. *Journal of Internal Medicine*, **230**, 293–7.

Anderson, J. W., Story, L., Sieling, B. *et al.* (1984). Hypocholesterolemic effects of oat-bran or bean intake for hypercholesterolemic men. *American Journal of Clinical Nutrition*, **40**, 1146–55.

Anderson, J. W., Zettwoch, N., Feldman, T. *et al.* (1988) Cholesterol-lowering effects of psyllium hydrophilic mucilloid for hypercholesterolemic men. *Archives of Internal Medicine*, **148**, 292–6.

Aro, A., Kostiainen, E., Huttunen, J. K., Seppala, E. & Vapaatalo, H. (1985). Effects of coffee and tea on lipoproteins and prostanoids. *Atherosclerosis*, **57**, 123–8.

Ashley, F. W. & Kannel, W. B. (1974). Relation of weight change to changes in atherogenic traits: the Framingham Study. *Journal of Chronic Disease*, **27**, 103–14.

Austin, M. A., Breslow, J. L., Hennekens, C. H. *et al.* (1988). Low-density lipoprotein subclass patterns and risk of myocardial infarction. *Journal of the American Medical Association*, **260**, 1917–21.

Bak, A. A. A. & Grobbee, D. E. (1989). The effect on serum cholesterol levels of coffee brewed by filtering or boiling. *New England Journal of Medicine*, **321**, 1432–7.

Baraona, E. & Lieber, C. S. (1979). Effects of ethanol on lipid metabolism. *Journal of Lipid Research*, **20**, 289–315.

Bell, L. P., Hectorne, K., Reynolds, H., Balm, T. K. & Hunninghake, D. B. (1989). Cholesterol-lowering effects of psyllium hydrophilic mucilloid. *Journal of the American Medical Association*, **261**, 3419–23.

Berry, E. M. (1992). The effects of nutrients on lipoprotein susceptibility to oxidation. *Current Opinion in Lipidology*, **3**, 5–11.

Bonaa, K., Arnesen, E., Thelle, D. S. & Forde, O. H. (1988). Coffee and cholesterol: is it all in the brewing? The Tromso study. *British Medical Journal*, **297**, 1103–4.

Bonanome, A. & Grundy, S. M. (1988). Effect of dietary stearic acid on plasma, cholesterol and lipoprotein levels. *New England Journal of Medicine*, **318**, 1244–8.

Brinton, E. A., Eisenberg, S. & Breslow, J. L. (1990). A low fat diet decreases high density lipoprotein (HDL) cholesterol levels by decreasing HDL apolipoprotein transport rates. *Journal of Clinical Investigation*, **85**, 144–51.

Brown, B. G., Zhao, X.-Q., Sacco, D. E. & Albers, J. J. (1993). Arteriographic view of treatment to achieve regression of coronary atherosclerosis and to prevent plaque disruption and clinical cardiovascular events. *British Heart Journal*, **69**, S48–53.

Brown, S. A., Morrisett, J., Patsch, J. R. *et al.* (1991). Influence of short term dietary cholesterol and fat on human plasma Lp(a) and LDL levels. *Journal of Lipid Research*, **32**, 1281–9.

Brunzell, J. D. (1989). Familial lipoprotein lipase deficiency and other causes of the chylomicronemia syndrome. In *The Metabolic Basis of Inherited Disease*, 6th edn, pp. 1165–80, ed. C. R. Scriver, A. L. Beaudet, W. S. Sly & D. Valle, 1. McGraw-Hill, New York.

Buchwald, H., Varco, R. L., Matts, J. P. *et al.* (1990). Effect of partial ileal bypass surgery on mortality and morbidity from coronary heart disease in patients with hypercholesterolemia. *New England Journal of Medicine*, **323**, 946–55.

Burr, M. L. (1992). Fish food, fish oil and cardiovascular disease. *Clinical and Experimental Hypertension*, **14**, 181–92.

Castelli, W. P., Doyle, J. T., Gordon, T. *et al.* (1977). Alcohol and blood lipids. The Cooperative Lipoprotein Phenotyping Study. *Lancet*, **ii**, 153–5.

Chait, A., Mancini, M., February, A. & Lewis, B. (1972). Clinical and metabolic study of alcoholic hyperlipidaemia. *Lancet*, **ii**, 62–4.

Committee on Medical Aspects of Food Policy. (1991). *Dietary Reference Values for Food Energy and Nutrients for the United Kingdom*. HMSO, London. 210 pp.

Connor, W. E. (1990). Dietary fiber – nostrum or critical nutrient? *New England Journal of Medicine*, **322**, 193–5.

Davignon, J., Gregg, R. E. & Sing, C. F. (1988). Apolipoprotein E polymorphism and atherosclerosis. *Arteriosclerosis*, **8**, 1–21.

Denke, M. A. & Grundy, S. M. (1991). Effects of fats high in stearic acid acid on lipid and lipoprotein concentrations in men. *American Journal of Clinical Nutrition*, **54**, 1036–40.

Denke, M. A., Sempos, C. T. & Grundy, S. M. (1990). Excess body weight: an unrecognised cause of high blood cholesterol. *Circulation*, **82** (III), 228.

Despres, J.-P. (1991). Obesity and lipid metabolism: relevance of body fat distribution. *Current Opinion in Lipidology*, **2**, 5–15.

Despres, J.-P., Moorjani, S., Lupien, P. J. *et al.* (1990). Regional distribution of body fat, plasma lipoproteins, and cardiovascular disease. *Arteriosclerosis*, **10**, 497–511.

Dormandy, T. L. (1989). Free-radical pathology and medicine. *Journal of the Royal College of Physicians of London*, **23**, 221–7.

Edington, J., Geekie, M., Carter, R. *et al.* (1987). Effect of dietary cholesterol on plasma cholesterol concentration in subjects following reduced fat, high fibre diet. *British Medical Journal*, **294**, 333–6.

Flynn, M. A., Nolph, G. B., Flynn, T. C., Kahrs, R. & Krause, G. (1979). Effect of dietary egg on human serum cholesterol and triglycerides. *American Journal of Clinical Nutrition*, **32**, 1051–7.

Frankel, E. N., Kanner, J., German, J. B., Parks, E. & Kinsella, J. E. (1993). Inhibition of oxidation of human low-density lipoprotein by phenolic substances in red wine. *Lancet*, **341**, 454–7.

Frick, M. H., Elo, O., Haapa, K., Heinonen, O. P., Heinsalmi, P. *et al.* (1987). Helsinki heart study: primary prevention trial with gemfibrozil in middle-aged men with hyperlipidemia. *New England Journal of Medicine*, **317**, 1237–45.

Fruchart, J. C. (1992). High-density lipoprotein particles, nutrition and arteriosclerosis. In *Nutrition and Cardiovascular Risks*, ed. J. C. Somogyi, Gy Biro & D. Hötzel, No. 49, pp. 66–78, Karger, Basel.

Fumeron, F., Brigant, L., Parra, H.-J. *et al.* (1991). Lowering of HDL2-cholesterol and lipoprotein A-I particle levels by increasing the ratio of polyunsaturated to saturated fatty acids. *American Journal of Clinical Nutrition*, **53**, 655–9.

Ginsberg, H. N., Le, N.-A. & Gibson, J. C. (1985). Regulation of the production and catabolism of plasma low density lipoproteins in hypertriglyceridaemic subjects. Effect of weight loss. *Journal of Clinical Investigation*, **75**, 614–23.

Glueck, C. J., Taylor, H. L., Jacobs, D. *et al.* (1980). Plasma high-density lipoprotein cholesterol: association with measurements of body mass. *Circulation*, **62** (Suppl. IV), 62–9.

Goldstein, J. L. & Brown, M. S. (1989). Familial hypercholesterolemia. In *The Metabolic Basis of Inherited Disease*, 6th edn, pp. 1215–50, ed. C. R. Scriver, A. L. Beaudet, W. S. Sly & D. Valle, 1. McGraw-Hill, New York.

Gordon, T., Kagan, A., Garcia-Palmieri, M. *et al.* (1981). Diet and its relation to coronary heart disease and death in three populations. *Circulation*, **63**, 500–18.

Grundy, S. M. (1992). How much does diet contribute to premature coronary heart disease? In *Atherosclerosis IX*, pp. 471–8, ed. O. Stein, S. Eisenberg, Y. R. Stein & L. Stein. Creative Communications, Tel Aviv.

Grundy, S. M. & Denke, M. A. (1990). Dietary influences on serum lipids and lipoproteins. *Journal of Lipid Research*, **31**, 1149–72.

Harris, W. S. (1990). Omega-3 fatty acids: effects on lipid metabolism. *Current Opinion in Lipidology*, **1**, 5–11.

Hegsted, D. M. (1986). Serum-cholesterol response to dietary cholesterol: a re-evaluation. *American Journal of Clinical Nutrition*, **44**, 299–305.

Hegsted, D. M. & Ausman, L. M. (1988). Diet, alcohol and coronary heart disease in men. *Journal of Nutrition*, **118**, 1184–9.

Hjermann, I., Velve Byre, K., Holme, I. & Leren, P. (1981). Effect of diet and smoking intervention on the incidence of coronary heart disease. *Lancet*, **ii**, 1303–10.

Holme, I. (1993). Relation of coronary heart disease incidence and total mortality to plasma cholesterol reduction in randomised trials: use of meta-analysis. *British Heart Journal*, **69**, S42-7.

Jackson, R., Scragg, R. & Beaglehole, R. (1991). Alcohol consumption and risk of coronary heart disease. *British Medical Journal*, **303**, 211–16.

Jenkins, D. J. A., Leeds, A. R., Newton, C. & Cummings, J. H. (1975). Effect of pectin, guar gum, and wheat fibre on serum-cholesterol. *Lancet*, **i**, 1107–17.

Kaplan, N. M. (1989). The deadly quartet. Upper-body obesity, glucose intolerance, hypertriglyceridemia, and hypertension. *Archives of Internal Medicine*, **149**, 1514–20.

Katan, M. B. & Beynen, A. C. (1987). Characteristics of human hypo- and hyperresponders to dietary cholesterol. *American Journal of Epidemiology*, **125**, 387–99.

Katan, M. B., Beynen, A. C., De Vries, J. H. M. & Nobels, A. (1986). Existence of consistent hypo- and hyperresponders to dietary cholesterol in man. *American Journal of Epidemiology*, **123**, 221–34.

Kern, F. (1991). Normal plasma cholesterol in an 88-year-old man who eats 25 eggs a day. *New England Journal of Medicine,* **324**, 896-9.

Kesaniemi, Y. A. & Grundy, S. M. (1983). Increased low density lipoprotein production associated with obesity. *Arteriosclerosis,* **3**, 170–7.

Kesaniemi, Y. A., Enholm, C. & Miettinen, T. A. (1987). Intestinal cholesterol absorption efficiency in man is related to apoprotein E phenotype. *Journal of Investigation,* **80**, 578–81.

Kestin, M., Clifton, P. M., Rouse, I. L. & Nestel, P. J. (1989). Effect of dietary cholesterol in normolipidemic subjects is not modified by nature and amount of dietary fat. *American Journal of Clinical Nutrition,* **50**, 528–32.

Kita, T. (1991). Oxidized lipoproteins and probucol. *Current Opinion in Lipidology,* **2**, 35–8.

Knuiman, J. T., Hermus, R. J. J. & Hautvast, J. G. A. J. (1980). Serum total and high density lipoprotein (HDL) cholesterol concentrations in rural and urban boys from 16 countries. *Atherosclerosis,* **36**, 529–37.

Kok, F. J., van Poppel, G., Melse, J. *et al.* (1991). Do antioxidants and polyunsaturates have a combined association with coronary atherosclerosis? *Atherosclerosis,* **31**, 85–90.

LaCroix, A. Z., Mead, L. A., Liang, K.-Y., Thomas, C. B. & Pearson, T. A. (1986). Coffee consumption and the incidence of coronary heart disease. *New England Journal of Medicine,* **315**, 977–82.

Leaf, A. & Weber, P. C. (1988). Cardiovascular effects of *n*-3 fatty acids. *New England Journal of Medicine,* **318**, 549–57.

Lieber, C. S. (1991). Hepatic, metabolic and toxic effects of ethanol: 1991 update. *Alcoholism: Clinical and Experimental Research,* **15**, 573–92.

Lindahl, B., Johansson, I., Huhtasaari, F., Hallmans, G. & Asplund, K. (1991). Coffee drinking and blood cholesterol – effects of brewing method, food intake and life style. *Journal of Internal Medicine,* **230**, 299–305.

Losowsky, M. S., Jones, D. P., Davidson, C. S. & Lieber, C. S. (1963). Studies of alcoholic hyperlipemia and its mechanism. *American Journal of Medicine,* **35**, 794–803.

Lunec, J. & Blake, D. (1990). Oxygen free radicals: their relevance to disease processes. In *The Metabolic and Molecular Basis of Acquired Disease,* 1st edn, ed. R. D. Cohen, B. Lewis, K. G. M. M. Alberti & A. M. Denman, pp. 189–212, 1. Baillière Tindall, London.

Marmot, M. & Brunner, E. (1991). Alcohol and cardiovascular disease: the status of the U shaped curve. *British Medical Journal,* **303**, 565–8.

MBewu, A. D. & Durrington, P. N. (1990). Lipoprotein (a): structure, properties and possible involvement in thrombogenesis and atherogenesis. *Atherosclerosis,* **85**, 1–14.

McNamara, D. J. (1987). Effects of fat-modified diets on cholesterol and lipoprotein metabolism. *Annual Reviews of Nutrition,* **7**, 273–90.

McNamara, D. J. (1990*a*). Dietary cholesterol: effects on lipid metabolism. *Current Opinion in Lipidology,* **1**, 18–22.

McNamara, D. J. (1990*b*). Relationship between blood and dietary cholesterol. *Advances in Meat Research,* **6**, 63–87.

McNamara, D. J., Kolb, R., Parker, T. S. *et al.* (1987). Heterogeneity of cholesterol homeostasis in man. *Journal of Clinical Investigation,* **79**, 1729–39.

Meade, T. W., Chakrabarti, R., Haines, A. P., North, W. R. S. & Stirling, Y. (1979). Characteristics affecting fibrinolytic activity and plasma fibrinogen concentrations. *British Medical Journal,* **1**, 153–6.

Mensink, R. P. & Katan, M. B. (1987). Effect of monounsaturated fatty acids versus complex carbohydrates on high density lipoproteins in healthy men and women. *Lancet*, **i**, 122–5.

Mensink, R. P. & Katan, M. B. (1989). Effect of a diet enriched with monounsaturated or polyunsaturated fatty acids on levels of low-density and high-density lipoprotein cholesterol in healthy women and men. *New England Journal of Medicine*, **321**, 436–41.

Mensink, R. P. & Katan, M. B. (1990). Effect of dietary trans fatty acids on high-density and low-density lipoprotein cholesterol levels in healthy subjects. *New England Journal of Medicine*, **323**, 439–45.

Miesenbock, G. & Patsch, J. R. (1992). Postprandial hyperlipidemia: the search for the atherogenic lipoprotein. *Current Opinion in Lipidology*, **3**, 196–201.

Miettinen, T. A., Naukkarinen, V., Huttunen, J. K., Mattila, S. & Kumlin, T. (1982). Fatty-acid composition of serum lipids predicts myocardial infarction. *British Medical Journal*, **285**, 993–6.

Miettinen, T. A., Gylling, H., Vanhanen, H. & Ollus, A. (1992). Cholesterol absorption, elimination, and synthesis related to LDL kinetics during varying fat intake in men with different apoprotein E phenotypes. *Arteriosclerosis and Thrombosis*, **12**, 1044–52.

Mikhailidis, D. P., Jeremy, J. Y., Barradas, M. A., Green, N. & Dandona, P. (1983). Effect of ethanol on vascular prostacyclin (prostacyclin I_2) synthesis, platelet aggregation, and platelet thromboxane release. *British Medical Journal*, **287**, 1495–8.

Miller, J. P. (1992). Nutrition and therapeutics: editorial comment. *Current Opinion in Lipidology*, **3**, III 1–2.

Miller, J. P., Heath, I. D., Choraria, S. K. *et al.* (1988). Triglyceride lowering effect of MaxEPA fish lipid concentrate: a multicentre placebo controlled double blind study. *Clinica Chimica Acta*, **178**, 251–60.

Mistry, P., Miller, N. E., Laker, M., Hazzard, W. R. & Lewis, B. (1981). Individual variation in the effects of dietary cholesterol on plasma lipoproteins and cellular cholesterol homeostasis in man. *Journal of Clinical Investigation*, **67**, 493–502.

Moore, R. D. & Pearson, T. A. (1986). Moderate alcohol consumption and coronary artery disease. *Medicine*, **65**, 242–67.

Newman, W. P., Middaugh, J. P., Propst, M. T. & Rogers, D. R. (1993). Atherosclerosis in Alaska natives and non-natives. *Lancet*, **341**, 1056–7.

Nicoll, A., Duffield, R. & Lewis, B. (1981). Flux of plasma lipoproteins into human arterial intima. *Atherosclerosis*, **39**, 229–42.

Oh, S. Y. & Miller, L. T. (1985). Effect of dietary egg on variability of plasma cholesterol levels and lipoprotein cholesterol. *American Journal of Clinical Nutrition*, **42**, 421–31.

Oh, S. Y. & Monaco, P. A. (1985). Effect of dietary cholesterol and degree of fat unsaturation on plasma lipid levels, lipoprotein composition, and fecal steroid excretion in normal adult young men. *American Journal of Clinical Nutrition*, **42**, 399–413.

Oliver, M. F., Riemersma, R. A., Thomson, M. *et al.* (1989). Linoleic acid and coronary heart disease. *British Journal of Hospital Medicine*, **42**, 298–302.

Ornish, D., Brown, S. E., Scherwitz, L. W. *et al.* (1990). Can lifestyle changes reverse coronary heart disease? The lifestyle heart trial. *Lancet*, **336**, 129–33.

Packard, C. J., McKinney, L., Carr, K. & Shepherd, J. (1983). Cholesterol feeding increases low density lipoprotein synthesis. *Journal of Clinical Investigation*, **72**, 45–51.

Porter, M. W., Yamanaka, W., Carlson, S. D. & Flynn, M. A. (1977). Effect of dietary egg on human serum cholesterol and triglyceride of human males. *American Journal of Clinical Nutrition*, **30**, 490–5.

Ramsay, L. E., Yeo, W. W. & Jackson, P. R. (1991). Dietary reduction of serum cholesterol concentration: time to think again. *British Medical Journal*, **303**, 953–7.

Reaven, P., Parthasarathy, S., Grasse, B. J. *et al.* (1991). Feasibility of using an oleate-rich diet to reduce the susceptibility of low density lipoprotein to oxidative modification in humans. *American Journal of Clinical Nutrition*, **54**, 701–6.

Regnstrom, J., Nilsson, J., Tornvall, P., Landou, C. & Hamsten, A. (1992). Susceptibility to low-density lipoprotein oxidation and coronary atherosclerosis in man. *Lancet*, **339**, 1183–6.

Renaud, S. & De Lorgeril, M. (1992). Wine, alcohol, platelets, and the French paradox for coronary heart disease. *Lancet*, **339**, 1523–6.

Rimm, E. B., Giovannucci, E. L., Willett, W. C. *et al.* (1991). Prospective study of alcohol consumption and risk of coronary heart disease in men. *Lancet*, **338**, 464–8.

Rimm, E. B., Stampfer, M. J., Ascherio, A. *et al.* (1993). Vitamin E consumption and the risk of coronary heart disease in men. *New England Journal of Medicine*, **328**, 1450–6.

Rose, G. & Day, S. (1990). The population mean predicts the number of deviant individuals. *British Medical Journal*, **301**, 1031–4.

Sacks, F. M. & Willett, W. W. (1991). More on chewing the fat. *New England Journal of Medicine*, **325**, 1740–2.

Savolainen, M. J., Hannuksela, M., Seppanen, S., Kervinen, K. & Kesaniemi, Y. A. (1990). Increased high-density lipoprotein cholesterol concentration in alcoholics is related to low cholesteryl ester transfer protein activity. *European Journal of Clinical Investigation*, **20**, 593–9.

Savolainen, M. J., Rantala, M., Kervinen, K. *et al.* (1991). Magnitude of dietary effects on plasma cholesterol concentration: role of sex and apolipoprotein E phenotype. *Atherosclerosis*, **86**, 145–52.

Schmitz, G. & Williamson, E. (1991). High-density lipoprotein metabolism, reverse cholesterol transport and membrane protection. *Current Opinion in Lipidology*, **2**, 177–89.

Schonfeld, G., Patsch, W., Rudel, L. L. *et al.* (1982). Effects of dietary cholesterol and fatty acids on plasma lipoproteins. *Journal of Clinical Investigation*, **69**, 1072–80.

Shaper, A. G., Wannamethee, G. & Walker, M. (1988). Alcohol and mortality in British men: explaining the U-shaped curve. *Lancet*, **ii**, 1267–73.

Shepherd, J., Packard, C. J., Grundy, S. M. *et al.* (1980). Effects of saturated and polyunsaturated fat diets on the chemical composition and metabolism of low density lipoproteins in man. *Journal of Lipid Research*, **21**, 91–9.

Spady, D. K. & Dietschy, J. M. (1988). Interaction of dietary cholesterol and triglycerides in the regulation of hepatic low density lipoprotein transport in the hamster. *Journal of Clinical Investigation*, **81**, 300–9.

Stamler, J. & Shekelle, R. (1988). Dietary cholesterol and human coronary heart disease. *Archives of Pathological and Laboratory Medicine*, **112**, 1032–40.

Stampfer, M. J., Hennekens, C. H., Manson, J. E. *et al.* (1993). Vitamin E consumption and the risk of coronary heart disease in women. *New England Journal of Medicine*, **328**, 1444–9.

Standing Medical Advisory Committee to the Secretary of State for Health. (1990). *Blood Cholesterol Testing*. Department of Health, London.

Steinberg, D. (1989). The cholesterol controversy is over, Why did it take so long? *Circulation*, **80**, 1070–8.

Steinberg, D. (1993). Antioxidant vitamins and coronary heart disease. *New England Journal of Medicine*, **328**, 1487–9.

Steinberg, D., Parthasarathy, S., Carew, T. E., Khoo, J. C. & Witztum, J. L. (1989). Beyond cholesterol. Modifications of low-density lipoprotein that increase its atherogenicity. *New England Journal of Medicine*, **320**, 915–24.

Superko, H. R., Bortz, W., Williams, P. T., Albers, J. J. & Wood, P. D. (1991). Caffeinated and decaffeinated coffee effects on plasma lipoprotein cholesterol, apolipoproteins, and lipase activity: a controlled randomized trial. *American Journal of Clinical Nutrition*, **54**, 599–605.

Swain, J. F., Rouse, I. L., Curley, C. B. & Sacks, F. M. (1990). Comparison of the effects of oat bran and low-fiber wheat on serum lipoprotein levels and blood pressure. *New England Journal of Medicine*, **322**, 147–52.

Talmud, P. J., Boerwinkle, E., Xu, C.-F. et al. (1992). Dietary intake and gene variation influence the response of plasma lipids to dietary intervention. *Genetic Epidemiology*, **9**, 249–60.

Taskinen, M.-R., Valimaki, M., Nikkila, E. A. et al. (1982). High density lipoprotein subfractions and postheparin plasma lipases in alcoholic men before and after ethanol withdrawl. *Metabolism*, **31**, 1168–74.

Thelle, D. S. (1991). Coffee and cholesterol: what is brewing? *Journal of Internal Medicine*, **230**, 289–91.

Thompson, G. R., Miller, J. P. & Breslow, J. L. (1985). Improved survival of patients with homozygous familial hypercholesterolaemia treated with plasma exchange. *British Medical Journal*, **291**, 1671–3.

Tikkanen, M. J., Huttunen, J. K., Enholm, C. & Pietinen, P. (1990a). Apolipoprotein E4 homozygosity predisposes to serum cholesterol elevation during high fat diet. *Arteriosclerosis*, **10**, 285–8.

Tikkanen, M. J., Xu, C.-F., Hamalainen, T. et al. (1990b). Xbal polymorphism of the apolipoprotein B gene influences plasma lipid response to diet intervention. *Clinical Genetics*, **37**, 327–34.

Todd, P. A., Benfield, P. & Goa, K. L. (1990). Guar gum. A review of its pharmacological properties and use as a dietary adjunct in hypercholesterolaemia. *Drugs*, **39**, 917–28.

Topping, D. L. (1991). Dietary fibre and cholesterol metabolism. *Current Opinion in Lipidology*, **2**, 20–3.

Tuomilehto, J., Silvasti, M., Manninen, V., Uusitupa, M. & Aro, A. (1989). Guar gum and gemfibrozil – an effective combination in the treatment of hypercholesterolaemia. *Atherosclerosis*, **76**, 71–7.

Tuomilheto, J. & Pietinen, P. (1991). Coffee and cardiovascular disease. *Cardiovascular Risk Factors*, **1**, 165–73.

Turner, P. R., Tuomilehto, J., Happonen, P. et al. (1990). Metabolic studies on the hypolipidaemic effect of guar gum. *Atherosclerosis*, **81**, 145–50.

Tverdal, A., Stensvold, I., Solvoll, K. et al. (1990). Coffee consumption and death from coronary heart disease in middle aged Norwegian men and women. *British Medical Journal*, **300**, 566–9.

Ulbricht, T. L. V. & Southgate, D. A. T. (1991). Coronary heart disease: seven dietary factors. *Lancet*, **338**, 985–92.

van Dusseldorp, M., Katan, M. B. & Demacker, P. N. M. (1990). Effect of decaffeinated versus regular coffee on serum lipoproteins. *American Journal of Epidemiology*, **132**, 33–40.

Watts, G. F., Lewis, B., Brunt, J. N. H. et al. (1992). Effects on coronary artery disease of lipid-lowering diet, or diet plus cholestyramine, in the St Thomas' Atherosclerosis Regression Study (STARS). *Lancet*, **339**, 563–9.

Wilson, P. W. F., Abbott, R. D. & Castelli, W. P. (1988). High density lipoprotein cholesterol and mortality. *Ateriosclerosis*, **8**, 737–41.

Witztum, J. L. (1993). Role of oxidised low density lipoprotein in atherogenesis. *British Heart Journal*, **69**, S12–18.

Wolf, R. N. & Grundy, S. M. (1983). Influence of weight reduction on plasma lipoproteins in obese patients. *Arteriosclerosis*, **3**, 160–9.

Wood, P. D., Stefanick, M. L., Dreon, D. M. *et al.* (1988). Changes in plasma lipids and lipoproteins in overweight men during weight loss through dieting as compared with exercise. *New England Journal of Medicine*, **319**, 1173–9.

Xu, C.-F., Boerwinkle, E., Tikkanen, M. J. *et al.*, (1990). Genetic variation at the apolipoprotein gene loci contribute to response of plasma lipids to dietary change. *Genetic Epidemiology*, **7**, 261–75.

Yano, K., Rhoads, G. G. & Kagan, A. (1977). Coffee, alcohol and risk of coronary heart disease among Japanese men living in Hawaii. *New England Journal of Medicine*, **297**, 405–9.

Zilversmit, D. B. (1979). Atherogenesis: a postprandial phenomenon. *Circulation*, **60**, 473–85.

Zock, P. L., Katan, M. B., Merkus, M., van Dusseldorp, M. & Harryvan, J. L. (1990). Effect of a lipid-rich fraction from boiled coffee on serum cholesterol. *Lancet*, **335**, 1235–7.

20

Diet and blood pressure

J. D. SWALES

The value most frequently quoted for the environmental contribution to blood pressure is 70%. In isolation, however, this statement is simplistic since it ignores the complex interaction between genetic and environmental factors. The well-known Dahl sensitive strain of rat for instance only develops sustained hypertension if given large quantities of dietary sodium (Dahl, 1972). The powerful influence of calorie intake on blood pressure is dependent upon the conversion of calorie excess to increased body mass which is regulated by genetic factors. Nevertheless the paramount importance of environmental factors is clearly shown by the effect of migration on blood pressure. Some cultures show little or no hypertension and fail to exhibit the normal rise in blood pressure with age which is seen in Westernised societies (Glieberman, 1973). When individuals migrate to an urban environment blood pressure rises and they exhibit the characteristic change in blood pressure with age observed in the host culture. The difficulty with such studies is identifying cause and effect. In one study for instance the rise in blood pressure was associated with weight increase, increased urinary sodium-potassium ratio and higher pulse rates (Poulter et al., 1990). A complex change involving diet and social stress had occurred. Which particular components of diet were responsible for the blood pressure change and whether social stress made a contribution cannot be ascertained. Precisely the same problem arises in interpreting studies which have been directed at reversing the undesirable features of Westernised lifestyle. Stamler et al. (1987) adopted a multifactorial approach to the control of blood pressure in a large population of hypertensive patients involving intensive advice on weight reduction, dietary control of lipids, physical activity, electrolyte intake and alcohol intake. Significant blood pressure lowering was achieved and it was possible to reduce antihypertensive medication. The study conclusively demonstrated the blood pressure lowering effects of non-pharmacological therapy but unfortunately its design could not demonstrate the benefits of specific manoeuvres.

The blood pressure lowering action of some dietary manoeuvres is well established. In other cases controversy still reigns. The evidence we have for each dietary component is largely based upon epidemiological association and intervention trial. Despite occasional controversy, the evidence from these two sources in most cases is surprisingly concordant.

Obesity

There is a close relationship between body weight and blood pressure level which extends across the complete spectrum of body mass. Indeed, in population studies weight has consistently proved to be the best predictor of blood pressure. In a screening survey of over one million Americans the prevalence of hypertension (diagnosed by a diastolic blood pressure equal to or more than 95 mmHg) was 19% in subjects regarded as underweight, 24.1% in subjects regarded as being of normal weight and 37.1% in overweight subjects aged 40–64 (Stamler *et al.*, 1979). In a Norwegian study each 10 kg increase in body weight was associated with a 3 mm rise in systolic and a 2 mm rise in diastolic pressure (Boe *et al.*, 1957). Change in weight in longitudinal studies is related even more strongly to blood pressure. In the Framingham survey each 10% weight gain over 17 years was associated with a 6.5 mmHg increase in systolic blood pressure (Ashley & Kannel, 1974). In most Westernised countries body weight exceeds the desirable weight calculated from actuarial tables. Obesity thus makes a powerful contribution to the overall incidence of essential hypertension. In the Australian National study, where obesity was defined as a body mass index of more than 25.5%, it was estimated that up to 60% of hypertension (defined by a blood pressure in excess of 150/90 mmHg) in subjects aged less than 45 years could be attributed to obesity (MacMahon *et al.*, 1984).

The relationship between body weight and blood pressure is not only one of cause and effect, although dietary weight reduction undoubtedly lowers blood pressure (see below). There is now strong evidence for complex genetic linkage. Thus, hypertensive subjects in population studies tend to have higher body mass index than normotensive subjects and exhibit insulin resistance and hyperinsulinaemia (Ferrannini *et al.*, 1987). This is not simply attributable to the effect of obesity on blood pressure. Thus lean hypertensives were twice as likely to become overweight as normotensive subjects in the Framingham study (Ashley & Kannel, 1974). In addition, subjects with a positive family history of hypertension have increased body weight and body mass index. The Utah family study has defined a subset of hypertensive patients with insulin resistance, obesity and an unfavourable lipid profile (Williams *et al.*, 1992). These traits are highly familial and associated with a much higher mortality from ischaemic heart disease. There are other associations between carbohydrate metabolism and hypertension which have not been adequately explained but which may be of relevance. Thus, there is an association between insulin resistance, hyperinsulinaemia and hypertension which is independent of body mass.

Intervention studies

Despite the complexity of the association between body mass and blood pressure, there is unequivocal evidence that dietary weight reduction lowers blood pressure. Indeed weight reduction is the most effective of all non-pharmacological manoeuvres. Many studies suffer from defects in design such as absence of control groups or failure to randomise patients so that the results may be confounded by a placebo blood pressure lowering effect. Of the five randomised control trials four were reported as positive and one negative. However, the one negative study produced a relatively small fall in weight (4.1 kg) whilst the positive studies reported weight losses of between 5.1 and 8.8 kg (Swales, 1990*a*). This is not to conclude, of course, that a weight loss of more than 5 kg is necessary to produce a fall in blood pressure, since the published trials were probably of insufficient statistical power to demonstrate a small fall in blood pressure. Overall, from a pooled analysis of the trials Hovell concluded that a weight loss of 12 kg would lower blood pressure by 21/13 mmHg and a weight loss of 3 kg by 7/4 mmHg (Hovell, 1982).

Mechanisms

Dietary weight loss is associated with reduced nervous system activity manifest by decreased heart rate, circulating catecholamines and plasma renin (Reisen *et al.*, 1983). It is likely therefore that the reduction in circulating insulin levels results in a downward resetting of sympathetic nervous system activity. The role of changes in sodium balance is still controversial. The blood pressure response to calorie restriction however can occur without reduction in sodium intake (Reisen *et al.*, 1983). In one study, however, calorie restriction restored the sensitivity of blood pressure to sodium restriction (Rocchini *et al.*, 1989).

Alcohol

Blood pressure is higher and the prevalence of hypertension greater amongst heavy drinkers. This may account for the higher incidence of disturbed parenchymal liver function tests in hypertensive patients. The positive relationship between self-reported alcohol intake and blood pressure has been almost universally found in different cultures and amongst different ethnic groups. In the largest study of 83 947 healthy subjects, it was possible to demonstrate that the association between alcohol and blood pressure was independent of such potential confounders as age, sex, race, smoking, coffee, educational attainment and adiposity (Klatsky *et al.*, 1977). The magnitude of the contribution of alcohol intake to the prevalence of hypertension was well demonstrated in the careful study carried out by Arkwright *et al.* (1982) in 491 working men aged 20 to 44 years. This study indicated that heavy drinking contributed as much to blood pressure elevation as obesity (8.5 mmHg systolic blood pressure). The prevalence of hypertension (i.e. blood pressure in excess of 140/90 mmHg) was 2–3% in non-drinkers and rose to 9–12% in individuals consuming three or more units of alcohol per day. The causal nature of the relationship has been conclusively demonstrated by cohort studies, in which heavy drinking was associated with later development of high blood pressure and in which change in alcohol consumption was associated with change in blood pressure (Beilin, 1988).

Approximately half the studies of alcohol intake and blood pressure have reported that blood pressures of non-drinkers are greater than blood pressures of those consuming 2–3 drinks per day, i.e. there is a J-shaped relationship between blood pressure and alcohol intake (Friedman *et al.*, 1983). The major difficulty in elucidating the nature of the putative J-shaped relationship is the heterogenous nature of the non-drinkers. In addition to total abstainers this category may also include individuals who have been advised not to drink on health grounds and heavy drinkers who deny their problem. Nevertheless whether the relationship between alcohol intake and blood pressure is linear, J-shaped or whether there is a threshold, it is likely that only an alcohol intake of more than 2–3 units a day makes a significant contribution to blood pressure elevation. Above these levels as a rough approximation one unit of alcohol increases systolic blood pressure by 1 mmHg.

Intervention studies

A limited number of controlled studies has examined the effect of alcohol withdrawal on the blood pressure of heavy drinkers, using parallel groups of crossover design. Thus Potter and Beevers (1984) admitted a group of heavy drinking hypertensive patients to hospital and withdrew alcohol from half for three days and retained the other half on normal alcohol intake. Alcohol was removed from the latter group and given to the former group for the next four days. The period of alcohol withdrawal in both groups was associated with significant lowering of blood pressure. Puddey *et al.* (1985, 1987) also used a crossover design but extended the intervention period for six weeks. In addition, subjects were blinded to the level of alcohol intake by being given a low alcohol lager with or without the addition of alcohol. Significant blood pressure lowering occurred when alcohol was restricted amongst heavy drinkers and this effect was seen in both hypertensive and normotensive subjects. The fall in blood pressure induced in these studies is of a similar order of magnitude to that which would be predicted from population associations if these were attributable to a genuinely causal effect. As in the case of obesity therefore epidemiological and intervention studies together make an extremely powerful case for the hypertensive effects of heavy consumption of alcohol.

Mechanisms

Alcohol and its active metabolite acetaldehyde are biologically extremely active with the physico-chemical properties and biological function of the cell membrane as a prime target (Knochel, 1983). Acute alcohol intake has a vasodilator, blood pressure lowering action. It seems probable therefore that chronic alcohol administration has actions upon the cardiovascular system which are not evident in acute studies. The nature of this pressor effect is unknown although decreased cell membrane fluidity perhaps at the vascular smooth muscle level has been implicated (Knochel, 1983). There is also some evidence for a neurogenic mechanism of blood pressure elevation in the form of reduced baroreflex sensitivity and resting tachycardia although plasma catecholamines are not elevated. In addition elevation of plasma renin activity and plasma cortisol has been reported amongst chronic drinkers. The relative importance of these fairly minor aberrations in the pathogenesis of hypertension is unknown at present (Howes & Reid, 1986).

Salt intake

The original hypothesis that there was a causal association between salt intake and the prevalent of hypertension was put forward by Dahl (1972). Later Glieberman (1973) in a review of 27 published studies reported a rather weaker association. These were inter-cultural comparisons of subjects with widely differing lifestyles. They were open studies and not rigorous in either measurement of blood pressure or of dietary salt. Other dietary components, body mass, chronic infection, ill-health, social and psychological stress could not be taken into consideration but are potential, powerful confounders. Nevertheless, it is notable that most of the regression of blood pressure on salt intake in Glieberman's meta-analysis is attributable to very low and very high salt intakes, i.e. daily intakes of sodium of less than 50 mmol and more than 250 mmol per day. Between these extremes there was little relationship between salt intake and blood pressure. These poorly controlled observations have been largely rendered obsolescent by the Intersalt Study which assessed salt intake in 52 centres in 32 countries (Intersalt Cooperative Research Group, 1988). Each recruited 200 subjects in which sodium intake was estimated from a single 24-hour urinary sodium excretion. Sodium excretion and systolic blood pressure were significantly and positively correlated in 15 centres and negatively in two. For the diastolic pressure these numbers were four and one respectively. The importance of confounding factors related both to blood pressure and salt intake was evident after adjustment for body mass index, alcohol consumption and urinary potassium. The number of significant positive associations fell to 8 for systolic blood pressure and to 3 for diastolic blood pressure after such adjustment. Significant negative associations remained at 2 and 3 respectively. After adjustment for these confounders, the rise in systolic blood pressure for 100 mmol increase in sodium excretion, was 2.2 mm and for diastolic blood pressure, 0.1 mm/Hg, the latter being non-significant. It is interesting in the light of Glieberman's analysis that, when four centres with very low sodium excretions were excluded, the relationship between the prevalence of hypertension or median blood pressure and sodium excretion disappeared. The Intersalt Study therefore provides a dramatic contrast with epidemiological studies linking body mass or alcohol to blood pressure, where consistent relationships have been found of approximately similar magnitude. One positive finding from the Intersalt Study is more difficult to interpret. There was a significant relationship between the slope of blood pressure with age and sodium intake. It is difficult to draw conclusions about longitudinal changes in blood pressure from a cross-sectional study since different cohorts will have had different lifetime's experience. It nevertheless remains a possibility that salt intake contributes secondarily to the rise in blood pressure with age seen in Western societies. This is consistent with biochemical data demonstrating that exchangeable sodium is reduced in younger hypertensives but rises with age and is positively correlated with blood pressure in older hypertensive patients.

Single centre studies have in the main produced negative results. By far the largest was the Scottish Heart Health Study which recruited a healthy population of 7354 subjects (Smith *et al.*, 1988). A weakly positive correlation between blood pressure and sodium excretion disappeared when adjusted for body mass index, alcohol consumption and urinary potassium. This again emphasises the importance of taking potential confounders into account before inferring causal associations.

Some authors have argued that the relationship between sodium intake and blood pressure is underestimated by taking a single 24-hour urinary sodium excretion, since there is considerable intra- as well as inter-variability in sodium intake (Law *et al.*, 1991a). On these grounds much more powerful associations have been inferred by 'correcting' the correlation for variability in sodium intake. Such 'corrections' depend of course on the fundamental assumption that a genuine causal association is present which has been underestimated through inaccuracy in estimation of sodium intake. Without independent confirmation such an assumption cannot be made. Such confirmation depends critically upon the results of intervention studies.

Intervention studies

The effect of changing sodium intake on blood pressure must remain the gold standard in analysing population effects of salt intake on blood pressure. One difficulty is the limited duration of intervention studies. It has been argued that if the slow rise in blood pressure extending over several decades observed in Western societies is due to high salt intake, this effect could not be detected in intervention trials lasting a few weeks. If correct, this belief would remove the salt-blood pressure relationship from the field of scientific testability. However, the greater part of the rise in blood pressure observed when subjects move from a rural to urban environment occurs within weeks of migration (Poulter *et al.*, 1990). At the same time, individuals undergo a radical change in diet and social stress. It should therefore be possible to detect blood pressure effects of a cultural change in diet by means of short-term trials.

A large number of trials have been carried out with conflicting results (Swales, 1990*b*). One cause in discrepancy is failure to distinguish between trials in hypertensive patients and normotensive individuals. It is not valid to extrapolate from one group to the other. Thus, the mechanisms which protect blood pressure against volume depletion (particularly the renin-angiotensin system), may be under-active in hypertensive patients producing a larger fall in blood pressure. Further, falls in blood pressure produced by other manoeuvres (e.g. drug treatment) are usually related to the baseline blood pressure and are therefore greater in hypertensive patients. The major problem in this field however results from poorly controlled intervention studies (Swales, 1991). Thus, when measured by conventional methods, blood pressure falls over the first four to eight weeks of repeated measurement. This may create an apparent depressor response to dietary manoeuvres. Dietary salt restriction also alters other components of diet which may have an effect upon blood pressure. The optimal design therefore is a double-blind randomly allocated trial in which patients are all placed on the salt restricted diet and after a run-in period, receive either sodium supplements or placebo. Whilst some such studies in hypertensive patients have shown a modest fall in blood pressure (Australian National Health and Medical Research Council 1989) it has not been possible to show any impact on blood pressure in normotensive volunteers using this trial design (Watt *et al.*, 1985). Adherence to dietary sodium restriction has also created difficulties. The most carefully conducted prolonged study of salt restriction (three years), only succeeded in producing a marginally significant reduction in sodium intake and produced no impact on blood pressure in patients with borderline hypertension (Hypertension Prevention Trial Research Group, 1990). Other long term studies of large groups of mildly hypertensive patients have proved equally disappointing (Langford *et al.*, 1991). These observations contrast with the meta-analysis carried out by Law *et al.* (1991*b*) on 78 studies of sodium restriction, which calculated that 100 mmol reduction in sodium intake (e.g. from 150–50 mmol) a day, would produce a fall in blood pressure of 10 mm systolic blood pressure and 5 mm diastolic blood pressure in subjects over 50 years of age. This analysis however included 47 non-randomised studies (i.e. effectively uncontrolled investigations) which failed to distinguish between a placebo effect on blood pressure and a genuine response to salt restriction. Thus, the mean fall in systolic blood pressure in the non-randomised studies (hypertensives and normotensives) was twice that reported in investiga-tions using a random allocation design (Swales, 1991). While moderate salt restriction probably produces a modest blood pressure lowering in some sub-groups of hypertensive subjects there is little evidence that moderate salt restriction produces significant effects on blood pressure in normotensive individuals, unless intake is reduced to below 50 mmol a day (Figs. 20.1 and 20.2). Such a reduction in sodium intake is unlikely to be feasible and the adverse consequences in the shape of compromised cardiovascular response to stress cannot be calculated in the absence of relevant data. For the general population however the evidence for a link between salt intake and blood pressure, whether one looks at population associations or intervention trials, is extremely weak compared with comparable evidence on body mass, alcohol intake and physical exercise.

Potassium intake

Some of the inter- and intra-population studies of the relationship between urinary electrolyte excretion and blood pressure have shown a negative correlation between 24 hour urinary potassium and blood pressure (e.g. Khaw & Barrett-Connor, 1998).

In some cases, by combining the sodium and potassium data, it has been possible to show a stronger correlation between urinary sodium/ potassium ratio and blood pressure. The critical importance of confound-ing variables in analyses of this type, is well shown in the Intersalt Study (Intersalt Cooperative Research Group, 1988). There was a small positive correlation between urinary potassium and blood pressure adjusting for age and sex but when further adjustment was made for body mass index, alcohol intake and sodium excretion, the relationship became negative and significant, both for systolic and diastolic blood pressure. The relationship was however comparatively weak. A 50 mmol alteration in potassium excretion was associated with a 2.2 mmHg change in systolic blood pressure. In the largest single population study, the Scottish Heart Health Study (Smith *et al.*, 1988) there was again a weak negative correlation between urinary/potassium and systolic and diastolic blood pressure, which remained after adjustment for age, pulse rate, body mass index and alcohol consumption. In both the major interpopulation and intrapopulation investigations therefore, the negative relationship of potassium and blood pressure, was slightly stronger than the sodium/ blood pressure relationship. Even the weakly negative relationship between potassium and blood pressure does not of course necessarily imply

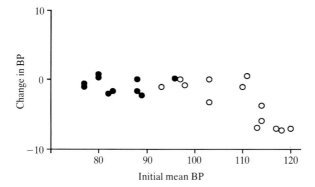

Fig. 20.1. Change in mean blood pressure induced by moderate salt restriction in controlled intervention trials in normotensive subjects (closed circles) and hypertensive subjects (open circles).

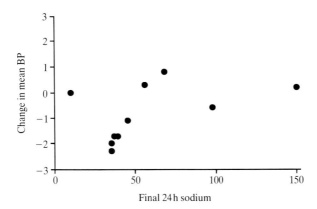

Fig. 20.2. Change in blood pressure observed in trials of sodium restriction in normotensive subjects. Note fall in blood pressure was only observed when sodium intake was reduced below about 50 mmol/d (data for both figures from Swales 1991).

causality, as potassium excretion could simply be acting as a marker for some other dietary component, which had a direct effect on blood pressure. Alternatively, potassium intake could reflect social factors related to blood pressure. Intervention studies are necessary to clarify this relationship.

Intervention studies

A number of trials have been designed to investigate the effect of potassium supplementation on blood pressure in normotensive and hypertensive subjects. The results have been discrepant: in some cases, a significant fall in blood pressure was observed and in other cases potassium supplementation had no impact on blood presure. In a meta-analysis of published trials, Cappuccio and MacGregor (1991) concluded that potassium supplementation overall produced a fall in supine blood pressure of 5.9/3.4 mmHg. The fall in blood pressure was greater in trials carried out in hypertensive subjects. In normotensive individuals, falls on average of 2.0/1.2 mmHg were reported. The degree of potassium supplementation was substantial, i.e. 63 mmol a day. This would be difficult to achieve with changes in dietary intake as opposed to potassium supplementation of the diet. In addition, meta-analysis of published studies have to be treated with caution, since there is a strong possibility of publication bias in favour of positive investigations. Whilst it seems possible therefore that an increase in dietary potassium would have a small blood pressure lowering effect, only trivial blood pressure lowering could be achieved in healthy people as a result of dietary advice.

Dietary lipids

Diets high in oleic acid (e.g. the characteristic 'Mediterranean diet') have been shown to produce small blood pressure lowering effects (Strazzullo *et al.*, 1986). On the other hand, other unsaturated fats (e.g. linoleic acid) in carefully conducted trials have had no effect upon blood pressure (Sacks *et al.*, 1987). In contrast, the omega-3 unsaturated fish-oils have been demonstrated to lower blood pressure in untreated hypertensives (Bonaa *et al.*, 1990). This effect seems to be related to the basal consumption of these oils and is only observed where basal consumption is low. It seems likely therefore that there are specific-lipid effects upon blood pressure which are not simply a reflection of the degree of saturation of dietary fats. More precise definition of these effects and their mechanism still waits elucidation, although both direct effects upon the bio-physical properties of vascular smooth muscle or indirect effects mediated by prostanoids have been postulated.

Vegetarian diet

It has been shown repeatedly that vegetarians have a lower blood pressure and show less of a rise in blood pressure with age than the general population (Rouse & Beilin, 1984). These effects are still seen when subjects are matched for other aspects of lifestyle. Differences of 6–9 mmHg systolic and 3–5 mmHg diastolic blood pressure have been found after adjustment for body mass index. Intervention trials have shown small but highly significant blood pressure lowering effects of the vegetarian diet in normotensive and untreated hypertensive omnivores (Rouse & Beilin, 1984; Margetts *et al.*, 1986). In an extensive series of investigations, Beilin and co-workers were unable to relate the blood pressure fall to changes in dietary fats, fibre, protein or electrolytes (Beilin, 1988). It is possible that a combination of nutrient changes is involved, with each single component making only a small contribution to the net fall in blood pressure. Nevertheless the strong epidemiological data on blood pressure in vegetarians, indicates the potential value of long-term dietary change in preventing hypertension.

Conclusions

There is an impressive concordance of epidemiological and intervention trial evidence in favour of significant dietary effects on blood pressure. Thus, in the case of body mass, alcohol intake and vegetarianism epidemiological studies have consistently shown associations and carefully conducted intervention trials have shown significant effects which are of similar order of magnitude (Tables 20.1 and 20.2). Smaller effects may be seen with sodium restriction and potassium supplementation although these are only persuasive when applied to hypertensive individuals and even then there appears to be some heterogeneity of response. An important question is how far are the effects of dietary components upon blood pressure additive? Few studies have examined this possibility. However, Puddey *et al.* used a two-way factorial study to investigate the combined effects of weight reduction and alcohol restriction in overweight male drinkers (Puddey *et al.*, 1992). The combined measures had additive effects giving in total a fall of 10.2/7.5 mmHg supine blood pressure. By contrast, the same group were unable to detect any further reduction in blood pressure when salt restriction was combined with a decrease in alcohol intake in hypertensive drinkers (Parker *et al.*, 1990). Although there have been claims that weight reduction lowers blood pressure

Table 20.1. *Epidemiological data*

	Systolic	Diastolic
Weight	−3.5 kg	−2.3 kg
Alcohol	−1 unit/d	−1 unit/day
Sodium	−45 mmol/d	−1000 mmol/d
Potassium	+22 mmol/d	+35 mmol/d
Vegetarian diet	20%	33%

Changes in nutritional components needed to produce a 1 mmHg fall in blood pressure on basis of epidemiological associations.

Table 20.2. *Intervention trial data*

	Systolic	Diastolic
Weight (obese subjects)	−0.5 kg	−0.7 kg
Alcohol (heavy drinkers)	−1.5 unit/d	—
Sodium[a]	−66 mmol/d	−73 mmol/d
Potassium[a]	+11 mmol/d	+19 mmol/d
Vegetarian diet	(16%)	(25%)

Changes in nutritional components needed to produce a 1 mmHg fall in blood pressure on basis of controlled intervention trials.

[a] Data from pooled analyses of controlled trials in hypertensive and normotensive subjects. (Data from Swales, 1991 and Cappuccio & MacGregor, 1991.)

through reduction in salt intake, one rigorously controlled study reported independent effects of the two manoeuvres in hypertensive subjects (Reisen *et al.*, 1978). Rose (1981) has pointed to the importance of quite small downwards shifts in the population blood pressure distribution. The need for population advice as well as the possible role of dietary blood pressure lowering in the treatment of hypertension has led to increased interest in the role of diet on blood pressure control. The evidence we have is sufficiently persuasive to support relevant population advice with confidence that it will be effective.

References

Arkwright, P. D., Beilin, L. J., Rouse, I., Armstrong, B. K. & Vandongen, R. (1982). Effects of alcohol use and other aspects of life-style on blood pressure levels and prevalence of hypertension in a working population. *Circulation*, **66**, 60–6.

Ashley, F. W. & Kannel, W. B. (1974). Relation of weight change to changes in atherogenic traits. The Framingham Study. *Journal of Chronic Diseases*, **27**, 103–14.

Australian National Health and Medical Research Council (1989). Dietary Salt Study Management Committee. Fall in blood pressure with modest reduction in dietary salt intake in mild hypertension. *Lancet*, **i**, 399–402.

Beilin, L. J. (1988). Epitaph to essential hypertension – a preventable disorder of known aetiology. *Journals of Hypertension*, **6**, 85–94.

Boe, J., Humerfelt, S., Wedervang, F. & Oecon, C. (1957). The blood pressure in a population: blood pressure readings and height and weight determinations in the adult population in the city of Bergen. *Acta Medica Scandinavia*, **157**, 202–6.

Bonaa, K. H., Bjerve, K. S., Straume, B., Gram, I. T. & Thelle, D. (1990). Effect of eicospentaenoic and docasahexaenoic acids on blood pressure in hypertension. A population-based intervention trial from the Tromso study. *New England Journal of Medicine*, **322**, 795–801.

Cappuccio, F. P. & MacGregor, G. A. (1991). Does potassium supplementation lower blood pressure? A meta-analysis of published trials. *Journal of Hypertension*, **9**, 465–73.

Dahl, L. K. (1972). Salt and hypertension. *American Journal of Clinical Nutrition*, **25**, 231–44.

Ferrannini, E., Buzzigoli, G., Bonadonna, R. *et al.* (1987). Insulin resistance in essential hypertension. *New England Journal of Medicine*, **317**, 350–7.

Friedman, G. D., Klatsky, A. L. & Siegelaub, A. B. (1983). Alcohol intake and hypertension. *Annals of Internal Medicine*, **98**, 846–9.

Glieberman, L. (1973). Blood pressure and dietary salt in human populations. *Ecology of Food and Nutrition*, **2**, 143–56.

Hovell, M. F. (1982). The experimental evidence for weight loss treatment of essential hypertension: a critical review. *American Journal of Public Health*, **72**, 359–68.

Howes, L. G. & Reid, J. L. (1986). The effects of alcohol on local, neural and humoral cardiovascular regulation. *Clinical Science*, **71**, 9–15.

Hypertension Prevention Trial Research Group (1990). The Hypertension Prevention Trial: Three year effects of dietary changes on blood pressure. *Annals of Internal Medicine*, **150**, 153–6.

Intersalt Cooperative Research Group. Intersalt (1988). An international study of electrolyte excretion and blood pressure. Results for 24 hours urinary sodium and potassium excretion. *British Medical Journal*, **2**, 97, 319–28.

Khaw, K-T. & Barrett-Connor, E. (1988). The Association between blood pressure, age and dietary sodium and potassium: a population study. *Circulation*, **77**, 53–61.

Klatsky, A. L., Friedman, G. D., Siegelaub, A. B. & Gerald, M. J. (1977). Alcohol consumption and blood pressure. *New England Journal of Medicine*, **296**, 1194–200.

Knochel, J. P. (1983). Cardiovascular effects of alcohol. *Annals of Internal Medicine*, **98**, 849–54.

Langford, H. G., Davis, B. R., Blaufox, D. *et al.* (1991). Effect of drug and diet treatment of mild hypertension on diastolic blood pressure. *Hypertension*, **17**, 210–17.

Law, M. R., Frost, C. D. & Wald, N. J. (1991*a*). By how much does dietary salt reduction lower blood pressure? 1. Analysis of observational data among populations. *British Medical Journal*, **302**, 811–15.

Law, M. R., Frost, C. D. & Wald, N. J. (1991*b*). By how much does dietary salt reduction lower blood pressure. III. Analysis of data from trials of salt reduction. *British Medical Journal*, **302**, 819–24.

MacMahon, S. W., Blacket, R. B., MacDonald, G. J. & Hall, W. (1984). Obesity, alcohol consumption and blood pressure in Australian men and women. The National Heart Foundation of Australia Risk Factor Prevalence Study. *Journal of Hypertension*, **2**, 85–91.

Margetts, B. M., Beilin, L. J., Vandongen, R. & Armstrong, B. K. (1986). Vegetarian diet in mild hypertension: a randomised controlled trial. *British Medical Journal*, **29**, 3, 1468–71.

Parker, M., Puddey, I. B., Beilin, L. J. & Vandongen, R. (1990). Two-factorial study of alcohol and salt restriction in treated hypertensive men. *Hypertension*, **16**, 398–406.

Potter, J. F. & Beevers, D. G. (1984). Pressor effect of alcohol in hypertension. *Lancet*, **i**, 119–22.

Poulter, N. R., Khaw, K. T., Hopwood, B. E. C. *et al.* (1990). The Kenyan Luo migration study: observations on the initiation of a rise in blood pressure. *British Medical Journal*, **300**, 967–72.

Puddey, I. B., Beilin, L. J., Vandongen, R., Rouse, I. L. & Rogers, P. (1985). Evidence for a direct effect of alcohol consumption on blood pressure in normotensive men: A randomized controlled trial. *Hypertension*, **7**, 707–13.

Puddey, I. B., Beilin, L. J. & Vandongen, R. (1987). Regular alcohol use raises blood pressure in treated hypertensive subjects. *Lancet*, **i**, 647–51.

Puddey, I. B., Parker, M., Beilin, L. J., Vandongen, R. & Masarei, J. R. L. (1992). Effects of alcohol and calorie restrictions on blood pressure and serum lipids in overweight men. *Hypertension*, **20**, 533–41.

Reisen, E., Rachel, A., Modan, M., Siverberg, D. S., Eliahou, H. E. & Modan, B. (1978). Effect of weight loss without salt restriction on the reduction of blood pressure in overweight hypertensive patients. *New England Journal of Medicine*, **298**, 1–6.

Reisen, E., Frohlich, E. D., Messerli, F. H. (1983). Cardiovascular changes after weight reduction in obesity hypertension. *Annals of Internal Medicine*, **98**, 315–19.

Rocchini, A. P., Key, J., Bondie, D., Chico, R., Moorehead, C., Katch, V. & Martin, M. (1989). The effect of weight loss of the sensitivity of blood pressure to sodium in obese adolescents. *New England Journal of Medicine*, **321**, 580–5.

Rouse, I. L. & Beilin, L. J. (1984). Vegetarian diet and blood pressure. *Journal of Hypertension*, **2**, 231–40.

Rose, G. (1981). Strategy of prevention: lessons learned from cardiovascular disease. *British Medical Journal*, **282**, 1847–51.

Sacks, F. M., Rouse, I. L., Stampfer, M. J., Bishop, L. M., Lenherr, C. F. & Walthier, R. J. (1987). Effect of dietary fats and carbohydrate on blood pressure of mildly hypertensive patients. *Hypertension*, **10**, 452–60.

Smith, W. C. S., Crombie, I. K., Tavendale, R. T., Gulland, S. K. & Tunstall-Pedoe, H. D. (1988). Urinary electrolyte excretion, alcohol consumption and blood pressure in the Scottish heart health study. *British Medical Journal*, **297**, 329–30.

Stamler, R., Grimm, R., Gosch, F. C. *et al.* (1987). Control of high blood pressure by nutritional therapy. Final report of a 4-year randomised controlled trial – The Hypertension Control Program. *Journal of the American Medical Association*, **257**, 1484–91.

Stamler, R., Stamler, J., Riedlinger, W. F., Algera, G. & Roberts, R. H. (1979). Weight and blood pressure: Findings in hypertension. Screen of one million Americans. *Journal of the American Medical Association*, **240**, 1607–10.

Strazzullo, P., Ferro-Luzzi, A., Siani, A. *et al.* (1986). Changing the Mediterranean diet: effects on blood pressure. *Journal of Hypertension*, **4**, 407–12.

Swales, J. D. (1990a). Non-drug therapy: salt, weight, alcohol, exercise and tobacco. In *Handbook of Hypertension*. Vol. 13. *The Management of Hypertension*, ed. F. R. Buhler & J. H. Laragh, pp. 334–50. Elsevier, Amsterdam.

Swales, J. D. (1990b). Dietary sodium restriction in hypertension. In *Hypertension: Pathophysiology, Diagnosis and Management*, ed. J. H. Largah and B. M. Brenner, pp. 2011–19. Raven Press Ltd., New York.

Swales, J. D. (1991). Dietary salt and blood pressure: the role of meta-analyses. *Journal of Hypertension*, **9** (suppl. 6), s42–6.

Watt, G. C. M., Foy, C. J. W., Hart, J. T. *et al.* (1985). Dietary sodium and arterial blood pressured: evidence against genetic susceptibility. *British Medical Journal*, **291**, 1525–8.

Williams, R. R., Hunt, S. C., Schumacher, M. C. *et al.* (1992). Genes, hypertension and coronary heart diease: evidence for shared metabolic pathophysiology. In *Hypertension as an Insulin Resistant Disorder. Genetic Factors and Cellular Mechanisms*, ed. U. Smith *et al.*, pp. 89–101. Elsevier Science Publishers, Amsterdam.

21

Definition and prevalence of obesity and overweight

J. GARROW

Life insurance companies publish tables of 'desirable weight', based on the mortality experience of people they have insured. As more data become available for analysis, it emerges that this desirable range corresponds closely to the range of Quetelet's Index (QI, also known as body mass index, BMI) from 20–25. The index is calculated by dividing the individual's weight (kg) by the square of his or her height (m). Thus a person who weighed 65 kg and who was 1.73 m tall would have a QI of $65/(1.73 \times 1.73) = 21.7$, which is in the desirable range. In practice, it is usually more convenient to use a chart such as that shown in Fig. 21.1 which shows the boundaries of QI 20, 25, 30 and 40.

It is arbitrary to choose a value for QI above which a person is deemed obese: mortality starts to increase significantly somewhere between 25 and 30, and increases rapidly at values of QI above 30. Very thin people also show decreased longevity, so below 20 there is increased mortality. Therefore, there is an international consensus that 20–24.9 is a 'desirable range', 25–29.9 is overweight, over 30 is obese, and over 40 very obese. Garrow (1988) used the terms Grade O, Grade I, Grade II and Grade III for the ranges of desirable , overweight, obese and very obese, respectively: this notation will be used hereafter in this chapter. The life insurance data are based mainly on mortality experience with insured men, but other epidemiological surveys have shown that these weight ranges predict disease risk among uninsured populations, and also among women (Manson *et al.*, 1990).

The prevalence of overweight and obesity in the adult population of the UK was determined in 1980 in a survey of a representative sample of 5000 men and 5000 women aged 16–64 years. At that time, the proportion of men in Grades I, II and III were 34%, 6% and 0.1%, while for women they were 24%, 8% and 0.3% respectively. The prevalence was higher

460

Table 21.1. *Prevalence* (%) *of obesity* (*QI* > 30) *in a representative sample of men and women aged 16–64 years in the UK*

Age (years)		16–24	25–34	35–49	50–64
Men	1980	2.5	4.5	8.0	7.7
	1987	3.0	6.0	11.0	9.0
Women	1980	3.5	4.5	9.9	14.3
	1987	6.0	11.0	10.0	18.0

Data for 1980 from Rosenbaum *et al.* (1985) and for 1987 from Gregory *et al.* (1990).

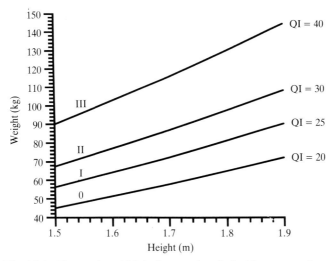

Fig. 21.1. The region 'O' indicates the desirable range of weight for height in adults. Below this is underweight, and grades of overweight are indicated by the bands I, II and III which begin at Quetelet's Index (QI) values of 25, 30 and 40, respectively (see text).

among the older subjects. Another survey was done in 1987 using the same methodology, which showed an alarming increase in the prevalence of obesity (QI > 30) which overall had increased from 6% to 8% in men and from 8% to 12% in women. The increase occurred in all age-groups, but particularly among women aged 25–34 years, in whom the prevalence appears to have doubled over the 7-year interval. This change is shown in Table 21.1.

Table 21.2. *Prevalence (%) of obesity*
(QI > 30) among men and women
aged 40–60 years in Europe and the
USA (Seidell, 1992)

Area	Men	Women
Northern Europe	10	15
Western Europe	13	16
Mediterranean	16	30
Eastern Europe	q8	30
USSR (formerly)	14	44
USA (whites)	15	18
USA (blacks)	20	37

It is difficult to make accurate comparisons of the prevalence of obesity in other countries, since the survey methodologies differ and, as shown above for the UK, the prevalence in a country may change greatly in a few years. A recent review of the prevalence of obesity (QI > 30) in different regions of Europe, among men and women aged 40–60 years, yields average results shown in Table 21.2 (Seidell, 1994).

Usually in affluent countries the prevalence of obesity is inversely related to social class, but there is no satisfactory explanation for this observed association. Although Grade I (QI 25–29.9) is usually commoner among men than among women of the same age, obesity (QI > 30) is commoner among women, and the preponderance of women increases with increasing severity of obesity. Men tend to reach maximum prevalence of obesity about age 45 years, but in women the prevalence increases to age 65 years and then starts to decline. People who smoke cigarettes tend to be lighter than non-smokers, and ex-smokers tend to gain weight. It must be emphasised, however, that the fear of weight gain is not a good reason for continuing smoking: weight gain is not inevitable, and the man or woman who stops smoking 20 cigarettes per day would have to gain about 20 kg in weight in order to lose the health benefit of stopping smoking.

Treatment by diet

Advice for reducing dietary energy intake

The rate of weight loss shown in Fig. 21.2 is usually found to be satisfactory for the treatment of severely obese patients. It is achieved with

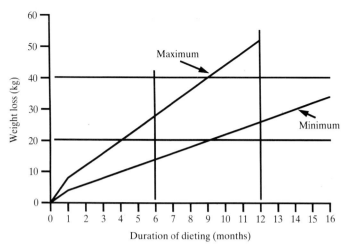

Fig. 21.2. This Figure indicates the limits of the range of desirable rates of weight loss in overweight and obese people. An average energy deficit of 1000 kcal/day will cause weight loss at the upper limit of the zone, and 500 kcal/day at the lower limit. Younger, taller, male and more overweight patients should aim at the upper line, while the lower line is more appropriate for older, shorter, female and less overweight patients.

an energy deficit of 500–1000 kcal/day. It may appear necessary, therefore, to assess the present energy intake of the patient by means of a dietary history, and then prescribe a diet which provides 500–1000 kcal/day less than estimated habitual intake. In practice, this is not useful, since it is so difficult to obtain a reliable estimate of habitual energy intake in obese patients. A rule of thumb is to start with a diet supplying 1000 kcal/day for an average obese woman (say age 30 years, weight 80 kg, height 1.6 m) and to increase this up to 1500 kcal/day for men, or for younger, taller women, or decrease to 800 kcal/day for older, shorter women. This estimate can be revised if the observed rate of weight loss is too high or too low. It is never necessary to prescribe a reducing diet outside the range of 800–1500 kcal/day.

The diet must provide the essential nutrients, so it is logical especially to seek to restrict those food items which provide energy but little else of nutritional importance, such as sucrose and alcohol. It is desirable to restrict intake of fat, and particularly saturated fat. This is partly because this policy is helpful in decreasing the risk of atheromatous heart disease, partly because fat is a concentrated energy source, and partly because there is some evidence that fat has a lower satiating capacity than iso-energetic quantities of carbohydrate or protein. The foods which are not restricted are fruit, vegetables and whole-grain cereals, since these are important sources of micronutrients and non-starch polysaccharides. It is important that protein intake should be adequate to avoid unnecessary loss of lean tissue, but extremely high protein diets are expensive and have not been shown to be particularly effective or acceptable. Within these guidelines, it is possible to construct an infinite variety of nutritionally sound reducing diets which can be adapted to the requirements of individual patients.

Very-low-calorie diets (VLCD)

Commercial diets which provide the recommended daily amounts of micronutrients with minimal energy, are heavily advertised and are attractive to patients wishing to lose weight rapidly. The disadvantages are that the rapid weight loss may signify excessive loss of lean tissue, the commercial aspects may cause the product to be given to people for whom weight loss is not appropriate, and the prospects for maintaining weight loss are not good for people who have not learned the principles on which reducing diets should be based. Despite these anxieties some authorities believe that VLCD have a place in the treatment of severe obesity. The author does not (Garrow, 1989).

Acceptability of reducing diets

It is very difficult to predict which diet will prove most acceptable to a given obese patient. Presumably the diet which the patient prefers is the one on which obesity developed, so a willingness to change from this is a necessary condition for successful weight loss. Some patients prefer exactly specified diets, whereas others prefer more flexibility. Patients may say that they find dieting difficult because they get hungry, but on closer questioning this may mean that they long for a particular forbidden item of food, such as chocolate. It is not clear if a small ration of chocolate (in this instance) is helpful or not: people differ. For some patients a monotonous bland diet (such as milk only) is easier to keep to than a varied diet, but for others it is intolerable.

Probably the factors which most help people to keep to a reducing diet are clear instructions about a diet appropriate for their weight, tastes and social circumstances, together with a realistic forecast of the rate of weight loss which this diet should provide. Good dietitians have the skill to provide this information: there is much more to it than simply handing out a standard diet sheet.

Frequency and timing of meals

Traditionally, patients are advised to have small meals evenly spaced throughout the day, and probably this advice is sound, although there is no impressive evidence of efficacy based on randomised controlled trials. In a cross-over protocol in a metabolic ward where obese patients were fed 800 kcal as either one or 5 meals per day, the patients were much hungrier, and lost more lean tissue, on the one-meal phase of the study, than when they were receiving five meals per day (Garrow *et al.*, 1981). However, there is no evidence that meal frequency affects total energy output. It is probably useful for patients to establish a formal pattern of eating meals at specified times, since continuous snacking or 'grazing' makes it very difficult to establish any control over total energy intake (Booth, Campbell & Chase, 1970).

Behaviour therapy

In the last decade psychologists have greatly increased our understanding of dieting behaviour. Most of us eat more or less automatically. If a patient's eating behaviour is to be altered, it is first necessary to become aware of what is being eaten, and the circumstances which tend to trigger inappropriate eating. The mere recording of a food diary is associated with some weight loss in most people, which suggests that we eat less when we are required to pay attention to what we eat, and such a food diary is also useful for the dietitian to assess the patient's habitual diet. There may be recurrent domestic situations which tend to precipitate binge eating: if these can be identified and that situation can be avoided, it increases the chance of compliance with the diet. It is also very helpful if other members of the patient's household provide intelligent co-operation with dieting efforts: ignorant nagging or ridicule from other members of the family will defeat all but the most determined dieter.

The central premise of behavioural therapy for obesity is that eating behaviour is not instinctive, but learned. In obesity, eating behaviour is inappropriate, so it should be re-learned. This approach is very effective, and should be in the repertoire of every dietitian. However it is a mistake to suppose that the treatment of obesity can be achieved by teaching the patient to eat 'normally'. It is true that control of abnormal eating binges is necessary if worthwhile weight loss is to be achieved, but that alone will not cause the weight loss. Severely obese patients are being asked to eat abnormally over quite a long time: if they have excess energy stores amounting to (say) 140 000 kcal, they are being asked to eat 140 000 kcal less than their requirements over a period of several months. Certainly it is a mistake to imagine that behaviour therapy somehow avoids the need to restrict energy intake: what it does is to make the restriction of energy intake easier to achieve.

Weight-loss groups

It is probably useful for the obese patient to have an initial assessment one-to-one with a dietitian, so the necessary information described above can be collected. However, for follow-up sessions there are several advantages in working with groups of about 10–15 patients. It is a more efficient use of the dietitian's time to talk to a group of patients, than to repeat almost the same message many times to the members of the group individually. Provided that the group is skilfully and sensitively led, the patients benefit from being associated with other people in a similar situation, and hearing answers to problems raised by other members of the group. This is particularly true for diffident patients who would not have had the courage to raise the problem themselves. However, group treatment is not a panacea, and may be disastrous if there is a particularly assertive or destructive personality within the group (Bush et al., 1988).

Long-term efficacy of dietary treatment

There are few, good, long-term controlled studies of the efficacy of purely dietary intervention in obesity, and the studies which have been published show rather poor results (Geppert & Splett, 1991). Programmes which tried to follow participants for 12 months always have high drop-out rates. This is not surprising, because long before 12 months the participants have learned the essentials of dieting, and there is no great incentive to attend a clinic to be weighed, when they could as easily weigh themselves at home.

In one study which initially enrolled 95 women and 20 men, only 13 women and 4 men were still attending for monthly visits up to one year, but 80 women and 18 men were traced and weighed at home visits (Gilbert & Garrow, 1983). In this study, the patients were randomly assigned to one of three treatment methods: diet alone, or diet with behaviour modification, or diet with an anorectic drug. Among the women traced after one year, for those on diet alone the weight loss (mean ± s.d.) was 1.6 ± 7.6 kg, those on anorectic drug 6.3 ± 8.3 kg, and behaviour therapy 7.6 ± 10.5 kg. A striking feature of the trial was the large variability in response within each treatment group. This underlines the point already made: that different obese patients have different requirements for treatment.

Exercise as a treatment for obesity

Physical activity increases energy expenditure, physical fitness, and sensitivity to the action of insulin, all of which are valuable effects for obese people. Although elite athletes can maintain very high levels of energy expenditure for sustained periods the maximum rate of work of the average non-athlete is about 6 kcal (25 kJ)/min over one hour. The average resting metabolism is about 1 kcal (4 kJ)/min, so after 1 hour the jogger will have used about 360 kcal, while his twin who remained at rest used 60 kcal, so the net cost of an hour jogging is about 300 kcal. This is probably the upper limit of the increase in energy expenditure which it is realistic to expect overweight people to achieve by exercise. At this level of exercise intensity there is no measurable elevation of metabolic rate when the exercise has stopped (Pacy *et al.*, 1985, Freedman-Akabas *et al.*, 1985).

It is often claimed that physical training can selectively increase the fat-free mass of the body, so although the obese person may not experience weight loss, some fat is being replaced by an equal weight of muscle. A recent review of the evidence by Forbes (1992) did not find evidence to support this claim. Certainly obese patients should be encouraged to take exercise within the limitations of their exercise tolerance, and they will benefit in physical fitness by doing so. However, exercise alone is not an effective method for achieving weight loss, nor of significantly altering the proportions of fat and lean tissue in the body.

Surgical procedures

It is outside the scope of this chapter to give a detailed account of surgical procedures for the treatment of obesity, but general physicians may be asked to give guidance to severely obese patients about surgery as an option 'instead of dieting'

The most important point is that surgical treatment of obesity (with one minor exception) is not an alternative to dieting, but a method for trying to enforce dieting. The minor exception is apronectomy: it is possible for the surgeon to cut away fat hanging in a fold of anterior abdominal wall, but this is really only applicable in severely obese patients, and preferably those who have already lost a considerable amount of their excess fat. Cutting, or sucking, fat from subcuntaneous sites is advertised as a cosmetic procedure, but the amount of fat which can be removed is trivial in comparison with the total excess fat in a patient who has medically important obesity. In many cases, the cosmetic result from an attempt to remove significant quantities of subcutaneous fat is very unsatisfactory.

Gastric bypass

This is an operation in which the gut is cut and rejoined to provide a relatively short exposure of the food to the action of digestive enzymes, while the majority of the bowel is short-circuited. The objective is to produce some degree of malabsorption, so that some of the energy in the food is not absorbed, and also so that a large energy intake provokes severe diarrhoea. The weight loss caused by operations of this kind depends more on the aversive consequences if the patient overeats than on failure to absorb what is eaten.

Gastric stapling

In this operation a line of staples closes off all but a small pouch at the fundus, which empties through a small stoma into the main body of the stomach, so only about 50 ml of food can be taken at a time. Typically patients lose about one-third of their excess weight in the year after operation, but there is then a tendency for weight regain. Weight loss is somewhat greater after the bypass than the stapling operation, but at the cost of greater metabolic complications, and a greater risk of nutrient deficiencies. Both operations are technically reversible, but weight gain after reversal is rapid and almost universal.

The relative advantages and disadvantages of these two operations have been reviewed in a Consensus Statement (1991): the main points which were agreed are set out below.

1. Patients seeking therapy for severe obesity for the first time should be considered for treatment in a non-surgical programme, with integrated components of a dietary regimen, appropriate exercise, and behavioural modification and support.

2. Gastric restrictive or bypass procedures could be considered for well-informed and motivated patients with acceptable operative risks.
3. Patients who are candidates for surgical procedures should be selected carefully after evaluation by a multi-disciplinary team with medical, surgical, psychiatric and nutritional expertise.
4. The operation should be performed by a surgeon substantially experienced with the appropriate procedures and working in a clinical setting with adequate support for all aspects of management and assessment.
5. Lifetime medical surveillance after surgical therapy is a necessity.

These are views with which experts in the field would agree: the problem in real life is what to do with the severely obese patient who is not well-motivated, or is not a good operative risk, or in whom the careful evaluation reveals some other reason why he/she is not ideally suited for surgery. The answer is that surgery is often selected because it seems to be the best choice at the time, but this decision may later be regretted by those who inherit the task of lifelong medical supervision.

Gastric balloon

Balloons have been inserted into the stomach to reduce gastric capacity without the hazards associated with abdominal operations in obese people. The results have been disappointing: weight loss is small and not sustained, and the risk of ulcerating the gastric mucosa is significant.

Jaw wiring

It is standard orthodontic practice to wire upper and lower jaws together for treatment of jaw fractures, or when it has been necessary to resect part of the lower jaw. With this procedure the patient can drink, but not chew, and since liquid diets tend to have a low energy density they often lose weight. Advantage was taken of this effect in the treatment of obesity (Garrow, 1974) but although weight loss of about 36 kg in 9 months was achieved it was not sustained when the wires were removed. The procedure is not justified unless it is combined with some method for helping the patient to maintain the weight loss (see below).

Maintenance of weight loss

If a patient manages to keep to a reducing diet for many months and achieves massive weight loss, it must not be assumed that the weight loss will be automatically maintained when the intense dieting effort is over. On the contrary, it should be assumed that a patient who reduces from, say, 100 kg will revert to 100 kg unless something is done to maintain the weight at 70 kg. After weight loss, energy requirements are reduced (Garrow, 1988), so if the patient goes back to eating 'normally' (that is, to the diet which previously supported a weight of 100 kg) then that is the weight which will be regained before equilibrium is re-established. We do not know what keeps people of desirable weight at their desirable weight, but whatever this characteristic may be, it clearly is not possessed by the formerly obese person.

Most people in affluent countries control their weight at least in part by noting unacceptable increases in weight, and altering energy intake (or output) to compensate. To a person who has never been more than 70 kg an increase to 80 kg is a new experience, which will cause some alarm, but this is not true of a person who was previously 100 kg. Reduced obese people benefit from a device which warns them of weight gain, which may be a spouse, or flatmate, or favourite pair of jeans. Alternatively, this monitoring function can be performed by a nylon cord fixed round the waist which becomes very tight if excessive weight is gained. A disadvantage with earlier versions of the waist cord was that it was either too loose to provide a sensitive monitor of unwanted weight gain, or else too tight to accommodate fluctuations in weight such as might occur premenstrually, or at an occasional celebratory meal. An alternative version can be shortened by taking a turn or two around a perspex rod for normal use, but these can be released to accommodate temporary weight gain. The patient must remember to lose the weight, and regain room for manoeuvre, before the next episode of temporary weight gain (Garrow, 1992).

Refractory obesity

Hospital obesity clinics are often called upon to investigate the metabolism of an obese person who inexorably gains weight while apparently keeping rigorously to a diet supplying only 800 kcal/day. This implies that the energy expenditure of the patient must be less than 800 kcal/day, but when this is checked in those centres which are fortunate to have facilities for 24-hour calorimetry, the observed energy output is always far in excess of 800 kcal/day (Garrow, 1988). The only conclusion compatible with thermodynamic principles which can be drawn from these observations is that the calculated diet was wrong: there may have been periods during which it was only 800 kcal/day, but on average it must have been much more, or prolonged weight gain would not have occurred. It should be emphasised that these cases of refractory obesity are not deliberately lying about their dietary intake: they are reporting what they believe to be true. These unfortunate people may be driven to try all sorts of drastic treatments with starvation, drugs or abdominal surgery because they believe that conventional diets are ineffective in their case, so it is important to establish the truth. In places where there are no facilities for calorimetry it may be useful to ask the patient to keep to a daily diet consisting solely of 2 pints of full-fat milk (or 3 semi-skimmed) for 3 weeks (which provides 800 kcal/day), and to observe weight change over this period. If a weight loss of more than 2 kg is observed (as almost always happens) then an error in the calculation of the diet must be sought, but if no weight loss occurs and the degree of obesity warrants it then then patient should be referred for calorimetry, if possible.

References

Booth, D. A., Campbell, H. T. & Chase, A. (1970). Temporal bounds of post-ingestive glucose induced satiety in man. *Nature*, **228**, 1104.

Bush, A., Webster, J., Chalmers, G. *et al.* (1988). The Harrow Slimming Club: report on 1090 enrolments in 50 courses, 1977–1986. *Journal of Human Nutrition and Dietetics*, **1**, 429–36.

Consensus Statement (1991). Gastrointestinal surgery for severe obesity. NIH Consensus Development Conference, March 25–27, 1991.

Forbes, G. B. (1992). Exercise and lean weight: the influence of body weight. *Nutrition Reviews*, **50**, 157–61.

Freedman-Akabas, S., Colt, E., Kissilef, H. R. & Pi-Sunyer, F. X. (1985). Lack of sustained increase in metabolic rate following exercise in fit and unfit subjects. *American Journal of Clinical Nutrition*, **41**, 545–9.

Garrow, J. S. (1974). Dental splinting in the treatment of hyperphagic obesity. *Proceedings of the Nutrition Society*, **33**, 29A.

Garrow, J. S. (1988). *Obesity and Related Diseases*, p. 329. Churchill Livingstone, London.

Garrow, J. S. (1989). Very low calorie diets should not be used. *International Journal of Obesity*, **13**, suppl. 2, 145–7.

Garrow, J. S. (1992). The management of obesity. Another view. *International Journal of Obesity*, **16**, 2, S59–S63.

Garrow, J. S., Durrant, M. L., Blaza, S., Wilkins, D., Royston, P. & Sunkin, S. (1981). The effect of meal frequency and protein concentration on the composition of the weight lost by obese subjects. *British Journal of Nutrition*, **45**, 5–16.

Geppert, J. & Splett, P. L. (1991). Summary document of nutrition intervention in obesity. *Journal of the American Dietetic Association* suppl: S31–5.

Gilbert, S. & Garrow, J. S. (1983). A prospective controlled trial of outpatient treatment for obesity. *Human Nutrition: Clinical Nutrition*, **37C**, 21–9.

Gregory, J., Foster, K., Tyler, H. & Wiseman, M. (1990). *The Dietary and Nutritional Survey of British Adults.* HMSO, London.

Manson, J. E., Colditz, G. A., Stamfer, M. J. *et al.* (1990). A prospective study of obesity and risk of coronary heart disease in women. *New England Journal of Medicine,* **322,** 822–9.

Pacy, P. J., Barton, N., Webster, J. D. & Garrow, J. S. (1985). The energy cost of aerobic exercise in fed and fasted normal subjects. *American Journal of Clinical Nutrition,* **42,** 764–8.

Rosenbaum, S., Skinner, R. K., Knight, I. B. & Garrow, J. S. (1985). A survey of heights and weights of adults in Great Britain. *Annals of Human Biology,* **12,** 115–27.

Seidell, J. C. (ed.) (1994). *Obesity in Europe: Prevalence and Public Health Implications.* Copenhagen, WHO, in press.

22

Eating disorders

L. F. PIERI AND A. C. P. SIMS

'What is food to one is bitter poison to others'
(Lucretius – *de Rerum Natura*).

Introduction

The term Eating Disorder incorporates a group of conditions whose central feature is abnormal eating behaviour. According to the International Classification of Diseases 10th Revision (I.C.D. 10, WHO, 1992): anorexia nervosa, bulimia nervosa, obesity and vomiting with psychological disturbances should be included. Vomiting is a frequent symptom of both anorexia and bulimia and will be mentioned only in that context. This chapter does not give further consideration to obesity, which may result as a reaction to distressing events or be a cause of further psychological disturbance.

Not only are food and eating necessary for our existence, they also have a central role in many important aspects of our lives, for instance, religious and social gatherings. Despite such a pivotal role being long recognised, it was not until 1689 that the first unmistakable account of anorexia nervosa was documented by Richard Morton, when he reported the first two cases of what he called 'nervous atrophy', showing them to be different from consumption. The name 'anorexia nervosa' was given to the syndrome by Sir William Gull, in 1874 (Gull, 1874). Bulimia nervosa has only emerged as a separately described and distinctive syndrome in the last 15 years (Russell, 1979).

Over the years there has been debate concerning the aetiologies of both anorexia and bulimia nervosa, and whether the conditions were purely psychological, purely biological or a combination of both (Hsu, 1983).

Definitions

Anorexia nervosa is characterised by extreme weight loss, body image disturbance and a 'pursuit of thinness' (Bruch, 1973). In bulimia nervosa

473

there is frequent consumption of large quantities of food in a short space of time (bingeing), followed by self-induced vomiting. A 'fear of fatness' accompanies the disorder. Extreme preoccupation with food is common to both syndromes.

Diagnostic guidelines for anorexia nervosa (I.C.D. 10)

For a definite diagnosis, all the following are required:

(a) Body weight is maintained at least 15% below that expected (either lost or never achieved), or Quetelet's body mass index is 17.5 or less (where Quetelet's body mass index = weight (kg)/height (m)^2). Prepubertal patients may show failure to make the expected weight gain during the period of growth.

(b) The weight loss is self-induced by avoidance of what are considered to be fattening foods and one or more of the following: self-induced vomiting; self-induced purging; excessive exercise; use of appetite suppresssants and/or diuretics.

(c) There is body-image distortion, in that dread of fatness persists as an intrusive, overvalued idea and the patient imposes a low weight threshold on himself or herself.

(d) A widespread endocrine disorder involving the hypothalamic–pituitary–gonadal axis is manifest in women as amenorrhoea and in men as a loss of sexual interest and potency. An apparent exception is the persistence of vaginal bleeds in anorexic woemen who are receiving replacement hormonal therapy, most commonly taken as a contraceptive pill. There may also be elevated levels of growth hormone, raised levels of cortisol, changes in the peripheral metabolism of thyroid hormone, and abnormalities of insulin secretion.

(e) If onset is prepubertal, the sequence of pubertal events is delayed or even arrested. Growth ceases; in girls the breasts do not develop and there is a primary amenorrhoea; in boys the genitals remain juvenile. With recovery, puberty is often completed normally, but the menarche is late.

Diagnostic guidelines for bulimia nervosa (I.C.D. 10)

For a definite diagnosis, all the following are required:

(a) There is a persistent pre-occupation with eating, and an irresistible craving for food; the patient succumbs to episodes of overeating in which large amounts of food are consumed in short periods of time.

(b) The patient attempts to counteract the 'fattening' effects of food by one or more of the following: self-induced vomiting; purgative abuse, alternating periods of starvation; use of drugs such as appetite suppressants, thyroid preparations or diuretics. When bulimia occurs in diabetic patients, they sometimes neglect their insulin treatment.

(c) The psychology consists of a morbid dread of fatness and the patient sets herself a sharply defined weight threshold, well below the premorbid weight that constitutes the optimum or healthy weight in the opinion of the physician. There is often, but not always, a history of an earlier episode of anorexia nervosa, the interval between the two disorders ranging from a few months to several years. This earlier episode may have been fully expressed, or may have assumed a minor cryptic form with a moderate loss of weight and/or a transient phase of amenorrhoea.

Clinical description

Anorexia nervosa

Characteristically, the onset of the condition occurs in late adolescence, though rarely it begins before puberty. Onset may be abrupt with an apparent trigger identifed, or conversely it may gradually develop over months or years. A period of dieting often precedes development of the overt condition. Anorexia nervosa is more common in girls than boys; the ratio being approximately 19:1 (Garfinkel & Garner, 1983).

Food and weight control dominate the patient's life. There is a single-minded avoidance of food that can result in so much weight being lost that the skin lies loosely over the patient's bones (Fig. 22.1). The consumption of a meal can take up to two hours; food may be concealed about the person or hidden amongst belongings and calorie counting is common. The term 'anorexia' is a misnomer, as the anorexic may be ravaged by hunger whilst vigorously resisting eating. She may para-doxically become pre-occupied with all aspects of food, start collecting recipes, prepare food for others, read cookery books voraciously and choose to work in food-related industries. The anorexic develops the idea of somehow being 'special' consequent upon her slimness and her sense of worth is based upon her low weight and her ability to control her eating. Besides restricting food, the anorexic may induce vomiting after meals, abuse laxatives or indulge in excess exercise in an attempt to burn off calories.

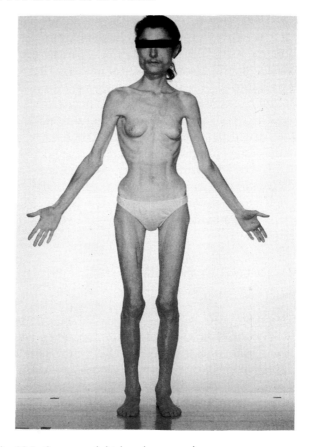

Fig. 22.1. Severe weight loss in anorexia nervosa.

The patient also develops a distorted body image in which she sees herself as much broader (i.e. fatter) than she really is, but not taller. The distortion of one's own body size is not limited to anorexia, but anorexics are more liable to greater distortion (Slade, 1988). Interestingly, anorexics judge themselves fatter immediately after a carbohydrate meal (Crisp & Kalucy, 1974).

Amenorrhoea is a constant feature and is directly related to the weight loss; in approximately 20%, the cessation of menses precedes weight reduction. Hypothermia is common and is secondary to loss of body fat and altered temperature regulation. This is usually accompanied by uncomplaining tolerance in the patient. The skin becomes cold and dry and loses its normal suppleness and elasticity. The body's extremities are cold with acrocyanosis due to poor peripheral circulation. A fine growth of downy or lanugo hair is seen. Initially, it appears over the patient's face, but eventually it can coat the whole body. Bradycardia, hypotension and delayed tendon reflexes are common features (Herzog & Copeland, 1985).

At times, bingeing episodes punctuate the severe, restrictive regime; this is a poor prognostic indicator.

Bulimia nervosa

Usually, this condition occurs in late adolescent or young females who have attempted various diets with little success. It has these characteristics:

1. Episodes of excess bingeing associated with loss of control over eating. Perhaps through friends, by reading magazines or occasionally accidentally, an individual learns of self-induced vomiting as a means of controlling weight. Vast quantities of food, sometimes more than 15 000 calories, may be consumed over short periods of time. Binges may be planned, with the individual shopping beforehand to select foods that they had previously forbidden themselves. On other occasions the binge is impulsive and any food that is available will be consumed irrespective of taste or consistency. The frequency of such episodes may vary from between two or three times weekly to many times a day. A binge is concluded when there is no longer food available, when the stomach becomes distended or painful, or if interrupted by a friend or relative. Vomiting, either self-induced or by reflex action will occur. Most patients experience feelings of guilt, shame or disgust after each episode. A characteristic symptom experienced by many during a binge is one of 'being out of control'. This pre-occupation with food and repeated bingeing may interfere with work, and severely restrict social activities. A binge can be precipitated by boredom, anxiety, depression and loneliness. The patient is almost invariably embarrassed by her symptoms and, as a result, energetically conceals her actions. In-between these bulimic episodes, the sufferer attempts to restrict her food intake.

2. In an attempt to control her weight, the bulimic introduces compensatory, and at times, extreme behaviours: excessive exercise, the consumption of large doses of laxatives in the mistaken belief that these will speed intestinal passage, diuretic abuse, strict dieting and various

mechanisms to induce vomiting using gastric irritants such as vinegar or ipecacuanha (Herzog & Copeland, 1985).

3. The third distinctive feature is a disturbed attitde towards weight and shape. Russell described this as 'a morbid fear of becoming fat' or in the Diagnostic and Statistical Manual, IIIR, 'a persistent over-concern with shape and weight' (American Psychiatric Association, 1987). These individuals may have a normal body weight but strongly dislike their bodily proportions. Low self-esteem is a common feature in bulimia, consequent upon negative feelings about weight and shape.

   In a distinctive sub-group of bulimics, impulsive eating is complemented by other chaotic behaviours such as alcohol and drug misuse, shop-lifting, stealing, disturbed relationships and suicidal behaviour.

Physical consequences

There are many harmful complications of anorexia and bulimia nervosa, some of which may be life threatening. The morbidity from these disorders is severe, and mortality of anorexia nervosa, if untreated, is high. Complications of anorexia nervosa arise through starvation, whereas for bulimia they are chiefly a consequence of bingeing and purging.

Anorexia nervosa

The most consistent consequences of anorexia nervosa are amenorrhoea and oestrogen deficiency (Warren & Vande Weile, 1975). Amenorrhoea results from weight-related suppression of the hypothalamic–pituitary axis. In approximately 20% of anorexics, however, amenorrhoea precedes the weight loss. Accompanying the oestrogen deficiency there is a paradoxical decrease in serum gonadotrophins: the luteinising hormone response is blunted and there is a slightly decreased response to follicle stimulating hormone, the same picture as in pre- or early puberty (Brown, 1983). With this profound reduction in oestrogen, loss of bone density, similar to that found in post-menopausal women, is common. Unfortunately, early adolescence is the principal time for the laying down of bone, and deficiency at this time is never totally rectified later (Rigotti et al., 1984).

There is a decreased peripheral conversion of thyroxine (T4) to triiodothyronine (T3) (Miyai et al., 1975). Thus, the picture of dry skin and hair, slowed relaxation of reflexes, cold intolerance, bradycardia and hypercarotenaemia, resembles that seen in the 'euthyroid sick'. This decrease in T3 is probably an adaptive mechanism in the starved state. Of anorexics, 50% have an elevated growth hormone level (Garfinkel *et al.*, 1975). This probably reflects the fact that the peptide, somatomedin C, which is synthesised in the liver and kidneys and has an intermediary role in the transport of growth hormone into bone, is deficient (Clemmons, Libanski & Underwood, 1981). Once calorific intake increases, the level of growth hormone returns to normal within a few days.

In patients with anorexia nervosa, vasopressin is secreted erratically in response to an osmotic challenge (Gold *et al.*, 1983). Some patients therefore cannot concentrate their urine in response to water deprivation and have vasopressin responses consistent with partial diabetes insipidus (Russell & Bruce, 1964). The urine can be concentrated when vasopressin is given.

Cardiovascular complications

Arrythymias, because of electrolyte disturbance, bradycardia and hypotension, because of decreased cardiac output, are common features. With time, thinning of the left ventricular wall and a decrease in cardiac chamber size may occur (Gottdiener *et al.*, 1978). Vasospasm, secondary to weight loss is seen. It is associated with thromboxane release and increased platelet aggregation (Mihkailidis, Barradas & DeSouza, 1986).

Haematological abnormalities

Leucopaenia, thrombocytopaenia and a normochromic, normocytic anaemia of moderate severity may be seen in the peripheral blood (Mant & Faragher, 1972). Altered red cell morphology can occur, for example acanthocytosis, macrocytosis, and anisopoikilocytosis with basophilic stippling (Amrein *et al.*, 1979). Leucopaenia occurs in up to fifty per cent of patients with anorexia nervosa and is secondary to a hypoplastic marrow (Silverman, 1983). Other bone marrow changes are gelatinous transformation, cell necrosis and increased histiocytes (Mant & Faragher, 1972).

Renal complications

The changes here largely result from dehydration and decreased glomerular filtration rate. Raised blood urea, renal calculi and peripheral oedema can result. Although renal failure is recognised, it is rare and is secondary to plasma volume depletion consequent upon vomiting and diuretic abuse (Bhanji & Mattingly, 1988).

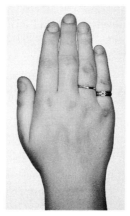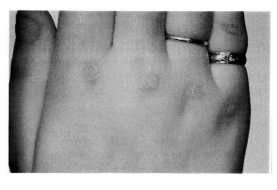

Fig. 22.2. Russell's sign.

Gastrointestinal tract

As the starved state continues, delayed gastric emptying may occur along with a decrease in intestinal motility (Dubois *et al.*, 1979). Constipation, because of laxative abuse, may result in colonic dilatation. Raised hepatic enzymes, of unknown aetiology, are found, but they usually revert to normal on re-feeding. Pancreatic disorders appear to be less frequent although an elevated serum amylase is seen in some patients. Hypoglycaemia is rare and secondary to severe malnutrition.

Severe weight loss associated with vomiting can be presenting features of achalasia of the oesophagus and as such can be a diagnostic problem (Duane *et al.*, 1992). In these cases, the abnormal psychopathology associated with anorexia nervosa is conspicuously lacking; correct diagnosis is thus essential for appropriate management.

Bulimia nervosa

The complications here are mostly due to the effects of bingeing and vomiting. Menstrual irregularities are common in bulimics but, since their weight remains either normal or slightly above normal, amenorrhoea is rare.

Vomiting is frequently induced by using the fingers to stimulate the gag reflex and as a result a characteristic distribution of calluses on the back of the hand (Fig. 22.2) can develop (Russell's sign). Hypertrophy of the salivary glands, especially the parotid, results in facial swelling. Dental erosion, at times to an extreme degree, is caused by this repeated vomiting. Oesophagitis, hiatus hernia, Mallory–Weiss tears and complete oeso-phageal rupture are all occasional consequences.

Gastric dilatation, secondary to ingestion of the vast amount of food is well documented, but should respond well to nasogastric aspiration and intravenous feeding.

The stomach may rupture with a very high ensuing mortality. Chronic laxative abuse may lead to constipation but in some a cathartic colon develops (Bo-Linn *et al.*, 1983). Here the large bowel becomes dilated, atonic and is unable to transport faeces. The normal haustration is lost and the mucosa becomes smooth and atrophic. Potassium depletion with cardiac complications is a major hazard in these patients. An aspiration pneumonia can result from the inhalation of regurgitated gastric contents.

Arrythymias secondary to hypokalaemia, hypocalcaemia and occasion-ally hypomagnesaemia do occur. Some bulimics use ipecacuanha to induce vomiting. This irritant may be absorbed across the gut with dangerous consequences; its frequent use can cause a cardiomyopathy (Adler *et al.*, 1980).

Treatment

For the management of eating disorders, a multidisciplinary team is required for the proper care of in-patients and some out-patients; the nurse, psychiatrist, general physician, occupational therapist, social worker, clinical psychologist, dietitian, and kitchen staff in the case of inpatients, all have distinctive roles to play. It is necessary, especially for patients with anorexia nervosa, to have a group of experts uniting their individual skills to aid the physical, psychological and social recovery of each patient. Anorectic inpatients are best sited on a psychiatric ward in a general hospital, although many variants are possible.

The view that anorexia nervosa and bulimia nervosa are different disorders with some shared pathology is supported by the fact that they each have distinct treatment programmes.

Milder cases of anorexia and bulimia nervosa may be managed successfully in general practice. Following diagnosis, regular appoint-ments are made to record eating behaviour and weight, to give advice concerning diet and lifestyle, and to deal with the family and other social problems. For patients who do not respond in a general practice setting and for those suffering more severe illnesses, especially the very emaciated individual, referral to a specialised unit with the potential for admission will be required. Both anorexia and bulimia nervosa are usually treatable conditions and most patients make substantial improvement with appropriate care.

Anorexia nervosa

When untreated, anorexia nervosa is a life-threatening illness with severe physical and psychosocial morbidity. Weight loss of the degree that occurs in anorexia nervosa, brings with it a catalogue of physiological and psychological changes that must be reversed before any meaningful psychotherapeutic relationship can be initiated (Garfinkel & Garner, 1983).

Many of the symptoms experienced in anorexia nervosa are due directly to the effects of starvation and a low body weight. A study by Keys vividly describes these effects (Keys *et al.*, 1950).

Treatment for the severely ill patient may be considered to take place in three stages:

Stage 1: Initiating treatment may be frustrated by the patient claiming nothing is wrong, by refusing to alter dietary and eating behaviour, or by refusing admission to hospital. Occasionally, compulsory admission under the Mental Health Act will be required.

Stage 2 Correction of profound emaciation necessarily involves the absorption of adequate nutrition, especially calories, and the reversal of any electrolyte imbalance. Immediate treatment is essential at this stage especially if the weight is below 30 kg, although urgent treatment may well be required above this level. Psychiatric nursing is the bedrock upon which any treatment plan should be constructed and the psychiatric ward of a distric general hospital has many advantages in co-ordinating the overall management of these patients.

Bedrest is often required initially and possibly at other times during the treatment programme. No one patient is exactly the same as another and therefore flexibility, based on sound clinical practice, must be adopted. For most patients a 1500 calorie daily intake is sufficient, which is then gradually increased over the ensuing days and weeks. A weight gain of approximately 0.5 to 1.5 kg per week is seen to be acceptable and any issues arising from the treatment programme, such as the hiding of food, or food refusal should be dealt with firmly but compassionately. The services of a skilled dietitian should ensure maintenance of essential components of the diet. There is also danger of dehydration when the patient is severely ill and occasionally naso-gastric feeding may be required. Treatment with anti-depressants is indicated should depressive symptoms be prominent, although symptoms such as dysphoric mood, irritability, decreased concentration and early morning waking are all shown to be part of the starvation process that do improve as the patient gains weight.

Regular weighing is required and it needs to be remembered that patients may sabotage the recording of their weight, the administration of their meal and, in fact, their whole treatment programme. Treatment of severe anorexia nervosa requires the maximum co-operation between all those involved in the patient's care.

Stage 3 Learning to control weight and diet is often the most difficult stage and involves establishing a good therapeutic relationship. It is only when a satisfactory weight has been reached that these problems can be adequately tackled. Family therapy has proved beneficial, especially for sufferers under the age of 18, and various types of cognitive behavioural therapy have also proved useful. This stage will make demands upon the professional expertise and personal resources of all the staff from different disciplines involved with the patient. Thus, collaboration and the under-standing of each other's role, are essential.

Bulimia nervosa

In direct contrast to anorexia nervosa, the great majority of bulimics can be managed on an outpatient basis; for many individuals with the disorder inpatient treatment is contraindicated (Freeman, 1991). Pharmacotherapy and psychotherapy, especially cognitive behavioural therapy, are used.

Each of these presentations of bulimia nervosa requires a different treatment approach:

1. The condition may follow a period of normal dieting with gradually decreasing body weight;
2. Some of these may, in fact, meet the criteria for anorexia nervosa but with bulimic symptoms dominant;

3. Others may present with bingeing initially and subsequent obesity;
4. Bulimia may alternate with relatively normal eating behaviour;
5. There may be multi-impulsive behaviour with drug misuse, shoplifting, self mutilation and alcohol abuse in addition to bulimia.

Cognitive therapy has proved especially useful in the treatment of bulimia (Fairburn, 1981). In 1967, Beck showed that patients diagnosed as suffering from certain types of psychiatric illness exhibited ways of thinking that resulted in poor decision-making and negative attitudes to life (Beck, 1967). He introduced cognitive therapy which aimed at identifying these abnormal conditions and, with the help of the therapist, altering these previously fixed attitudes (Beck, 1976). Fairburn adapted this method with good results for bulimia nervosa (Fairburn, 1981). Treatment involves the keeping of an 'eating diary' recording all food, vomiting, laxative abuse and resulting cognitions. More recently inter-personal psychotherapy has been used, successfully in the treatment of bulimia; this does not require focussing on the patient's eating habits.

There has also been considerable work of late on the use of serotonin re-uptake inhibitors in the treatment of bulimia nervosa. Controlled studies have shown that fluoxetine in a starting dose of 60 mg per day may be effective in correcting symptoms (Fluoxetine B. N. Collaborative Study Group, 1992). Its antidepressant properties are also useful as depressive symptoms are common during the course of bulimia nervosa. It is not considered a first-line anti-bulimic treatment.

Prognosis

Anorexia nervosa

Untreated, anorexia nervosa is a dangerous condition with an unfavour-able prognosis. Outcome studies of treated adolescent anorexia nervosa verify the good prognosis of this group (Kreipe, Churchill & Strauss, 1989). In hospitalised patients, however, although the short-term outcome is favourable, initial response to treatment does not predict continued improvement. If treated, approximately one-third recover fully; one-third improve adequately and approximately one-third show little or no improvement. The mortality rate with anorexia nervosa is approximately 5% (Hsu, 1980).

Most factors associated with poor outcome are older age of onset, longer duration of illness, severe weight loss, bulimic episodes, vomiting, poor childhood social adjustment and poor parental relationships (Hsu, Crisp & Harding, 1979).

Bulimia nervosa

Those factors which predict outcome in some studies of bulimia nervosa are not replicated in others. Thus, prognostic indicators remain uncertain.

A study by King (1991), followed a group of subjects with an eating disorder over a 30-month period. They had been identified as attending their general practitioners but, apart from that, had been prescribed no treatment intervention. Those suffering from bulimia nervosa showed no change in symptoms over the time-scale of the study. King concluded that, without treatment, bulimia nervosa tends to chronicity.

In general, however, the short-term outcome after treatment in bulimia nervosa is favourable, with reports of a 77–81% success rate at the end of treatment (Freeman *et al.*, 1988; Fairburn, 1981; Lacey, 1983).

Summary

The two conditions discussed in this chapter clearly illustrate that psychological and medical factors interact in aetiology and pathogenesis. This psycho-biological interface cogently demonstrates the need to view these disorders from a broad perspective. Social factors are also important in the aetiology, precipitation and propagation of both anorexia and bulimia nervosa. The psychological and physical morbidity resulting from eating disorders is amongst the highest for any psychiatric condition. Consequently, the need for a multi-disciplinary approach to the management and treatment of these conditions is paramount.

References

Adler, A. G., Walinsky, P., Krall, R. A. & Cho, S. Y. (1980). Death resulting from ipecac syrup poisoning. *Journal of the American Medical Association*, **243**, 1927–8.

American Psychiatric Association (1987). *Diagnostic and Statistical Manual of Mental Disorders* (Third Edition – Revised).

Amrein, P. C., Friedman, R., Kosinki, K. & Ellman, L. (1979). Haematologic changes in anorexia nervosa. *Journal of the American Medical Association*, **241**, 2190–1.

Beck, A. T. (1967). *Depression: Clinical, Experimental, and Theoretical Aspects.* Harper & Row, New York.

Beck, A. T. (1976). *Cognitive Therapy and Emotional Disorders.* International Universities Press, New York.

Bhanji, S. & Mattingly, D. (1988). *Medical Aspects of Anorexia Nervosa.* Butterworth & Co. (Publishers) Ltd.

Bo-Linn, G. W., Santa Ann, C. A., Morawski, S. G. & Fordtran, J. S. (1983). Purging and calorie absorption in bulimic patients and normal women. *Annals of Internal Medicine*, **99**, 14–26.

Brown, G. M. (1983). Endocrine abnormalities in anorexia nervosa. In *Anorexia Nervosa: Recent Developments in Research*, pp. 231–47. Alan R. Liss, Inc., New York.

Bruch, H. (1962). *Perceptual and conceptual disturbances in anorexia nervosa. Psychomatic Medicine*, **24**, 187–94.

Bruch, H. (1973). *Eating Disorders: Obesity, Anorexia Nervosa and the Person Within.* Basic Books, New York.

Clemmons, D. R., Libanski, A. & Underwood, L. E. (1981). Reduction of plasma immunoreactive Somatomedin C during fasting in humans. *Journal of Clinical Endocrinological Metabolism*, **53**, 1247–50.

Crisp, A. & Kalucy, R. (1974). Aspects of the perceptual disorder in anorexia nervosa. *British Journal of Medical Psychology*, **47**, 349–61.

Duane, P. D., Magee, T. M., Alexander, M. S., Heatley, R. V. & Losowsky, M. S. (1992). Oesophageal achalasia in adolescent women mistaken for anorexia nervosa. *British Medical Journal*, **305**, 43.

Dubois, A., Gross, H. A., Ebert, M. H. & Castell, D. O. (1979). Altered gastric emptying and secretion in primary anorexia nervosa. *Gastroenterology*, **77**, 319–23.

Fairburn, C. (1981). A cognitive behavioural approach to the treatment of bulimia. *Psychological Medicine*, **11**, 707–11.

Fluoxetine Bulimia Nervosa Collaborative Study Group: (1922). Fluoxetine in the treatment of bulimia nervosa. *Archives of General Psychiatry*, **49**, 139–47.

Freeman, C. P. L., Barry, F., Dunkeld-Turnbull, J. & Henderson, A. (1988). Controlled trial of psychotherapy for bulimia nervosa. *British Medical Journal*, **296**, 521–5.

Freeman, C. P. (1991). A practical guide to the treatment of bulimia nervosa. *Journal of Psychosomatic Research*, Suppl. 1, 41–9.

Garfinkel, P. E., Brown, G. M., Stancer, H. C. & Moldofsky, H. (1975). Hypothalamic pituitary function in anorexia nervosa. *Archives of General Psychiatry*, **32**, 739–44.

Garfinkel, P. E. & Garner, D. M. (1983). The multidetermined nature of anorexia nervosa. In *Anorexia Nervosa: Recent Developments in Research*, pp. 3–14. Alan R. Liss, Inc., New York.

Gold, P. W., Kaye, W., Robertson, G. L. & Ebert, M. (1983). Abnormalities in plasma and cerebrospinal fluid arginine vasopressin in patients with anorexia nervosa. *New England Journal of Medicine*, **308**, 1117–23.

Gottdiener, J. S., Gross, H. A., Henry, W. L., Borer, J. S. & Ebert, M. H. 1978). Effects of self-induced starvation on cardiac size and function in anorexia nervosa. *Circulation*, **58**, 426–33.

Garfinkel, P. E. & Garner, D. M. (1983). The multidetermined nature of anorexia nervosa. In *Anorexia Nervosa: Recent Developments in Research*, pp. 3–14. Alan R. Liss, Inc., New York.

Gull, W. W. (1874). Apepsia hysterica. *Clinical Society Transactions*, **7**, 22–8.

Herzog, D. B. & Copeland, P. M. (1985). Eating disorders. *New England Journal of Medicine*, **313**, 295–303.

Hsu, L. G. K., Crisp, A. H. & Harding, B. (1979). Outcome of anorexia nervosa. *Lancet*, **i**, 61–5.

Hsu, L. G. K. (1980). Outcome of anorexia nervosa. *Archives of General Psychiatry*, **37**, 1041–6.

Hsu,. L. G. K. (1983). The aetiology of anorexia nervosa. *Psychological Medicine*, **13**, 231–8.

Keys, A., Brozek, J., Henschel, A., Mickelson, O. & Taylor, H. L. (1950).

The Biology of Human Starvation. University of Minnesota Press, Minneapolis.

King, M. B. (1991). The natural history of eating pathology in attenders to primary medical care. *International Journal of Eating Disorders*, **10**, 379–88.

Kreipe, R. E., Churchill, B. H. & Strauss, J. (1989). Long-term outcome of adolescents with anorexia nervosa. *American Journal of Diseases of Children*. **143**, 1322–3.

Lacey, J. H. (1983). Bulimia nervosa: binge eating and psychogenic vomiting; a controlled treatment study and long term outcome. *British Medical Journal*, **286**, 1609–13.

Mant, M. J. & Faragher, B. S. (1972). The haematology of anorexia nervosa. *British Journal of Haematology*, **23**, 737–49.

Mikhailidis, D. P., Barradas, M. A. & DeSouza, V. (1986). Adrenalin-induced hyperaggregability of platelets and enhanced thromboxane release in anorexia nervosa. *Prostaglandins, Leukotrienes and Medicine*, **4**, 27–34.

Miyai, K., Yamamoto, T., Azukizawa, M., Ishibashi, K. & Kumahara, Y. (1975). Serum thyroid hormones and thyrotrophin in anorexia nervosa. *Journal of Clinical Endocrinology Metabolism*, **40**, 334–8.

Morton, R. (1689). *Phthisiologica:or a Treatise of Consumptions*. Sam Smith and Benjamin Walford, London.

Rigotti, N. A., Nussbaum, S. R., Herzog, D. B. & Neer, R. M. (1984). Osteoporosis in women with anorexia nervosa. *New England Journal of Medicine*, **300**, 1601–6.

Russell, G. F. M. & Bruce, T. (1964). Capillary-venous glucose differences in patients with disorders of appetite. *Clinical Science*, **26**, 157–63.

Russell, G. F. M. (1979). Bulimia nervosa: an ominous variant of anorexia nervosa. *Psychological Medicine*, **7**, 363–7.

Silverman, J. A. (1983). Medical consequences of starvation; the malnutrition of anorexia nervosa: Caveat Medicus. In *Anorexia Nervosa: Recent Developments in Research*, pp. 293–9. Alan R. Liss, Inc., New York.

Slade, P. D. (1988). Body image in anorexia nervosa. *British Journal of Psychiatry*, **153** (Suppl. 2), 20–2.

Warren, M. P. & Vande Weile, R. L. (1975). Clinical and metabolic features of anorexia nervosa. *American Journal of Obstetrics and Gynaecology*, **117**, 435–49.

World Health Organization (1992). *The ICD – 10 Classification of Mental and Behavioural Disorders: Clinical Descriptions and Diagnostic Guidelines*.

Index

Page numbers in italics refer to tables

absorption, nutrient, enteral diets
  fat, 117
  physiology, 95–129; concept of nutrient
    load, 97–8; intestinal nitrogen
    assimilation, 99–104; protein, 98–9
  see also carbohydrate absorption: enteral
    diets: fat absorption: malabsorption:
    protein absorption
acrodermatitis enteropathica, 75
adolescence, and micronutrient deficiency,
  58
adrenaline, activity after trauma and sepsis,
  320
ageing individuals, see elderly people
AIDS
  enteral feeding, 130
  parenteral nutrition, 144–5
alanine, requirements, 46
albumin, serum
  in cystic fibrosis, 397
  effect of nutritional support, 167, 168
alcohol
  coronary heart disease, and serum
    lipoproteins, 430–3; and
    hypertriglyceridaemia, 432–3;
    protective effect of moderate alcohol,
    430–3
  excess intake, and micronutrient
    deficiency, 58
alcoholic liver disease
  enteral feeding, 130
  immunocompetence, 84–5
  nutritional causes, 334
  TPN peri-operatively, 290
all-in-one delivery system for parenteral
  nutrition, 286
Amanita phalloides causing liver disease,
  336
amennorrhoea in anorexia nervosa, 474,
  476, 478

amino acids
  branched chains, see branched
    chain amino acids
  dibasic, transport, 101
  effect on immune function, 78
  essential: conditionally, 44–6; in cystic
    fibrosis, 400; and dietary intake, 43;
    estimates for maintenance, 42–4; for
    growth, gestation and lactation, 44,
    45; rate of oxidation, 43; required for
    maintenance, 41–4
  losses: obligatory: from skin and
    gastrointestinal tract, 41; oxidation,
    41; routes, 38–42
  precursors and non-protein pathways,
    38, 39
  profile for neonatal solutions, 233–4
  recovery in casein hydrolysates, 108–9
  requirements, 38–55; needs during
    illness, 46–51; non-essential, 44–6;
    physiological basis, 38–42
  solutions, in parenteral preparations,
    145
  transport, enteral diets; difference from
    peptide transport, 103–4; individual
    residues, 104; and nitrogen
    assimilation, 101
alpha-amylase inhibitor and starch
  absorption, 113–14
anabolism
  maintenance in adults, 63
  micronutrient requirements, 60
anaemia in IBD, 354
anaphylaxis and food intolerance, 209
Annatto causing urticaria, 207
Anorexia nervosa
  clinical description, 475–7
  definition, 473–4
  diagnostic guidelines (ICD10), 474
  enteral feeding, 130

historical background, 473
indications for enteral feeding in
    children, 193, *200–1*
physical consequences, 478–80
plasma proteins, 313
prognosis, 484
treatment, 481, 482–3; in general
    practice, 481; stages in severely ill
    patient, 482–3;   tube feeding, 315
anti-diarrhoeal drugs following
    jejunostomy, 373–4
see also diarrhoea
antibiotics in IBD, 357
antioxidants
    and nutrition in surgical patients, 250–51
    role in lipid and lipoprotein activity,
        429–30
    see also free radicals: oxidation
anxiety, and TPN peri-operatively, 290
aphthous ulcers and food intolerance, 207
apolipoproteins AI, B, E concentration,
    genetic factors, 428, 429
arginine
    dietary supplements, biological
        responses, 50
    enteral supplements after surgery, 249
    requirement in trauma, infection and
        cancer, 49–51
    role in cancer treatment, 50–1
    role in special diet formulations, 134
Ascites
    in chronic liver disease, 346
    and energy expenditure in liver disease,
        344
aspartate, requirements, 46
aspirin causing urticaria, 207
asthma, food intolerance, 208, 209
azo dyes
    causing urticaria, 207
    intolerance, and migraine, 209

B cells, role, 72–3
basophil histamine release and food
    allergy, 210
behaviour, diet affecting, 208–9
behaviour therapy and obesity/overweight,
    465–6
beta carotene
    metabolism in smokers, 66
    as nutrient antioxidant, 60
    requirements, and smoking, 59
bile salts, loss, and short bowel syndrome,
    376–7
biliary fistula, losses of micronutrients, 61
biliary sludging caused by TPN, 336
bingeing in bulimia nervosa, 477
blood pressure and diet, 444–59
    alcohol, 447–8; heavy drinkers, 447;

intervention studies, 448; J-shaped
        relationship, 447–8; mechanism, 448
    dietary lipids, 454
    environmental/genetic factors, 444
    mechanisms, 446
    obesity, 445–6
    potassium intake, 449–52
    vegetarian diet, 455
    weight loss, associated factors, 446–7
body composition measurement, 1–22
    accuracy, 15–16
    bedside techniques, 8–14; comparison
        with reference methods, 13–14;
        impedance/resistance, 10–12;
        inter-observer measurement
        variability, 17–18; near infra-red
        interactance, 12–13; skinfolds, 9–10,
        13; weight–height, 9
    comparison of methods, 13–14
    density, 3–4
    dual energy X-ray absorptiometry, 6–8
    in vivo neutron activation analysis, 8
    observer error, 17–18
    precision, 8, 9, 15–16
    reasons for, 1–2
    'reference man', 2–8
    total body potassium, 5–6
    total body water, 4–5
body density, measurement, 3–4
body mass and composition
    assessment, critical illness, 325–6
    in multiple organ failure, 328
body mass index, 460
body weight, *see* weight, body: obesity:
        overweight
bone disease and parenteral nutrition, 154–5
bowel rest, TPN peri-operatively, 294
brain, development, fetal and neonatal, and
        nutrition, 225
    pre-term infants, 225
    protein-energy malnutrition, 225
    see also neonatal intravenous feeding
brain, infant, and long chain
        polyunsaturated fatty acids, 226–7
branched chain amino acids
    in hepatic encephalopathy treatment, 346
    parenteral, 161
    requirement during illness, 47–8; and
        muscle wasting, 47
breast milk, long-term nutritional effect in
        pre-term babies, 225–6
bronchopulmonary dysplasia, and
        parenteral lipid, neonatal, 232
brush-border oligosaccharidases and
        membrane digestion, 111–13
Bulimia nervosa
    clinical description, 477–8
    definition, 473–4

Bulimia nervosa (*continued*)
  diagnostic guidelines (ICD10), 474–5
  historical background, 473
  physical consequences, 480–1
  prognosis, 485
  treatment, 481, 483–4; cognitive therapy,
    484; in general practice, 481
burns
  enteral feeding, 131
  micronutrient skin losses, 62
  resting metabolic expenditure,
    peri-operative, *263*
  TPN peri-operatively, 289
'Bush tea' causing liver disease, 336
butylated hydroxyanisole causing urticaria,
    207

caffeine, effect on serum lipids, 434
calcium supplements in neonatal
    intravenous feeding, 235
calorie intake in short bowel syndrome,
    381–2
calorie to nitrogen ratio, 264
calorimetry for assessing energy
    requirements, 23–31
  after trauma and sepsis, 323–5
  comparison, direct/indirect, 30–1
  direct methods, 23–4
  indirect methods, 24–31; limitations,
    27
cancer
  amino acid requirements during, 46–51
  cellular immunity, 81
  childhood, enteral feeding, 197
  contraindications of parenteral nutrition,
    162–3, 164–5
  effect of nutritional replenishment, 81
  enteral feeding, 130
  immunocompetence, 81
  parenteral nutrition, 145
  parenteral nutrition formulation, *287*
  reduced NK activity, 81
  role of arginine, 50
  role of beta carotene, 66
  role of carotenoids, 66
  therapy, summary of trials for
    nutritional support, 167–72, *181–91*
  TPN peri-operatively, 290, 291;
    guidelines, *292*
carbohydrate
  absorption, enteral diets, 110–16;
    digestion and absorption, 110–11;
    HPLC analysis of maltodextrins,
    114–15; hydrolysis of starch, 111–13;
    membrane digestion and brush-border
    oligosaccharidases, 111–13;
    rate-limiting steps in carbohydrate
    assimilation, 113–14; sucrose, 116–17

altered metabolism causing liver disease,
    339
  content of enteral feed in cystic fibrosis,
    404
  and fat powders and liquids, in cystic
    fibrosis, 402
  intestinal assimilation, enteral diet,
    perspective, 120
  malabsorption, in IBD, 354
  oxidation, 26
  polymer liquids, in cystic fibrosis, 402
  polymer powders, as supplements in
    cystic fibrosis, 401–2
  requirements for neonatal feeding, 229–30
cardiac surgery, guidelines for TPN
    peri-operatively, *293*
cardiovascular complications in anorexia
    nervosa, 479
carnitine in neonatal parenteral nutrition,
    233
carotenoids, role in lung cancer, 66
casein, enteral diets based on, 105–10
  preparation, *110*
casein hydrolysates
  and infant food intolerance, 207, 214
  percentage recovery of amino acids, *109*
catheter(s)
  central venous, complications, 281–3
  in neonatal intravenous feeding, 235
  four parenteral nutrition, 147–56;
    catheter care, 149; catheter-related
    complications, 150–3; central vein
    thrombosis, 151–3; infection, 150–1;
    occlusion, 151; effect on other organs,
    153–5; fracture of external catheter,
    153
  parenteral nutrition, peri-operative,
    277–83; maintenance protocol, 279
  sepsis, 283
CD cell activity in protein-energy
    malnutrition, 79
CD nomenclature, 73
CD4+ cells
  and humoral responses, 74
  and zind deficiency, 75
cellular immunity
  in Crohn's disease, 83–4
  mechanism, 73–4
  and nutritional deprivation, 80–1
central vein thrombosis and parenteral
    nutrition, 151–3
central venous cannulation for parenteral
    nutrition, peri-operative, 278
  complications, 281–3
cerebral palsy, children, enteral feeding,
    194–6, *200–1*
  indications, 195
cerebrovascular disease, enteral feeding, 131

chamber methods
  for direct calorimetry, 23–4
  for indirect calorimetry: closed-circuit,
    28; collection, 28–9; open-circuit,
    29–30; respiration, 27–8
cheese, intolerance, and migraine, 209
chemically defined diets, enteral nutrition,
    133–4
  composition, 133
  elemental diets, 95
  indications for use, 133
  specific feeds, *133*
  use in food allergy or intolerance, 133–4
  see also elemental diets
chemotherapy
  effect of parenteral nutrition, 162–3,
    164–5
  TPN peri-operatively, 289
chocolate, interolerance, and migraine, 209
cholecalciferol, role in liver disease, 341–2
cholesterol
  absorption, enteral diets, 117–19
  dietary, 423–5; atherogenicity, 425; in
    determining serum cholesterol, 423–4;
    effect on saturated fatty acid, 424;
    genetic factors in responsiveness,
    428–9; reasons for minimising, 424–5;
    reduction in fractional absorption,
    424
  increase, and coffee consumption, 433–4
  reducing properties of dietary fibres,
    434–5
  serum, reduction, effect on coronary
    heart disease prevention, 421
cholestyramine in IBD, 357–8
chromium, requirements, provision and
    toxicity, *68*
chronic obstructive pulmonary disease,
    parenteral nutrition formulation, *287*
cirrhosis
  alcoholic and other nutritional causes,
    334, 335
  nutritional consequences, 337
closed-circuit indirect calorimetry, 28
closed head injury, guidelines for TPN
    peri-operatively, *292*
codeine phosphate following jejunostomy,
    373–4
coeliac disease
  fat malabsorption, 61
  vitamin deficiency, 61
coffee
  and coronary heart disease risk, 433–4
  intolerance, and migraine, 209
cognition, role of micronutrients, 67
cognitive therapy in bulimia nervosa, 484
cola intolerance in asthma, 208
colic, and cows' milk intolerance, 207

colitis, infantile, and milk intolerance, 206
collection method of indirect calorimetry,
    28–9
computerised axial tomography in body
    composition measurement, 8
congenital heart disease, enteral feeding,
    children, 193–4, *200–1*
congestive cardiac failure, parenteral
    nutrition formulation, peri-operative,
    288
constipation and food intolerance, 207
copper
  defects in liver disease, 343
  requirements, provision and toxicity, *68*
coronary artery surgery patients,
    post-operative complications, 296
coronary heart disease
  action of antioxidants, 429–30
  alcohol, and serum lipoproteins, 430–3
  body weight and serum lipids, 421–3
  effect of cholesterol serum reduction, 421
  and fat distribution measurement, 7
  prevention, importance of diet, 421
  risk, and coffee, 433–4
corticosteroids in IBD, 357, 358
cortisol levels after trauma, 320
cost of peri-operative feeding, 297–8
cows' milk intolerance, 205, 206
  in asthma, 208
  causing urticaria, 207
  in cystic fibrosis, 405
  double-blind challenge, 213
  incidence, 205
  and protein hydrolysate formulas, 199,
    214
critical care, guidelines for TPN
    peri-operatively, *292*
critical illness
  energy requirements, peri-operative,
    262–3
  see also intensive care management
Crohn's disease
  anaemia, 354
  children: elemental feeds, 199–202;
    protein hydrolysate formula, 199–202
  electrolyte deficiencies, 354–5
  elemental diet and steroid treatment
    compared, 166
  enteral diets v. prednisolone, 359
  enteral feeding, 130, 131
  fat malabsorption, 61
  immunocompetence, 83–4
  medical therapy, 359
  mineral deficiencies, 355–6
  parenteral nutrition, 144
  prevalence of nutritional insufficiency,
    351
  protein-calorie malnutrition, 352–3

Crohn's disease (*continued*)
TPN, 358, 359; peri-operatively, 294;
versus enteral diets, 359
vitamin deficiencies, 61, 356–7
see also Inflammatory bowel disease
Crotolaria spp. causing liver disease, 336
cysteine, requirements, 51
cysteinensulfinic acid decarboxylase,
hepatic, activity, in infancy, 234
cystic fibrosis
comprehensive assessment, 419
dietary assessment, 393–4
enteral feeding, children, 196–7
essential fatty acids, 400
laboratory investigations, 395–400
minerals and trace elements, 400
nutrition, 388–419; additional strategies
to improve absorption, 408–9;
administration of pancreatic enzymes,
406–7; ensuring adequate energy
intake, 401; enteral feeding, 403–5;
evaluation and monitoring, 393; and
growth, 388; infant feeding, 405;
management, 401–8, 417–18;
carbohydrate polymer powders,
401–2; supplements, 401–3; parenteral
nutrition, 405; reasons for nutritional
and growth problems, 389; reasons for
poor energy intake, 389–93; regular
dietetic counselling, 401; vitamin
supplements, 405–6
nutritional state assessment, 394–5
cystine, requirements, 46
cytokines
activity after trauma and sepsis, 322
activity in IBD, 353
cytotoxic test, diagnostic test for food
allergies, *211*

demispan as measurement guide in
starvation, 311
depression, and TPN peri-operatively, 290
dextran assimilation, enteral diet, 114
dextrose
infusions, in fulminant hepatic failure,
347
in parenteral preparations, 145–6
diabetes mellitus
parenteral nutrition formulation,
peri-operative, *288*
prevalence with cystic fibrosis, 392
specific enteral diets, 273, *276*
diarrhoea
anti-diarrhoeal drugs following
jejunostomy, 373–4
caused by cows' milk intolerance, 206
caused by drug treatment, IBD, 357
complicating enteral feeding, 143

protein hydrolysate formula, 0–2 years,
199
diet(s), dietary
absorption, *see* carbohydrate absorption:
fat absorption: malabsorption:
nitrogen, intestinal assimilation:
protein hydrolysates: protein,
intestinal assimilation
affecting behaviour and learning ability,
208–9
assessment in cystic fibrosis, 393–4
and blood pressure, 444–59; *see also*
blood pressure and diet
causes of liver disease, 334–7
in coronary heart disease prevention,
importance, 421
factors, influence on lipids and
lipoprotein s, 420–43
fibre, cholesterol-reducing properties,
434–5
for food allergies, 211–15; double-blind
placebo-controlled challenge tests,
212–13; empirical, 212; exclusion, 211;
few food, *see* few food diet; food
reintroduction, 212; oligo-antigenic,
212; specific therapies, 213–15
habits, poor, and micronutrient deficiency,
58
intake, impaired, and malnutrition, in
surgical patients, 241
polymeric, *see* polymeric diets
see also elemental diets: enteral diets:
special formulations
dilution techniques for total body water
measurement, 5
diphenoxylate following jejunostomy, 373–4
disaccharides, digestion, 111–12, 113
distorted body image in anorexia nervosa,
476
double-blind placebo-controlled challenge
tests for food allergies, 212–13
doubly labelled water method of indirect
calorimetry, 31
Down's syndrome, zinc levels, 76
Dowsing, diagnostic test for food allergies,
211
dual energy X-ray absorptiometry in body
composition measurement, 6–8
duodenum, role in fat absorption, 117–18
DXA *see* dual energy X-ray absorptiometry

E numbers, intolerance, 205
eating disorders, 473–87
definitions, 473–4
historical background, 473
see also Anorexia nervosa: Bulimia
nervosa
ebb phase after trauma or sepsis, 319–21

eczema, and food intolerance, 207
egg(s)
    and anaphylaxis, 209
    free diets for food allergies, 215
    intolerance, 206; in asthma, 208; causing
        urticaria, 207; and migraine, 209
elderly people
    healthy, nutritional supplements, 82–3
    immunocompetence, 82–3
    and micronutrient deficiency, 59
electrolytes
    balance after major small bowel
        resection, 379–80
    in cystic fibroses, 397
    deficiencies in IBD, 354–5
    excretion, and blood pressure, 452
    infusions in short bowel syndrome, 383;
        indications, 383
    loss after jejunostomy, 370
    requirements, peri-operative, 261–2
elemental diets
    chemically defined, 95
    for children, 199–202
    composition, physiological rationale,
        95–6
    in Crohn's disease, 360; childhood,
        199–202; compared with steroid
        treatment, 166
    in cystic fibrosis, 404
    early work, 95
    in severe eczema, 208
encephalopathy
    and BCAA supplementation, 47, 48
    benefits of parenteral nutrition, 161
endocrine symptoms in anorexia nervosa,
    478–9
energy balance
    negative, causing liver disease, *338*
    responses to trauma and sepsis, 323
energy equivalents for fuel use, 26
energy expenditure, 323–5
    after trauma and sepsis, 321
    in liver disease, 340
    resting, increased, in cystic fibrosis,
        392–3
    in ventilated patients, 327–8
energy intake
    adequate, ensuring, in cystic fibrosis, 401
    in cystic fibrosis, 389
    poor, reasons, 389–93, 418
    inadequate, in children, enteral feeding,
        193
    measurement, critical illness, 326
    responses to trauma and sepsis, 323
energy metabolism and fat free mass
        estimates, 1
energy requirements
    assessment, 22–37; methods; 23–33:

direct calorimetry, 24–31; oxidation of
    fuels, 26–7; protein oxidation rate,
    25–6; relation to basal metabolic rate,
    22; relation to body weight, 22;
    respiratory gas exchange and fuel use,
    25
    due to oxidation of fuels, 26–7
    for neonatal feeding, 229
    peri-operative, 261–4
    in surgical patients, 243–4
energy supplements, nutritionally complete,
    in cystic fibrosis, 402–3
enteral diets
    for animals, 105–6
    carbohydrate absorption, 110–16
    categories, 132–5
    chemically-defined, 133–4
    disease specific, 273, 276
    examples of specific feeds, *133*
    malabsorption, 96
    nitrogen assimilation, 99–104
    polymeric, 132–3
    protein absorption, 98–9
    protein assimilation, 104–9
    special formulations, 134–5
    types of diets, 273–7: acute and chronic
        renal patient, 273, *276*; diabetes, 273,
        276; hepatic failure, 273, *276*; immune
        compromised patient, 273, *276*;
        stressed patients, 273, *276*
    see also protein hydrolysates
enteral feeding and nutrition, 130–43
    after surgery, 248
    chemically defined diets, 133–4
    clinical trials, 160–1; appendix (*tables*),
        181–91; results, 162
    contra-indications, 130–2
    cyclical/continuous feeding, 141–2
    in cystic fibrosis, 403–5
    diagnostic groups, 130, *131*
    disease specific diets, 273, 276
    effect on cancer patients undergoing
        chemotherapy, 162–3, 164–5
    equipment for patients, 141–2
    gastrointestinal complications, 143
    in IBD, 358, 359, 360
    indications, 130–2
    jejunal tubes, 137–42
    methods, 135–43
    nasogastric, 135–6
    in the newborn, 227–9;
        gastro-oesophageal reflux, 228–9;
        necrotising enterocolitis, 227, 229;
        parenteral or enteral?, 227–8; very low
        birthweight infant, 227–8
    nutrient delivery complications, 142–3
    nutrient solution, 132
    nutritional and metabolic problems, 143

enteral feeding and nutrition (*continued*)
  in paediatrics: choice of feeds, 198–204;
    choice of route, 202–4; complications,
    204; continuous or intermittent, 204;
    history, 192–204; indications, 192–8:
    specific clinical conditions, 193–8,
    200–1; modular feeds, examples of
    ingredients, 202, 203; nutritional
    requirements, 198, 200–1; oral–motor
    stimulation after, 204
percutaneous endoscopic gastronomy,
    135–6, 137
  polymeric diets, 132–3
  special formulations, 134–5
  standardised order forms, 273, 274, 275
  see also nutritional support,
    worthwhileness
enterocyte, mammalian, amino acid
    transport, 101
enzyme activity, maintenance and
    micronutrient adequacy, 64
Epilepsy and food intolerance, 208–9
essential fatty acids
  in cystic fibrosis, 400
  required for maintenance, 41–4
Ewing's sarcoma, childhood, enteral
    feeding, 197
exercise as treatment for obesity, 467

failure to thrive, enteral feeding, children,
    193, 200–1
fat
  absorption: defective, causing liver
    disease, 339–40; enteral diets, 117–19:
    perspective, 120–1
  dietary, genetic factors in responsiveness,
    428–9
  -free mass, 'reference man', 2
  malabsorption, in IBD, 354
  oxidation, 26
  restriction, in short bowel syndrome, 382
fatigue, and TPN peri-operatively, 290
fatty acids
  dietary: and cholesterol levels, 426–28;
    polyunsaturated, 426–8; saturated,
    426–8
  short chain, enteral supplements in
    surgical patients, 250
  trans, effect of lipoproteins, 427
fatty liver, 335
femoral fracture, TPN peri-operatively, 290
  guidelines, 293
few food diet
  and eczema, 207–8
  in epilepsy, 209
  in hyperactivity, 209
fibre, dietary, cholesterol-reducing
    properties, 434–5

fish
  and anaphylaxis, 209
  intolerance, 206; causing urticaria, 207
fish oils and coronary heart disease, 427
fistula, gastrointestinal, TPN
    peri-operatively, 291, 293, 295
flow phase after trauma or sepsis, 319–22
flow-through method of indirect
    calorimetry, 29–30
fluid
  balance after major small bowel
    resection, 379–80
  losses, peri-operative, 261
  without nutrient infusion: in short bowel
    syndrome, 383: indications, 383
folate deficiency
  causing liver disease, 340, 341
  in elderly, 59
folate intake and neural-tube defects, 63
folic acid IBD, 354, 355
food additives
  causing urticaria, 207
  incidence of intolerance, 205–6
  intolerance, and asthma, 208
food allergens, 209–10
food allergy and intolerance
  causing eczema, 207
  children, 204–17; definitions, 205;
    incidence and natural history,
    205–6;
    outgrow, 206; symptoms, 206–9
  definition of an allergen, 209–10
  diagnostic techniques, 210–11;
    unorthodox, 211
  diets, 211–15
  egg free diets, 215
  life threatening, 206, 209
  milk substitutes, 214
  nutritional adequacy of diets, 215
  specific allergens, 205–10
  wheat free diets, 215
food avoidance in IBD, 361–2
food, dilution by exocrine digestive
    secretions after jejunostomy, 371,
    373
food preferences in starvation, 314
free radicals
  and micronutrient activity, 67
  and micronutrient adequacy, 64
  and nutrition in surgical patients,
    250–1
  role in lipid and lipoprotein activity,
    429–30
  scavenging mechanisms in disease,
    59–60
  see also antioxidants: oxidation
fructose uptake, enteral diets, 114
fruit, intolerance, causing urticaria, 207

fulminant hepatic failure, nutritional therapy, 347
fungi containing hepatotoxins causing liver disease, 336–7

gallstones caused by TPN, 336
gastric
  balloon for weight reduction, 469
  bypass for weight reduction, 468
  dilatation in bulimia nervosa, 481
  luminal protein digestion, 98–9
  stapling for weight reduction, 468–9
gastrointestinal
  cancer, TPN peri-operatively, 290
  complications from enteral feeding, 143
  disease: causing malnutrition, surgical patients, 241–2; in children, enteral feeding, 193
  fistulas, TPN peri-operatively, guidelines, *293*
  losses of micronutrients, 61
  malabsorption: causing liver disease, *338*; causing poor energy intake in cystic fibrosis, 390–2, 418
  symptoms of food intolerance, 206–7
  tract in anorexia nervosa, 480
gastrostomy for peri-operative feeding, 268–9
gastro-oesophageal reflux and enteral nutrition, 228–9
gastrostomy feeding
  for children, 202; contraindications, 202–3
  in cystic fibrosis, 403–5
  in starvation, 315
genetic factors in responsiveness to dietary cholesterol and fat, 428–9
gestation, amino acid requirements, 44, *45*
glucose
  infusions, effects, 263
  intolerance, and sepsis in surgical patients, 243–4
  metabolism, after trauma and sepsis, 321
  requirements in surgical patients, 244
  and sodium solution, to promote absorption after jejunostomy, 374–5
  uptake, enteral diets, 113, 114
glutamate, requirements, 46
glutamine, 46
  in Crohn's disease, 361
  enteral supplements after surgery, 248–9
  and muscle protein metabolism, 48–9
  in parenteral preparations, 145
glutathione peroxidase, and removal of hydrogen peroxide, 60
glycine, requirements, 46

glycogen, myocardial, and post-operative complications, 296
growth
  amino acid requirements, 44, *45*
  micronutrient requirements, 60
  retardation, enteral feeding, 194, 200–1

H2 receptor antagonists, inhibiting effects, 99
haematological abnormalities in anorexia nervosa, 479
haematology investigations in cystic fibrosis, 395–6
hair analysis, diagnostic test for food allergies, *211*
Haldane transformation, 324
Harris–Benedict equation, 262
heart conditions, children, enteral feeding, *200–1*
  see also congenital heart disease
heart, effects of parenteral nutrition, 155
heart rate and energy expenditure, 31
height measurement for body composition, 10
hepatic disease, parenteral nutrition formulation, peri-operative, *288*
hepatic encaphalopathy and BCAA supplementation, 47–8
hepatic failure, specific enteral diets, 273, *276*
hepatitis A, causes, 337
hepatobiliary complications of parenteral nutrition, 154
hepatocellular carcinoma, sequel to alcoholic cirrhosis, 334
hepatotoxins causing liver disease, 336
high density lipoprotein cholesterol, 421–3
hip fractures in elderly, effect of nutritional supplements, 166
histidine, daily requirements, *45*
hormonal activity after trauma and stress, 320, 322
hostility, and TPN peri-operatively, 290
humoral immunity in ageing individuals, 82
humoral responses, action, 73
hunger strike, percentage weight loss against time, 309
hydration factor in total body water measurement, 5, 7
hydrolysates, see protein hydrolysates
hydrolysis of dietary fats, 117
25-hydroxyvitamin D
  serum levels after jejunostomy, 376
  in short bowel syndrome, 382
hyperactivity and food intolerance, 208–9
hyperglycaemia
  in cystic fibrosis, 404

hyperglycaemia (*continued*)
  in surgical patients, 243
  in very low birthweight infant receiving
    parenteral glucose, 230
hypermetabolism after trauma and sepsis,
    321
hyperosmolar states in surgical patients,
    243–4
hypertension
  effects of alcohol, 477; compared with
    obesity, 477; heavy drinkers, 447;
    intervention studies, 448; J-shaped
    relationship, 447; mechanisms, 448
  relation to obesity, 445–6
hypertriglyceridaemia, alcohol-related, 433
hypoproteinaemia in surgical patients, 256
hypothalamic–pituitary–adrenal axis,
    activation following trauma, 320

IgE-mediated food allergy
  life threatening, 206, 209
  specific test, 210
illness, micronutrient requirements, 60–1
  see also critical illness: intensive care
    management; immune compromised
    patients; specific enteral diets, 273, *276*
immune function
  micronutrient activity, 65–6
  and single nutrient deficiencies, 74–8
immune response
  malnutrition, and surgery, 240
  in protein-energy malnutrition in
    children and adults, 79–81
immunity, altered, associated clinical
    situations, 78–9
immunocompetence
  in ageing individuals, 82
  alcoholic liver disease, 84–5
  in Crohn's disease, 83–4
  and liver disease. 344
  in specific clinical conditions, 81–5
immunology
  nutritional, 72–94
  overview, 72–4
impedance, whole body, for body
    composition measurement, 10–11
in vivo neutron activation analysis in body
    composition measurement, 8
  precision, *9*
infant feeding in cystic fibrosis, 405
infection
  amino acid requirements during, 46–51
  catheter-related: in neonatal intravenous
    feeding, 235; parenteral nutrition, 150–1
  complicating peri-operative feeding, 272
and malnutrition in surgical patients, 242–3
  and parenteral lipid, neonatal, 233
  and parenteral nutrition, 165

infectious diseases, and vitamin A
    supplements, 66
inflammatory bowel disease
  definitions, 350
  malnutrition, and surgery, 240
  nutritional deficiencies, 350–69; anaemia,
    354; dietary restrictions, 361–2; effects
    of drugs, 357–8; effects of drugs,
    357–8; electrolyte deficiencies, 354–5;
    fat and carbohydrate absorption, 354;
    minerals and trace elements, 355–6;
    protein-calorie malnutrition, 352–4;
    treatment, 358–2; vitamins, 356–7
  pathogenesis of malnutrition, 351–2
  summary of trials for nutritional
    support, 167–72, *181–91*
  TPN peri-operatively, 290; guidelines,
    293, 294
inflammatory disease, parenteral nutrition,
    144
infra-red interactance in body composition
    measurements, 12–13
infra-red thermography for direct
    calorimetry, 24
inositol in neonatal intravenous feeding, 231
inotropic support of myocardium during
    multiple organ systems failure, 327
insulin resistance after trauma and sepsis,
    322
intensive care management, 319–32
  body mass and composition, 325–6
  endocrinological events following
    trauma and sepsis, 319–22
  energy balance, 323
  energy expenditure, 323–5
  energy intake, 323
  energy and nitrogen intake, 326
  multiple organ systems failure, 327–9
  physiological events following trauma
    and sepsis, 319–22
intermittent positive pressure ventilation in
    critical illness, 327–8
  energy expenditure, 327–8
intestinal
  adaptation, short bowel syndrome, 378–9
  complications of parenteral nutrition, 154
  lipase, role in enteral diets, 118
  malabsorption in cystic fibrosis, 418
  transplantation in short bowel
    syndrome, 384
intravenous feeding, neonatal, *see* neonatal
    intravenous feeding
ipecacuanha to induce vomiting in bulimia
    nervosa, adverse effects, 481
iron
  deficiency: in elderly, 59; in IBD, 354,
    355; protein-energy malnutrition and
    immunity, 76

injections, in short bowel syndrome, 383
overload, in liver disease, 343–4
requirements, provision and toxicity, *68*
supplements: and copper absorption, 61;
and zinc absorption, 61
isoleucine
daily requirements, *45*
requirements after trauma, 47
isotopes
in total body potassium measurement, 6
in total body water measurement, 5
IVNAA, *see in vivo* neutron activation
analysis

jaw wiring for weight reduction, 469
jejunal tubes, enteral feeding, 137–42
method of placing, 137–9
relative merits, *135*, 139
jejunostomy
decreasing output, effect of drugs, 373–4
early post-operative management, 379–80
enteral feeding for children, 204
feeding, in cystic fibrosis, 403
long-term management, 380–3
nutrient absorption, 376
optimum concentrations of glucose and
sodium to promote absorption, 374–5
for peri-operative feeding, 269–70;
mechanical complications, 270
physiological consequences, 370–6
potassium and divalent cations, 375–6

killer cells, role, 73
Kwashiorkor and immunodysfunction, 80

lactation, amino acid requirements, 44, *45*
D-lactic acidosis and short bowel
syndrome, 378
lactose intolerance in IBD, 362
lauric acid and cholesterol level, 426
laxative abuse
in anorexia nervosa, 475, 480
in bulimia nervosa, 477–8
learning ability, diet affecting, 208–9
leucine
daily requirements, *45*
requirements after trauma, 47
lingual lipase, role in enteral diets, 117
lipid(s)
alternative substrates, enteral
supplements after surgery, 249–50
assimilation in enteral diets, 117–19
and blood pressure, 455
effect on immune function, 78
in fulminant hepatic failure, 347
in neonatal intravenous feeding, 231;
and bronchopulmonary dysplasia, 232;
and infection, 233

in parenteral preparations, 145–6
requirements in surgical patients, 244
sludge on catheter walls, 151
lipoproteins
effect of dietary fibre, 434, 435
serum, alcohol, and coronary heart
disease, 430–3
liver disease alcohol-related, 334
benefits of parenteral nutrition, 161
caused by altered carbohydrate
metabolism, 339
caused by contaminants, 337
caused by decreased dietary intake, *338*
caused by defective fat absorption, 339
caused by defective protein balance,
337–9
caused by hepatotoxins, 336–7
children, enteral feeding, *200–1*
chronic, nutritional therapy, principles,
345–7
with cystic fibrosis, 392
dietary causes, 334–7
energy expenditure, 340
infective agents, 337
mineral metabolism, 342–4
nutritional assessment, 344
nutritional consequences, 337–44
summary of trials for nutritional
support, 167–72, *181–91*
vegetable protein diets, 346
vitamin deficiencies, 340–2
see also alcoholic liver disease
liver failure
enteral feeding, 130
TPN peri-operatively, 290; guidelines, 294
liver function tests in cystic fibrosis, 397
liver, role in nutrition, 333–49
biological activity, 333
dietary causes of liver disease, 334–7
long-chain triglycerides, absorption, enteral
diets, 117–19
loperamide following jejunostomy, 373–4
low birth weight infants, summary of trials
for nutritional support, 167–72, *181–91*
low density lipoprotein cholesterol, effect
of weight loss and gain, 421–3
low density lipoprotein oxidation, 429–30
low-residue diets in IBD, 362
lung cancer, role of carotenoids, 66
lysine, daily requirements, *45*

magnesium supplements
after jejunostomy, 376
in short bowel syndrome, 381
malabsorption
of micronutrients, 61
of nutrients: definition, 96–37; 'rate
limiting', 96; 'safety margin' (reserve

malabsorption (*continued*)
  capacity) of gastrointestinal tract,
    96–7
  syndromes, enteral feeding, 131
  see also carbohydrate absorption: fat
    absorption
malnutrition
  causing liver disease, 335
  in hospital patients, 80
  in IBD, pathogenesis, 351–2
  long-stay elderly patients, 308
  as nutritional consequence of liver
    disease, 337
  and peri-operative feeding, 259–60
  in specific clinical conditions, enteral
    feeding, children, 193–8
  and the surgical patient, 239–55; *see also*
    surgery and nutrition
maltases, enteral diets, membrane
  digestion, 112–13
maltodextrins in enteral diets, 110–17
  HPLC analysis, 114–15
maltose uptake, enteral diet, 113, 114
manganese, requirements, provision and
  toxicity, *68*
measurement, body composition, 1–22
  see also body composition measurement
medium chain triglycerides
  absorption, enteral diets, 117–19
  parenteral feeding in neonates, 232
metabolic
  complications: enteral nutrition,
    peri-operative, 271–2; in TPN, 283
  demand, altered, and malnutrition,
    surgical patients, 242
  disease, in children, enteral feeding,
    193
  events after trauma and sepsis, 319–32
  homeostasis, normal, disturbance,
    causing liver disease, *338*
  problems of enteral feeding, 143
metal, excessive ingestion causing liver
  disease, 337
metallothionein, as general antioxidant,
  60
methionine
  + cystine, daily requirements, *45*
  daily requirements, *45*
  functions in the body, 40–1
microdiet computer program assessment in
  cystic fibrosis, 394
micronutrients
  as cofactors in metabolism, 59
  deficiency: development, 56–8; effects of
    disease on likelihood, 59–62; 'healthy'
    individual at risk, 58–9; sub-clinical
    effects, 63; subclinical, 57
  malabsorption, 61

  optimisation of intake, 62–7; anabolism
    maintenance in adults, 63; biochemical
    markers of micronutrient adequacy,
    64; optimal biochemical and
    physiological function, 63; optimal
    substrate utilisation, 62–3;
    physiological markers of
    micronutrient adequacy, 65;
    prevention of clinical symptoms, 62
  recommended intake, 67
  requirements due to growth and
    anabolism, 60
  toxicity, 68–9
migraine and food intolerance, 208–9
milk
  and anaphylaxis, 209
  -free diets, 213–14
  intolerance: *see* cows' milk intolerance
    and migraine, 209
  substitutes for food allergies, 214
minerals
  in cystic fibrosis, 400
  deficiencies, development, 56–8
  in IBD, 355–6
  metabolism, in liver disease, 342–4
  requirements due to growth and
    anabolism, 60
  supplements, toxicity, 68–9
mitogen responsiveness in elderly people,
  82
mitogen transformation, effect of vitamin
  C, 77
modular feeds for children, 202
molybdenum, requirements, provision and
  toxicity, *68*
monitoring of artificial nutritional support,
  155–6
monounsaturates
  and cholesterol levels, 426–8
  oxidation, 430
  protective effect, 431–2
mood states, and TPN peri-operatively,
  290
motility disorders, parenteral nutrition,
  144–5
motility disturbances in short bowel
  syndrome, 378
motor neurone disease
  enteral feeding, 131
  tube feeding, 315
multiple organ failure, and malnutrition in
  surgical patients, 242–3
multiple organ systems failure, intensive
  care management, 327–9
  appearance of patient, 327
  body composition changes, 328
  energy expenditure, 327–8
  feeding patients, 328–9

muscle
  activity, in multiple organ failure, 327
  protein metabolism, and glutamine, 48–9
  wasting, and BCAA requirements, 47
  see also skeletal muscle
mushroom toxins causing liver disease, 336
mycotoxins causing liver disease, 336
myocardial infarction, and TPN peri-operatively, 290
myristic acid and cholesterol level, 426

nasogastric feeding, 135–6
  after surgery, 247, 248
  for children, 202; contraindications, 202–3
  in cystic fibrosis, 403
  peri-operative, 267–8; disadvantages, 267–8; method for placing, 267
  relative merits, *135*
  in starvation, 315
  of thin, very thin and normal patients, 307–8
  tubes used, 135–6
natural killer cells, role, 73
near infra-red interactance in body composition measurement, 12–13
necrotising enterocolitis and parenteral nutrition, 227, 229
neonatal intravenous feeding, 224–38
  enteral nutrition and gastro-oesophageal reflux, 228–9
  indications for parenteral nutrition, 227–35
  macronutrient requirements, 229–35
  nutritional vulnerability, 224
  venous access, 235–6
  very low birthweight infants, 224–5; enteral or parenteral?, 227–9
neural-tube defects, folate intake during pregnancy, 63
neuro-development and nutrition, 225
neuroblastoma, childhood, enteral feeding, 197
neurological symptoms of food intolerance, 208–9
nitrogen
  balance, effect of nutritional support, 167, *168*
  intake, measurement, critical illness, 326
  intestinal assimilation, enteral diets, 99–104; amino acids derived from non-dietary sources, 100–1; dietary and endogenous protein, 99–100; free amino acid transport, 101; peptide transport, 101–4; urea recycling, 100–in parenteral feeding, neonatal, 233–4
  requirement, peri-operative, 264

nuclear magnetic resonance imaging in body composition measurement, 8
  precision, *9*
null cells, role, 73
nutritional disorders, sequence of events to disease, 255–60
nutritional support, timing, 167
nutritional support, worthwhileness, 158–80
  background, 158
  conclusions, 172–3
  effect on clinical outcome, 161–7
  effect on nutritional outcome, 167–72
  evidence, 159–60
  methodologic considerations, 160–1
  nutritional outcome, 167–72
  prospective randomised clinical trials: appendix (*tables*), *181–91*; clinical outcome, 161–7; effect on mortality and morbidity, 161–7, 171–2; methods, 160–1; summary, 162
nuts
  and anaphylaxis, 209
  intolerance: in asthma, 208; causing urticaria, 207

oat bran and decrease in serum cholesterol, 434–5
obese subjects, potassium concentration, 6
obesity, 460–72
  acceptability of reducing diets, 464
  advice for reducing dietary energy intake, 462–4
  behaviour therapy, 465–6
  and blood pressure, 445–6; compared with alcohol intake, 447; Framingham studies, 445; interventional studies, 446; Utah family study, 446
  calorie-controlled, 462–4
  as cause for liver disease, 335
  definition, 460
  desirable range of weight for height, 460
  exercise as treatment, 467
  forbidden items, attitudes, 464
  frequency and timing of meals, 465
  long-term efficacy of dietary treatment, 466–7
  maintenance of weight loss, 469–70
  prevalence, 460–2
  refractory, 470–1
  surgical procedures, 467–9
  treatment by diet, 462–8
  very-low-calorie diets, 464
  weight-loss groups, 466
obstetrics, guidelines for TPN peri-operatively, *293*
occlusion, catheter, in parenteral nutrition, 151

octreotide, after jejunostomy, 373
oedema
    in chronic liver disease, 346
    and food intolerance, 207
oesophagostomy for peri-operative feeding,
    268
    mechanical complications, 270
oleic acid, effect on blood pressure, 454
oligo-entigenic diet for food allergies, 212
olsalazine in IBD, 357
oncotherapy, and nutritional support,
    summary of trials, 161–7, *181–91*
open-circuit method of indirect
    calorimetry, 29–30
oral feeding in starvation, 314
oral–motor stimulation after tube feeding, 204
oranges, intolerance, and migraine, 209
order form for enteral nutrition, 273, *274,
    275*
    disease specific diets, 273, *276*
order form for total parenteral nutrition,
    284–6
oropharyngeal neoplasia, enteral feeding,
    131
osteomalacia
    in cystic fibrosis, 397–8
    in IBD, 356, 357–8
    osteoporosis
    bone mineral assessment, 1–2
    in cystic fibrosis, 398
overweight, 460–72
    acceptability of reducing diets, 464
    advice for reducing dietary energy
        intake, 462–4
    behaviour therapy, 465–6
    calorie-controlled, 462–4
    definition, 460
    exercise as treatment, 467
    forbidden items, attitudes, 464
    frequency and timing of meals, 465
    long-term efficacy of dietary treatment,
        466–7
    maintenance of weight loss, 469–70
    prevalence, 460–2
    surgical procedures, 467–9
    treatment by diet, 462–8
    very-low-calorie diets, 464
    weight-loss groups, 466
oxidation rates of fuel and energy
    requirements, 26–7
oxygen consumption after trauma and
    sepsis, 320
    measurement, 323–5

paediatrics
    enteral feeding, 192–204; *see also* enteral
        feeding, in paediatrics
    TPN peri-operatively, guidelines, *294*

palmitic acid and cholesterol level, 426
pancreatic damage in cystic fibrosis
    effect, 390–2; enzyme insufficiency, 390
pancreatic endopeptidases for hydrolysis in
    diets, 107–8
pancreatic enzyme administration in cystic
    fibrosis, 406–7
    acid resistance microspheres, 407
    determination of dose, 407
    higher lipase content, 407
    infants, 407
    young children, 407
pancreatic enzyme supplements in cystic
    fibrosis, 404–5
pancreatic function, impaired, protein
    assimilation, 107
pancreatic lipase, role in enteral diets,
    117–18
pancreatitis, TPN peri-operatively, 289,
    291
    guidelines, *293*
parenteral feeding in neonates, medium
    chain triglycerides, 232
parenteral formations, types, 286–7
parenteral nutrition, 144–56
    all-in-one delivery system, 286
    catheter-related complications, 150–3
    clinical trials, 160–1; appendix (*tables*),
        181–91; results, 162
    complications, 281–3
    contra-indications, 145
    in cystic fibrosis, 405
    effect on cancer patients undergoing
        chemotherapy, 162–3, 164–5
    effect on other organs, 153–5
    equipment for patients, 147–8
    indications, 144–5
    methods, 147–9
    monitoring, 155–6
    neonatal, *see* neonatal intravenous
        feeding in the newborn: indications,
        227–8;
        macronutrient requirements, 229–35;
        very low birthweight infants, 227–35
    nutrient solutions, 145–7
    nutritional complications, 149–50
    peri-operatively, guidelines, *292–4*
    standardised order form, 284–6
    support team, 283–4
    terminology, 144
    venous access, 277–83
    see also nutritional support,
        worthwhileness: total parenteral
        nutrition
peanuts, intolerance, 206
peptide(s)
    assimilation, effect of chain-length, 104;
        profile of hydrolysates, 108

non-nutritional, non-absorptive aspects, clinical nutrition, 107–10
in parenteral preparations, 145
transport, enteral diets, 101–4; characteristics of uptake, 102–3; di-, tri- and tetra-peptides, *1022*, 103–4; difference from amino acid transport, 103–4; low and high affinity, 103; structural requirements of high-affinity, 103–4
percutaneous endoscopic gastrostomy complications, 137
in feeding for starvation, 315
method, 137
for peri-operative feeding, 269; mechanical complications, 270
relative merits, *135*
tubes used, 136
peri-operative feeding, 256–306
advantages, 289–97
baseline water requirements to meet obligatory fluid losses, 261
complications of enteral nutrition, 270–2
disadvantages, 297–8
effect of parenteral nutrition, 163–6
enteral nutrition, types of diets, 273–7
enteral route, 267
gastrostomy, 268–9
guidelines, *293–4*
infectious complications, 272
jejunostomy, 269–70; mechanical complications, 270
mechanical complications, 270–1
metabolic complications, 271–2
nasogastric route, 267–8; disadvantages, 267–8; method for placing, 267
oesophagostomy, 268; mechanical complications, 270
patients' nutrient requirements, 261–6
percutaneous endoscopic gastronomy, 269; mechanical complications, 270
peripheral vein cannulation, 277–8
pharyngostomy, 268; mechanical complications, 270
post-operative complications, 296
safety, 297
standardized enteral order forms, 273
summary of trials for nutritional support, 167–72, *181–91*
venous access for parenteral nutrition, 277–83
peripheral vein cannulation for parenteral nutrition, peri-operative, 277–8
peripherally inserted central catheters for peri-operative feeding, 281–1
indications, 281

pharyngostomy for peri-operative feeding, 268
mechanical complications, 270
phenylalanine
daily requirements, *45*
+ tyrosine, daily requirements, *45*
phosphate supplements in neonatal intravenous feeding, 235
physical characteristics and energy expenditure, 31–2
phytohaemaglutinin, in Crohn's disease, 83
phytohaemaglutinin transformation
in Crohn's disease, 84
in protein-energy malnutrition, 79
and vitamin C, 77
plants containing hepatotoxins causing liver disease, 336–7
plasma concentration and micronutrient adequacy, 64–5
polymeric diets, enteral nutrition
composition, 132
in Crohn's disease, *359*, 360
indications for use, 132
paediatric: 0–5 years, 198–9; over 5 years, 199
specific feeds, *133*
polyunsaturated fatty acids
and cholesterol levels, 426–8
enteral supplements in surgical patients, 250
long chain, and the infant brain, 226–7
peroxidation in LDL-lipids, 429
port, subcutaneous implantable injection, for catheters, peri-operative feeding, 280
potassium after jejunostomy, 375–6
potassium intake and blood pressure, 452–4
Intersalt Study, 452
intervention studies, 454
Scottish Heart Health Study, 452
potassium, total body, measurement, 5–6
pre-term babies, nutritional effect of mothers' milk, 225–6
proline
in severely burned patients, 51
in skin collagen, 51
prospective randomised clinical trials in nutritional support
appendix (*tables*), *181–91*
effect on mortality and morbidity, 161–7
methods, 160–1
nutritional outcome, 167–72
summary, 162
protein absorption, enteral diets, 98–9
gastric luminal protein digestion, 98–9
poor solubilisation, 99
protein-calorie malnutrition in IBD, 352–4

protein, dietary, assimilation, quantitative
  aspects, 104–7
  animal feeding studies, 105–6; diets
    based on casein, 105–6; hydrolysates
    v. free amino acid diets, 106; loss of
    nitrogen, 106; trials, 105
  and endogenous, 99–100
  feeding studies in man, 106–7
  impaired pancreatic function, 107
  intestinal, enteral, 119–20
  normal or moderately impaired gut
    function, 106
  severely reduced absorptive area, 107
protein-energy malnutrition and
  immunodeficiency, 72
  effect of zinc deficiency, 77
protein-energy malnutrition and
  neuro-development, 225
protein hydrolysate formulas in enteral diets
  for amino acid absorption, 104
  cascade hydrolysis, 108–9
  for children, 199–202
  effect of pancreatic enzymes, 108
  in food allergies, 214
  peptide chain length profile, 108
  percentage of amino acid recovery, 108–9
  preparation of intravenous use, *110*
  reducing bitterness, 108
  sequence and hydrophobicity, 104
  taste, 108
protein intake in short bowel syndrome,
  381–2
protein in liver disease
  imbalance, 337–9
  intake decrease, 337–9
protein oxidation rate, 25–6
protein, plasma
  concentration in sepsis, and nutritional
    repletion, surgical patients, 244
  rise after injury, 320–1
  and treatment of starvation, 313
protein supplements, nutritionally
  complete, in cystic fibrosis, 402–3
protein turnover after surgery or trauma,
  321
proton-dependence, 103
pulmonary failure, TPN peri-operatively,
  290
pulmonary ventilation and energy
  expenditure, 31
pulse test, diagnostic test for food allergies,
  211
purgative abuse in bulimia nervosa, 475

Quetelet's Index, 460

radiation enteritis, parenteral nutrition,
  144

radioallergosorbent test for food
  intolerance, 210
radionics, diagnostic test for food allergies,
  211
red wine intolerance
  in asthma, 208
  and migraine, 209
refeeding syndrome, 143
'reference man', body composition, 2–8
renal complications in anorexia nervosa,
  479
renal disease, parenteral nutrition
  formulation, peri-operative, *288*
renal failure
  enteral feeding, 130
  TPN peri-operatively, 290; guidelines,
    293
  renal patients, acute and chronic, specific
    enteral diets, 273, *276*
renal stones, liability to, in short bowel
  syndrome, 377
respiration chamber calorimetry method,
  27–8
respiratory distress syndrome
  intravenous feeding, 224; *see also*
    neonatal intravenous feeding
  neonatal, inositol in parenteral feeding,
    231
respiratory gas exchange and fuel use, 25
respiratory symptoms of food intolerance,
  208
riboflavin deficiency causing liver disease,
  340, 341
rickets, in cystic fibrosis, 397–8
right atrial catheters for parenteral
  nutrition, peri-operative, 278
  inferior vena cava, 279–80
  superior vena cava, 278–9
Russell's sign in bulimia nervosa, 480

saccharides, digestion, 111–12
salicylates causing asthma, 208
salt intake and blood pressure, 449–52
  confounding factors, adjustment, 449
  effect of changing intake, 450–1
  Intersalt Study, 449–50
  intervention studies, 450–2
  other trial results, 450–2
  Scottish Heart Health Study, 452
  see also sodium
saturated fatty acid
  and cholesterol levels, 426–8; replacing
    with carbohydrate, 427–8
  dietary, effect of cholesterol intake, 424
selenium
  deficiency in liver disease, 343
  requirements, provision and toxicity, *68*
Senecio spp. causing liver disease, 336

sepsis
  and altered metabolic demand, 242
  energy requirements, peri-operative, *263*
  and malnutrition in surgical patients,
    242–3
  physiological and endocrinological
    events, 319–22; ebb and flow phases,
    319–22
serotonin re-uptake inhibitors in bulimia
  nervosa, 484
short bowel syndrome, 370–87
  by-passing the gut, 383
  children, enteral feeding, *200–1*
  D-lactic acidosis, 378
  early post-operative management of the
    short gut, 379–80; assess major
    deficiencies, 380; complete transfer to
    enteral feeding, if possible, 380; fluid
    and electrolyte balance, 379–80;
    gaining stability and assessment of
    needs, 379; gradual transfer to oral
    fluids and nutrients, 380; plan for
    future care, 380
  enteral feeding, 131
  general metabolic consequences of major
    small bowel resection, 377–8
  interruption of entero-hepatic
    circulation, 377–8
  intestinal adaptation, 378
  long-term management, 380–83; oral
    supplements, 381–2
  long-term TPN causing liver disease, 336
  metabolic consequences of major
    resection with enterocolic
    anastomosis, 376–7
  motility disturbances, 378
  parenteral nutrition, 144–5
  physiological consequences of
    jejunostomy, 370–6; *see also*
    jejunostomy
  protein hydrolysate formula, 0–2 years,
    199
  restriction of oral intake, 382–3
  surgical treatment, 384
  TPN peri-operatively, 290; guidelines,
    294
  vitamins and iron by injection, 383
single nutrient deficiencies and immune
  function, 74–8
skeletal muscle, activity after trauma and
  sepsis, 322
skeleton, complications of parenteral
  nutrition, 154–5
skin
  appearance in anorexia nervosa, 476–7
  losses of micronutrients through, 62
  symptoms of food intolerance, 207
  tests for food intolerance, 210

skinfold measurements, 10–11
  critical illness, 325
  precision, *9*
skinfold thickness, effect of nutritional
  support, 167, *168*
sleep disturbance complicating enteral
  feeding, 204
small intestine, carbohydrate assimilation,
  110–17
smoking
  and beta carotene metabolism, 66
  and micronutrient deficiency, 59
sodium
  benzoate, causing asthma, 208
  depletion after jejunostomy, 370–1;
    magnitude, 371
  and glucose solution, to promote
    absorption after jejunostomy, 374–5
  intake and blood pressure, 449–52; *see
    also* salt intake and blood pressure
  solutions, dilute, effect on stomal loss
    after jejunostomy, 371, *372*
  supplements, in short bowel syndrome,
    381
soya milk substitutes, *217*
special formulations, enteral nutrition,
  134–5
starch
  hydrolysis in small intestine, 111–13;
    brush-border, 111–12; maltase/sucrase
    classification, 112–13
  uptake, enteral diet, 113
starvation, 307–18
  before surgery, 311–12
  biochemical adjustments, 323
  definition, 307
  in eating disorders, 475, 478, 482
  how to treat, 314–16
  inability to withstand, neonate, 224–5
  inadequate oral nutrient period, 313
  long-stay elderly patients, 308
  making clinical decision to support, 313,
    314
  measurement, 310
  nasogastric feeding trials on fractured
    femur patients, 307–8; normal, thin
    and very thin, 307–8
  oral intake, 314–15
  other impairments, 309–10
  partial, return to normal, 308
  physiological consequences, 310
  plasma proteins, 313
  progressive deterioration in function, 309
  progressive weight loss against time, 309
  sequence of events, 256, *258*
  tube feeding, 315–16
  voluntary oral intake, 311–13
  weight and anthropometrics, 310–11

stearic acid and cholesterol level, 426
stomach rupture in bulimia nervosa, 481
stomal loss, effect of water or dilute
    sodium solutions, 371
stressed patients, specific enteral diets, 273;
    276
sucrases, enteral diets, membrane digestion,
    112–13
sucrose and enteral nutrition, 116–17
suit method for direct calorimetry, 24
sulphasalazine in IBD, 357
sulphur dioxide causing asthma, 208
superoxide dismutase, and removal of
    superoxide radicals, 60
surgery and nutrition, 239–55
    due to impaired intake, 241; due to
        gastrointestinal disease, 241–2
    intravenous nutrition, 246–7
    nutritional support: indications, 245–8;
        influence on disease, 246–8;
        post-operative, 245–6; pre-operative,
        245; route and timing, 246–8
    practical considerations, 248
    prevalence of malnutrition, 239–40;
        adverse effects, 240–1; causes, 241–2
    recovery, role of arginine, 50
    specific nutrients, 248
sympathetic activity after trauma and
    sepsis, 320

T cells
    activity in protein-energy malnutrition, 79
    in Crohn's disease, 83
    role, 72–3
tartrazine causing asthma, 208
taurine in neonatal intravenous feeding,
    234–5
tea, intolerance, and migraine, 209
thermoregulatory changes after trauma
    and sepsis, 320
thiamine deficiency causing liver disease,
    340, 341
threonine, daily requirements, 45
thrombosis, and superior vena cava
    catheterisation, 279
tomatoes, intolerance
    causing urticaria, 207
    and migraine, 209
total body water measurement, 4–5
total enteral nutrition in Crohn's disease,
    358, 359, 360–1
    see also enteral nutrition
total parenteral nutrition
    as cause of liver disease, 335–6
    complications, 281–3
    in IBD, 358–9
    monitoring, peri-operative, 288–9

peri-operatively, guidelines, *292–4*
standardised order form, 284–6
support team, 283–4
    see also parenteral nutrition
trace elements
    and cognition, 67
    in cystic fibrosis, 400
    deficiencies, development, 56–8
    in IBD, 355–6
    peri-operative requirements, 264–6
    provision, *68*
    recommended intake, 67
    requirements, *68*
    in short bowel syndrome, 382
    toxicity, 68
trans-fatty acids, effect on lipoproteins, 427
trauma
    amino acid requirements, peri-operative,
        263
    physiological and endocrinological
        events, 319–22; ebb and flow phases,
        319–22
tricarboxylic acid cycle, 46
triglycerides
    absorption, enteral diets, 117–19
    dietary intake, 426–8
    effect of weight loss and gain, 421–3
    medium chain, parenteral feeding in
        neonates, 232
tryptophan, daily requirements, *45*
tube feeding in starvation, 315–16
tubes, feeding, difficulties with children, 204
tubes used in nasogastric feeding, 135–36
tyrosine, requirements, 51

ulcerative colitis
    TPN support, 358–9
    see also inflammatory bowel disease
urea in cystic fibrosis, 397
urticaria and food intolerance, 207

valine
    daily requirements, *45*
    requirements after trauma, 47
vasopressin responses in anorexia nervosa,
    479
vegetable protein diets in liver disease,
    346
vegetarian diet, and blood pressure, 455
venous access
    neonatal intravenous feeding, 235–6
    for parenteral nutrition, 277–83
ventilation in multiple organ failure, 327–8
    energy expenditure, 327–8
ventricular arrhythmias, TPN
    peri-operatively, 290

very low birthweight infant, intravenous feeding, 224, 229–35
see also neonatal intravenous feeding
vitamin A
  causing liver damage, 337
  deficiency: causing liver disease, 341; in Crohn's disease, 357
  effect on immune function, 77–8
  levels in cystic fibrosis, 397; to avoid deficiency, 418
  metabolism: in adolescence, 58; and excess alcohol intake, 58
  supplements, in infectious diseases, 66
vitamin B
  deficiency in IBD, 356
  intake, and micronutrient deficiency, 58
vitamin B6
  in cystic fibrosis, 400
  deficiency causing liver disease, 340, 341
vitamin B12
  deficiency causing liver disease, 340; 341
  in IBD, 354, *355*, 356
  loss, and short bowel syndrome, 376–7, 383
vitamin C
  and the common cold, 66
  effect on immune function, 76–7; lymphocytes, 77; mitogen transformation, 77
  levels in cystic fibrosis, 400
  as nutrient antioxidant, 60
  plasma concentration during illness, 65
  requirements of elderly, 59
  requirements and smoking, 59
  supplements, in IBD, 356
vitamin D
  deficiency: causing liver disease, 341–2; in IBD, 356
  levels in cystic fibrosis, 397–8; to avoid deficiency, 418
  in short bowel syndrome, 382
vitamin E
  deficiency, causing liver disease, 342
  effect on immune function, 77–8
  requirements and smoking, 59
  supplements, and coronary heart disease, 430
vitamin F as nutrient antioxidant, 60
vitamin K
  deficiency, causing liver disease, 342
  levels in cystic fibrosis, 398, 399; to avoid deficiency, 418
vitamins
  and cognition, 67
  consequences of inadequate intake, 56–8
  deficiencies, in IBD, 356–7
  deficiencies in liver disease, 340–42
  peri-operative requirements, 264–6

recommended intake, 67
requirements due to growth and anabolism, 60
requirements during illness, 59
in short bowel syndrome, 382
supplements, in cystic fibrosis, 405–6
toxicity, requirements and provision, 68–9
water soluble, in cystic fibrosis, 399–400
vomiting
  in anorexia nervosa, 475, 480
  in bulimia nervosa, 475, 477, 480
  caused by cows' milk intolerance, 206

water
  body, *see* body composition, measurement: total body water
  effect on stomal loss after jejunostomy, 371, *372*
  loss, after jejunostomy, 370
  requirements, peri-operative, 261
  restriction, in short bowel syndrome, 381
weight, body
  and blood pressure, 445–6
  effect of nutritional support, 167, *168*
  gain: inadequate, enteral feeding, children, 194; increase in serum cholesterol, 423
  loss: effects on triglycerides and LDL-C and HDL-C, 421–3; lipids, and coronary heart disease, 421–3; maintenance, 469–70
  -loss groups, 466
  measurement, during critical illness, 325–6
  measurements for body composition, 10
  reduction, and body composition measurement, 1
  'reference man', 2
  serum lipids and coronary heart disease prevention, 421
  value in starvation, 310–11
  see also obesity: overweight
wheat free diets for food allergies, 215
whey protein intolerance, 214
whey protein powder and colic, 207
whole body impedance for body composition measurement, 10–11
Wilms tumour, childhood, enteral feeding, 197
wine, coronary heart disease, and serum lipoproteins, 431–2
wound healing, TPN peri-operatively, 290

yeast intolerance causing urticaria, 207

zinc
    absorption: and copper supplements, 61;
      and excess alcohol intake, 58; and
      iron supplements, 61
    deficiency: in alcoholic liver disease, 85;
      in cystic fibrosis, 400; effect on
      immune function, 75–6; impairment to
      wound healing, 63; in liver disease,
      342–3

as immunostimulant, 75–6
maintenance of anabolism, 63
metabolism in disease, 75
requirements, provision and toxicity,
  68
status in elderly, 59
supplements, in healthy people, 76

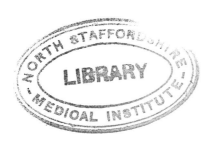